Pediatric and Adolescent Gynecology

SECOND EDITION

Pediatric and Adolescent Gynecology

SECOND EDITION

EDITORS

SUE ELLEN KOEHLER CARPENTER, M.D.
Department of Reproductive Endocrinology
Crawford Long Hospital
Emory Clinic;
Assistant Professor
Department of Gynecology and Obstetrics
Emory University School of Medicine
Atlanta, Georgia

JOHN A. ROCK, M.D.
Professor and Chairman
Department of Gynecology and Obstetrics
Emory University School of Medicine
Atlanta, Georgia

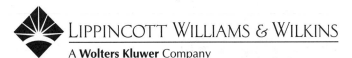

LIPPINCOTT WILLIAMS & WILKINS
A **Wolters Kluwer** Company
Philadelphia • Baltimore • New York • London
Buenos Aires • Hong Kong • Sydney • Tokyo

Acquisitions Editor: Lisa McAllister
Developmental Editor: Gina Gerace
Production Editor: Melanie Bennitt
Manufacturing Manager: Colin Warnock
Cover Designer: Mark Lerner
Compositor: Lippincott Williams & Wilkins Desktop Division
Printer: Edwards Brothers

© 2000 by LIPPINCOTT WILLIAMS & WILKINS
530 Walnut Street
Philadelphia, PA 19106 USA
LWW.com

Printed in the USA

Library of Congress Cataloging-in-Publication Data
Pediatric and adolescent gynecology / editors, Sue Ellen Koehler Carpenter, John A. Rock — 2nd ed.
        p. ; cm.
    Includes bibliographical references and index.
    ISBN 0-7817-1781-7
        1. Pediatric gynecology. 2. Adolescent medicine. I. Carpenter, Sue Ellen Koehler.
II. Rock, John A.
        [DNLM: 1. Genital Diseases, Female—Adolescence. 2. Genital Diseases, Female—Child. 3. Adolescent Medicine. WS 360 P3705 2000]
    RJ478.P43 2000
    618.92′098—dc21

                                                                                        00-036096

10 9 8 7 6 5 4 3 2 1

To our families

Contents

Contributing Authors

Robert A. Ambros, M.D. *Associate Professor, Department of Pathology and Laboratory Medicine, The Albany Medical College, Albany, New York 12208*

Jean Anderson, M.D. *Associate Professor, Department of Gynecology and Obstetrics, Johns Hopkins University School of Medicine, Baltimore, Maryland 21205*

Ricardo Azziz, M.D., M.P.H. *Professor, Departments of Gynecology and Obstetrics and Medicine, University of Alabama at Birmingham, Birmingham, Alabama 35233*

G. William Bates, M.D. *Clinical Professor, Department of Gynecology and Obstetrics, Vanderbilt University Medical Center, Nashville, Tennessee 37240*

Gary D. Berkovitz, M.D. *Department of Pediatrics, Johns Hopkins University School of Medicine, Baltimore, Maryland 21205*

Lesley L. Breech, M.D. *Instructor, Department of Gynecology and Obstetrics, Washington University School of Medicine, St. Louis, Missouri 63110*

Sue Ellen Koehler Carpenter, M.D. *Department of Reproductive Endocrinology, Crawford Long Hospital, Emory Clinic; Assistant Professor, Department of Gynecology and Obstetrics, Emory University School of Medicine, Atlanta, Georgia 30322*

Sandra Ann Carson, M.D. *Professor, Department of Gynecology and Obstetrics; Chief, Baylor Assisted Reproductive Technology, Baylor College of Medicine, Houston, Texas 77030*

Carol M. Choi, M.D. *Attending Physician, Department of Gynecology and Obstetrics, The University Hospital; Assistant Professor, Department of Gynecology and Obstetrics, University of Cincinnati, Cincinnati, Ohio 45267*

Andrew S. Cook, M.D. *Private practice, Metairie, Louisiana 70002*

Vanessa E. Cullins, M.D., M.P.H. *Vice President and Medical Director, Department of Technical Resources, AVSC International, New York, New York 10001*

Mark A. Damario, M.D. *Consultant and Assistant Professor, Department of Gynecology and Obstetrics, Mayo Clinic, Rochester, Minnesota 55905*

David L. Dudgeon, M.D. *Director, Pediatric Surgery, Department of Surgery, Rainbow Babies and Children's Hospital; Professor, Department of Surgery and Pediatrics, Case Western Reserve University, Cleveland, Ohio 44106*

Peter J. Fagan, M.D. *Sexual Behaviors Consultation Unit, Baltimore, Maryland 21205*

Nancy N. Fajman, M.D., M.P.H. *Medical Director, Egleston Child Protection Program, Egleston Children's Hospital; Assistant Professor, Department of General Pediatrics, Emory University School of Medicine, Atlanta, Georgia 30322*

Mark R. Feneley, M.D., F.R.C.S.(Urol.) *The James Buchanan Brady Urological Institute, Johns Hopkins University School of Medicine, Baltimore, Maryland 21287*

John P. Gearhart, M.D.   *Chief, Department of Pediatric Urology, The James Buchanan Brady Urological Institute; Professor, Department of Urology, Johns Hopkins University School of Medicine, Baltimore, Maryland 21287*

Gary A. Glasser, M.D.   *Atlanta Gynecology and Obstetrics, Decatur, Georgia 30030; Clinical Assistant Professor, Department of Gynecology and Obstetrics, Emory University School of Medicine, Atlanta, Georgia 30303*

Enrique R. Grisoni, M.D.   *Director, Pediatric Trauma, Department of Pediatric Surgery, Rainbow Babies and Children's Hospital; Associate Professor, Departments of Surgery and Pediatrics, Case Western Reserve University, Cleveland, Ohio 44106*

Sarah E. Herbert, M.D.   *Director, Psychiatry Obstetrics Consultation/Liaison Service, Department of Psychiatry, Grady Health System; Assistant Professor, Department of Psychiatry and Behavioral Sciences, Emory University School of Medicine, Atlanta, Georgia 30322*

John S. Hesla, M.D.   *Portland Center for Reproductive Medicine, Portland, Oregon 97210*

Ira R. Horowitz, M.D.   *Director, Department of Gynecology and Obstetrics, Emory University Hospital; Professor and Vice Chairman, Department of Gynecology and Obstetrics, Emory University School of Medicine, Atlanta, Georgia 30322*

George R. Huggins, M.D.   *Professor and Chairman, Department of Gynecology and Obstetrics, Johns Hopkins Bayview Medical Center, Baltimore, Maryland 21224*

Eugene Katz, M.D.   *Director, The GBMC Fertility Center, The Greater Baltimore Medical Center; Assistant Professor, Department of Gynecology and Obstetrics, University of Maryland, Baltimore, Maryland 21204*

William R. Keye, Jr., M.D.   *Director, Department of Gynecology and Obstetrics, William Beaumont Hospital, Royal Oak, Michigan 48073; Clinical Associate Professor, Department of Gynecology and Obstetrics, University of Michigan, Ann Arbor, Michigan 48109*

Joel S. Krasnow, M.D.   *Department of Gynecology and Obstetrics, Women's Endocrine Division, University of Wisconsin, Madison, Wisconsin 53792*

Robert J. Kurman, M.D.   *Director, Gynecologic Pathology, Department of Pathology, Johns Hopkins Hospital; Richard Te Linde Distinguished Professor, Gynecologic Pathology, Departments of Gynecology and Obstetrics and Pathology, Johns Hopkins University School of Medicine, Baltimore, Maryland 21287*

Bhagirath Majmudar, M.D.   *Chief, Department of Pathology, Grady Health System; Professor, Department of Pathology, Associate Professor, Department of Gynecology and Obstetrics, Emory University Hospital, Atlanta, Georgia 30322*

Claude J. Migeon, M.D.   *Director, Department of Pediatrics, Division of Endocrinology, Johns Hopkins University School of Medicine, Baltimore, Maryland 21287*

John E. Niederhuber, M.D.   *Department of Surgery, Stanford University Medical Center, Stanford, California 94305*

Wilberto Nieves-Neira, M.D.   *Clinical Fellow, Department of Gynecology and Obstetrics, Jackson Memorial Hospital; Clinical Assistant, Department of Gynecology and Obstetrics, University of Miami School of Medicine, Miami, Florida 33136*

Leslie Plotnick, M.D. *Associate Professor, Department of Pediatrics, Johns Hopkins University School of Medicine, Baltimore, Maryland 21287*

Thomas M. Price, M.D. *Director, Department of Reproductive Endocrinology, Greenville Hospital System, Greenville, South Carolina 29605; Associate Professor, Department of Gynecology and Obstetrics, University of South Carolina, Columbia, South Carolina 29203*

Janet S. Rader, M.D. *Associate Professor, Department of Gynecology and Obstetrics, Washington University School of Medicine, St. Louis, Missouri 63110*

Spencer S. Richlin, M.D. *Fellow, Reproductive Endocrinology and Infertility, Department of Gynecology and Obstetrics, Emory University School of Medicine, Atlanta, Georgia 30322*

John A. Rock, M.D. *Professor and Chairman, Department of Gynecology and Obstetrics, Emory University School of Medicine, Atlanta, Georgia 30322*

Ricardo Sainz De La Cuesta, M.D. *Formerly at Department of Gynecology and Obstetrics, Emory University Hospital and Emory University School of Medicine, Atlanta, Georgia 30322*

Joseph S. Sanfilippo, M.D. *Chairman, Department of Gynecology and Obstetrics, Allegheny General Hospital; Professor, Department of Gynecology and Obstetrics, MCP Hahnemann School of Medicine, Pittsburgh, Pennsylvania 15212*

Betsy Schroeder, M.D. *Director, Division of Pediatric and Adolescent Gynecology, Department of Gynecology and Obstetrics, MCP Hahnemann School of Medicine, Allegheny General Hospital, Pittsburgh, Pennsylvania 15212*

Sander S. Shapiro, M.D. *Director, Department of Reproductive Endocrine Service, University Hospital; Professor, Department of Gynecology and Obstetrics, University of Wisconsin, Madison, Wisconsin 53792*

Joe Leigh Simpson, M.D. *Ernst W. Bertner Chairman and Professor, Department of Gynecology and Obstetrics, Baylor College of Medicine, Houston, Texas 77030*

Melinda B. Stein, M.D. *Francis Scott Key Medical Center, Baltimore, Maryland 21244*

Ulun Uluğ, M.D. *Attending Physician, IVF Unit, Department of Gynecology and Obstetrics, German Hospital at Istanbul, Taksim, Istanbul, Turkey*

Eric A. Wiebke, M.D. *Associate Professor, Department of Surgery, Indiana University School of Medicine, Indianapolis, Indiana 46202*

Michele D. Wilson, M.D. *Assistant Physician and Clinical Associate Professor, Department of Pediatrics, Children's Hospital of Philadelphia, Philadelphia, Pennsylvania 19104*

Preface

This book brings a multidisciplinary approach to the gynecologic care of infants, children, and adolescents. The editors are truly fortunate to have outstanding contributors from the fields of pediatrics, urology, psychology, surgery, and gynecology, who discuss the recognition and treatment of medical illness in these specific age groups. The pathophysiology of disease is stressed. Knowledgeable handling of pediatric patients requires a background in genetics and developmental biology. Genital examination requires forethought and gentleness, particularly in children, so variations from a standard examination are discussed. Ultrasonography and laparoscopy have enhanced our ability to diagnose routine gynecologic complaints of children and adolescents, but new norms for their use must be established.

Since the publication of our first edition, the field of pediatric and adolescent gynecology has matured. New contributions to our understanding of this patient population have been made, clinical experience has grown and been documented, and exciting improvements in preventive care have occurred. Nonetheless, this population still tends to be underserved. The demands for quality care affect many specialties, including family practice, pediatrics, urology, pediatric surgery, and pediatric and reproductive endocrinology.

The fertility potential and gynecologic and psychosexual health of our youngest patients must be protected; it is essential that we provide quality care for a wide variety of complaints. We hope that this book will assist those who are called upon to deliver expert care for gynecologic complaints in infants, children, and adolescents.

Acknowledgments

We acknowledge the assistance of Glenda Walker in the preparation of this manuscript. We also thank Lisa McAllister and Gina Gerace of Lippincott Williams & Wilkins. We are especially grateful to the many fine contributors whose experience and research is represented in this book.

Sue Ellen Koehler Carpenter
John A. Rock

1

Genetics of Sexual Differentiation

Joe Leigh Simpson

REPRODUCTION EMBRYOLOGY

Primordial germ cells originate in the endoderm of the yolk sac and migrate to the genital ridge to form the indifferent gonad. 46,XY and 46,XX gonads are initially indistinguishable. Indifferent gonads develop into testes if the embryo, or more specifically the gonadal stroma, is 46,XY. This process begins about 43 days after conception. Testes become morphologically identifiable 7 to 8 weeks after conception (9 to 10 weeks gestational or menstrual weeks).

Testicular Differentiation

Sertoli cells are the first cells to become recognizable in testicular differentiation, or-

ganizing the surrounding cells into tubules. Both Leydig cells (1) and Sertoli cells (2) function in dissociation from testicular morphogenesis, consistent with these cells directing gonadal development rather than the converse. These two cell types secrete different hormones, which in aggregate direct subsequent male differentiation (Fig. 1.1).

Fetal Leydig cells produce an androgen—testosterone—that stabilizes wolffian ducts and permits differentiation of the vasa deferentia, epididymides, and seminal vesicles. After conversion by 5α-reductase to dihydrotestosterone (DHT), external genitalia are virilized. These actions can be mimicked by the administration of testosterone to female or castrated male embryos, as proven by exis-

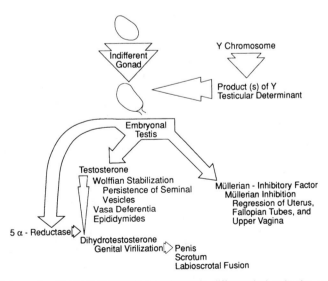

FIG. 1.1. Schematic diagram illustrating embryonic differentiation in the normal male.

tence of teratogenic forms of female pseudo-hermaphroditism. Fetal Sertoli cells produce anti-müllerian hormone (AMH) (müllerian inhibitory substance [MIS]), a glycoprotein that diffuses locally to produce regression of müllerian derivatives (uterus and fallopian tubes). This hormone is important for gonadal development. When AMH is chronically expressed in XX transgenic mice, oocytes fail to persist, tubule-like structures develop in gonads, and müllerian differentiation is abnormal (3). AMH also has an inhibitor effect on oocyte meiosis and plays a role in the descent of the testes (4). AMH is detectable in the serum of males throughout life but is not measurable in females until the second decade of life; thus, the presence of AMH can serve as a sensitive marker for the presence of testicular tissue in pseudohermaphroditism or true hermaphroditism (5).

Ovarian Differentiation

In the absence of a Y chromosome, the indifferent gonad develops into an ovary. Transformation into fetal ovaries begins at 50 to 55 days of embryonic development. Germ cells are initially present in 46,X embryos (6) but undergo atresia at a rate more rapid than that occurring in normal 46,XX embryos. Ovarian maintenance determinants can be localized to specific regions of the X, as will be discussed later. Certain autosomal genes also must remain intact for normal ovarian development and gametogenesis.

Ductal and Genital Differentiation

Independent of gonadal differentiation is the process of ductal and external genital development. In the absence of testosterone and AMH, external genitalia develop in female fashion. Müllerian ducts form the uterus and fallopian tubes; wolffian ducts regress. Such changes occur in normal XX embryos as well as in XY animals castrated embryonically before testicular differentiation.

GENETIC CONTROL OF SEX DIFFERENTIATION

Both sex chromosomes (X and Y) as well as autosomes contain loci that must remain intact for normal sexual development. The chromosomal location of these loci is important for clinical management, because autosomal factors influencing sexual development would be predicted to be perturbed by autosomal translocations and deletions.

Genetics of Testicular Development

Y Chromosome

That 46,X,i(Yq) individuals were female in appearance was the first indication that the major testicular determinants (testis-determining factor) were localized to the Y short arm (Yp). Since those observations were first made 30 years ago, various candidate genes have been proposed as the testis-determining factor. The testes determinants were localized to the distal Y short arm just below the pseudoautosomal boundary. Initially H-Y antigen (HYA) and later ZFY were considered strong candidates. However, the gene SRY (sex-determining region Y) is the testicular determinant (7,8).

Identification of SRY came as result of mapping in 46,XX males and sporadic 46,XY phenotype females (gonadal dysgenesis). The etiology of most (80%) 46,XX males involves interchange of not just the usual pseudoautosomal regions of Xp and Yp, but also the contiguous proximal nonpseudoautosomal region. In XX males, SRY was present in the smallest translocated region compatible with male differentiation. That SRY, and not ZFY, was pivotal was shown by some 46,XX males showing SRY but not ZFY. Moreover, 10% to 15% of sporadic XY gonadal dysgenesis shows point mutations within SRY (9). SRY is expressed before testicular differentiation is manifested (7). Transgenic XX mice with SRY predictably show testicular differentiation (10).

The SRY gene is composed of two open reading frames consisting of 99 and 273

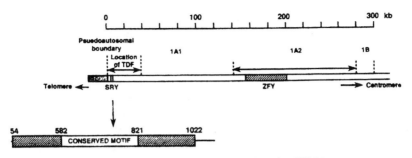

FIG. 1.2. Schematic diagram illustrating the SRY gene.

amino acids (Fig. 1.2), respectively. On the basis of females with XY gonadal dysgenesis who have mutations involving SRY (9,11–13), the key sequence involves a high-mobility group (HMG) box that shares characteristics in common with other DNA-binding sequences. When XY gonadal dysgenesis is associated with a point mutation or deletion in SRY, the mutant sequence has always proved to be located in the HMG box.

X Chromosome

In addition to genes on the Y chromosome, various clinical disorders indicate that testicular differentiation also requires loci on X. The importance of genes on the X has long been evidenced by existence of an X-linked recessive form of XY gonadal dysgenesis (14,15). Xp also contains a region that, if duplicated, suppresses testicular development despite the presence of SRY. This phenomenon was first recognized by Bernstein et al. (16), and since then other cases have been reported (16–20). The duplicated region responsible for this phenomenon (21) has been called dose-sensitive sex reversal (DSS), and the actual gene DAX-1. The sex reversal (male to female) appears to be the result of duplication and not disruption, given molecular analysis showing breakpoints encompassing the entire region believed to include the gene. The locus is near that of adrenal hypoplasia congenita (AHC), but the exact relationship between AHC and DSS remains obscure.

Autosomes

Autosomal loci are pivotal for testicular differentiation. Several autosomal regions have generated special interest: 9p, 10q, 11p, and 17q. The gene responsible for campomelia dysplasia and XY gonadal dysgenesis (sex reversal) is localized to 17q24.3→q25.1) (22). Pathogenesis involves SOX9. Like SRY, SOX9 is DNA binding and has an HMG box (23); however, analysis of SOX9 in campomelia dysplasia has not always shown correlations with sex reversal (24), suggesting genetic heterogeneity. The Wilms' tumor suppressor gene (WT-1), located on 11p, is associated with gonadal and genital abnormalities (male pseudohermaphroditism) (25,26); however, WT-1 apparently is rarely, if ever, deleted in XY gonadal dysgenesis (27). Deletions of 10q also have been associated with XY gonadal dysgenesis (28). No candidate gene is identified.

An autosomal region that seems pivotal could be 9p (29,30). Approximately 70% of 46,XY cases with del(9p) show sex reversal (31), and an increasing number of XY gonadal dysgenesis cases show this deletion (30,32,33). Vegetti et al. (30) found that five of nine cases of XY gonadal dysgenesis showed 9p deletions.

Other syndromes deleteriously affecting testicular differentiation are heritable and act in autosomal fashion, but they have not been localized to a specific chromosomal region. These include agonadia (34), rudimentary testes syndrome (35), and the syndrome of germ cell hypoplasia in both males (germinal cell aplasia) and females (streak gonads) (36–40). In addition, autosomal genes must influence XX true hermaphroditism. Familial aggregates occur, and SRY usually is not present.

Genetics of Ovarian Development

In the absence of a Y chromosome, the indifferent gonad develops into an ovary. Germ cells exist in 45,X human fetuses (6) and 39,X mice (41); thus, presumably the pathogenesis of germ cell failure involves increased germ cell attrition, not failure of formation. If two intact X chromosomes are not present, 45,X ovarian follicles usually degenerate by birth. Therefore, the second X chromosome is responsible for ovarian *maintenance* rather than ovarian *differentiation*.

Ovarian maintenance determinants can be deduced (phenotypic-karyotypic correlations) to exist on both the X short arm and the X long arm (42–48). Each arm probably has several distinct regions of differential importance for ovarian development. The number and location will be discussed later at length. In addition to regions on the X chromosome, autosomal loci are essential for normal ovarian development.

MONOSOMY X (TURNER'S SYNDROME)

The complement most frequently associated with ovarian dysgenesis is 45,X. The proportion of 45,X individuals in a given sample will depend on the method of ascertainment. Fewer 45,X individuals will be detected if primary amenorrhea is the presenting complaint than if short stature or various somatic anomalies are the presenting complaints. Primary amenorrhea is more likely to be the presenting complaint in women ascertained by gynecologists, whereas short stature is likely in children ascertained by pediatricians. Overall, about 50% of all patients with gonadal dysgenesis have a 45,X complement; 25% have sex chromosomal mosaicism with a structural ab-

normality (e.g., 45,X/46,XX). Far fewer have a structurally abnormal X or Y chromosome (49,50).

In 80% of cases, the paternally derived X has been lost (51). The phenotype does not in general differ between $45,X^m$ and $45,X^p$ cases (X^m,X of maternal origin; X^p,X of paternal origin). In structurally abnormal X chromosomes, it is also the paternal X that is lost (52,53). This suggests that X^m and X^p chromosomes are lost at random (54). Assuming 45,Y is lethal, the theoretical percentage of $45,X^m$ cases would be 67%, which is not greatly different from the 80% actually observed.

Gonads

In most 45,X adults with gonadal dysgenesis, the normal gonad is replaced by a white fibrous streak, 2 to 3 cm long and about 0.5 cm wide, located in the position ordinarily occupied by the ovary (Fig. 1.3). A streak gonad is characterized histologically by interlacing waves of dense fibrous stroma, indistinguishable from normal ovarian stroma (Fig. 1.4). That germ cells usually are completely absent in adults but present in 45,X embryos is the basis for the belief that the pathogenesis of germ cell failure is increased atresia, not failure of germ cell formation. Ovarian rete tubules, which probably originate from either

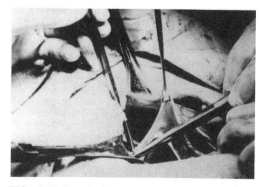

FIG. 1.3. A streak gonad. (From Simpson JL. *Disorders of sexual differentiation: etiology and clinical delineation.* New York: Academic Press, 1976:1–466, with permission.)

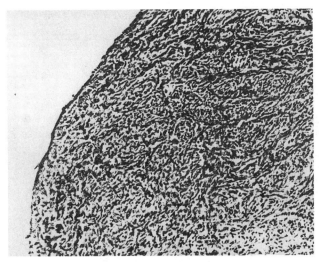

FIG. 1.4. Histologic appearance of a streak gonad showing lack of oocytes. (From Simpson JL. *Disorders of sexual differentiation: etiology and clinical delineation.* New York: Academic Press, 1976:1–466, with permission.)

mesonephric tubules or medullary sex cords, are present in the medial portion of most streak gonads. Hilar cells usually are detected in streak gonads of patients past the age of expected puberty.

That 45,X humans manifest streak gonads is not as obvious as one might expect, with relatively normal ovarian development occurring in many other monosomy X mammals (e.g., mice). The more likely explanation is that, in humans, not all loci on the normal heterochromatic (inactive) X are inactivated. In addition, X-inactivation never exists in oocytes; X-reactivation of germ cells occurs before entry in meiotic oogenesis (55). X-inactivation also can occur only after some crucial time of differentiation, beyond which only a single euchromatic (active) X is necessary for continued oogenesis.

Secondary Sexual Development

Although streak gonads usually are present in 45,X individuals, about 3% of adult cases menstruate spontaneously and 5% show breast development (Table 1.1). Occasionally,

the interval between menstrual periods appears normal in 45,X patients, and fertile patients have been reported. Although an undetected 46,XX cell line should always be suspected in menstruating 45,X patients, it is plausible that a few 45,X individuals could be fertile, inasmuch as germ cells are present in 45,X embryos.

The rare offspring of 45,X women probably are not at greatly increased risk for chromosomal abnormalities (56,57), although theoretically they should be. Some authors disagree with this statement (58), and recent work using X-specific fluorescence *in situ* hybridization probes suggests low-grade 45,X/46, XX mosaicism in some women experiencing repeated abortions (59). Irrespective, menstruation and fertility occur so rarely that 45,X patients should be counseled to anticipate primary amenorrhea and sterility. After hormone therapy is initiated in such women, uterine size becomes normal. This permits 45,X women to carry pregnancies in their own uterus after receiving donor embryos or donor oocytes and fertilization in vitro with their husband's sperm.

TABLE 1.1. *Somatic features associated with 45,X chromosomal complement*

Growth
  Decreased birth weight
  Decreased adult height (141–146 cm)
Intellectual function
  Verbal IQ > performance IQ
  Cognitive deficits (space-form blindness)
Craniofacial
  Premature fusion of sphenooccipital and other sutures, producing brachycephaly
  Abnormal pinnae
  Retruded mandible
  Epicanthal folds (25%)
  High-arched palate (36%)
  Abnormal dentition
  Visual anomalies, usually strabismus (22%)
  Auditory deficits; sensorineural or secondary to middle ear infections
Neck
  Pterygium coli (46%)
  Short broad neck (74%)
  Low nuchal hair (71%)
Chest
  Rectangular contour (shield chest) (53%)
  Apparent widely spaced nipples
  Tapered lateral ends of clavicle
Cardiovascular
  Coarctation of aorta or ventricular septal defect (10% to 16%)
Renal (38%)
  Horseshoe kidneys
  Unilateral renal aplasia
  Duplication of ureters
Gastrointestinal
  Telangiectasias
Skin and lymphatics
  Pigmented nevi (63%)
  Lymphedema (38%) due to hypoplasia of superficial vessels
Nails
  Hypoplasia and malformation (66%)
Skeletal
  Cubitus valgus (54%)
  Radial tilt of articular surface of trochlear
  Clinodactyly V
  Short metacarpals, usually IV (48%)
  Decreased carpal arch (mean angle 117 degrees)
  Deformities of medical tibial condyle
Dermatoglyphics
  Increased total digital ridge count
  Increased distance between palmar triradii a and b
  Distal axial triradius in position t′

Modified from Simpson JL. Gonadal dysgenesis and abnormalities of the human sex chromosomes. *Birth Defects* 1975;11(4):23, with permission.

Somatic Anomalies

45,X individuals not only are short (less than 4 feet 10 inches), but often they exhibit many features of Turner's stigmata (Table 1.1). No single feature of Turner's stigmata is pathognomonic, but in aggregate a character-istic spectrum exists that is more likely to occur in those with a 45,X complement than in individuals with most other sex chromosomal abnormalities. Assessment of renal, vertebral, cardiac, and auditory function is obligatory.

The molecular basis for short stature in Turner's stigmata is uncertain, although the distal X short arm has long been known to be integral for normal somatic development. Fisher et al. (60) suggested that absence of a specific DNA sequence may cause features of "Turner's stigmata." Sequence RPS4Y is present on the Y short arm, and homologous sequence RPS4X is present on the X. These sequences differ at only 19 of 263 amino acid residues. RPS4X is not inactivated; thus, monosomy X individuals would be deficient at this locus. Fisher et al. (60) believe the number of ribosomes per cell is reduced if a RPS4X sequence is lacking, as it is in monosomy X.

Growth

45,X is associated with decreased birth weight (61). Total body length at birth sometimes is less than normal, but often close to the 50th percentile. Height velocity before puberty generally lies in the 10th to 15th percentile (62), however, and the mean height of 45,X adults (16 years and older) lies between 141 and 146 cm (50,63).

Various treatments for short stature in 45,X patients have been considered: growth hormone, anabolic steroids, and low-dose estrogen. Growth hormone abnormalities have long been proposed; however, their existence is contentious and abnormalities might only be secondary to lack of gonadal activity (64). All the treatment regimens listed show ostensible benefit, especially in the first few years of therapy. The effect on ultimate height is less uncertain, but the consensus is that final height is increased by no more than 6 to 8 cm (65). Most pediatric endocrinologists now appear to favor use of human recombinant DNA-derived human growth hormone. Limited efficacy of growth hormone treatment may be unavoidable, however, because epiphyses in patients with a 45,X complement are structurally abnormal. Not only are long bones abnormal, but so are the teeth (66) and skull (67). Thus, those with a 45,X karyotype could be said to have a skeletal dysplasia.

Intelligence

Most 45,X patients have normal intelligence, but any given 45,X patient has a slightly higher probability of being retarded than a 46,XX person (50). Performance IQ is lower than verbal IQ, the latter being similar to 46,XX matched controls. 45,X individuals also may have a cognitive defect characterized by poor spatial processing skills (space-form blindness). Predictable psychosocial deficits occur, primarily involving immaturity and blunted social relationships (68,69).

X CHROMOSOMAL MOSAICISM: 45,X/46,XX AND 45,X/47,XXX

The most common form of mosaicism associated with gonadal dysgenesis is 45,X/ 46,XX. Individuals with a 45,X/46,XX complement predictably show fewer anomalies than do 45,X individuals. Simpson (49) tabulated that 12% of 45,X/46,XX individuals menstruate compared with only 3% of 45,X individuals. Among 45,X/46,XX individuals, 18% undergo breast development compared with 5% of 45,X individuals. Mean adult height is greater with a 45,X/46,XX complement than with 45,X; more mosaic (25%) than nonmosaic (5%) patients reach adult heights greater than 152 cm (49). Somatic anomalies are less likely to occur in 45,X/46,XX than in 45,X.

45,X/47,XXX is less common but phenotypically similar to 45,X/46,XX. Individuals with 45,X/46,XY also may show bilateral streak gonads; however, more often they show a unilateral streak gonad and a contralateral dysgenetic testis (mixed gonadal dysgenesis).

PITFALLS IN LOCALIZING OVARIAN MAINTENANCE GENES TO SPECIFIC REGIONS OF THE X

Delineating the region (genes) on the X responsible for ovarian maintenance is the first step in understanding normal ovarian differentiation and producing gene products of therapeutic benefit. Until the last decade, phenotypic-karyotypic correlations to deduce location of gonadal and somatic determinants relied solely on metaphase analysis. Prometaphase karyotypes allow 1,200 band analysis (traditional GTG banding 400 to 500), but each band still contains considerable DNA. More refined analysis now is possible using polymorphic DNA markers that allow precise resolution far beyond the capacity of light microscopy.

Progress has been slow compared to that achieved in delineating the regions of the Y necessary for testicular differentiation (SRY) or spermatogenesis (DAZ). Several impediments have led to a relative lack of progress. One is that the incidence of X-deletions in the general population is very low. Analyzing only cases ascertained by population-based methods is impractical because no individuals with X-deletions were recovered among 50,000 consecutively born neonates (70). Most del(Xp) or del(Xq) individuals have been identified only because they manifested clinical abnormalities. Exceptions were familial cases or cases detected at prenatal genetic diagnosis for advanced maternal age. Doubtless many less severely affected individuals escape detection. Mode of ascertainment should ideally be considered in phenotypic-karyotypic analysis, but in reality this is impractical because sample sizes are too small. Inevitably biases of selection arise.

Another pitfall impeding molecular analysis of X-ovarian maintenance genes is that analysis is not always derived from individuals who are well studied cytogenetically. Mosaicism in nonhematogenous tissues has not always been excluded to the extent reasonably possible. Individuals with unstable aberrations (e.g., rings, dicentrics) probably should be excluded from phenotypic-karyotypic deductions because monosomy X and other cell lines may arise secondarily.

X SHORT ARM DELETIONS

46,X,del(Xp) or 45,X/46,X,del(Xp) Deletions

Deletions of the short arm of the X chromosome show variable phenotype, depending on the amount of Xp persisting. The most common breakpoint for terminal deletions is Xp11 (Fig. 1.5). In 46,X,del(X)(p11) only proximal Xp remains; the del(Xp) chromosome thus appears acrocentric or telocentric. Chromosomes characterized by progressively more distal breakpoints have been reported: Xp21, 22.1, 22.3. Availability of polymorphic DNA markers now allow precise determinations of breakpoints in terminal deletions to be determined, but still relatively few cases have been subjected to refined molecular analysis.

Approximately half the reported 46,X, del(Xp)(p11) individuals show primary amenorrhea and gonadal dysgenesis. Others menstruate and usually show breast development. In one early tabulation by Simpson (71) of 27 reported del(X)(p11.2→11.4) individuals, 12

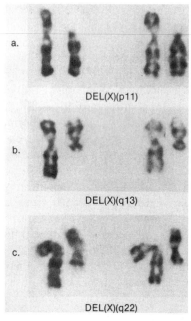

FIG. 1.5. A normal X chromosome and deletions of the X chromosome derived from three different persons. (From Simpson JL, LeBeau MN: Gonadal and statural determinants on the X chromosome and their relationship to *in vitro* studies showing prolonged cell cycles in 45,X, 46,X,del(X)(p11), 46,X,del(X)(q13), and q(22) fibroblasts. *Am J Obstet Gynecol* 1981;141:930, with permission.)

menstruated spontaneously; however, menstruation rarely was normal. More recent tabulations have not materially altered these conclusions (45,46,48,72). Ogata and Matsuo (54) estimate that 50% of del(X)p11 cases show primary amenorrhea, with 45% showing secondary amenorrhea. Ovarian function thus is observed more often in individuals with del(Xp11) than 45,X. Women with more distal deletions [del(X)(p21.1 to p22.1.22)] menstruate more often, but many are infertile or even have secondary amenorrhea (Fig. 1.6) Thus, Xp [X(pter→p21)] retains a role in ovarian development (45,46,48,72). The distal region of importance must involve Xp21,22.1 or 22.2, because del(X) (p22.3) cases do not show primary amenorrhea.

Most women with deletions of Xp are short in stature. Thus, statural determinant(s), i.e., regions with genes, must exist on Xp. Given that del(Xp) women may menstruate but still be short, regions on Xp responsible for ovarian and statural determinants must be distinct (45,48,72–75). Clinically it is important to realize that del(Xp) women may be short despite manifesting normal ovarian function.

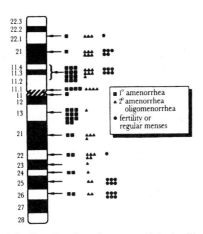

FIG. 1.6. Ovarian function associated with simple deletions of the X chromosome. All cases are characterized by banding studies and reasonable exclusion of mosaicism. (From Simpson JL. *Genetic control of ovarian development.* In: Lobo R, Menopause. San Diego, CA: Academic Press (in press); 77–94, with permission.)

Isochromosomes for Xq

Division of the centromere in the transverse rather than the longitudinal plane results in an isochromosome, a metacentric chromosome consisting of isologous arms. Both arms are structurally identical and contain the same genes. An isochromosome for the X long arm [i(Xq)] differs from a terminal deletion of Xp in that not just the terminal portion but all of the Xp is deleted. In reality, many isochromosomes for Xq are isodicentrics, the clinical significance of which is that a minute portion of Xp is duplicated and retained in addition to duplication of the entire Xq. An isochromosome for the X long arm is the most common X-structural abnormality, but coexisting 45,X cell lines (mosaicism) are typical. Nonmosaic cases are relatively uncommon.

46,X,i(Xq) individuals almost always have streak gonads and primary amenorrhea. Occasionally menstruation is observed, but surveys continue to agree with those published by Simpson (49) over 25 years ago in showing rarity of menstruation (54). The near-complete lack of gonadal development in 46,X, i(Xq) contrasts to that in 46,X, del(X)(p11) individuals, about half of whom menstruate or develop breasts.

Almost all reported 46,X,i(Xq) patients are short. Their mean height seems to be less than in 45,X (Table 1.1). The mean height of nonmosaic 46,X,i(Xq) patients is 136 cm (49), and many somatic features of the Turner's stigmata are observed (49). Somatic anomalies occur as frequently in 46,X,i(Xq) as in 45,X, and the spectrum of anomalies associated with the two complements generally is similar.

X LONG ARM DELETIONS

46,X,del(Xq) and 45,X/46,X,del(Xq) Deletions

Deletions of the X long arm are well known (43,45,48,72) and, like del(Xp), vary in composition (Fig. 1.5).

Almost all deletions originating at Xq13 are associated with primary amenorrhea, lack of breast development, and complete ovarian failure (48). Thus, Xq13 seems to be an important region for ovarian maintenance. Key loci could lie in proximal Xq21, but not more distal given that del(X)(q21) to (q24) individuals menstruate far more often (Fig. 1.6). Menstruating del(X)(q21) women might have retained a region that contained an ovarian maintenance gene, whereas del(X)(q13 or 21) women with primary amenorrhea might have lost such a locus (48).

Molecular attempts at mapping the region of Xq most integral for ovarian development have begun. Sala et al. (76) studied seven X/autosome translocations involving Xq21-22. Five of the seven had primary amenorrhea. A region of Xq spanning 15 mb encompassed breakpoints in all seven cases. Breakpoints in four other X/autosome translocations studied by Philippe et al. (77) also were localized to the same region. The YAC contig encompassing these breakpoints spanned most of the Xq21 region and extended between DXS233 and DXS1171 (78). That breakpoints associated with ovarian failure spanned the entire Xq21 region, making it unlikely that a single gene causes ovarian failure, unless in these balanced X/autosome translocations ovarian failure is the result not of disruption of a gene per se, but rather is reflective of generalized cytologic perturbation.

In more distal Xq deletions, the more common phenotype is not primary amenorrhea but premature ovarian failure (POF) (45,72,79,80). Distal Xq seems less important for ovarian maintenance than proximal Xq, but the former still must have regions important for ovarian maintenance.

Although there is no clear demarcation into discrete regions, it is heuristically useful to stratify terminal deletions into those occurring in regions Xq 13→21, Xq22-25, and Xq 26-28. Table 1.2 shows the extent of ovarian function tabulated by Ogata and Matsuo (54) using such stratification. Figure 1.6 shows Simpson's tabulation using a different format. Both estimates are based on pooled cases, and both are generally consistent.

Distal Xq deletions may be familial. Some familial Xq deletions are a derivative of Xq autosome translocations, but familial terminal or interstitial deletions also exist (47). Familial Xp terminal or interstitial deletions have been characterized by various breakpoints ranging between Xq25 and Xq28. Some families have been ascertained for reasons other than POF. A case reported by our group was ascertained after amniotic fluid analysis in a fetus (47). This suggests that additional fami-

TABLE 1.2. *Ovarian function based on cases reviewed by Ogata and Matsuo*

	Ovarian failure (percentage) in X-deletions		
	Complete (primary amenorrhea or streak gonads)	Partial (secondary amenorrhea or abnormal menses)	None (presumed normal)
Monosomy X (45,X)	88%	12%	0
Short-arm deficiency			
del (X)(p11)	50	45	5
del (X)(p21–22.2)	13	25	62
del (X)(p22.3)	0	0	100
i(Xq)	91	9	0
idic(Xq)	80	20	0
Long-arm deficiency			
del(X)(q13–21)	69	31	0
del(X)(q22–25)	31	56	13
del(X)(q26–28)	8	67	25
idic(Xp)	73	27	0

Ogata and Matsuo (54) provided data in the first two columns, with the assumption that the remainder of cases have normal ovarian function [e.g., 5% in del(X)(p11)]. Publications surveyed overlap in large part those used for analysis of Simpson.

lies would be detected if prometaphase analysis or polymorphic molecular studies were performed more routinely performed in POF.

Distal Xq deletions seem to have a less severe effect on stature than proximal deletions. Somatic anomalies of Turner's stigmata are uncommon and perhaps no more common than in the general population.

NATURE OF X-OVARIAN MAINTENANCE DETERMINANTS

Clearly the X chromosome is necessary for ovarian maintenance, preventing premature germ cell attribution and permitting progression beyond meiotic pachytene.

Ultimately both the number of individual genes and their gene product(s) will be determined. This would have both prognostic as well as potential therapeutic value, given that recombinant technology allows synthesis of a protein gene product(s) once the DNA sequence is known. At present little is known about the nature of ovarian maintenance gene products. Jones et al. (81) proposed that a key gene product is DFFRX, located on Xp11.4 and homologous to a locus on Yq11.2. Both genes escaped inactivation in two *de novo* (X)(p11.2) deletions. James et al. (53) considered DFFRX an unlikely candidate after observing ovarian function despite haploinsufficiency; however, neither of the two cases of James et al. (53) were completely normal clinically, for which reason a role for DFFRX in gonadal development is not categorically excluded.

A candidate gene for a role in ovarian maintenance is the human homologue of the *Drosophila melanogaster* gene *diaphanous* (*dia*). This gene causes sterility in male and female *Drosophila* (82). Sequence comparisons between *dia* and the relevant human expressed sequence tag (EST) DRE25 show significant homology. DRE25 in turn maps to human Xq22 (82). As already noted, Xq22 is a key region for ovarian maintenance. *Drosophila dia* is a member of a family of proteins that help establish cell polarity, govern cytokinesis, and reorganize the actin cytoskeleton. Studying familial POF, an Xq21/autosome translocation alluded to earlier (83) was found to be associated with disruption of DRE25 (84).

A broader biologic question can be posed concerning X-ovarian maintenance determinants. Do the various regions contain gene(s) coding for different gene products? If so, all these genes might be either essential or at least contribute to normal ovarian differentiation. If different genes exist, the prospect of alternative therapeutic options is raised, given that various gene products eventually will all be synthesized. However, it would seem hazardous evolutionarily if perpetuation of the species were to depend on transcription and translation of an entire cascade of ovarian differentiation genes, perturbation of any of which would be deleterious if not lethal (genetically). Moreover, ovarian disturbance associated with many X-deletions is rarely complete. Proximal deletions involving either Xp or proximal Xq may be associated with complete ovarian failure, but more distal deletions are more likely to be associated with POF or normal ovarian function.

Teleologically, it might be more attractive if all X-ovarian maintenance determinants were to produce the same gene product or perhaps products capable of interaction (e.g., dimerization). This would seem to be more conservative evolutionarily, for mutation or deletion of a single locus would not be singularly catastrophic. If such a scenario were true, an ineluctable corollary would be that the X-ovarian genes act in threshold fashion and thus exert their primary effect through an autosomal gene. One mode of action might involve transcriptional or translational regulation of DNA-binding proteins.

AUTOSOMAL GENES CAUSING OVARIAN DYSGENESIS

XX Gonadal Dysgenesis

Gonadal dysgenesis histologically similar to that occurring in individuals with an abnormal sex chromosomal complement may be present in 46,XX individuals, as shown by Simpson et al. (14) over 25 years ago. Mosaicism has been reasonably excluded in affected individuals. The general term *XX gonadal dysgenesis* is applied to those individuals.

Many different forms of 46,XX gonadal dysgenesis exist, but the form of XX gonadal dysgenesis not associated with somatic anomalies is clearly inherited in autosomal recessive fashion. Affected individuals are normal in stature (mean height 165 cm) (85), and Turner's stigmata usually are absent. Frequent reports of consanguinity have long made it clear that autosomal recessive genes are responsible. More recent segregation analysis by the author and colleagues revealed the segregation ratio to be 0.16 for female siblings. Thus, two thirds of gonadal dysgenesis cases in 46,XX individuals are genetic (86). The one third of cases that are nongenetic (phenocopies) could be due to infection, infarction, or infiltrative or autoimmune phenomena.

Of clinical interest is the variable expressivity. In some families, one sibling has streak gonads, whereas another affected individual had primary amenorrhea and extreme ovarian hypoplasia (presence of a few oocytes) (14,87–90). If the mutant gene responsible for XX gonadal dysgenesis is capable of variable expression, the gene may be responsible for some sporadic cases of POF.

The mechanism underlying failure of germ cell persistence in XX gonadal dysgenesis is unknown, but several hypotheses seem reasonable. One is perturbation of meiosis, which would be manifested as ovarian failure and infertility in otherwise normal women. Other possibilities include interference with germ cell migration, abnormal connective tissue milieu, or gonadotropin receptor perturbation.

In the absence of candidate genes, identifying autosomal genes responsible for the various forms of XX gonadal dysgenesis is more difficult. A fortuitous family might arise in which an autosomal translocation cosegregates with XX gonadal dysgenesis. Sporadic cases of gonadal dysgenesis have long been associated with reciprocal autosomal translocations, but for years there seemed to be little consistency in the chromosome involved. An alternate approach is a "brute force" genome-wide search for relevant gene(s), utilizing sib-pair analysis with the polymorphic DNA markers readily available throughout the genome. Using sib-pair analysis, as few as 50 to 100 families should identify chromosomal region(s) worthy of sequencing. This method has been applied successfully in Finland to elucidate the form of XX gonadal dysgenesis due to follicle-stimulating hormone receptor (FSHR) mutation (see section on XX Gonadal Dysgenesis due to FSHR Mutation).

Perrault Syndrome (XX Gonadal Dysgenesis with Neurosensory Deafness)

A distinct variant of XX gonadal dysgenesis is that associated with the neurosensory deafness. This condition is called Perrault syndrome. Like XX gonadal dysgenesis without deafness, Perrault syndrome is autosomal recessive (85,91–94).

XX Gonadal Dysgenesis due to Follicle-Stimulating Hormone Receptor Mutation

In Finland, Aittomaki (89) and Aittomaki et al. (90) searched hospitals and cytogenetic laboratories to identify 75 patients countrywide having XX gonadal dysgenesis, defined as 46,XX women with primary or secondary amenorrhea and serum FSH greater than 40 mIU/mL. These 75 patients included 57 sporadic cases and 18 cases having affected relatives (seven different families). Most cases were found in north central Finland, a sparsely populated part of the country. The overall frequency of the disorder in Finland was one per 8,300 liveborn females, a relatively high incidence attributed to a founder effect. Segregation ratio of 0.23 for female siblings was consistent with autosomal recessive inheritance, as was the high consanguinity rate (12%). Sib-pair analysis using polymorphic DNA markers localized the gene to chromosome 2p, a region that was known to contain genes for both the FSHR and the luteinizing hormone receptor (LHR). One specific mutation in exon 7 (C566T: yielding alanine rather than valine) was observed in six families (90,95).

C566T was not found in all Finnish XX gonadal dysgenesis cases. The C566T-negative cases in Finland could represent the same disorder discussed previously (XX gonadal dysgenesis with no somatic anomalies). This would be consistent with the C566T mutation only rarely being detected in women with 46,XX ovarian failure who reside outside Finland. Layman et al. (96) found no mutations in the FSHR gene in 35 46,XX women having hypergonadotropic hypogonadism (15 with primary amenorrhea and 20 with secondary amenorrhea). Liu et al. (97) found no sequence abnormalities in one multigeneration POF family, four sporadic POF cases, and two cases of hypergonadotropic hypogonadism cases.

When Aittomaki et al. (95) contrasted the phenotype of C566T XX gonadal dysgenesis with non-C566T XX gonadal dysgenesis, the former was more likely to have ovarian follicles on ultrasound. C566T XX gonadal dysgenesis thus showed some features expected for gonadotropin resistance (Savage syndrome); however, FSH level clearly was elevated, and the phenotype was far more reminiscent of the bilateral streak gonads and prototypal XX gonadal dysgenesis.

Inactivating Luteinizing Hormone Receptor Mutations

Another trophic hormone receptor gene in which a mutation causes gonadal dysgenesis is the LHR. Most LHR mutations have occurred in 46,XY cases, but 46,XX cases occurred in sibships in which an affected 46,XY male had Leydig cell hypoplasia (98).

Latronico et al. (99) reported primary amenorrhea in a 22-year-old woman. In that family, three males and one female had a homozygous nonsense (stop) mutation at codon 554 (C554X). The resulting stop codon produced a truncated protein having five rather than seven transmembrane domains. The affected female had breast development but only a single episode of menstrual bleeding at age 20 years; LH was 37 mIU/mL and FSH was 9 mIU/mL. The mutation reduced signal transduction activity of the LHR gene. In another 46,XX case reported by Toledo et al. (100), secondary amenorrhea occurred; LH and FSH were 10 and 9 mIU/mL, respectively; the mutation was Ala 593Pro.

Activating LHR mutations seems to have little effect in females, although in males precocious puberty occurs (98).

XX Gonadal Dysgenesis and Multiple Malformation Syndromes

Mutant genes that act on multiple organ systems are called pleiotropic. The pleiotropic gene causing XX gonadal dysgenesis and neurosensory deafness (Perrault syndrome) has already received comment. Other syndromes include XX gonadal dysgenesis and cerebellar ataxia (101); XX gonadal dysgenesis, microcephaly, and arachnodactyly (102); XX gonadal dysgenesis and epibulbar dermoid (103); and XX gonadal dysgenesis, short stature, and metabolic acidosis (104). These four disorders presumably are distinct and autosomal recessive in nature, based on presence of multiple affected siblings.

An autosomal dominant syndrome of relevance is the blepharophimosis-ptosis syndrome, recognized as associated with ovarian failure (105,106). Sib-pair analysis using polymorphic DNA variants localized the gene for blepharophimosis-ptosis to chromosome 3 (3q21-24), a region that contains no obvious candidate gene (107). Surprisingly, Fraser et al. (108) reported that ovaries in one blepharophimosis-ptosis case were unresponsive to gonadatropins.

In each of the multiple malformation syndromes associated with ovarian failure, underlying biologic questions must be posed. Does the seemingly pleiotropic gene cause both the somatic anomalies and the ovarian failure? Do the somatic and nonsomatic phenotypes involve only closely linked genes, i.e., contiguous gene syndrome? Could an unrecognized parental chromosomal rearrangement exist? In turn, do any of these genes play pivotal roles in normal ovarian differentiation and maintenance? Or, is perturbation of ovarian development merely secondary, perhaps occurring through generalized disturbance of connective tissue?

Other Causes of 46,XX Ovarian Failure

A more complete discussion of this topic is provided elsewhere (48). Of note, however, are the several disorders that need to be considered in differential diagnosis: 17α-hydroxylase deficiency, aromatase defects, and galactosemia.

GERM CELL FAILURE IN BOTH SEXES

In several sibships, male and female siblings each have shown germinal cell failure. Affected females show streak gonads, whereas males show germ cell aplasia (Sertoli-cell only syndrome or del Castillo phenotype) (see later). In two of these families, parents were consanguineous, and in each no somatic anomalies were associated (37,38). In three other families, characteristic patterns of somatic anomalies coexisted, suggesting distinct entities. Hamet et al. (36) reported germ cell failure, hypertension, and deafness. Al-Awadi et al. (39) reported germ cell failure and alopecia. Mikati et al. (40) reported germ cell failure, microcephaly, short stature, and minor anomalies.

These families demonstrate that a single autosomal gene can deleteriously affect germ cell development in both sexes. Presumably the gene(s) acts at a site common to early germ cell development or through a mechanism producing meiotic abnormalities. Elucidating such genes could have profound implications for an understanding of normal developmental processes.

XY GONADAL DYSGENESIS

Gonadal dysgenesis may occur in individuals with apparently normal male (46,XY) chromosomal complements. Loss of testicular tissue before 7 to 8 weeks of embryogenesis would be expected to produce such a phenotype, as originally shown by Jost (109) in rabbits. In at least some cases, the gonads of these individuals were embryologically ovaries (110).

Individuals with XY gonadal dysgenesis show female external genitalia, a uterus, and fallopian tubes. At puberty, secondary sexual development fails to occur. Height is normal and somatic anomalies usually are absent. However, a relationship exists between XY gonadal dysgenesis and renal failure (111–113).

Approximately 20% to 30% of XY gonadal dysgenesis patients develop a dysgerminoma or gonadoblastoma (114). Often the neoplasia arises in the first or second decade. A still intriguing observation is that two thirds of XY gonadal dysgenesis individuals were HYA positive, and that HYA-positive cases were far more likely to develop neoplasia than HYA-negative cases (115). Because of the relatively high likelihood of undergoing neoplastic transformation, gonads should be extirpated from individuals with XY gonadal dysgenesis. However, uterus and fallopian tubes should not be removed, because retention of the uterus could allow pregnancy through donor oocytes or donor embryos. Laparoscopic removal of gonads and/or sometimes even a gonadoblastoma usually is possible (116,117).

As noted, the XY gonadal dysgenesis phenotype may result from a mutation within the SRY HMG box (12,13). However, only 10% to 15% of sporadic cases show perturbations of SRY (9). Another form of XY gonadal dysgenesis segregates in the fashion expected of an X-linked recessive (14,56,85,118–120). A third form of XY reversal is the X-linked gene is related in any way to the postulated DSS region (DAX-1 locus) on Xp21. One of 27 "46,XY sex-reversal females" studied by Bardoni et al. (21) showed a submicroscopic duplication of the region [Xp21.2→22.1] that contains DSS.

Genetic heterogeneity (111) is illustrated further by the existence of at least four syndromes: (a) XY gonadal dysgenesis and compomelic dwarfism (121,122); (b) XY gonadal dysgenesis and ectodermal anomalies (123); (c) genito-palato-cardiac (Gardner-Silengo-Wachtel) syndrome (124) and (d) XY gonadal dysgenesis, spastic paraplegia, optic atrophy, and microcephaly (125).

FEMALE PSEUDOHERMAPHRODITISM

In female pseudohermaphrodites, 46,XX individuals have external genitalia that fail to develop as expected for normal females. By far the most common cause is congenital adrenal hyperplasia, resulting from deficiencies of the various enzymes required for steroid biosynthesis (Fig. 1.7) 21-hydroxylase, 11β-hydroxylase, and 3β-ol-dehydrogenase. The common pathogenesis involves decreased production of adrenal cortisol, which regulates secretion of adrenocorticotropic hormone (ACTH) through a negative feedback inhibition mechanism. If cortisol production is decreased, ACTH secretion is not inhibited. Elevated ACTH levels lead to increased quantities of steroid precursors, from which androgens can be synthesized.

The syndromes of adrenal hyperplasia must be excluded quickly when assessing an individual with genital ambiguity, because cortisol and corticosterone deficiencies result in sodium wasting that may be life threatening. Even if cortisol administration is begun immediately after birth, patients with adrenal hyperplasia usually only attain heights between the 3rd and 15th percentiles (126). If cortisol is not administered, affected individuals initially experience increased growth during early childhood; however, premature epiphyseal closure leads to decreased final adult height.

Deficiency of 21-Hydroxylase

Clinical

Deficiency of 21-hydroxylase is the most common cause of genital ambiguity. 21-Hydroxylase deficiency is the result of a cytochrome P450 enzyme fails to convert 17α-hydroxyprogesterone (17α-OHP) to 11-deoxycortisol (Fig. 1.7). Serum cortisol and deoxycortisol are decreased; 17α-OHP, androstenedione, estrone, and testosterone are increased. Increased 17α-OHP in either serum

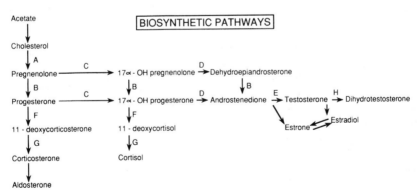

FIG. 1.7. Important adrenal and gonadal biosynthetic pathways. Letters designate enzymes required for the appropriate conversions. A, 20α-hydroxylase and 20,22-desmolase; B, 3β-ol-dehydrogenase; C, 17α-hydroxylase; D, 17,20-desmolase; E, 17-ketosteroid reductase; F, 21-hydroxylase; G, 11β-hydroxylase. (From Simpson JL. *Disorders of sexual differentiation: etiology and clinical delineation.* New York: Academic Press, 1976:1–466, with permission.)

(affected neonate) or amniotic fluid (affected fetus) provides the basis for diagnosis.

Females deficient for 21-hydroxylase or 11β-hydroxylase show clitoral hypertrophy, labioscrotal fusion, and displacement of the urethral orifice to a location more nearly approximating that expected of a male. The extent of virilization may vary among individuals having the same enzyme deficiency. Wolffian derivatives (vasa deferentia, seminal vesicles, epididymides) are rarely present, probably because fetal adrenal function begins too late in embryogenesis to stabilize the wolffian ducts. Müllerian derivatives develop normally, as would be expected in the absence of AMH (MIS). Ovaries develop normally. Scrotal and areolar hyperpigmentation may occur, presumably because ACTH has melanocyte stimulating properties. Increased synthesis of proopiomelanocortin, the parent hormone of both melanocyte-stimulating hormone and ACTH, also occurs. In fact, hyperpigmentation suggests the diagnosis of 21-hydroxylase or 11β-hydroxylase deficiencies in males whose genitalia are normal at birth. If not ascertained by birth, these enzyme deficiencies may pass undetected until the child is 2 years of age or older. At that time, genital enlargement, pubic hair, and prematurely increased height are noted.

Sodium wasting may or may not occur in 21-hydroxylase. In the form of 21-hydroxylase deficiency not associated with sodium wasting (nonsodium-wasting 21-hydroxylase deficiency), it is assumed that increased ACTH secretion results in levels of aldosterone and cortisol sufficient to prevent sodium wasting. Mineralocorticoid and sodium chloride must be administered to correct hyperkalemia and restore fluid-electrolyte balance. If untreated, hyponatremia, hyperkalemia, dehydration, and death may occur. Cortisol administration must be continued into adulthood, although after infancy requirements per unit weight may diminish. Long-term replacement with sodium-retaining hormone (e.g., fluorinated hydrocortisone) may be necessary.

Molecular

21-Hydroxylase is a P450 enzyme and thus located in mitochondria. Its gene (CYP21) is located on chromosome 6p21, closely linked to human leukocyte antigen (HLA). This linkage facilitates heterozygote identification and antenatal diagnosis. The CYP21 gene is unusual in that it is tandemly arranged with the gene for the C4 component of complement. In addition, this entire arrangement is repeated. The actual order is C4A-CYP21P-C4B-CYP21, oriented with the sense strand reading left to right (see later for definition of CYP21P). It is presumed that this CYP21/C4 tandem configuration arose by gene duplication through recombination. The two complement genes (C4A and C4B) are both active, but only a single CYP21 gene is active. The other is a pseudogene (CYP21P), an 8-bp deletion in exon 3 having produced an altered reading forum and, hence, a truncated nonfunctional protein.

As result of the CYP21/C4 tandem arrangements, a predisposition exists to unequal crossing over due to chromosomal misalignment. This may lead to unusual molecular perturbations, specifically one chromosome having a further duplication and its homologue deficiency. A related phenomenon is gene conversion, in which nonreciprocal recombination results in CYP21 being "converted" to a CYP21/P. However, deletions (25%) and gene conversion (15%) are still less common than single nucleotide (point) mutations.

Simple virilizing 21-hydroxylase deficiency is associated with a nucleotide substitution, whereas the salt-wasting form is more likely to be associated with deletions, frame shifts, and nonsense mutations. However, phenotype cannot always be predicted from the mutation. Late onset 21-hydroxylase may produce hirsutism, especially in Ashkenazi Jews. In that ethnic group, one specific mutation is relatively common.

Deficiency of 11β-Hydroxylase

Less common than 21-hydroxylase deficiency, 11β-hydroxylase deficiency also is inherited in autosomal recessive fashion. In this disorder, there is decreased conversion of 11-deoxycortisol to cortisol and 11-deoxycorticosterone to corticosterone; therefore, the major metabolite of 11-deoxycortisol, tetrahydrocortisol, is increased. Because deoxycortisol and deoxycorticosterone are potent sodium-retaining hormones, increased levels may lead to hypervolemia and, hence, hypertension. In 11β-hydroxylase deficiency, infants manifest not only the genital virilization characteristic of 21-hydroxylase deficiency, but also hypertension.

The gene for 11β-hydroxylase is located on chromosome 8 (127). Actually there are two 11β-hydroxylase genes coding for the mitochondrial cytochrome P450 enzymes CYP11B1 and CYP11B2. The latter is expressed only in zona glomerulosa and is important for aldosterone synthesis. The gene responsible for female pseudohermaphroditism is CYP11B1. The gene is located on 8q22, and its most common perturbations are point mutations (128–130).

Deficiency of 3β-Hydroxysteroid Dehydrogenase

In 3β-ol-dehydrogenase (Fig. 1.7) deficiency, the principal androgen synthesized is dehydroepiandrosterone (DHEA). This relatively weak androgen cannot be converted to either androstenedione or testosterone. Females with 3β-ol-dehydrogenase deficiency are less virilized than females with 21-hydroxylase or 11β-hydroxylase deficiencies. On the other hand, DHEA is such a weak androgen that males with 3β-ol-dehydrogenase deficiency fail to masculinize completely (male pseudohermaphroditism). Therefore, 3β-ol-dehydrogenase deficiency is the only form of adrenal hyperplasia in which both males and females show genital ambiguity. In embryonic testes, 3β-ol-dehydrogenase activity reaches its maximum capacity earlier in embryogenesis (third month) than the adrenals and ovaries (fourth month). Otherwise, the external genitalia might be identical in affected males and affected females.

Complete deficiency of 3β-ol-dehydrogenase results in severe sodium wasting secondary to deficiency of sodium-retaining hormones. Sodium wasting often is so pronounced that affected infants die precipitously. However, less severe deficiencies are compatible with long-term survival, and cases are being detected increasingly in older infants (131).

3β-ol-Dehydrogenase deficiency is inherited in an autosomal recessive fashion. It is best diagnosed on the basis of serum steroids measured before and after ACTH stimulation (131). The gene is located on chromosome 1, but, unlike CYP21 and CYP11B, it is not mitochondrial but microsomal. That is, 3β-ol-dehydrogenase is not a cytochrome P450 enzyme. There are two 3β-ol-dehydrogenase genes (I and II) both located on chromosome 1 (p11-13) and both consisting of four exons. Type II is expressed in gonads and adrenals. Point mutations have been described in individuals with 3β-ol-dehydrogenase deficiency (132–134).

17α-Hydroxylase/17,20-Lyase (CYP17) Deficiency

If the cytochrome P450 enzyme 17α-hydroxylase/17,20-lyase is deficient, pregnenolone could not be converted to 17α-hydroxypregnenolone. If the enzyme defect were complete, then cortisol, androstenedione, testosterone, and estrogens could not be synthesized; however, 11-deoxycorticosterone and corticosterone could. As ACTH secretion compensatorily increases, 11-deoxycorticosterone and corticosterone increase. This results in hypernatremia, hypokalemia, and hypervolemia. Clinically, hypertension is evident. Aldosterone levels are decreased, presumably because hypervolemia suppresses the renin-angiotensin system.

Females with 17α-hydroxylase deficiency have normal external genitalia, but at puberty they fail to undergo normal secondary sexual development (primary amenorrhea). Women ordinarily are encountered in differential diagnosis of XX gonadal dysgenesis. Hypertension is a major diagnostic clue. Oocytes appear incapable of reaching a diameter greater than 2.5 mm (135). Affected males usually have genital ambiguity (male pseudohermaphroditism). Oocytes are capable of responding to exogenous gonadotropins (136).

17α-Hydroxylase deficiency is inherited in an autosomal recessive fashion. This cytochrome P450 enzyme is produced by a gene (CYP17) localized to 10q24-25. A single gene is responsible for the action of 17α-hydroxy compounds to 17,20-desmolase (lyase). Because most individuals with 17α-hydroxylase mutations are male pseudohermaphrodites, discussion of molecular aspects of the CYP17α gene is deferred until the section on male pseudohermaphroditism, starting on page 19.

Teratogenic Forms

To interfere with genital differentiation, a teratogen also must exert its action during organogenesis. Before that time, no organ-specific structure can be affected. In humans, the genital tubercle first becomes evident at about 5 weeks of embryogenesis (7 weeks of gestation). If an androgenic teratogen is administered before 12 weeks of gestation, labioscrotal fusion may occur. After 12 weeks, an androgenic teratogen may cause clitoral enlargement but not labioscrotal fusion.

Female pseudohermaphroditism can result from administration of androgens or certain progestins during pregnancy. These forms of female pseudohermaphroditism are rare, but they are important because these causes are preventable. Testosterone and other androgens may masculinize the female offspring of pregnant women, producing phallic enlargement, labioscrotal fusion, and displacement of the urogenital sinus invagination. Excessive androgen production does not affect müllerian differentiation or ovarian differentiation.

Androgen-induced female pseudohermaphroditism was more common decades age, when women more frequently were treated during pregnancy with high doses of synthetic progestins. Not infrequently viril-

ized female offspring resulted (137,138). Administration of progestins during pregnancy, especially in high doses, now rarely is indicated (139), so the problem arises only rarely.

Testosterone, ethinyl testosterone, norethindrone acetate, norethindrone, and danocrine remain potent teratogens. In doses administered therapeutically for conditions such as endometriosis, female pseudohermaphroditism may result (50,137). Norethynodrel, medroxyprogesterone, and 17α-OHP caproate have rarely been implicated. With these latter agents, high doses are required to produce virilization; a single oral contraceptive pill daily should not produce teratogenic female pseudohermaphroditism.

Fetal masculinization has been reported in pregnancies associated with Sertoli cell tumors (arrhenoblastoma), Leydig cell tumors, luteomas of pregnancy, and certain adenocarcinomas that metastasize to the ovary (e.g., Krukenberg tumor). Frequently cited in texts as a cause for masculinizing female fetuses, androgen-secreting tumors in pregnant women are actually a very rare cause of female pseudohermaphroditism. Moreover, patients with preexisting androgen-secreting tumors rarely become pregnant. In 1973, Verhoeven et al. (140) collected only 45 reports in which virilizing tumors were associated with pregnancy. Among the offspring were 18 females whose external genitalia were described; nine had clitoral or labial hypertrophy, but only one had labioscrotal fusion.

Marked clitoral enlargement of unexplained origin sometimes results from hemangiomas, neurofibromas, or tumors. The enlargement seems to be idiopathic in some cases, and may reflect end-organ hyperresponsiveness.

Other Forms of Female Pseudohermaphroditism

Two siblings had clitoral hypertrophy, a single perineal orifice leading anteriorly to a urethra and posteriorly to a vagina, and numerous skeletal anomalies (hypoplasia of the mandible and maxilla, brachycephaly, narrow vertebral bodies, relatively long slender bones, dislocation of fusion of the radial heads leading to abnormal-appearing elbows, coxa valga, and phalangeal fusion of several toes) (141,142). Müllerian derivatives and ovaries were normal. Both siblings developed breasts and pubic hair but failed to menstruate. Their parents were consanguineous; thus, autosomal recessive inheritance seems probable.

Female pseudohermaphroditism of unknown origin can be associated with one or more of the following anomalies: absence or duplication of the uterus; renal absence, duplication, or hydronephrosis; and imperforate anus (143). Short stature, mental retardation, deafness, ear and nasal malformation, and a blindly ending colon are less often associated; the ovaries usually are normal.

Genital abnormalities may result from maldevelopment of the genital tubercle, cloacal membrane, urogenital membrane, or the entire hind end of the embryo (i.e., caudal regression syndrome). In some of these malformations, the external genitalia may be so abnormal that the sex of rearing is in doubt. These rare disorders include exstrophy of the bladder, exstrophy of the cloaca, and sirenomelia (50).

MALE PSEUDOHERMAPHRODITISM

In male pseudohermaphroditism, individuals with a Y chromosome have external genitalia that fail to develop as expected for normal males. This implies external genitalia sufficiently ambiguous to confuse the sex of rearing. Cytogenetic forms of male pseudohermaphroditism (45,X/46,XY and variants) are discussed here to contrast their phenotype with those of genetic male pseudohermaphroditism.

Teratogenic Forms

If given in sufficiently high doses in the first trimester to a woman pregnant with a male fetus, several drugs would be expected to produce female external genitalia. These include cyproterone acetate, whose mode of action involves blocking androgen receptor, and finisteride, whose mode of actions involves inhibiting 5α-reductase. The consequence of mutations affecting such functions will become clear later. Both agents are approved in the United States for treatment of hirsutism.

Controversy still exists about whether administration of progestins or progesterones to women having male fetuses can produce hypospadias. In my opinion, the weight of evidence is that these agents do not produce this defect (144).

Cytogenetic Forms

45,X/46,XY individuals have both a 45,X cell line and at least one cell line containing a Y chromosome. Based on cohort studies of 45,X/46,XY cases detected without bias *in utero* (prenatal genetic diagnosis), well over 90% of cases are normal males (145). However, cases ascertained postnatally differ, manifesting a variety of phenotypes: almost normal males with cryptorchidism or penile hypospadias, and genital ambiguity females indistinguishable from those with 45,X Turner's syndrome (50,146,147). Different phenotypes presumably reflect different tissue distributions of the various cell lines. A structurally abnormal Y chromosome may be present. Because many structurally abnormal chromosomes (e.g., dicentric) are unstable, it is likely that the 45,X line arises secondarily after loss of the structurally abnormal Y.

45,X/46,XY Unambiguous Female External Genitalia

45,X/46,XY individuals may have Turner's stigmata and thus be clinically indistinguishable from 45,X individuals. Such individuals usually are normal in stature and show no somatic anomalies. As in other types of gonadal dysgenesis, the external genitalia, vagina, and müllerian derivatives remain unstimulated because of the lack of sex steroids. Breasts fail to develop, and little pubic or axillary hair develops. If breast development occurs in a

45,X/46,XY individual, an estrogen-secreting tumor such as gonadoblastoma or dysgerminoma should be suspected (148). Virilization also has been claimed to result from gonadotropin stimulation of streak gonads (149).

Although streak gonads of 45,X/46,XY individuals may be histologically indistinguishable from those of 45,X individuals, gonadoblastomas or dysgerminomas develop in about 15% to 20% of 45,X/46,XY individuals (114). Neoplasia may develop in the first or second decade of life. Despite the possibility that a locus on Yq may protect against neoplasia (150), gonadal extirpation is recommended for all 45,X/46,XY individuals having female external genitalia. The uterus should be retained because pregnancy may be achieved through donor oocytes or donor embryos. Gonadectomy usually can be accomplished by laparoscopy (117). It is preferable to remove only gonads, but technically it may be necessary to remove the adnexa as well. Laparotomy should only rarely prove necessary.

45,X/46,XY Ambiguous External Genitalia

The term *asymmetric* or *mixed gonadal dysgenesis* is applied to individuals with one streak gonad and one dysgenetic testis. These individuals usually have ambiguous external genitalia and a 45,X/46,XY complement, and usually they have a uterus. Occasionally only 45,X or only 46,XY cells are demonstrable. Many investigators believe that the phenotype invariably is associated with 45,X/46,XY mosaicism. Nonmosaic cases most likely reflect merely the inability to sample enough tissues.

45,X/46,XY individuals with ambiguous external genitalia usually have müllerian derivatives (e.g., a uterus). Presence of a uterus is a very important diagnostic sign, because that organ is absent in almost all the genetic (mendelian) forms of male pseudohermaphroditism discussed elsewhere in this section. If an individual has ambiguous external genitalia, bilateral testes, and a uterus, it is reasonable to infer that individual actually has 45,X/46,XY mosaicism, regardless of whether both lines can be demonstrated cytogenetically. Occasionally the uterus may be rudimentary, or a fallopian tube may fail to develop ipsilateral to a testis.

45,X/46,XY Nearly Normal Male External Genitalia

45,X/46,XY mosaicism may be detected in individuals with nearly normal male external genitalia. This phenotype has the highest incidence, based on follow-up of most 45,X/46,XY fetuses ascertained at amniocentesis; most (90%) have a normal male phenotype (151). That 45,X/46,XY neonates are far more common postnatally showing genital ambiguity reflects biases of ascertainment.

45,X/46,XY individuals having almost normal male external genitalia do not seem to develop neoplasia as often as 45,X/46,XY individuals with female or frankly ambiguous genitalia (114). Gonadal extirpation may not be necessary if a male sex of rearing is chosen, provided gonads can be assessed periodically within the scrotum by ultrasound or palpation (114).

Male Pseudohermaphroditism in Multiple Malformation Syndromes

Genital ambiguity may occur in individuals with various multiple malformation syndromes. Coexistence of genital ambiguity with the Meckel-Gruber syndrome, Smith-Lemli-Opitz type I syndrome, brachio-skeletal-genital syndrome (152), and esophageal-facial-genital syndrome (153) has long been recognized. These disorders are inherited in either autosomal recessive or X-linked recessive fashion.

Drash syndrome is an appellation applied to individuals with Wilms' tumor, aniridia, and male pseudohermaphroditism. This disorder is associated with deletion of chromosome 11p13 (154,155), for which reason 11p is implicated as an autosomal region integral for male development. Smith-Lemli-Opitz syndrome is an autosomal recessive syndrome in which 46,XY individuals show genital abnormalities (male pseudohermaphroditism). In type II Smith-Lemli-Opitz syndrome, external genitalia may be female (sex reversal) (156). The molecular explanation is mutation involving the gene responsible for converting 7-hydroxycholesteral cannot be converted to cholesterol. The usual molecular explanation is a defect in exon-intron splicing.

In the genito-palato-cardiac (Gardner-Silengo-Wachtel) syndrome, 46,XY individuals show phenotypic variability, not only in external genitalia but also in gonads (124). Complete sex reversal can even occur in 46,XY individuals who have ovaries. A recently described sex reversal syndrome is that characterized by 46,XY female siblings having spastic paraplegia, optic atrophy, and normal intelligence despite microcephali (125). General implications of these syndromes for the autosomal control of sex determination has long been recognized by Simpson (157).

Deficiencies in Testosterone Biosynthesis

Male pseudohermaphroditism may result from deficiencies of 17α-hydroxylase, 3β-ol-dehydrogenase, or 17-ketosteroid reductase 17,20-desmolase. These enzymes are required to convert cholesterol to pregnenolone (congenital adrenal lipoid hyperplasia) (Fig. 1.7). Deficiencies of 21-hydroxylase or 11β-hydroxylase, the most common causes of female pseudohermaphroditism, do not cause male pseudohermaphroditism. Males (46,XY) show precocious masculinization.

Adrenal biosynthetic defects should be suspected if levels of testosterone or its metabolites are decreased. Diagnosis of the various conditions, to be discussed later, is not difficult in older children, but detection may be difficult during infancy because neonatal testosterone levels are physiologically low. Provocative tests (i.e., human chorionic gonadotropin stimulation) may facilitate diagnosis.

Congenital Adrenal Lipoid Hyperplasia

In congenital adrenal lipoid hyperplasia, male pseudohermaphrodites show ambiguous or female-like external genitalia and severe sodium wasting. Adrenals are characterized by foamy-appearing cells filled with cholesterol (158,159). Accumulation of cholesterol has long indicated that cholesterol cannot be converted to pregnenolone (Fig. 1.7). Inheritance has been presumed to be autosomal recessive on the basis of increased parental consanguinity.

The cytochrome P450 enzyme responsible for converting cholesterol to pregnenolone is P450scc (side chain cleavage); the gene is CYP11A. P450scc converts cholesterol to pregnenolone via 20α-hydroxylase, 22α-hydroxylase, and 20,22-desmolase. A large gene located on chromosome 15, CYP11A is 20 kb long and has nine exons.

Surprisingly, perturbations of this gene have never been shown in congenital adrenal lipoid hyperplasia (160). Rather, congenital adrenal lipoid hyperplasia results from perturbation of the steroidogenic acute regulatory (StAR) protein. The StAR protein delivers precursors for cholesterol side chain cleavage, and predictably its perturbation would have major effects of hormone action in gonads and adrenals. Mapped to 8p11.2, the gene spans 8 kb and consists of seven exons interrupted by six introns. Mutations in StAR have been reported in congenital lipoid hyperplasia (161), producing a nonfunctional protein. Typically a point mutation produces stop codons or exon/intron splicing errors that yield large deletions or truncated gene products.

3β-Hydroxysteroid Dehydrogenase (3β-ol-Dehydrogenase Deficiency)

This enzyme deficiency is inherited in autosomal recessive fashion. Decreased synthesis of both androgens and estrogens occurs (Fig. 1.7). The major androgen produced is DHEA, as already discussed. DHEA is a weaker androgen than testosterone and as such is not capable of adequately virilizing the male fetus. Diagnosis usually is established on the basis of serum DHEA levels before and after ACTH stimulation. In addition to genital abnormalities, 3β-ol-dehydrogenase deficiency is associated with severe sodium wasting, given that both aldosterone and cortisol are decreased.

Incompletely developed external genitalia of males with 3β-hydroxysteroid dehydrogenase (3β-HSD) deficiency are clinically similar to the external genitalia of most other male pseudohermaphrodites: small phallus, urethral opening proximal on the penis, and incomplete labioscrotal fusion. Testes and wolffian ducts differentiate normally. Given that affected females (46,XX) also show genital ambiguity, 3β-ol-dehydrogenase (3β-HSD) is the only enzyme that, when deficient, produces male pseudohermaphroditism in males and female pseudohermaphroditism in females.

3β-HSD is a microsomal enzyme, unlike 21-hydroxylase or 11β-hydroxylase. The gene is located on 1p13.1. Type I is expressed in placenta, skin, and breasts; type II is expressed in adrenal cortex and gonads. Male pseudohermaphroditism results from type II mutations, usually due to point mutations (133).

17α-Hydroxylase and 17,20-Desmolase (Lyase) Deficiency

17α-Hydroxylase is another cytochrome P450 gene (CY17), located on 10q24-25. The gene product also possesses 17,20-desmolase (lyase) activity.

Males deficient in 17α-hydroxylase/17,20-desmolase (lyase) usually show ambiguous external genitalia and may even show female external genitalia (162). Wolffian duct development and testicular development are normal. Although affected females (46,XX) show hypertension (see earlier), males deficient in 17α-hydroxylase typically display normal blood pressure. Both males and females are affected; thus, inheritance has long been considered to be autosomal recessive.

When it became evident that a single enzyme serves both 17α-hydroxylase and 17,20-desmolase functions, considerable genetic and nosologic confusion was generated (163). That a single gene/enzyme is responsible for both these functions was a surprise,

because enzyme studies had suggested two genetically distinct conditions involving two separate genes. That mutations recently have been reported in which only the 17,20-lyase function was affected has partially elucidated the confusion (164,165). This perhaps may help explain the family reported by Zachmann et al. (166). In this family, two maternal cousins had genital ambiguity, bilateral testes, and no müllerian derivatives; a maternal "aunt" was said to have abnormal external genitalia and bilateral testes. The deficient enzyme was considered to be 17,20-desmolase (lyase), based on both cousins showing low plasma testosterone and DHEA levels despite normal urinary excretion of pregnanediol, pregnanetriol, and 17-hydroxycorticoids. In testicular tissue, testosterone could be synthesized from androstenedione or DHEA, excluding 17-ketosteroid reductase deficiency (see later) but suggesting isolated 17,20-desmolase deficiency.

This P450c17 enzyme is coded by a gene (CYP17) on chromosome 10q24-25. This gene (CYP17) consists of eight exons. It is structurally reminiscent of its CYP21 cousin, 21-hydroxylase, but no pseudogene exists. Deletions and gene conversions are uncommon; point mutations are the more typical molecular perturbation (167–169).

Deficiency of 17β-Hydroxysteroid Dehydrogenase (17-Ketosteroid Reductase)

Inability to convert DHEA to testosterone is the result of deficiency of this microsomal enzyme (Fig. 1.7) (170). Plasma testosterone usually is decreased; and androstenedione and DHEA are increased. Affected males show ambiguous external genitalia, bilateral testes, and no müllerian derivatives. Breast development may or may not be present, apparently reflecting the estrogen-to-testosterone ratio (171). Pubertal virilization is greater than in many other enzyme deficiencies, and sometimes gynecomastia is not even evident (172). In one report, the sex of rearing of an affected individual was changed from female to male after puberty (171).

The 17β-hydroxysteroid dehydrogenase gene (17HSD-3) is located on chromosome 9 and consists of 11 exons. This gene is microsomal, like 3β-HSD reflecting action on gonads rather than adrenals. Molecular perturbations typically involve single amino-acid substitutions (173,174), but disruption of the splice junction involving intron 3 is not uncommon. Although exon or intron 3 is most commonly involved, mutations also may occur in exons 2, 8, 9, 10, 11, and 12. Missense mutations may result in negligible levels of testosterone due to complete impairment of the enzyme.

Complete Androgen Insensitivity (Complete Testicular Feminization)

In complete androgen insensitivity (CAI; or complete testicular feminization), 46,XY individuals show bilateral testes, female external genitalia, a blindly ending vagina, and no müllerian derivatives (Fig. 1.8). These findings are entirely predictable, given the underlying pathogenesis involving inability to respond to testosterone. AMH is synthesized, as in the normal testis. The body responds normally to AMH, for which reason no uterus is present. As predicted on the basis of testes synthesizing estrogens in unimpeded fashion, affected individuals manifest breast development and pubertal feminization.

Despite pubertal feminization, some individuals with androgen insensitivity show clitoral enlargement and labioscrotal fusion. The term *incomplete* or *partial androgen insensitivity* (PAI) (*incomplete testicular feminization*) is applied to these patients. The mildest end of the spectrum consists of males only manifesting gynecomastia and oligospermia/azoospermia. Complete, incomplete (partial), and mild androgen insensitivity are all inherited in X-linked recessive fashion. All result from mutations of the androgen receptor gene present on the X long arm (Xq11).

As adults, individuals with CAI may be quite attractive and show excellent breast development. Despite this traditional textbook description, most cases are actually similar in appearance to unaffected females in the general population. Breasts contain normal ductal and glandular tissue, but areolae often are pale and underdeveloped. Pubic hair and axillary hair (terminal) usually are sparse (only vellus hair present), but scalp hair is normal. The vagina terminates blindly, and sometimes vaginal length is shorter than usual. Occasionally, the vagina is only 1 to 2 cm long or is represented merely by a dimple. Surgery to create a neovagina or use of dilations may be necessary, but usually vaginal length is adequate without intervention. Neither a uterus nor fallopian tubes are ordinarily present, but there may be fibromuscular remnants, rudimentary fallopian tubes, or, rarely, even a uterus (175).

Testes usually are normal in size. They may be located in the abdomen, inguinal canal,

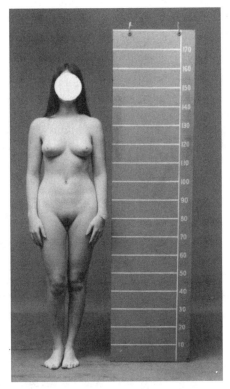

FIG. 1.8. Patient with complete testicular feminization. (From Simpson JL. *Disorders of sexual differentiation: etiology and clinical delineation.* New York: Academic Press, 1976:1–466, with permission. Courtesy of Dr. Charles Hammond.)

labia, or anywhere along the path of embryonic testicular descent. If located in the inguinal canal, the testes may produce inguinal hernias. One half of all individuals with testicular feminization develop inguinal hernias. Therefore, it is worthwhile to determine the cytogenetic status of prepubertal girls with inguinal hernias, although most will be 46,XX. Height is slightly increased compared with normal women but unremarkable compared to 46,XY males.

Frequency of gonadal neoplasia is increased, but not so much as once assumed (176). The actual risk is probably no greater than 5% (114,148). The risk of malignancy is low before 25 to 30 years of age. Benign tubular adenomas (Pick adenomas) are common in postpubertal patients, probably as a result of increased LH secretion. Orchiectomy eventually is necessary, but it is acceptable to leave the testes *in situ* until after spontaneous pubertal feminization. However, if a herniorrhaphy proves necessary before puberty, most surgeons perform the orchiectomy at the same time. There also may be some psychological benefit in prepubertal orchiectomies.

The androgen receptor gene is localized to Xq11-12. This gene consists of eight exons; exons 2 and 3 are the DNA-binding domains, whereas exons 4 through 8 are androgen-binding domains (Fig. 1.9) (177). Many different mutations have been reported and tabulated yearly (178). No single perturbation has proved paramount. Deletions and insertions are rare (179); point mutations are far more common. These include deletion of three nucleotides with preservation of an open reading frame, or single nucleotide changes resulting in either substitution of an unscheduled amino acid or changes generating a stop codon that would result in premature message termination and production of a nonfunctional protein.

Mutations are found throughout the gene, but particularly in exons 4 through 8 (the androgen-binding domain). In exons 5 through 8, the preponderance of mutations are missense, and again both PAI and CAI arise. Mutations in exon 1 usually cause CAI, and mutations in exons 2 and 3 (the DNA-binding domain) produce either CAI and PAI. In general, large deletions and mutations resulting in premature termination (stop codon) predictably produce no functional receptor and cause CAI (180). Point mutations resulting from single nucleotide substitutions have a similar phenotype but also may be compatible with production of some androgen receptor. Irrespective, the receptor may be unstable or display poor binding (180).

Exons, Binding Domains of the hAR

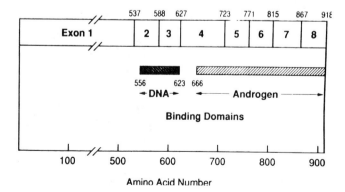

FIG. 1.9. Schematic diagram showing androgen-binding gene. Exons 2 through 4 relate to DNA binding, whereas exons 5 through 7 confer androgen binding. Sites of some reported mutations are noted. (Adapted from a diagram by Dr. Leonard Pinsky, Montreal, Quebec, Canada.)

Partial Androgen Insensitivity (Incomplete Testicular Feminization) and Reifenstein's Syndrome

At puberty, certain 46,XY individuals feminize (develop breasts) and their external genitalia are characterized by phallic enlargement and partial labioscrotal fusion (Fig. 1.10). These individuals have PAI (incomplete testicular feminization). PAI and CAIs share many features: bilateral testes with Leydig cell hyperplasia, no müllerian derivatives, pubertal breast development, lack of pubertal virilization, normal (male) plasma testosterone, and failure to respond to androgen (181). The cellular pathogenesis of PAI may involve decreased numbers or qualitative defects of androgen receptors (182–184).

First, it is worth recounting to avoid nosologic confusion that incomplete (partial) androgen insensitivity is an X-linked recessive condition that encompasses several entities historically considered separate (i.e., the erstwhile Lubs syndrome, Gilbert-Dreyfus syndrome, and Reifenstein's syndrome). In 1974, Wilson et al. (185) reported a single kindred that had both the Reifenstein's phenotype and

PAI as traditionally defined. In 1984, the same group confirmed PAI in two individuals with the Lubs syndrome phenotype (186). Thus, the traditional separation among Reifenstein's syndrome, Lubs syndrome, and incomplete androgen insensitivity was not valid. All three disorders merely represent different spectrums of a single X-linked recessive disorder, herein called *incomplete (partial) androgen insensitivity.*

The clinical significance of PAI (incomplete androgen insensitivity) is that this disorder must be excluded before a male sex of rearing can be assigned. Demonstration of response by androgen receptors or finding of a clinical response to exogenous androgen excludes the condition. Demonstration of a specific molecular defect in the androgen receptor gene would be useful only if an index case were already known or the phenotype of that specific nucleotide change known.

As in CAI, molecular analysis reveals mutations throughout the gene. Molecular analysis has revealed many different mutations in the DNA-binding and androgen-binding domains. Other than generalizations already made, correlation is poor between phenotype and the exon or sequence involved.

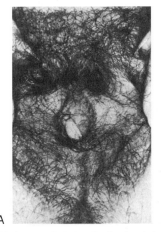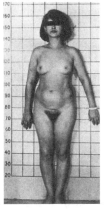

A　　　　　　　　　　　　　　　　B

FIG. 1.10. Individual with incomplete testicular feminization. Despite the enlarged phallus and labioscrotal fusion **(A)**, breast development occurred at puberty **(B)**. (From Park IJ, Jones HW. Familial male hermaphroditism with ambiguous external genitalia. *Am J Obstet Gynecol* 1970;108:1197, with permission.)

5α-Reductase Deficiency (Pseudovaginal Perineoscrotal Hypospadias)

For decades it has been recognized that some genetic males show ambiguous external genitalia at birth, but at puberty they undergo virilization like normal males. They experience phallic enlargement, increased facial hair, muscular hypertrophy, and voice deepening, but no breast development. Their external genitalia consist of a phallus that resembles a clitoris more than a penis, a perineal urethral orifice, and usually a separate, blindly ending, perineal orifice that resembles a vagina (pseudovagina) (Fig. 1.11).

Initially called *pseudovaginal perineoscrotal hypospadias* (PPSH), this trait was shown in 1971 to be inherited in an autosomal recessive fashion (187,188). This disorder later proved to result from deficiency of the enzyme 5α-reductase (189–191), an enzyme that converts testosterone to DHT. That intracellular 5α-reductase deficiency results in the PPSH phenotype is consistent with virilization of the external genitalia during embryogenesis requiring DHT; wolffian differentiation requires only testosterone. Pubertal virilization also can be accomplished by testosterone alone. 46,XX females deficient in 5α-reductase show normal ovarian function (192).

Diagnosis is made most easily on the basis of an elevated testosterone-to-DHT ratio after administration of human chorionic gonadotropin or testosterone propionate (193). The ratio of the respective urinary metabolites of testosterone and DHT (i.e., etiocholanolone and androsterone) also is elevated. In infants, baseline levels of testosterone and DHT are so low that distinguishing normal from affected individuals may be difficult. An elevated ratio of urinary tetrahydrocortisol to 5α-tetrahydrocortisol also can serve as the basis for diagnosis (194).

It is preferable to assay cells derived from genital tissue (e.g., foreskin). Considerable variability exists in 5α-reductase activity among control genital tissues, with near overlap between controls and individuals recog-

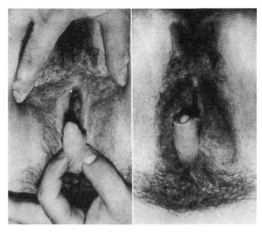

FIG. 1.11. External genitalia of an individual with pseudovaginal perineoscrotal hypospadias. At puberty, phallic enlargement occurred but breast development did not. Some individuals with this phenotype have 5α-reductase deficiency. (From Opitz JM, Simpson JL, Sarto GE, et al. Pseudovaginal perineoscrotal hypospadias. *Clin Genet* 1972;3:1, with permission.)

nized on other grounds to be deficient for 5α-reductase. Presence of 5α-reductase in cultured genital fibroblasts thus excludes 5α-reductase deficiency, whereas absence of 5α-reductase offers less confidence in confirming the diagnosis. Diagnosis may be especially difficult in infants, because baseline levels of testosterone and DHT are so low. Distinguishing normal from affected individuals may be difficult.

Two 5α-reductase (SRD5) genes exist. The type I gene (SRD5A1) is located on chromosome 5, and the type II gene (SRD5A2) is located on chromosome 2p23. Only type II is expressed in gonads; thus, of the two isoforms, type II is deficient in male pseudohermaphroditism. Consisting of five exons (195), the SRD5A2 gene has been shown to have undergone deletions far less often (196) than point mutations (197). Different ethnic groups show different mutations (founder effect), scattered among the five exons. Molecular studies can be exploited for prenatal diagnosis and genetic counseling in kindreds, but usually only after one affected case has been detected.

Aromatase Mutations (CYP19)

Conversion of androgens (Δ4-androstenedione) to estrogens (estrone) requires cytochrome P450 aromatase, an enzyme that is the gene product of a single 40-kb gene located on chromosome 15q21.1 (198). The gene consists of ten exons. Although Ito et al. (199) reported a mutation in this CYP19 (P450 arom) gene in a 18-year-old 46,XX woman with primary amenorrhea and cystic ovaries, deficiency of the aromatase enzyme more often is associated with genital ambiguity. Shozu et al. (200) detected *placental* aromatase deficiency manifesting as maternal virilization during the third trimester. The 46,XX infant was born with genital ambiguity (female pseudohermaphroditism). Adrenal enzyme defects were not evident. The molecular basis of the mutation was a 87-bp insert in exon 6 of the aromatase gene, altering the splice junction site to produce a novel protein with 29 additional amino acids. Aromatase mutations in 46,XX female infants have been associated with genital ambiguity (199) or clitoromegaly (201). Clitoral enlargement occurred at puberty, but breast development did not. Multiple ovarian follicular cysts were evident. FSH was elevated; estrone and estradiol were low. Estrogen and progesterone therapy resulted in a growth spurt, decreased FSH, decreased androstenedione and testosterone, breast development, menarche, and fewer follicular cysts. Molecular studies demonstrated compound heterozygosity for CYP19 point mutations.

Estrogen Receptor Defects

The estrogen receptor gene consists of eight exons and is coded on chromosome 6q24→27. Analogous to the androgen receptor gene, there is a DNA-binding region (exons 2 and 3) and an estrogen-binding domain (exons 4 though 8).

An estrogen receptor mutation was found by Lubahn et al. (202) in a 28-year-old man who showed normal male sexual development. Incomplete epiphyseal closure led to tall stature. Serum gonadotropin and estrogen levels were elevated; neither decreased after exogenous estrogen administration. The molecular basis proved to be a homozygous transition in exon 2 that resulted in a premature stop codon (203).

Agonadia (Testicular Regression Syndrome)

In agonadia, gonads are absent, external genitalia are normal, and all but rudimentary müllerian or wolffian derivatives are absent. External genitalia usually consist of a phallus about the size of a clitoris, underdeveloped labia majora, and nearly complete labioscrotal fusion. Persistent urogenital sinus often is present. By definition, gonads are undetectable. Neither normal müllerian derivatives nor normal wolffian derivatives ordinarily are present; however, rudimentary structures may be present along the lateral pelvic wall. Somatic anomalies (craniofacial or vertebral anomalies or mental retardation) may coexist (204).

The pathogenesis of agonadia must take into account not only absence of gonads but also abnormal external genitalia and absence of internal ducts. Two explanations seem plausible:

1. Fetal testes functioned long enough during development to inhibit müllerian development but not long enough to allow complete normal male sexual differentiation. Believing this explanation to be valid, some prefer the appellation *testicular regression syndrome.*
2. Alternatively, gonadal, ductal, and genital systems all could have developed abnormally as a result of either defective primordium, defective connective tissue, or teratogenic action. Coexistence of somatic anomalies is most consistent with this second hypothesis.

Several sibships of affected males have been reported (34). SRY is present, indicating that pathogenesis does not involve gross perturbation of that gene (9,205,206). Kwok et al. (205) found no mutations in the sequence 2-kb 5' to the SRY coding region.

Leydig Cell Hypoplasia (Luteinizing Hormone Receptor Mutation)

In complete absence of Leydig cells (207,208), 46,XY cases have female external genitalia, no uterus, and bilateral testes devoid of Leydig cells. Epididymides and vasa deferentia are present, and serum LH is elevated. Affected siblings have been reported (209,210) and parental consanguinity observed (211). Thus, autosomal recessive inheritance has long been accepted.

The molecular basis involves mutation in the LHR gene, located on chromosome 2. Kremer et al. (212) reported two siblings of consanguineous parents; homozygosity for a missense mutation (Ala$^{(593)}$→Pro) existed. In another case, Salameh et al. (213) detected a deletion in exon 11. Leydig cells presumably fail to develop because LH cannot exert its effect during embryogenesis. This is reminiscent of ovarian failure due to FSHR mutation.

In contrast to the *inactivating* LHR mutations, *activating* mutations cause precocious puberty in males. In females, LHR activating receptor mutations do not seem to exert the same effect.

TRUE HERMAPHRODITISM

True hermaphrodites have both ovarian and testicular tissue. They may have a separate ovary and a separate testis or, more often, one or more ovotestes. Most true hermaphrodites (60%) have a 46,XX chromosomal complement; however, a minority have 46,XX/46,XY, 46/XY, 46,XX/47,XXY, or other complements (214). Phenotype probably reflects karyotype (214), but it is preferable here only to generalize about the phenotype of all true hermaphrodites.

If there is no medical intervention (obviously now a rarity in most venues), two thirds of true hermaphrodites would be raised as males (50). By contrast, external genitalia usually are ambiguous or predominantly female. Breast development usually occurs at puberty, even with predominantly male external genitalia. Gonadal tissue may be located in the ovarian, inguinal, or labioscrotal regions. A testis or an ovotestis is more likely to be present on the right than on the left. Spermatozoa are rarely present (215); however, apparently normal oocytes often are present, even in ovotestes (Fig. 1.12). 46,XX true hermaphrodites have even become pregnant (216,217), usually but not always after removal of testicular tissue.

The greater the proportion of testicular tissue in an ovotestis, the greater the likelihood of gonadal descent. In 80% of ovotestes, testicular and ovarian components are juxtaposed end to end (218). Thus, an ovotestis may be detectable by inspection or palpation, because testicular tissue is softer and darker than ovarian tissue. Accurate identification by ultrasound or magnetic resonance imaging is particularly necessary if the inappropriate portion of the ovotestis is to be extirpated. Both gonadal neoplasia and breast carcinoma have been reported (148,214). The former may reflect risks associated with the intraabdominal location of testicular tissue.

A uterus usually is present, although sometimes it is bicornuate or unicornuate. Absence of a uterine horn usually indicates ipsilateral testis or ovotestis. The fimbriated end of the fallopian tube may be occluded ipsilateral to an ovotestis, and squamous metaplasia of the endocervix may occur (218). Menstruation is not uncommon and may be manifested as cyclic hematuria.

Presence of a uterus is diagnostically useful in true hermaphroditism and is particularly invaluable in the rare 46,XY cases. Of individuals with genital ambiguity having a chromosome, only 46,XY hermaphrodites and 45,X/46,XY mosaics have a uterus.

Diagnosis usually is made only after excluding male and female pseudohermaphroditism. If a female sex of rearing is chosen, extensive surgery may or may not be necessary. If a male sex of rearing is chosen, geni-

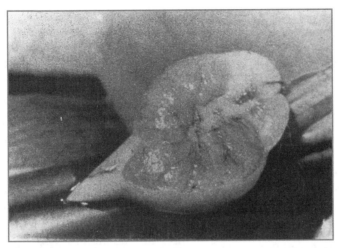

FIG. 1.12. Bisected ovotestis from a patient of Van Niekerk. The patient had a 46,XX complement. The ratio of ovarian to testicular tissue is about 1:4; ovarian tissue is present in the *upper right.* The testicular portion appeared yellowish brown, whereas the ovarian portion was white, although color differentiation cannot be appreciated in this photograph. The ovarian portion was firmer than the testicular portion. In 80% of ovotestes, just as in this patient, ovarian and testicular tissues are arranged end to end. (From Van Niekerk WA. *True hermaphroditism.* New York: Harper & Row, 1974, with permission.)

tal reconstruction and selective gonadal extirpation are invariably indicated.

46,XX/46,XY AND 46,XY

True hermaphroditism is heterogeneous in origin. 46,XX/46,XY true hermaphroditism usually is caused by chimerism, the presence in a single individual of two or more cell lines, each derived from different zygotes. 46,XY cases may be unrecognized chimeras (214). However, chimerism is not the likely explanation for 46,XX true hermaphrodites. Explanations for the presence of testes in individuals who ostensibly lack a Y have focused on (a) translocation during paternal meiosis of SRY from the Y to an X, (b) translocation of SRY from the Y to an autosome, (c) undetected mosaicism or chimerism, and (d) autosomal sex-reversal genes.

46,XX

46,XX true hermaphrodites fail to show DNA sequences from their father's Y (219). This contrasts with 46,XX males, 80% of whom show SRY. Unexplained is why HYA was reported present in almost all 46,XX true hermaphrodites (115). Detection of the SRY sequence in one 46,XX true hermaphrodite and a 46,XX male sibling gave a strong clue that Y/X translocation can be involved (13), but overall mendelian factors seem more likely explanation for the several reported sibships with XX true hermaphroditism (214).

Occurrence of 46,XX males and 46,XX true hermaphrodites in the same kindred has been reported. 46,XX males in these kindreds usually show genital ambiguity, unlike the typical 46,XX male. Familial true hermaphroditism is more likely to be characterized by bilateral ovotestes and uterine absence than nonfamilial true hermaphroditism. That both gonads are morphologically similar (213) favors a central basis for gonadal perturbation, as opposed to chimerism. Thus, it could be postulated that perturbation (derepression) of an ordinarily dormant autosomal gene induces inappropriate (testicular) gonadal development in 46,XX individuals. This argument has been developed in detail elsewhere

(42–44). Once seemingly iconoclastic, the plausibility that various autosomal regions (9p, 10p, 17q) could undergo activating mutations and lead to testes in 46,XX individuals now seems high.

GENITAL DUCT DISORDERS

Surgical management of genital duct malformations is discussed in detail elsewhere is this volume. Here we shall confine our remarks to the embryologic and genetic aspects of selected disorders.

Fusion of the Labia Minora

Fusion of the labia minora is often the sequela of infection or sexual abuse. However, congenital fusion apparently unassociated with these factors has been observed in siblings (220) and in more than one generation (221,222).

Imperforate Hymen

Ordinarily the central portion of the hymen is patent (perforate), thereby allowing outflow of mucus and blood. If the hymen is imperforate, mucus and blood accumulate in the vagina or uterus (hydrocolpos or hydrometrocolpos). An imperforate hymen is easily corrected by surgical incisions, preferably cruciform. McIlroy and Ward (223) reported affected siblings. Recently, Stelling et al. (224) reported two monozygotic twins concordant for imperforate hymen. One twin had an affected daughter.

Transverse Vaginal Septa and the McKusick-Kaufman Syndrome

Transverse vaginal septa occur at several locations and may be complete or incomplete. These septa usually are about 2 cm thick and located near the junction of the upper third and lower two thirds of the vagina (50,225, 226). Septa may be present in the middle or lower third of the vagina (226). Perforations usually are central, but they may be eccentric

in location (227–230). If no perforation is present, mucus and menstrual fluid cannot exit; thus, hydrocolpos or hydrometrocolpos develop. Pelvic organs otherwise usually are normal, although occasionally the uterus is bicornuate.

Vaginal septa presumably result from failure of urogenital sinus derivatives and müllerian duct derivatives to fuse or canalize. This explanation is deduced from location of the septa, namely at the predicted sites of urogenital sinus and müllerian fusion. Cranial surfaces of septa typically are lined by columnar (müllerian) epithelium, whereas caudal surfaces are lined by squamous epithelium (urogenital sinus invagination).

If transverse vaginal septa is associated with postaxial polydactyly and cardiac defects (231), the eponymous McKusick-Kaufman syndrome is applied (231). The original description of this syndrome and most cases reported since have been in the Amish. A single pleiotropic gene causing transverse vaginal septa could exist, or transverse vaginal septa could be genetically heterogeneous.

A single pleiotropic gene was the assumption underlying analysis of 54 Amish cases studied by Chitayat et al. (232). Hydrometrocolpos was estimated to be present in 95% of female cases, polydactyly in 93%, and cardiovascular malformations in 9%. Individuals were observed with all three anomalies, various combinations of two anomalies, and only one anomaly (233). Stone et al. (234) estimated penetrance to be 70% for hydrometrocolpos in females, 60% for polydactyly in both sexes, and 15% for cardiovascular defects. Given these probabilities, one would expect 9% of males and 3% of females to have the gene in the completely nonpenetrant state. In the Amish, the transverse vaginal septa gene has been localized to chromosome 20p12.

Longitudinal Vaginal Septa

Isolated longitudinal vaginal septa reflects a different etiology than transverse vaginal septa. In the former, heritable tendencies have

TABLE 1.3. *Syndromes associated with longitudinal vaginal septa*

Syndrome	Somatic anomalies	Etiology
Edwards-Gale (camptobrachydactyly)	Flexion contractures of distal interphalangeal joints, brachydactyly, polydactyly, syndactyly, urinary incontinence	Autosomal dominant
Johanson-Blizzard	Scalp defects, deafness, hypoplastic alae nasi, microdontia, primary hypothyroidism, malabsorption, mental retardation, hypotonia, short stature	Autosomal recessive

not been discerned. However, longitudinal septa may be part of several multiple malformation syndromes (Edwards-Gale, Fraser) (Table 1.3).

Müllerian Aplasia

Aplasia of the müllerian ducts leads to absence of the uterine corpus, uterine cervix, and upper portion of the vagina (Fig. 1.13). The foreshortened 1- to 2-cm vagina presumably is derived exclusively from invagination of the urogenital sinus. Individuals with müllerian aplasia usually consult physicians because of primary amenorrhea. Secondary sexual development is normal, no uterine structures are palpable, but uterine remnants may exist in the form of bilateral cords. The term *Rokitansky-Küster-Hauser syndrome* often is applied, sometimes only if remnants persist and sometimes synonymously with müllerian aplasia.

Only one other disorder ordinarily needs to be considered in the differential diagnosis of CAI. Müllerian aplasia is about twice as common. Androgen insensitivity can be excluded on the basis of chromosomal studies and gonadal composition (testes rather than ovaries). Pubertal patients with müllerian aplasia invariably show pubic hair, whereas those with androgen insensitivity usually do not. Renal (pelvic kidney, renal ectopia, and unilateral aplasia), skeletal, and vertebral anomalies are not uncommon.

Müllerian Aplasia   Vaginal Atresia

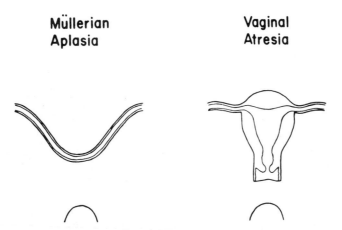

FIG. 1.13. Diagrammatic representation of two distinct entities, müllerian aplasia and vaginal atresia. Each sometimes is designated as "congenital absence of the vagina." (From Sarto GE, Simpson JL. Abnormalities of the Müllerian and Wolffian duct systems. In: Summitt RL, Bergsma D, eds. *Sex differentiation and chromosomal abnormalities* / Sponsored by the National Foundation-March of Dimes, New York: A.R. Liss Publishers. *Birth Defects Orig Artic Ser* 14(6C):37–54, 1978, with permission.)

Affected siblings with müllerian aplasia have been reported (235–239). However, Lischke and associates (240) observed three sets of discordant monozygotic twin. Thus, autosomal recessive inheritance is not the explanation for all cases. In 1978, autosomal dominant inheritance was proposed by Shokeir (239) based on 16 Saskatchewan families. In 13 of 16 families, the proband showed complete absence of the uterine cervix and corpus; in the remaining three, uterine remnants were present. None of the three individuals with uterine remnants had an affected relative, but ten of the 13 with complete absence of the uterine cervix and corpus did. Two of these ten had affected siblings, whereas the other eight had other affected paternal relatives (aunts, first cousins, second cousins, or great-aunts). These observations suggest sex-limited (female) autosomal dominant inheritance. Females with the postulated mutant would manifest müllerian abnormalities, whereas males would show no deleterious effect.

In contrast to the conclusions of Shokeir were the findings of Carson and co-workers (241). Not a single relative was affected in 23 U.S. families, encompassing 30 postpubertal sisters, 31 paternal aunts, and 41 maternal aunts. This makes sex-limited autosomal dominant inheritance unlikely; absence of affected siblings and lack of paternal consanguinity speaks against autosomal recessive inheritance.

The data of Carson et al. (241) are consistent with those of Petrozzi et al. (242), who studied women with müllerian aplasia who underwent assisted reproductive technologies (ART). Because women with müllerian aplasia have normal ovaries, one strategy is to obtain oocytes from affected women, perform fertilization *in vitro* with their husband's sperm, and transfer fertilized embryos to a surrogate uterus of another woman in hormonal synchrony. Offspring would reflect genetic constitution of the woman with müllerian aplasia. Petrozza et al. (242) surveyed U.S. ART programs and collected 34 pregnancies involving oocytes of women with müllerian aplasia. Of the 34 offspring, 17 were female. None were affected; one male child had a middle ear defect and hearing loss.

The most logical explanation for müllerian aplasia is polygenic/multifactorial inheritance, the usual mode of inheritance for malformations affecting either a single organ system or embryologically related systems. Polygenic/multifactorial inheritance is consistent with the occasional reports of multiple affected siblings. After the birth of one child with a polygenic/multifactorial disorder, the recurrence risk for first-degree relatives of affected probands approximates the square root of the incidence of the trait in the population. Given that müllerian aplasia is rare, one would expect the recurrence risk in siblings to be low. Failure to detect affected siblings in a relatively small sample is consistent with polygenic/multifactorial inheritance and a low (1% to 2%) recurrence risk for first-degree relatives.

No significant progress has been reported in the molecular elucidation of müllerian aplasia. Reindollar and colleagues have searched for perturbations in several potential candidate genes. Large deletions, insertions, or rearrangements have not been detected in the genes WT-1 (Wilms' tumor) (243), PAX 2 (244), HOXA13 (245), and AMH (MIS) (246). There is no increase in the N314 allele of galactose-1-phosphate uridyl transferase (247).

In several multiple malformation syndromes, müllerian aplasia is one component. The etiology presumably reflects perturbation of genes different from those responsible for müllerian aplasia in otherwise normal individuals.

Incomplete Müllerian Fusion

Familial aggregates of incomplete müllerian fusion include multiple affected siblings, as well as affected mother and daughter (248–256). In some families, affected relatives show different forms of incomplete müllerian fusion (257).

The only one formal genetic study is that of Elias et al. (257), who found only one of 37 (2.7%) sisters of probands to have a clinically symptomatic uterine anomaly; no (0/24) mothers, no (0/44) maternal aunts, and no (0/50) paternal aunts were affected. The prevalence of 2.7% in siblings should be considered a minimum frequency, because relatives might have a minor uterine anomaly in asymptomatic form. If female relatives have not attempted pregnancy, the opportunity to manifest symptoms that would suggest an anomaly would be limited. Performing hysteroscopy, hysterosalpingography, or laparoscopy on relatives would be ideal but impractical. Even with these inherent limitations, however, the likelihood of first-degree female relatives being similarly affected with müllerian fusion anomalies would seem too low to be compatible with autosomal dominant or autosomal recessive etiology.

That approximately 3% of female siblings were affected in the one formal study is most consistent with predictions based on polygenic/multifactorial etiology.

TABLE 1.4. *Syndromes associated with incomplete müllerian fusion*

Syndrome	Somatic anomalies	Etiology
Bardet-Biedl	Retinal pigmentary degeneration (retinitis pigmentosa), polydactyly, obesity, mental deficiency	Autosomal recessive
Beckwith-Wiedemann	Macroglossia, omphalocele, macrosomia	Autosomal dominant, after uniparental disomy
Donohue (leprechaunism)	Elfin facies with thick lips; large, low-set ears; prominent breasts and external genitalia; hirsutism; abnormal carbohydrate metabolism; failure to thrive; motor and mental retardation	Autosomal recessive
Fraser	Cryptophthalmia, external ear and nose anomalies, laryngeal stenosis, syndactyly, skeletal defects, renal agenesis, large clitoris and labia majora, mental retardation	Autosomal recessive
Hand-foot-genital (HFG)	Metacarpal and metatarsal anomalies, malformed thumbs, displaced urethral meatus, urinary incontinence	Autosomal dominant
Johanson-Blizzard	Deafness, hypoplastic alae nasi, primary hypothyroidism, mental retardation	Autosomal recessive
Laryngeal atresia	Hydrocephaly, complete or partial laryngeal obstruction, tracheoesophageal fistula or atresia, renal hypoplasia, varus deformity of feet	Unknown
Meckel-Gruber	Microcephaly, posterior encephalocele, eye anomalies, cleft palate, polycystic kidneys, polydactyly	Autosomal recessive
Roberts	Sparse, silvery-blond hair; midfacial hemangioma; cleft lip with or without cleft palate; limb reduction defect; intrauterine growth retardation	Autosomal recessive
Rudiger	Bifid uvula, coarse facies, absent ear cartilage, hydronephrosis secondary to ureterovesical stenosis, short digits	Autosomal recessive
Thalidomide teratogenicity	Nasal hemangioma, neurosensory hearing loss, ear anomalies, limb reduction defects, visceral anomalies	Teratogen
Trisomy 18	Prominent occiput, malformed ears, micrognathia, short sternum, cardiac defects, horseshoe kidney, overlapping fingers, intrauterine growth retardation, severe development retardation	Chromosomal aneuploidy
Trisomy 13	Microcephaly, microphthalmia, malformed ears, cleft lip and palate, cardiac anomalies, polydactyly, intrauterine growth retardation, severe developmental retardation	Chromosomal aneuploidy
Urogenital adysplasia, hereditary (hereditary renal agenesis)	Oligohydramnios, flattened (Potter) facies, pulmonary hypoplasia, unilateral or bilateral absent kidneys, limb deformities	Autosomal dominant

Hand-Foot-Genital Syndrome

Hand-foot-genital (HFG) syndrome is an autosomal dominant disorder in which incomplete müllerian fusion is a major feature. First reported by Stern and associates (258), multiple kindreds have now been recognized (148,259–261). The HFG syndrome is characterized by skeletal (hand and foot) malformations and either incomplete müllerian fusion in females or hypospadias in males (thus, "hand-foot-genital" has replaced the original appellation "hand-foot-uterus") (261,262). Limb abnormalities include short first metacarpals, small distal phalanges on the thumbs, short middle phalanges on the small finger, and fusion of the wrist bones (263). The great toe is shortened due to a shortened metatarsal; the distal phalanx is small and pointed.

Urinary system anomalies in HFG syndrome include urinary incontinence in females, ventrally displaced urethral meatus (male and female), and malposition of the ureteral orifices in the bladder wall (females) (263). These urologic anomalies differ from those associated with isolated incomplete müllerian fusion. Moreover, vertebral anomalies do not seem characteristic of the HFG syndrome.

Even with a negative family history, HFG syndrome should be considered present if an individual with incomplete müllerian fusion has any of the skeletal or genital anomalies characteristic of HFG syndrome. Given that variable expressivity is characteristic of all autosomal dominant disorders, it also would be expected that some females with the HFG gene would manifest only uterine anomalies or only skeletal anomalies, whereas others in the same kindred show both.

HOXA13 is an attractive candidate gene for human HFG (264). A HOXA13 mutation was detected in a member of the original family reported by Stern et al. (258), and a HOXA13 nonsense mutant was found in other HFG families (265). The manner by which perturbation of HOXA13 produces HFG still is uncertain.

HFG is not the only multiple malformation syndrome associated with incomplete müllerian fusion. Table 1.4 provides a more complete list. Many different genes as well as nonmendelian factors must remain intact for normal müllerian development. Whether wild-type genes for these syndromes are integral for normal müllerian differentiation remains unclear. The uterine anomalies merely could arise secondary to connective tissue or vascular perturbations.

REFERENCES

1. Patsavoudi E, Magre S, Castinior M, et al. Dissociation between testicular morphogenesis and functional differentiation of Leydig cells. *J Endocrinol* 1985;28:235.
2. Magre S, Jost A. Dissociation between testicular morphogenesis and endocrine cytodifferentiation of Sertoli cells. *Proc Natl Acad Sci U S A* 1984;81:783.
3. Behringer RR, Cate RL, Froelick GJ, et al. Abnormal sexual development in transgenetic mice chronically expressing Müllerian inhibiting substance. *Nature* 1990;345:16.
4. Lee MM, Donahoe PK. Müllerian inhibiting substance: a gonadal hormone with multiple functions. *Endocr Rev* 1993;14:152.
5. Gustafson ML, Lee MM, Asmundson L, et al. Müllerian inhibiting substance in the diagnosis and management of intersex and gonadal abnormalities. *J Pediatr Surg* 1993;28:439.
6. Jirasek J. Principles of reproductive embryology. In: Simpson JL, ed. *Disorders of sexual differentiation.* San Diego: Academic Press, 1976:51.
7. Gubbay J, Collignon J, Koopman P, et al. A gene mapping to the sex-determining region of the mouse Y chromosome is a member of a novel family of embryonically expressed genes. *Nature* 1991;346:245.
8. Sinclair AH, Berta PH, Palmer MS, et al. A gene from the human sex-determining region encodes a protein with homology to a conserved DNA-binding motif. *Nature* 1990;346:240.
9. Pivnick EK, Wachtel S, Woods D, et al. Mutations in the conserved domain of SRY are uncommon in XY gonadal dysgenesis. *Hum Genet* 1992;90:308.
10. Koopman P, Gubbay J, Vivian N, et al. Male development of chromosomally female mice transgenic for Sry. *Nature* 1991;351:117.
11. Berta P, Hawkins JR, Sinclair AH, et al. Genetic evidence equating SRY and the testis-determining factor. *Nature* 1990;348:448.
12. Hawkins JR, Taylor A, Berta P, et al. Mutational analysis of SRY; nonsense and missense mutations in XY sex reversal. *Hum Genet* 1992;88:471.
13. Jager RJ, Anvret M, Hall K, et al. A human XY female with a frame shift mutation in the candidate testis-determining gene SRY. *Nature* 1990;348:452.
14. Simpson JL, Christakos AC, Horwith M, et al. Gonadal dysgenesis associated with apparently chromosomal complements. *Birth Defects* 1971;7(6):215.

15. German J, Simpson JL, Chaganti RSK, et al. Genetically determined sex-reversal in 46,XY humans. *Science* 1978;205:53.
16. Bernstein R, Jenkins, T, Dawson T, et al. Female phenotype and multiple abnormalities in siblings with a Y-chromosome and partial X-chromosomal duplication: H-Y antigen and Xg blood group findings. *J Med Genet* 1980;17:291.
17. Ogata T, Hawkins JR, Taylor A, et al. Sex reversal in a child with a 46,X,Yp+ karyotype: support for the existence of a gene, located in distal Xp, involved in testis formation. *J Med Genet* 1992;29:226.
18. Ogata T, Tomita K, Hida A, et al. Chromosomal localisation of a Y specific growth gene(s). *J Med Genet* 1995;32:572.
19. Arn P, Chen H, Tuck-Muller CM, et al. SRVX, a sex reversing locus in Xp21.2→p22.11. *Hum Genet* 1994;4:389.
20. Rao PN, Klinepeter K, Stewart W, et al. Molecular cytogenetic analysis of a duplication Xp in a male: further delineation of a possible sex influence region on the X chromosome. *Hum Genet* 1994;94:149.
21. Bardoni B, Xanaria E, Guioli S, et al. A dose sensitive locus at chromosome Xp21 is involved in male to female sex reversal. *Nat Genet* 1994;7:497.
22. Tommerup N, Schempp W, Meinecke P, et al. Assignment of an autosomal sex reversal locus (SRA1) and campomelic dysplasia (CMPD1) to 17q24.3-q25.1. *Nat Genet* 1993;4:170.
23. Foster JW, Dominguez-Steglich MA, Guioli S, et al. Campomelic dysplasia and autosomal sex reversal caused by mutations in an SRY-related gene. *Nature* 1994;372:525.
24. Meyer J, Sudbeck P, Held M, et al. Mutational analysis of the SOX9 gene in campomelic dysplasia and autosomal sex reversal: lack of genotype/phenotype correlations. *Hum Mol Genet* 1997;6:91.
25. Pelletier J, Bruening W, Li FP, et al. WT1 mutations contribute to abnormal genital system development and hereditary Wilm's tumour. *Nature* 1991;353:431.
26. Pelletier J, Bruening W, Kashtan CE, et al. Germline mutations in the Wilms' tumor suppressor gene are associated with abnormal urogenital development in Danys-Drash syndrome. *Cell* 1991;67:437.
27. Nordenskjold A, Fricke G, Anvret M. Absence of mutations in the WT1 gene in patients with XY gonadal dysgenesis. *Hum Genet* 1995;96:102.
28. Wilkie AOM, Campbell FM, Daubeney P, et al. Complete and partial XY sex reversal associates with terminal deletion of 10q: report of cases and literature review. *Am J Med Genet* 1993;46:597.
29. Bennett CP, Docherty Z, Robb SA, et al. Deletion 9p and sex reversal. *J Med Genet* 1993;30:518.
30. Vegetti W, Grazia Tibiletti M, Testa G, et al. Inheritance in idiopathic premature ovarian failure: analysis of 71 cases. *Hum Reprod* 1998;13:1796.
31. Schinzel A. Phocomelia and additional anomalies in two sisters. *Hum Genet* 1990;84:539.
32. Ferguson-Smith MA, Sanoudou D, Lee C. Microdeletion of DMT1 at 9p24.3 is the commonest cause of 46,XY females. *Am J Hum Genet* 1998;63:A162.
33. McDonald MT, Flejter W, Sheldon S, et al. XY sex reversal and gonadal dysgenesis due to 9p24 monosomy. *Am J Med Genet* 1997;73:321.
34. de Grouchy J, Gompel A, Salmon-Bernard Y. Embryonic testicular regression syndrome and severe mental retardation in sibs. *Ann Genet* 1985;28:154.
35. Najjar SS, Takla RJ, Nassar VH. The syndrome of rudimentary testes: occurrence in five siblings. *J Pediatr* 1974;84:119.
36. Hamet P, Kuchel O, Nowacynski JM, et al. Hypertension with adrenal, genital, renal defects, and deafness. *Arch Intern Med* 1973;131:563.
37. Smith A, Fraser IS, Noel M. Three siblings with premature gonadal failure. *Fertil Steril* 1979;32:528.
38. Granat M, Amar A, Mor-Yosef S, et al. Familial gonadal germinative failure: endocrine and human leukocyte antigen studies. *Fertil Steril* 1983;40:215.
39. Al-Awadi SA, Farag TI, Geebie AS, et al. Primary hypergonadism and partial alopecia in three sibs with Müllerian hypoplasia in the affected females. *Am J Med Genet* 1985;22:619.
40. Mikati MA, Samir SN, Sahil IF. Microcephaly, hypergonadotropic hypogonadism, short stature and minor anomalies. A new syndrome. *Am J Med Genet* 1985;22:599.
41. Burgoyne PS, Baker TG. Perinatal oocyte loss in XO mice and its implication for the etiology of gonadal dysgenesis in XO women. *J Reprod Fertil* 1987;75:633.
42. Simpson JL. Phenotypic-karyotypic correlations of gonadal determinants: current status and relationship to molecular studies. In: Sperling K, Vogel F, eds. *Proceedings of the 7th International Congress, Human Genetics, Berlin, 1986.* Heidelberg: Springer-Verlag, 1987:224.
43. Simpson JL. Genetic control of sexual development. In: Ratnam SS, Teoh ED, eds. *Advances in fertility and sterility: releasing hormones and genetics and immunology in human reproduction, vol. 3. Proceedings of the 12th World Congress on Fertility and Sterility, Singapore, 1986.* Lancaster, UK: Parthenon Press, 1987:165.
44. Simpson JL. Genetic control of sex determination. In: Iizuka R, Seem K, Ohno T, eds. *Human reproduction: current status, future prospects. Proceedings of the 6th World Congress on Human Reproduction, Tokyo, 1987.* Amsterdam: Elsevier Scientific, 1988:19.
45. Simpson JL. Genetics of female infertility. In: Filicori M, Flamigni C, eds. *Proceedings of the conference. Treatment of infertility: the new frontiers.* Boca Raton, FL: Communications Media for Education, Inc., 1998:37.
46. Zinn AR, Tonk VS, Chen Z, et al. Evidence for a Turner syndrome locus or loci Xp11.2-p22.1. *Am J Hum Genet* 1998;63:1757.
47. Tharapel AT, Anderson KP, Simpson JJ, et al. Deletion (X)(q26.1→q28) in a proband and her mother: molecular characterization and phenotypic-karyotypic deduction. *Am J Hum Genet* 1993;52:463.
48. Simpson JL. Genetics of oocyte depletion. In: Lobo RA, ed. *Perimenopause. Serono symposia USA Norwell, Massachusetts.* New York: Springer, 1998:36.
49. Simpson JL. Gonadal dysgenesis and abnormalities of the human sex chromosomes: current status of the phenotypic-karyotypic correlations. *Birth Defects* 1975;11:(4)23.
50. Simpson JL. *Disorders of sexual differentiation: etiology and clinical delineation.* New York: Academic Press, 1976:259.

51. Loughlin SAR, Redha A, McIver J, et al. Analysis of the origin of Turner's syndrome using polymorphic DNA probes. *J Med Genet* 1991;28:156.

52. James, RS, Dalton P, Gustashaw K, et al. Molecular characterization of isochromosomes of Xq. *Ann Hum Genet* 1997;61:485.

53. James RS, Coppin B, Dalton P, et al. A study of females with deletions of the short arm of the X chromosome. *Hum Genet* 1988;102:507.

54. Ogata T, Matsuo N. Turner syndrome and female sex chromosome aberrations: deduction of the principal factors involved in the development of clinical features. *Hum Genet* 1995;95:607.

55. Migeon BR, Jelalian K. Evidence for two active X chromosomes in germ cells of female before meiotic entry. *Nature* 1977;269:242.

56. Simpson JL. Pregnancies in women with chromosomal abnormalities. In: Schulman JD, Simpson JL, eds. *Genetic disease in pregnancy.* New York: Academic Press, 1981: 439.

57. Dewhurst J. Fertility in 47,XXX and 45,X patients. *J Med Genet* 1978;15:132.

58. Singh DN, Hara S, Foster HW, et al. Reproductive performance in women with sex chromosome mosaicism. *Obstet Gynecol* 1980;55:608.

59. Ishikawa M, Hidaka E, Wakui K, et al. Habitual abortion and low frequent X chromosome monosomy mosaicism: detection by interphase FISH analyses of buccal mucosa cells and lymphocytes. 48th Annual Meeting, American Society of Human Genetics. *Am J Hum Genet* 1998;63:A108.

60. Fisher EM, Beer-Romero P, Brown LG, et al. Homologous ribosomal protein genes on the human X and Y chromosomes: escape from X inactivation and possible implications for Turner syndrome. *Cell* 1990;63: 1205.

61. Chen YC, Woolley PV Jr. Genetic studies on hypospadias in males. *J Med Genet* 1971;8:153.

62. Brook CGD, Wagner H, Zachman M, et al. Familial occurrence of persistent Müllerian structures in otherwise normal males. *BMJ* 1973;1:771.

63. Ranke MB, Pfluger H, Rosendahl W, et al. Turner's syndrome: spontaneous growth in 150 cases and review of the literature. *Eur J Pediatr* 1983;181:141.

64. Ranke MB, Blum WF, Hang F, et al. Growth hormone, somatomedin levels and growth regulation in Turner's syndrome. *Acta Endocrinol (Copenh)* 1987;116:305.

65. Rosenfeld RG, Grumbach MM. *Turner syndrome.* New York: Marcel Dekker, 1990.

66. Filippson R, Lindsten J, Almqvist S. Time of eruption of the permanent teeth cephalometric and tooth measurement and sulphation factor activities in 45 patients with Turner syndrome with different types of X chromosome aberration. *Acta Endocrinol (Copenh)* 1965;48:91.

67. Lindsten J, Fraccaro M. Turner's syndrome. In: Rashad MN, Morton WRN, eds. *Genital anomalies.* Springfield, IL: Charles C Thomas Publisher, 1969:396.

68. McCauley E, Sybert VP, Ehrhardt A. Psychological adjustments of adult women with Turner syndrome. *Clin Genet* 1986;29:284.

69. McCauley E, Kay T, Ito I, et al. The Turner syndrome: cognitive defects, affective discrimination and behavior problems. *Child Dev* 1987;58:464.

70. Hook EB, Hamerton JL. The frequency of chromosome abnormalities detected by consecutive newborn studies differences between studies: results by sex and by severity of phenotypic involvement. In: Hook EB, Porter IH, eds. *Population cytogenetic studies in human.* New York: Academic Press, 1977:63.

71. Simpson JL. Genetic control of sexual development. In: Teoh ES, Ratnam SS, Goh VHH, eds. *Fertility and sterility series.* Lancaster, UK: Parthenon Press, 1987: 165.

72. Simpson JL. Ovarian maintenance determinants on the X chromosome and on autosomes. In: Coutifaris C, Mastroianni L, eds. *New horizons in reproductive medicine. Proceedings of the IXth World Congress on Human Reproduction, Philadelphia, 1996.* New York: The Pantheon Publishing Group, 1997:439.

73. Fraccaro M, Maraschio P, Pasquali F, et al. Women heterozygous for deficiency of the (Xpter→X21) region of the X chromosome are fertile. *Hum Genet* 1977;39:283.

74. Simpson JL, LeBeau MM. Gonadal and statural determinants on the X chromosome and their relationship to *in vitro* studies showing prolonged cell cycles in 45,X,46,X, del(X)(p11); 36,X,del(X)(q13) and q(22) fibroblasts. *Am J Obstet Gynecol* 1981;141:930.

75. Soyke A, Stumm M, Krebs P, et al. Familial occurrence of a del(Xp−) chromosome: pitfall in karyotype/phenotype correlation. *Am J Med Genet* 1998;80:436.

76. Sala C, Arrigo G, Torri G, et al. Eleven X chromosome breakpoints associated with premature ovarian failure (POF) map to a 15-Mb YAC contig spanning Xq21. *Genomics* 1997;40:123.

77. Philippe C, Arnould C, Sloan F, et al. A high-resolution interval map of the q21 region of the human X chromosome. *Genomics* 1995;27:539.

78. Willard HF, Cremers FP, Mandel JL, et al. Report of the fifth international workshop on human X chromosome mapping. *Cytogenet Cell Genet* 1994;67:295.

79. Krauss CM, Turkray RN, Atkins L, et al. Familial premature ovarian failure due to interstitial deletion of the long arm of the X chromosome. *N Engl J Med* 1987; 317:125.

80. Fitch N, de Saint, VJ, Richer CL, et al. Premature menopause due to small deletion in long arm of the X chromosome: a report of three cases and a review. *Am J Obstet Gynecol* 1982;142:968.

81. Jones MH, Furlong RA, Burkin H, et al. The Drosophila developmental gene fat facets has a human homologue in Xp11.4 which escapes X-inactivation and has related sequences on Yp11.2. *Hum Mol Genet* 1996;5:1695.

82. Castrillon DH, Wasserman SA. Diaphanous is required for cytokinesis in Drosophila and shares domains of similarity with the products of the limb deformity gene. *Development* 1994;120:3367.

83. Philippe C, Cremers FPM, Chery M, et al. Physical mapping of DNA markers in the q13-q22 region of the human X chromosome. *Genomics* 1993;17:147.

84. Bione S, Sala C, Manzini C, et al. A human homologue of the Drosophila melanogaster diaphanous gene is disrupted in a patient with premature ovarian failure: evidence for conserved function in oogenesis and implications for human sterility. *Am J Hum Genet* 1998; 62:533.

85. Simpson JL. Gonadal dysgenesis and sex chromosome abnormalities. Phenotypic/karyotypic correlations. In:

Vallet HL, Perter IH, eds. *Genetic mechanisms of sexual development.* New York: Academic Press, 1979: 365.

86. Meyers CM, Boughman JA, Rivas M, et al. Gonadal dysgenesis in 46,XX individuals: frequency of the autosomal recessive form. *Am J Med Genet* 1996;63:518.

87. Boczkowski K. Pure gonadal dysgenesis and ovarian dysplasia in sisters. *Am J Obstet Gynecol* 1970;106: 626.

88. Portuondo JA, Neyro JL, Benito JA, et al. Familial 46,XX gonadal dysgenesis. *Int J Fertil* 1987;32:56.

89. Aittomaki K. The genetics of XX gonadal dysgenesis. *Am J Hum Genet* 1994;54:844.

90. Aittomaki K, Dieguez Luccena JL, Pakarinen P, et al. Mutation in the follicle-stimulating hormone receptor gene causes hereditary hypergonadotropic ovarian failure. *Cell* 1995;82:959.

91. Christakos AC, Simpson JL, Younger JB, et al. Gonadal dysgenesis as an autosomal recessive condition. *Am J Obstet Gynecol* 1969;104:1027.

92. Pallister PD, Opitz JM. The Perrault syndrome: autosomal recessive ovarian dysgenesis with facultative, non sex-limited sensorineural deafness. *Am J Med Genet* 1979;22:629.

93. McCarthy DJ, Opitz JM. Perrault syndrome in sisters. *Am J Med Genet* 1985;22:629.

94. Nishi Y, Hamamoto K, Kajiyama M, et al. The Perrault syndrome: clinical report and review. *Am J Med Genet* 1988;31:623.

95. Aittomaki K, Herva, R, Stenman, UH, et al. Clinical features of primary ovarian failure caused by a point mutation in the follicle-stimulating hormone receptor gene. *J Clin Endocrinol Metab* 1996;81:3722.

96. Layman LC, Amede S, Cohen DP, et al. The Finnish follicles-stimulating hormone receptor gene mutation is rare in North American women with 46,XX ovarian failure. *Fertil Steril* 1998;69:300.

97. Liu JY, Gromoll J, Cedars MI, et al. Identification of allelic variants in the follicle-stimulating hormone receptor genes of females with or without hypergonadotropic amenorrhea. *Fertil Steril* 1998;70:326.

98. Sultan LH, Lumbroso S. LH receptor defects. In: Kempers RD, Cohen J, Haney AF, Younger JB, eds. *Fertility and reproductive medicine. Proceedings of the XVI World Congress on Fertility and Sterility.* Amsterdam: Elsevier Science, 1998:769.

99. Latronico AC, Anasti J, Arnhold IJ, et al. Brief report: testicular and ovarian resistance to luteinizing hormone caused by inactivating mutations of the luteinizing hormone-receptor gene. *N Engl J Med* 1996;334: 507.

100. Toledo SP, Brunner HG, Kraaij R, et al. An inactivating mutation of the luteinizing hormone receptor causes amenorrhea in a 46,XX female. *J Clin Endocrinol Metab* 1996;81:3850.

101. Skre H, Bassoe HH, Berg K, et al. Cerebella ataxia and hypergonadotropic hypogonadism in two kindreds. Chance concurrence, pleiotropism or linkage? *Clin Genet* 1976;9:234.

102. Maximilian C, Ionescu B, Bucur A. Deux soeurs avec dysgenesie gonadique majeure, hypotrophic staturale, microcephalie, arachondactylie et caryotype 46,XX. *J Genet Hum* 1970;10:26.

103. Quayle SA, Copeland KC. 46,XX gonadal dysgenesis with epibulbar dermoid. *Am J Med Genet* 1991;40:75.

104. Pober BR, Zemel S, Hisama FM. 46,XX gonadal dysgenesis, short stature and recurrent metabolic acidosis in two sisters. 48th annual meeting of the American Society of Human Genetics. *Am J Hum Genet* 1998; 63:652.

105. Zlotogora J, Sagi M, Cohen, T. The blepharophimosis-ptosis, and epicanthus inversus syndrome: delineation of two types. *Am J Hum Genet* 1983;33:1020.

106. Panidis D, Rousso D, Vavilis D, et al. Familial blepharophimosis with ovarian failure. *Hum Reprod* 1994;9:2034.

107. Harrar HS, Jeffrey S, Patton MA. Linkage analysis in blepharophimosis-ptosis syndrome confirms localisation to 3q21-24. *J Med Genet* 1995;32:774.

108. Fraser IS, Shearman RP, Smith A, et al. An association among blepharophimosis, resistant ovary syndrome, and true premature menopause. *Fertil Steril* 1988;50: 747.

109. Jost A. Problems of fetal endocrinology. The gonadal and hypophyseal hormones. *Recent Prog Horm Res* 1953;8:379.

110. Cussen LK, McMahon R. Germ cells and ova in dysgenetic gonads of a 46,XY female dizygote twin. *Arch Dis Child* 1979;133:373.

111. Simpson JL, Blagowidow N, Martin OA. XY gonadal dysgenesis: genetic heterogeneity based upon clinical observations. H-Y antigen status and segregation analysis. *Hum Genet* 1981;58:91.

112. Simpson JL, Chaganti RSK, Mouradian J, et al. Chronic renal disease myotonic dystrophy, and gonadoblastoma in an individual with XY gonadal dysgenesis. *J Med Genet* 1982;19:73.

113. Haning RV Jr, Chesney RW, Moorthy AV, et al. A syndrome of chronic renal failure and XY gonadal dysgenesis in young phenotypic females without genital ambiguity. *Am J Kidney Dis* 1985;6:40.

114. Simpson JL, Photopulos G. The relationship of neoplasia to disorders of abnormal sexual differentiation. *Birth Defects* 1976;12(1):15.

115. Wachtel SS. *H-Y antigen and the biology of sex determination.* New York: Grune & Stratton, 1983.

116. Wilson EE, Vuitch F, Carr BR. Laparoscopic removal of dysgenetic gonads containing a gonadoblastoma in a patient with Swyer syndrome. *Obstet Gynecol* 1992; 79:842.

117. Pisarska MD, Simpson JL, Zepeda DE, et al. Laparoscopic removal of streak gonads in 46,XY or 45,X/46,XY gonadal dysgenesis. *J Gynecol Tech* 1998;4:95.

118. Sternberg WH, Barclay DL, Kloepfer HW. Familial XY gonadal dysgenesis. *N Engl J Med* 1968;278:695.

119. Espiner EA, Veale AMO, Sands VE, et al. Familial syndrome of streak gonads and normal male karyotype in five phenotypic females. *N Engl J Med* 1970; 238:6.

120. Mann JR, Corkery JJ, Fisher HJW, et al. The X-linked recessive form of XY gonadal dysgenesis with high incidence of gonadal cell tumours: clinical and genetic studies. *J Med Genet* 1983;20:264.

121. Bricarelli FD, Fraccaro M, Lindsten J, et al. Sex-reversed XY females with campomelic dysplasia are H-Y negative. *Hum Genet* 1981;57:15.

122. Puck SM, Haseltine FP, Francke U. Absence of H-Y antigen in an XY female with campomelic dysplasia. *Hum Genet* 1981;57:23.

123. Brosnan PC, Lewandowski RC, Toguri AG, et al. A familial syndrome of the 46,XY gonadal dysgenesis with anomalies of ectodermal and mesodermal structures. *J Pediatr* 1981;97:586.

124. Greenberg F, Gresik MW, Carpenter RJ, et al. The Gardner-Silengo-Wachtel or genito-palato-cardiac syndrome: male pseudohermaphroditism with micrognathia, cleft palate, and conotruncal cardiac defects. *Am J Med Genet* 1987;26:59.

125. Teebi AS, Miller S, Ostrer H, et al. Spastic paraplegia, optic atrophy, microcephaly with normal intelligence, and XY sex reversal: a new autosomal recessive syndrome? *J Med Genet* 1998;35:759.

126. Riddick DH, Hammond CB. Long-term steroid therapy in patients with adrenogenital syndrome. *Obstet Gynecol* 1975;45:15.

127. Mornet E, White PC. Analysis of genes encoding steroid 11-betahydroxylase. *Cytogenet Cell Genet* 1989;15:1047(abst).

128. White PC, Dupont J, New MI, et al. A mutation in CYP11B1 (Arg-448---His) associated with steroid 11 beta-hydroxylase deficiency in Jews of Moroccan origin. *Clin Invest* 1991;87:1664.

129. Naiki Y, Kawamoto T, Mitsuuchi Y, et al. A nonsense mutation (TGG [Trp116]→TAG [Stop]) in CYP11B1 causes steroid 11 beta-hydroxylase deficiency. *Clin Endocrinol Metab* 1993;77:1677.

130. Skinner CA, Rumsby G. Steroid 11 beta-hydroxylase deficiency caused by a five base pair duplication in the CYP11B1 gene. *Hum Mol Genet* 1994;3:377.

131. Bongiovanni AM. Further studies of congenital adrenal hyperplasia due to 3β-hydroxysteroid dehydrogenase deficiency. In: Vallet HL, Porter IH, eds. *Genetic mechanisms of sexual development.* New York: Academic Press, 1979:189.

132. Rheaume R, Simard J, Morel Y, et al. Congenital adrenal hyperplasia due to point mutation in the type II 3β-hydroxysteroid dehydrogenase gene. *Nat Genet* 1992;1:239.

133. Simard J, Rheaume E, Sanchez R, et al. Molecular basis of congenital adrenal hyperplasia due to 3β-HSD deficiency. *Mol Endocrinol* 1993;7:716.

134. Sanchez R, Rheaume D, Laflamme N, et al. Detection and functional characterization of the novel missense mutation Y254D in type II 3β-HSD gene of a female patient with nonsalt-losing 3β-HSD deficiency. *J Clin Endocrinol Metab* 1994;78:561.

135. Araki S, Chikazawa K, Sekisuchi I, et al. Arrest of follicular development in a patient with 17 alphahydroxylase deficiency: folliculogenesis in association with a lack of estrogen synthesis in the ovaries. *Fertil Steril* 1987;47:169.

136. Rabinovici J, Blankenstein J, Goldman B, et al. In vitro fertilization and primary embryonic cleavage are possible in 17 alpha-hydroxylase deficiency despite extremely low intrafollicular 17 beta-estradiol. *J Clin Endocrinol Metab* 1989;68:693.

137. Carson SA, Simpson JL. Virilization of female fetuses following maternal ingestion of progestational and androgenic steroids. In: Mahesh VB, Greenblatt RB, eds. *Hirsutism and virilization.* Littleton, MA: PSG Publishing, 1994:177.

138. Grumbach MM, Ducharme JR, Moloshak RE. On fetal masculinizing action of certain oral progestins. *J Clin Endocrinol Metab* 1959;19:1369.

139. Simpson JL, Carson SA. Genetic and nongenetic causes of spontaneous abortion. In: Sciarra JJ, eds. *Gynecology and obstetrics, vol. III.* Philadelphia: JB Lippincott, 1998:1–29.

140. Verhoeven ATM, Mastboom JL, Van Leusden HAIM, et al. Virilization in pregnancy coexisting with an (ovarian) mucinous cystadenoma: a case report and review of virilizing ovarian tumors in pregnancy. *Obstet Gynecol Surv* 1973;28:597.

141. Jones HW, Park IJ. A classification of special problems in sex differentiation. *Birth Defects* 1971;7:113.

142. Park IJ, Jones HW, Melham RE. Nonadrenal familial female hermaphroditism. *Am J Obstet Gynecol* 1971;112:930.

143. Lubinsky MS. Female pseudohermaphroditism and associated anomalies. *Am J Med Genet* 1980;6:123.

144. Simpson JL, Kaufman R. Fetal effects of progestogens and diethylstilbestrol. In: Fraser I, Jansen RPS, Lobo RA, Whitehead MI, eds. *Estrogens and progestogens in clinical practice.* London: Churchill Livingstone, 1998:533.

145. Chang HJ, Clark RD, Bachman H. The phenotype of 45,X/46,XY mosaicism: an analysis of 92 prenatally diagnosed cases. *Am J Hum Genet* 1990;46:156.

146. McDonough PG, Tho PT. The spectrum of 45X/46,XY gonadal dysgenesis and its implications (a study of 19 patients). *Pediatr Adolesc Gynecol* 1983;1:1.

147. Rosenberg C, Frota-Pessoa O, Vianna-Morgante AM, et al. Phenotypic spectrum of 45,X/46,XY individuals. *Am J Med Genet* 1987;27:553.

148. Verp MS, Simpson JL. Abnormal sexual differentiation and neoplasia. *Cancer Genet Cytogenet* 1987;25:191.

149. Boscze P, Szamel I, Molnar F, et al. Non-neoplastic gonadal testosterone secretion as a cause of vaginal cell maturation in streak gonad syndrome. *Gynecol Invest* 1986;22:153.

150. Lukusa T, Fryns JP, Van den Berge H. Gonadoblastoma and Y-chromosome fluorescence. *Clin Genet* 1986;29:311.

151. Hsu LYF. Prenatal diagnosis of chromosome abnormalities through amniocentesis. In: Milunsky A, ed. *Genetic disorders and the fetus,* 3rd ed. Baltimore: Johns Hopkins Press, 1986:155.

152. Elshay AI, Waters WR. The brachio-skeleto-genital syndrome. *Plast Reconstr Surg* 1971;48:542.

153. Opitz JM, Howe JJ. The Meckel syndrome (dysencephalic splanchnocystica, the Gruber syndrome). *Birth Defects* 1969;5:167.

154. Eddy AA, Mauer M. Pseudohermaphroditism, glomerulopathy and Wilms tumor (Drash syndrome): frequency in end-stage renal failure. *J Pediatr* 1985;106:584.

155. Habib R, Loirat C, Gubler MC, et al. The nephropathy associated with male pseudohermaphroditism and Wilm's tumor (Dash syndrome): a distinctive glomerular lesion. Report of 10 cases. *Clin Nephrol* 1985;24:269.

156. Curry CRJ, Carey JC, Holland JS, et al. Smith-Lemli-Opitz syndrome-type II. Multiple congenital anomalies with male pseudohermaphroditism and frequent early lethality. *Am J Med Genet* 1987;26:45.

157. Simpson JL. Genetic heterogeneity in XY sex-reversal: potential pitfalls in isolating the testes-determining-factor: TDF. In: Wachtel SS, ed. *Evolutionary*

mechanisms in sex determination. Baton Rouge, LA: CRC Press, 1989:265.

158. Frydman M, Kauschansky A, Zamir R, et al. Familial lipoid adrenal hyperplasia: genetic marker data and an approach to prenatal diagnosis. *Am J Med Genet* 1986;25:319.

159. Chung BC, Matteson KJ, Voutilainen R, et al. Human cholesterol side-chain cleavage enzyme P450scc: cDNA cloning assignment of the gene to chromosome 15 and expression in the placenta. *Proc Natl Acad Sci U S A* 1986;83:8962.

160. Lin D, Gitelman SE, Saenger P, et al. Normal genes for the cholesterol side chain cleavage enzyme, P450scc, in congenital lipoid adrenal hyperplasia. *J Clin Invest* 1991;88:1955.

161. Bose HS, Sugawara T, Strauss JF 3rd, et al. The pathophysiology and genetics of congenital lipoid adrenal hyperplasia. International congenital lipoid adrenal hyperplasia consortium. *N Engl J Med* 1996;335:1870.

162. Heremans GFP, Moolenaar AJ, Van Gelderen HM. Female phenotype in a male child due to 17α-hydroxylase deficiency. *Arch Dis Child* 1976;51:721.

163. Nebert DW, Nelson DR, Adesnik M, et al. The P-450 superfamily: updated listing of all genes and recommended nomenclature for the chromosomal loci. *DNA* 1989;8:1.

164. Biason-Lauber A, Leiberman E, Zachmann M. A single amino acid substitution in the putative redox partner-binding site of P450c17 as cause of isolated 17,20-lyase deficiency. *J Clin Endocrinol Metab* 1997;82:3807.

165. Geller DH, Auchus RJ, Mendonca BB, et al. The genetic and functional basis of isolated 17,20-lyase deficiency. *Nat Genet* 1997;17:201.

166. Zachmann M, Vollmin JA, Hamilton W, et al. Steroid 17,20-desmolase deficiency: a new cause of male pseudohermaphroditism. *Clin Endocrinol* 1972;1:369.

167. Yanase T, Kagimoto M, Suzuki S, et al. Deletion of a phenylalanine in the N-terminal region of human cytochrome P-450 (17 alpha) results in partial combined 17 alpha-hydroxylase/17,20-lyase deficiency. *J Biol Chem* 1989;264:18076.

168. Kagimoto K, Waterman MR, Kagimoto M, et al. Identification of a common molecular basis for combined 17 alpha-hydroxylase/17,20-lyase deficiency in two Mennonite families. *Hum Genet* 1989;82:285.

169. Rumsby G, Skinner C, Lee HA, et al. Combined 17 alpha-hydroxylase/17,20-lyase deficiency caused by heterozygous stop codons in the cytochrome P450 17 alpha-hydroxylase gene. *Clin Endocrinol (Oxf)* 1993;39:483.

170. Balducci R, Toscano V, Wright F, et al. Familial male pseudohermaphroditism with gynecomastia due to 17β-hydroxysteroid dehydrogenase deficiency. A report of 3 cases. *Clin Endocrinol* 1985;23:439.

171. Imperato-McGinley J, Peterson RE, Stoller R, et al. Male pseudohermaphroditism secondary to a 17α-hydroxysteroid dehydrogenase deficiency: gender role with puberty. *J Clin Endocrinol Metab* 1979;49:391.

172. Caufriez A. Male pseudohermaphroditism due to 17-ketoreductase deficiency: report of a case without gynecomastia and without vaginal pouch. *Am J Obstet Gynecol* 1986;154:148.

173. Geissler W, Favis D, Wu L, et al. Male pseudohermaphroditism caused by mutations of testicular 17β-hydroxysteroid dehydrogenase 3. *Nat Genet* 1994;7:34.

174. Andersson S, Geissler W, Ling W, et al. Molecular genetics and pathophysiology of β-hydroxysteroid dehydrogenase 3 deficiency. *J Clin Endocrinol Metab* 1996;81:130.

175. Ulloa-Aguirre A, Mendez PJ, Chavez A, et al. Incomplete regression of Müllerian ducts in the androgen insensitivity syndrome. *Fertil Steril* 1990;53:1024.

176. Morris JM, Mahesh VB. Further observations on the syndrome "testicular feminization." *Am J Obstet Gynecol* 1963;87:731.

177. Gottlieb B, Trifiro M, Lumbroso R, et al. The androgen receptor gene mutations database. *Nucleic Acids Res* 1996;24:151.

178. Gottlieb B, Lehvaslaiho H, Beitel LK, et al. The androgen receptor gene mutations database. *Nucleic Acids Res* 1998;26:234.

179. Quigley CA, Friedman KJ, Johnson A, et al. Complete deletion of the androgen receptor gene: definition of the null phenotype of the androgen insensitivity syndrome and determination of carrier status. *J Clin Endocrinol Metab* 1992;74:927.

180. McPhaul MJ, Marcelli M, Zoppi S, et al. Genetic basis of endocrine disease. 4. The spectrum of mutations in the androgen receptor gene that causes androgen resistance. *J Clin Endocrinol Metab* 1993;76:17.

181. Park IJ, Jones HW. Familial male hermaphroditism with ambiguous external genitalia. *Am J Obstet Gynecol* 1970;108:1197.

182. Griffin JE, Punyashthiki K, Wilson JD. Dihydrotestosterone binding by culture human fibroblasts. Comparison of cells from control subjects and from patients with hereditary pseudohermaphroditism due to androgen resistance. *J Clin Invest* 1976;57:1342.

183. Pinsky L, Kaufman M. Genetics of steroid receptors and their disorders. *Adv Hum Genet* 1985;16:299.

184. Pinsky L, Kaufman M, Levitzky LL. Partial androgen resistance due to a distinctive qualitative defect of the androgen receptor. *Am J Med Genet* 1987;27:459.

185. Wilson JD, Harrod MJ, Goldstein JL, et al. Familial incomplete male pseudohermaphroditism type I. *N Engl J Med* 1974;290:940.

186. Wilson JD, Harrod MJ, Goldstein JL, et al. Familial incomplete male pseudohermaphroditism. *N Engl J Med* 1984;290:1097.

187. Simpson JL, New M, Peterson RE, et al. Pseudovaginal perineoscrotal hypospadias (PPSH) in sibs. *Birth Defects* 1971;7:140.

188. Opitz JM, Simpson JL, Sarto GE, et al. Pseudovaginal perineoscrotal hypospadias. *Clin Genet* 1971;3:1.

189. Imperato-McGinley J, Guerrero L, Gauiter T, et al. Steroid 5α-reductase deficiency: an inherited form of male pseudohermaphroditism. *Science* 1974;186:1213.

190. Walsh C, Madden JD, Harrod MJ, et al. Familial incomplete male pseudohermaphroditism, type 2. *N Engl J Med* 1974;291:944.

191. Peterson RE, Imperato-McGinley J, Gautier T, et al. Male pseudohermaphroditism due to steroid 5α-reductase deficiency. *Am J Med* 1977;62:170.

192. Wilson JD, Griffin JE, Russell DW. Steroid 5α-reductase 2 deficiency. *Endocrinol Rev* 1993;14:577.

193. Green S, Zachmann M, Mannella B. Comparison of two tests to recognize or exclude 5α-reductase defi-

ciency in prepubertal children. *Acta Endocrinol (Copenh)* 1987;114:113.

194. Imperato-McGinley J, Gautier T, Pichardo M, et al. The diagnosis of 5 alpha-reductase in infancy. *J Clin Endocrinol Metab* 1986;63:1313.

195. Labrie F, Sugimoto Y, Luu-The V, et al. Structure of human type II 5 alpha-reductase gene. *Endocrinology* 1992;131:1571.

196. Andersson S, Berman DM, Jenkins EP, et al. Deletion of steroid 5 alpha-reductase 2 gene in male pseudohermaphroditism. *Nature* 1991;354:159.

197. Thigpen AE, Davis DL, Milatovich A, et al. Molecular genetics of steroid 5α-reductase deficiency. *J Clin Invest* 1992;90:799.

198. Simpson ER, Michael MD, Agarwal VR, et al. Cytochromes P450 11: expression of the CYP19 (aromatase) gene: an unusual case of alternative promoter usage. *FASEB J* 1997;11:29.

199. Ito Y, Fisher CR, Conte FA, et al. Molecular basis of aromatase deficiency in an adult female with sexual infantilism and polycystic ovaries. *Proc Natl Acad Sci U S A* 1993;90:11673.

200. Shozu M, Akasofu K, Harada T, et al. A new cause of female pseudohermaphroditism: placental aromatase deficiency. *J Clin Endocrinol Metab* 1991;72:560.

201. Mullis PE, Yoshimura N, Kuhlmann B, et al. Aromatase deficiency in a female who is compound heterozygote for two new point mutations in the P450 arom gene: impact of estrogens on hypergonadotropic hypogonadism, multicystic ovaries, and bone densitometry in childhood. *Clin Endocrinol Metab* 1997;82:1739.

202. Lubahn DB, Moyer JS, Golding TS, et al. Alteration of reproductive function but not prenatal sexual development after insertional disruption of the mouse estrogen receptor gene. *Proc Natl Acad Sci U S A* 1993;90:11162.

203. Smith EP, Frank GR, Takahashi H, et al. Estrogen resistance caused by a mutation in the estrogen-receptor gene in a man. *N Engl J Med* 1994;331:1056.

204. Sarto GE, Opitz JM. The XY gonadal agenesis syndrome. *J Med Genet* 1973;10:288.

205. Kwok C, Tyler-Smith C, Mendonca B, et al. Mutation analysis of the 2 kb 5′ to SRY in XY females and XY intersex subjects. *J Med Genet* 1996;33:465.

206. Marcantonio SM, Fechner PY, Migeon CJ, et al. Embryonic testicular regression sequence: a part of the clinical spectrum of 46,XY gonadal dysgenesis. *Am J Med Genet* 1994;49:1.

207. Brown DM, Markland C, Dehner LP. Leydig cell hypoplasia: a case of male pseudohermaphroditism. *J Clin Endocrinol Metab* 1976;46:1.

208. Lee PA, Rock JA, Brown TR, et al. Leydig cell hypofunction resulting in male pseudohermaphroditism. *Fertil Steril* 1981;37:675.

209. Perez-Palacios G, Scaglia HE, Kofman-Afaro S. Inherited male pseudohermaphroditism due to gonadotrophin unresponsiveness. *Acta Endocrinol (Copenh)* 1982;98:148.

210. Saldanha PH, Arnhold IJP, Mendonca BB, et al. A clinico-genetic investigation of Leydig cell hypoplasia. *Am J Med Genet* 1987;26:337.

211. Schwartz M, Imperato-McGinley J, Peterson RE, et al. Male pseudohermaphroditism secondary to an abnormality in Leydig cell differentiation. *J Clin Endocrinol Metab* 1981;53:123.

212. Kremer H, Kraaij R, Toledo SP, et al. Male pseudohermaphroditism due to a homozygous missense mutation of the luteinizing hormone receptor gene. *Nat Genet* 1995;9:160.

213. Salameh W, Shoukair M, Keswani A, et al. Evidence for a deletion in the LH receptor gene in a case of Leydig cell aplasia. In: *77th annual meeting of Endocrine Society, June 14–17, Washington, DC.* 1995;abstract P2-150:328.

214. Simpson JL. True hermaphroditism. Etiology and phenotypic considerations. *Birth Defects* 1978;14(6C):9.

215. Aaronsen I. True hermaphroditism. A review of 41 cases with observations on testicular history and function. *Br J Urol* 1985;57:775.

216. Tegenkamp TR, Brazzell JW, Tegenkamp I, et al. Pregnancy without benefit of reconstructive surgery in a bisexually active true hermaphrodite. *Am J Obstet Gynecol* 1979;135:427.

217. Minowada S, Fukutani K, Hara M, et al. Childbirth in a true hermaphrodite. *Eur Urol* 1984;10:414.

218. Van Niekerk WA. *True hermaphroditism.* New York: Harper & Row, 1974:1–466.

219. Ramsay M, Bernstein R, Zwane E, et al. XX true hermaphroditism in South African blacks: an enigma of primary sexual differentiation. *Am J Hum Genet* 1988;43:4.

220. Simpson JL. Genetic aspects of gynecologic disorders occurring in 46,XX individuals. *Clin Obstet Gynecol* 1972;15:157.

221. Sueiro MM, Piloti R. Adrenica incomplete dos pequenos labios cam caracter familiar. *Arch Anat Antrop* 1964;32:187.

222. Klein VR, Willman SP, Carr BR. Familial posterior labial fusion. *Obstet Gynecol* 1987;73:500.

223. McIlroy DM, Ward IV. Three cases of imperforate hymen occurring in one family. *Proc R Soc Med* 1930;23:633.

224. Stelling JR, Gray MR, Davis AJ, et al. Familial transmission of imperforate hymen. *Fertil Steril* 1998;70:S47.

225. Jones HW Jr, Rock JA. *Reparative and constructive surgery of the female generative tract.* Baltimore: Williams & Wilkins, 1983.

226. Lodi A. Contributo clinico statistico sulle malformazioni della vagina osservate nella Clinica Obstetrica e Gineocologica di Milano del 1906 al 1950. *Ann Obstet Ginecol* 1951;73:1246.

227. Bowman JA Jr, Scott RB. Transverse vaginal septum: report of four cases. *Obstet Gynecol* 1954;3:441.

228. Deppisch LM. Transverse vaginal septum. *Obstet Gynecol* 1972;39:193.

229. Kanagasuntheran R, Dassanayake AGS. Nature of the obstructing membrane in primary cryptomenorrhea. *J Obstet Gynecol Br Common* 1958;65:487.

230. White AJ. Vaginal atresia: high transverse septum. *Obstet Gynecol* 1966;27:695.

231. Kaufman RL, Hartmann AF, McAlister WH. Family studies in congenital heart disease: II. A syndrome of hydrometrocolpos, postaxial polydactyly and congenital heart disease. *Birth Defects* 1972;8:85.

232. Chitayat D, Hahm SY, Marion RW, et al. Further delineation of the McKusick-Kaufman hydrometrocolpos-polydactyly syndrome. *Am J Dis Child* 1987;141:1133.

233. McKusick VA. The William Allen memorial award lecture: genetic nosology: three approaches. *Am J Hum Genet* 1978;30:105.

234. Stone DL, Agarwala R, Schaffer AA, et al. Genetic and physical mapping of the McKusick-Kaufman syndrome. *Hum Mol Genet* 1998;7:475.

235. Kupperman HJ. *Human endocrinology, vol. 1.* Philadelphia: FA Davis, 1963.

236. Anger D, Hamet J, Ensel J. Forme familiale du syndrome de Rokitansky-Kuster-Hauser. *Bull Fed Soc Gynecol Obstet Lang Fr* 1966;18:299.

237. Jones HW Jr, Mermut S. Familial occurrence of congenital absence of the vagina. *Am J Obstet Gynecol* 1972;114:1100.

238. Griffin JE, Edwards C, Madden JD, et al. Congenital absence of the vagina, the Mayer-Rokitansky-Kuster-Hauser syndrome. *Ann Intern Med* 1976;85:224.

239. Shokeir MHK. Aplasia of the Müllerian septum: evidence of probably sex-limited autosomal dominant inheritance. *Birth Defects* 1978;14(6C):147.

240. Lischke JH, Curtis CH, Lamb EJ. Discordance of vaginal agenesis in monozygotic twins. *Obstet Gynecol* 1973;41:920.

241. Carson SA, Simpson JL, Malinak LR, et al. Heritable aspects of uterine anomalies: II. Genetic analysis of Müllerian aplasia. *Fertil Steril* 1983;40:86.

242. Petrozza JC, Gray MR, Davis AJ, et al. Congenital absence of the uterus and vagina is not commonly transmitted as a dominant genetic trait: outcomes of surrogate pregnancies. *Fertil Steril* 1997;67:387.

243. van Lingen BL, Reindollar RH, Davis AJ, et al. Further evidence that the WT1 gene does not have a role in the development of the derivatives of the müllerian duct. *Am J Obstet Gynecol* 1998;179:597.

244. van Lingen BL, Eccles MR, Reindollar RH, et al. Molecular analysis of the PAX 2 gene in patients with congenital absence of the uterus and vagina. *Fertil Steril* 1998;70:S402.

245. Stelling JR, Bhagavath B, Gray MR, et al. HOXA13 homeodomain mutation analysis in patients with müllerian system anomalies. *J Soc Gynecol Invest* 1998;5:140A.

246. Resendes BL, Sohn SH, Tineo R, et al. The role for müllerian inhibiting substance in congenital absence of the uterus and vagina. *Am J Med Genet* (in press, 2000).

247. Bhagavath B, Stelling JR, van Lingen BL, et al. Congenital absence of the uterus and vagina (CAUV) is not associated with the N314D allele of the galactose-1-phosphate uridyl transferase (GALT) gene. *J Soc Gynecol Invest* 1998;5:140A.

248. Nykiforuk NE. Uterus didelphys. *Can Med Assoc J* 1938;38:175.

249. Tyler GT. Didelphys in sisters. *Am J Surg* 1939;45:337.

250. Polishuk WZ, Ron MA. Familial bicornuate and double uterus. *Am J Obstet Cynecol* 1974;119:982.

251. Verp MS, Simpson JL, Elias S, et al. Heritable aspects of uterine anomalies. I. Three familial aggregates with Müllerian fusion anomalies. *Fertil Steril* 1983;40:80.

252. Way S. The influence of minor degrees of failure of fusion of the Müllerian ducts on pregnancy and labor. *J Obstet Gynaecol Br Emp* 1945;52:325.

253. Holmes JA. Congenital abnormalities of the uterus and pregnancy. *Br Med J* 1956;1:1144.

254. Stevenson AC, Dudgeon MY, McCluire HI. Observations on the results of pregnancies in women resident in Belfast: II. Abortions, hydatidiform males, and ectopic pregnancies. *Ann Hum Genet* 1959;23:395.

255. Hay D. Uterus and unicollis and its relationship to pregnancy. *J Obstet Gynaecol Br Emp* 1961;68:361.

256. Ergun A, Pabuccu R, Atay V, et al. Three sisters with septate uteri: another reference to bidirectional theory. *Hum Reprod* 1997;12:140.

257. Elias S, Simpson JL, Carson SA, et al. Genetics studies in incomplete müllerian fusion. *Obstet Gynecol* 1984;63:276.

258. Stern AM, Gall JC Jr, Perry BL, et al. The hand-foot-uterus syndrome: a new hereditary disorder characterized by hand and foot dysplasia, dermatoglyphic abnormalities, and partial duplication of the female genital tract. *Pediatrics* 1970;77:109.

259. Posnanski AK, Kuhns LR, Lapides J, et al. A new family with the hand-foot-genital syndrome: a wider spectrum of the hand-foot-uterus syndrome. *Birth Defects Orig Art Ser* 1975;11:127.

260. Giedion A, Prader A. Hand-foot-uterus (HFU) syndrome with hypospadias: the hand-foot-genital (HFG) syndrome. *Pediatr Radiol* 1976;4:96.

261. Donnenfeld AE, Schrager DS, Corson SL. Update on a family with hand-foot-genital syndrome: hypospadias and urinary tract abnormalities in two boys from the fourth generation. *Am J Med Genet* 1992;44:482.

262. Fryns JP, Vogels A, Decock P, et al. The hand-foot-genital syndrome: on the variable expression in affected males. *Clin Genet* 1993;43:232.

263. Verp MS. Urinary tract abnormalities in hand-foot-genital syndrome. *Am J Med Genet* 1989;32:555.

264. Mortlock DP, Innis JW. Mutation of HOXA13 in hand-foot-genital syndrome. *Nat Genet* 1997;15:179.

265. Goodman F, Donnenfeld AE, Feingold M, et al. Novel HOXA13 mutations and the phenotypic spectrum of hand-foot-genital syndrome. *Am Soc Hum Genet* 1998;abstract SP69:S31.

2

Normal Growth and Development of the Genitalia in Infancy and Childhood

Andrew S. Cook

OVERVIEW

Changes that occur in the prepubertal female genitalia are a reflection of both the changes in the hormonal environment and the physical growth of the child. The genitalia of the newborn and child are hormonally responsive. At birth, the newborn is under the influence of estrogen via passive transmission across the placenta from the mother. The effects of this hormonal stimulation usually resolve within the first 6 to 8 weeks of life. The most common hormonally related changes include vulvar edema, vaginal discharge, vaginal bleeding, and breast enlargement. The external genitalia of the newborn are swollen and edematous. The hymen usually is thickened and prominent, protruding at the introitus. The hymen can remain thick and redundant as a result of hormonal stimulation for up to 2 years after birth (1). Changes occur in hymenal configuration in approximately two thirds of infants between birth and 3 years of age (2).

The vaginal epithelium of the newborn is thickened with glycogen-rich cells in response to estrogen stimulation. The estrogen response also is reflected in the increased number of superficial cells present on the maturation index (3). The newborn physiologic vaginal discharge is the same as that seen in women in the reproductive age group. About 10% of female infants will experience withdrawal vaginal bleeding in the newborn period (4). A significant number of newborn infants experience some enlargement of the breast tissue by the fifth or sixth day. Approximately two thirds of these infants will secrete a colostrum-like fluid followed by small amounts of milk (5). Secretion has been reported to persist up to 1 year.

These findings are much less pronounced in the premature infant. The most prominent feature of the female genitalia in the premature infant is the relatively large clitoris. This is a normal finding, but it is a potential cause for concern to the unsuspecting parent or physician.

Once out of the neonatal period, the child enters a time of relative quiescence until puberty approaches. This time period is influenced primarily by the physical growth of the patient. The uterus undergoes regression from its hormonally influenced size at birth. The initial size of the uterus is not regained until the patient is 5 years old.

PHYSICAL EXAMINATION OF THE PREPUBERTAL FEMALE GENITALIA

The request for examination of prepubertal female genitalia may be initiated as a result of suspected sexual abuse. It is crucial for the clinician to be able to differentiate normal congenital findings from posttraumatic changes (6). An examination that is initiated based on suspected sexual abuse will focus primarily on the external genitalia, including the hymen, labia, posterior fourchette, and perineal body. Examination of potential genital anomalies, masses, or nontraumatic pain usually will focus on the internal genitalia.

The physical examination of the prepubertal female genitalia is unique. Success of the physical examination is highly dependent on the rapport and interaction established with the patient. The physician should be sensitive to the child's emotions and fears, displaying gentleness, patience, and time. A lack of empathy toward the pediatric patient may, at minimum, adversely affect the ability to obtain adequate information from the physical examination and may, at worse, increase the potential risk of inadvertent nosocomial sexual abuse (7).

The office evaluation of the female prepubertal genitalia also requires both an understanding of the range of normal findings in a given age group and the advantages and disadvantages of the various examination techniques.

Examination Techniques in Evaluation of Prepubertal Female Genitalia

Explanation to both the mother and child of the examination process and the instruments (if any) used is an important precursor to the genital examination. The perception that the virginal introitus is completely covered by the hymen is not uncommon. Newborn hymenal configurations include annular hymen with a central or ventrally displaced orifice (80%), fimbriated hymen (19%), and a septated or cribriform hymen (1%) (8).

Reassurance that the examination will not alter the hymen should help to alleviate potential fears and increase the cooperation of both the patient and her mother. A great deal of information about the female genitalia can be gained during the office examination. The goal of the examination is to obtain the necessary information without causing long-term emotional sequelae. In many cases, the necessary information can be obtained in the office without instrumentation. Occasionally the use of general anesthesia will be necessary to per-

form an adequate examination. Use of the colposcope can provide detailed information not available without magnification (9). If vaginal instrumentation is necessary, the preferred type of instrument is dependent on the age of the patient. The Cameron-Miller vaginoscope is both financially economical and efficient (Fig. 2.1).

An initial evaluation of hormonally sensitive tissue will provide a guide of the patient's endocrine status. Stage of breast development, vaginal mucosal maturation index, pattern of hair growth, and apocrine gland activity will provide information as to sex steroid production. In the child, an ovarian cyst or mass will present as an abdominal rather than pelvic mass, underscoring the importance of a good abdominal examination. The inguinal areas should be examined for the presence of an inguinal hernia or gonad. An inguinal gonad may represent the undescended testes of an undiagnosed male pseudohermaphrodite (10).

A prepubertal gynecologic examination should include evaluation of the external genitalia, including the clitoris, labia, perineal body and hymen, vagina, and cervix. A rectoabdominal examination or sonographic evaluation may determine the presence and size of the uterus. The normal values and

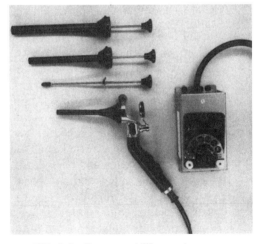

FIG. 2.1. Cameron-Miller vaginoscope.

findings of prepubertal female genitalia will be detailed subsequently.

Three different methods used in examination of the prepubertal female genitalia have been compared. Initially 172 children were each examined colposcopically using all three techniques (11). The examination techniques included (a) the supine position with labial separation, (b) the supine position with labial traction, and (c) the knee-chest position. Each technique was evaluated for the ability to open the vaginal introitus.

For examination in the supine position, the child is placed in a frog-leg position, with her legs abducted and the soles of her feet together. The supine separation method involves the examiner separating the labia with the fingertips in a lateral and downward direction until the introitus opens. The lower aspect of the labia majora are grasped between the thumb and index fingers and with gentle traction pulled, outward and slightly upward with the supine traction technique. The knee-chest examination technique uses the knee-chest position, with the child's chest on the table and knees separated by 6 to 8 inches. The introitus is opened by placing the examiner's thumbs on the gluteus maximus at the level of the introitus and lifting, moving the perineal body and posterior fourchette dorsally.

The ability of the three examination techniques to open the introitus was compared. The knee-chest and supine traction techniques (98% and 96%) were superior to the supine separation technique (86%) in the overall ability to open the vaginal introitus. The difference in the ability to open the introitus was especially marked in the younger children. The separation technique opened the introitus in only 29% of infants and 76% of preschoolers. The knee-chest examination method is most successful in opening the vaginal orifice and providing visualization of the cervix but requires an increased level of cooperation from the child. The vertical transhymenal diameters obtained with the knee-chest technique were consistently greater than with the other two techniques.

Normal Appearance and Values in the Examination of the Prepubertal Female Genitalia

A recent study by McCann et al. (1) details the normal values and appearance of the prepubertal female genitalia. Ninety-three nonabused girls 10 months to 19 years old were examined using the three examination techniques described. Examination of the prepubertal external female genitalia in the supine position (both traction and separation) yielded a greater incidence of positive findings than did examination in the knee-chest position. Labial adhesions, posterior fourchette raphe, and midline avascularity of the posterior fourchette are common findings, whereas isolated vascularity and friability of the posterior fourchette are uncommon. Vestibular erythema, periurethral bands, and follicles are seen in a significant portion of patients. The majority of the labial adhesions were less than 2 mm in length. The authors believed that these small adhesions accounted for the midline avascularity with traction (supine or knee-chest) and bleeding with further traction.

Labial adhesions, which probably are related to the hypoestrogenic state of the prepubertal female, usually are asymptomatic and do not require treatment. Most labial adhesions will resolve spontaneously with puberty. The patient may present to the physician as a result of maternal concern that the daughter has vaginal agenesis. The inferior half of the hymen is occluded by labial agglutination in 8% of 1-year-old children (6). Treatment is required if the labial adhesions impede urination or drainage of vaginal secretions. Application of an estrogen cream b.i.d. to the adhesion line should be performed by a parent for 2 weeks, then once a day at bedtime for another week or two, until there is complete resolution of the labial adhesions. Gentle traction on the adhesion line at the time of estrogen application is required. Subsequent application of an ointment (e.g., Vaseline) for a couple of weeks or months may help to prevent adhesion reformation.

All patients in the study by McCann et al. (1) had a hymen present. A crescent-shaped hymen was the most commonly observed hymenal shape, followed by the concentric hymen. The septate-, cribriform-, and imperforate-shaped hymens were rarely seen. Redundancy of the hymenal membrane was reduced and, as a result, visualization of the hymen was increased with the supine traction and knee-chest examination techniques.

The significance of a hymenal notch or cleft is dependent on both the location and extent of the lesion. Hymenal notches located between the 5 and 7 o'clock positions are considered suggestive of previous abuse or trauma (12). Superior and lateral notches should be considered normal and are found in 35% of newborns. Longitudinal intravaginal ridges are a normal finding. These can be found in all four quadrants of the hymen and may extend from the hymen into the vagina. Several studies suggest that less than 1 mm of hymenal tissue at the inferior rim (6 o'clock position) in prepubertal girls is evidence of prior abuse (13,14). Difficulty in obtaining accurate measurements may limit the usefulness of this finding.

The colposcopic transhymenal diameters were measured using the three different examination techniques in preschoolers (2 years to 4 years 11 months), early school age (5 years to 7 years 11 months), and preadolescent (8 years to Tanner II) (Table 2.1). On average, the transhymenal diameters increased with the age of the child. The greatest vertical transhymenal diameters were measured with the supine traction technique; the largest horizontal diameters were seen with the knee-chest method.

The percentage of the introitus that was covered by the hymen varied over a wide range and was dependent on the examination technique. Eighty-four patients were examined using the three examination techniques described. The ability to visualize the cervix was highly dependent on the examination technique used. The cervix was seen in 58 patients (69%) with the knee-chest examination technique, but it was seen in none of the patients using the supine traction or separation techniques (1).

Normal findings in nonabused children can include perianal redness, smooth areas, venous engorgement, skin tags, and hymenal ridges, bumps, tags, bands, and anterior notches.

TABLE 2.1. *Colposcopic transhymenal diameter means and ranges by age group and examination method*[a]

Age group	Method	Plane	n	Mean ± SD (mm)	Range (mm)
II: Preschool (2–4 $^{11}/_{12}$ years)	Separation	Vertical	21	5.5 ± 2.2	2.5–10.0
		Horizontal	21	3.9 ± 1.4	1.0–5.5
	Traction	Vertical	24	5.5 ± 1.7	3.0–8.5
		Horizontal	24	5.2 ± 1.4	2.0–8.0
	Knee-chest	Vertical	29	6.3 ± 1.7	3.0–10.0
		Horizontal	29	4.6 ± 1.3	2.5–7.5
III: Early school age (5–7 $^{11}/_{12}$ years)	Separation	Vertical	39	5.6 ± 2.3	1.0–11.0
		Horizontal	39	4.2 ± 1.7	1.0–8.0
	Traction	Vertical	43	6.1 ± 2.1	1.0 ± 10.0
		Horizontal	43	5.6 ± 1.8	1.0–9.0
	Knee-chest	Vertical	41	7.0–2.0	3.0–11.5
		Horizontal	41	56 ± 1.5	2.5–8.5
IV: Preadolescent (8 to Tanner II)	Separation	Vertical	19	8.4 ± 2.2	5.0–13.5
		Horizontal	19	5.7 ± 1.6	3.0–8.5
	Traction	Vertical	20	8.3 ± 2.8	2.0–15.0
		Horizontal	20	6.9 ± 2.0	2.5–10.5
	Knee-chest	Vertical	21	8.7 ± 2.6	5.0–15.0
		Horizontal	21	7.3 ± 1.7	4.0–11.0

[a]n = 72. Infant age group not included because of small n.
From McCann J, Wells R, Simon M, et al. Genital findings in prepubertal girls selected for nonabuse: a descriptive study. *Pediatrics* 1990;86:428, with permission.

NORMAL OVARIAN DEVELOPMENT AND FINDINGS

At birth, the infant has high levels of circulating sex steroids as a result of passive placental transfer. Gonodatropin levels begin to rise after birth as the infant clears the placental steroids and reach a peak in the first couple of months of life, with a slow return to low levels as the "gonadostat" is reset. This period of gonadotropin activity in the first year of life results in normal follicular activity and occasionally the formation of functional ovarian cysts. With suppression of the gonadotropins, follicular activity is reduced, but the ovary does not become quiescent. Continuous follicular growth and atresia occurs in both infancy and childhood (15). In contrast to the menstruating female who has cyclic follicular maturation and ovulation, the premenarcheal child rarely develops a dominant follicle or functional ovarian cyst.

Ovarian Morphology

Follicular growth in infancy and childhood has been documented by both morphologic and sonographic studies. An interesting study by Peters et al. (15) histologically evaluated 52 ovaries at autopsy of children who died in an accident or after an acute illness. The children ranged in ages from 2 months to 11 years. Ovarian growth was classified as (a) quiescent—small, resting follicles, with no growth; (b) early growth—preantral follicles present but not larger than 0.5 mm in diameter; and (c) actively growing—with antral follicles larger than 0.5 mm and evidence of degeneration and "scars." None of the ovaries were quiescent; three were in early growth and 49 of 52 were actively growing. Antral follicles measuring 3, 4, and 5 mm were commonly seen at all ages. The authors subjectively believed that both the number and size of antral follicles increased after the age of 6 years.

The ovarian architecture of infants and premenarcheal children has been evaluated sonographically. Ovaries can be classified as follows: the homogeneous ovary is void of cystic structures; the microcystic ovary has cysts smaller than 9 mm; and the macrocystic ovary has at least one cyst larger than 9 mm (16). Follicular activity is noted from early childhood, with an increasing percentage of children demonstrating microcystic ovaries with increasing age. Macrocystic ovaries were not observed before 12 years of age (16–18). Stanhope et al. (19) defined a megalocystic ovary as containing more than six follicles larger than 4 mm. They noted a progressive increase in the proportion of megalocystic ovaries in normal premenarcheal girls over the age of 8.5 years. This study considered as abnormal ovarian cysts larger than 9 mm in diameter in girls less than 12 years of age. Ovarian cysts larger than 9 mm are seen in 12- and 13-year-old girls, even if they are premenarcheal (17). In a more recent study, 155 ovaries in 101 children ages 2 to 12 years of age were evaluated sonographically (20). On average, 68% of ovaries were cystic, with no age group having less than 53% prevalence of cystic ovaries. Macrocystic ovaries were noted approximately 10% of the time. The highest incidence of macrocystic ovaries was observed in girls 3 and 8 years old. The author of this study believed that the discrepancy in the incidence of macrocystic ovaries might be a result of improved sonographic technologies and resolution.

Most large ovarian cysts up to the age of 2 years are functional cysts (21). Between the ages of 5 and 15 years, most complex ovarian masses are teratomas, 30% of which are malignant.

Computed tomographic (CT) evaluation of 125 normal girls revealed microcystic ovaries (cysts smaller than 9 mm) in 71% of ovaries visualized in girls under 8 years of age and 84% of ovaries in girls 8 years of age or older. Macrocystic ovaries (cyst larger than 9 mm) were seen in 12.5% of ovaries in girls 8 years of age or older (22).

Ovarian Size

Ovarian size has been evaluated sonographically in premenarcheal, menstruating, and postmenopausal women. These studies agree that the normal ovarian size is different in each group; however, the actual value is subject to controversy. The ovarian volume of menstruating women has been most widely studied and is the standard against which the premenarcheal and postmenopausal ovarian size is compared. Classically, the ovary of a menstruating woman was described as measuring $1 \times 2 \times 3$ cm (23). Using the mathematical formula to estimate the volume of a prolate ellipse (height $\times$ width $\times$ length $\times$ 0.523), this represents an ovarian volume, in menstruating women, of 3 cm^3. An ovarian volume, in menstruating women, of 6 cm^3 also has been quoted as normal. This corresponds to dimensions of $2 \times 2 \times 3$ cm^3. A range in ovarian volume from 4.4 to 9.8 cm^3 has been documented by sonographic evaluation (23).

Sonographic estimates of premenarcheal ovarian size have varied. Difficulty in sonographic visualization of the ovaries in young girls was experienced initially (24). Recent reports have visualized the majority of premenarcheal ovaries, including those in infants. Ivarson et al. (24) demonstrated an average ovarian volume of 0.7 cm^3 by sonographic evaluation. The authors also used the histologic data of Simkins (25) to calculate the ovarian volume using the prolate ellipsoid

formula. Patients 6 months to 2 years had an average ovarian volume of 0.41 cm^3, and patients 7 to 9 years had an average ovarian volume of 0.74 cm^3. Stanhope et al. (19) sonographically evaluated 40 premenarcheal girls age 6 months to 14 years. At 2 years of age, the average volume was 1 cm^3 and at 12 years the volume was 2 cm^3.

Cohen et al. (23) studied ovarian volume of 725 consecutive patients (1,157 ovaries) by ultrasound. The average volume of menstruating women in this study was 9.8 cm^3, which is on the upper end of normal values reported in the literature. The age of range of premenarcheal patients was 3 to 15 years (average 9.5 years). The average volume of 32 premenarcheal ovaries was 3.0 cm^3. The mean volume of patients in the first decade of life (19 ovaries) was 1.7 cm^3. Salardi et al. (17) sonographically measured the ovaries of 101 premenarcheal girls. The mean ovarian volume was determined for each year, from age 2 to 13 years (Table 2.2). Ovarian size is stable until about 5 years, when age-related growth begins.

The appearance of pediatric ovaries is documented in a study of 125 young girls and adolescents between 1 and 18 years of age without evidence of gynecologic abnormalities. The ovaries were visualized in only 6.3% of girls under 8 years of age. The mean ovar-

TABLE 2.2. *Ovarian volume*[a]

		Ovarian volume (cm^3)	
Age (yr)	Number of patients	By chronologic age	By bone age
2	5	0.75 ± 0.41	0.78 ± 0.38
3	6	0.68 ± 0.17	0.64 ± 0.18
4	14	0.82 ± 0.36	1.00 ± 0.45
5	4	0.86 ± 0.02	0.95 ± 0.52
6	9	1.19 ± 0.36	1.05 ± 0.65
7	8	1.26 ± 0.59	1.23 ± 0.47
8	10	1.05 ± 0.50	1.29 ± 0.33
9	11	1.98 ± 0.76	1.35 ± 0.71
10	12	2.22 ± 0.69	1.47 ± 0.56
11	12	2.52 ± 1.30	2.45 ± 0.86
12	6	3.80 ± 1.40	3.10 ± 1.29
13	4	4.18 ± 2.30	4.38 ± 2.74

[a]As determined by ultrasonography in 101 girls from age 2 to 13.
From Orsini LF, Salardi S, Pilu G, et al. Pelvic organs in premenarcheal girls: real-time ultrasonography, *Radiology* 1984;153–113, with permission.

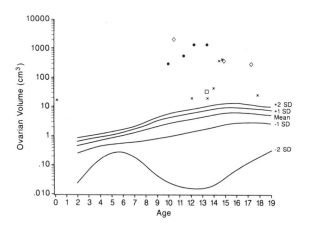

FIG. 2.2. Normal age-related mean ovarian volume and standard deviation values plotted on a logarithmic scale. The central line represents the age-related mean ovarian volume. The two adjacent inner lines represent 1 SD above and below the mean. The two outer lines represent 2 SD above and below the mean. Pathologic ovarian volumes are represented by the following symbols: x, cyst; ○, torsion; ◇, teratoma; ●, malignant tumor. (From Rigsby CK, Siegel MJ. CT appearance of pediatric ovaries and uterus. *J Comput Assist Tomogr* 1994; 18:72, with permission.)

ian volume of those ovaries visualized was 0.8 cm^3 or less in girls under 8 years. Ovaries were identified in 75% of the girls over 8 years of age. The mean ovarian volume in this group was 6.9 cm^3. The ovarian volume as determined by CT examination is similar to the volume measured sonographically. The increase in ovarian size was noted at a slightly older age (8 years) with CT evaluation than that noted sonographically (5 years). An increased rate of ovarian growth occurs during two periods. The first occurs at approximately 8 years of age, coinciding with an increase in androgen secretion by the adrenal gland, and the second occurs just before and during puberty (26). The ovarian volume of all pathologically proven ovaries in this study was more than 2 SD above that of age-related controls (Fig. 2.2).

Management of Premenarcheal Ovarian Cysts

Thind et al. (26) performed a retrospective study of 64 girls who were diagnosed with an ovarian cyst or tumor. Twenty-eight of these patients were managed surgically, 27 of which were benign and half were functional cysts. Fifty of the patients presented with pain or a palpable abdominal mass. The majority of these cysts were managed conservatively and resolved over a 6- to 8-week period. Management of ovarian cysts in premenarcheal girls is virtually the same as management of ovar-

ian cysts in the adult female. Sonographic findings that are suggestive of a malignancy or a cyst, which does not begin to resolve in 6 to 8 weeks, should be explored surgically. In addition, one must be aware that, in the pediatric population, an ovarian cyst more commonly results in torsion than in the adult or may cause ureteric compression with resulting hydronephrosis and persistent pyrexia may be confused with an undiagnosed appendiceal abscess.

Normal Uterine Development and Size

The fetal uterus enlarges in response to maternal hormonal stimulation. The infant experiences postnatal regression of uterine size. The size of the uterus remains stable until about 7 years of age. The cervix is larger than the corpus in the young child, resulting in an inverted pear shape of the uterus. The predominance of the cervix over the corpus persists until uterine growth begins at about age 7 years. Both the total uterine volume and the ratio of the corpus to the cervix begins to increase significantly between 6 and 8 years (9,10). The normal age-related values of the uterine dimensions, as determined by sonographic evaluation of 114 normal premenarcheal girls, are presented in Table 2.3 (16).

On CT examination, the uterus was identified in 66% of girls 8 years and under and was identified in 92% of girls over 8 years of age.

TABLE 2.3. *Uterine diameters and volume*[a]

Age (yr)	Numbers of patients	Uterine diameters (mm)				Uterine volume (cm³)	
		TUL	COAP	CEAP	COAP/ CEAP	By chronologic age	By bone age
2	7	33.1 ± 4.4	7.0 ± 3.4	8.3 ± 2.0	0.84 ± 0.29	1.98 ± 1.58	1.76 ± 0.72
3	8	32.4 ± 4.3	6.4 ± 1.3	7.6 ± 2.2	0.89 ± 0.29	1.63 ± 0.81	1.80 ± 0.74
4	15	32.9 ± 3.3	7.6 ± 1.8	6.6 ± 1.8	0.90 ± 0.22	2.10 ± 0.57	1.97 ± 0.74
5	7	33.1 ± 5.5	8.0 ± 2.8	8.4 ± 1.6	0.95 ± 0.28	2.36 ± 1.39	2.19 ± 1.16
6	9	33.2 ± 4.1	5.7 ± 2.9	7.5 ± 1.8	0.86 ± 0.18	1.80 ± 1.57	1.65 ± 0.93
7	9	32.3 ± 3.9	8.0 ± 2.2	7.7 ± 2.5	1.08 ± 0.26	2.32 ± 1.07	2.81 ± 1.44
8	11	35.8 ± 7.3	9.0 ± 2.8	8.4 ± 1.7	1.05 ± 0.20	3.12 ± 1.52	2.70 ± 1.43
9	11	37.1 ± 4.4	9.7 ± 3.0	8.8 ± 2.0	1.10 ± 0.24	3.70 ± 1.62	2.69 ± 1.83
10	13	40.3 ± 6.4	12.8 ± 5.3	10.7 ± 2.6	1.17 ± 0.31	6.54 ± 3.78	4.66 ± 3.03
11	13	42.2 ± 5.1	12.8 ± 3.1	10.7 ± 2.6	1.22 ± 0.26	6.66 ± 2.87	6.24 ± 3.07
12	6	54.3 ± 6.4	17.3 ± 5.3	14.3 ± 5.2	1.23 ± 0.16	16.18 ± 9.15	8.68 ± 3.65
13	5	53.8 ± 11.4	15.8 ± 4.5	15.0 ± 2.4	1.03 ± 0.15	13.18 ± 5.64	15.55 ± 5.98

[a]As determined by ultrasonography in 114 girls from age 2 to 13. Mean ± SD.
CEAP, anteroposterior diameter of the cervix; COAP, anteroposterior diameter of the corpus; TUL, total uterine length.
From Orisini LF, Salardi S, Pilu G, et al. Pelvic organs in premenarcheal girls: real-time ultrasonography. *Radiology* 1984;153:113, with permission.

The size of the uterus was stable until 8 years of age, when a dramatic increase in volume was noted. A range in volume from 0.5 to 1.3 cm³ was observed in the group 8 years and younger. Girls over 8 years of age averaged a uterine volume from 4.1 to 37.3 cm³. Uterine neoplasms in the younger group (rhabdomyosarcoma) and in the older group (hydatidiform mole) were far greater than 2 SD above the age-related controls (Fig. 2.3).

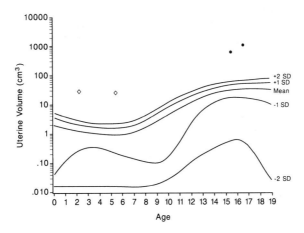

FIG. 2.3. Normal age-related mean uterine volume and standard deviation values plotted on a logarithmic scale. The central line represents the age-related mean uterine volume. The two adjacent inner lines represent 1 SD above and below the mean. The two outer lines represent 2 SD above and below the mean. The "–2 SD" uterine volume values for girls under age 10 years fall below zero, but because uterine volume cannot actually be less than zero, these values were plotted as a straight line just above the horizontal axis. Pathologic uterine volumes are represented by the following symbols: ◇, rhabdomyosarcoma; ●, hydatidiform mole. (From Rigsby CK, Siegel MJ. CT appearance of pediatric ovaries and uterus. *J Comput Assist Tomogr* 1994;18:72, with permission.)

REFERENCES

1. McCann J, Wells R, Simon M, et al. Genital findings in prepubertal girls selected for nonabuse: a descriptive study. *Pediatrics* 1990;86:428.
2. Berenson AB. A longitudinal study of hymenal morphology in the first 3 years of life. *Pediatrics* 1995;95:490.
3. Cowell CA. The gynecologic examination of infants, children, and young adolescents. *Pediatr Clin North Am* 1981;28247.
4. Edmonds DK. Patterns of childhood and adolescent gynaecology. In: *Dewhurst's practical paediatric and adolescent gynaecology,* 2nd ed. London: Butterworth & Co., 1989:1.
5. Bronstein IP, Cassorta E. Breast enlargement in pediatric practice. *Med Clin North Am* 1946;30:121.
6. Berenson AB. Appearance of the hymen at birth and one year of age: a longitudinal study. *Pediatrics* 1993;91:820.
7. Money J, Lamacz M. Genital examination and exposure experienced as nosocomial sexual abuse in childhood. *J Nerv Ment Dis* 1987;175:713.
8. Berenson AB. Appearance of the hymen in newborns. *Pediatrics* 1991;87:458.
9. Muam D, Jones CE. The use of video-colposcopy in the gynecologic examination of infants, children and young adolescents. *Adolesc Pediatr Gynecol* 1993:6:154.
10. Ernans SJH, Goldstein DP. *Pediatric and adolescent gynecology,* 2nd ed. Boston: Little, Brown and Company, 1982:1.
11. McCann J, Voris J, Simon M, et al. Comparison of genital examination techniques in prepubertal girls. *Pediatrics* 1990;85:182.
12. Berenson AB. The prepubertal genital exam: what is normal and abnormal. *Curr Opin Obstet Gynecol* 1994;6:526.
13. Berenson AB, Heger AH, Hayes JM, et al. Appearance of the hymen in prepubertal girls. *Pediatrics* 1992;89:387.
14. McCann J, Wells R, Simon M, et al. Genital findings in prepubertal girls selected for nonabuse: a descriptive study. *Pediatrics* 1990;86:428.
15. Peters H, Himelstein-Braw R, Faber M. The normal development of the ovary in childhood. *Acta Endocrinol* 1976;82:617.
16. Orsini LF, Salardi S, Pilu G, et al. Pelvic organs in premenarcheal girls: real-time ultrasonography, *Radiology* 1984;153:113.
17. Salardi S, Orsini LF, Cacciari E, et al. Pelvic ultrasonography in premenarcheal girls: relation to puberty and sex hormone concentrations. *Arch Dis Child* 1985;60:120.
18. Salardi S, Orsini LF, Cacciari E, et al. Pelvic ultrasonography in girls with precocious puberty, congenital adrenal hyperplasia, obesity, or hirsutism. *J Pediatr* 1988;112:880.
19. Stanhope R, Jacobs HS, Brook CGD. Ovarian ultrasound assessment in normal children, idiopathic precocious puberty, and during low dose pulsatile gonadotropin releasing hormone treatment of hypogonadotrophic hypogonadism. *Arch Dis Child* 1985;60:116.
20. Cohen HL, Eisenberg P, Mandel F, et al. Ovarian cysts are common in premenarchal girls: a sonographic study of 101 children 2–12 years old. *Am J Roentgenol* 1992;159:89.
21. Fleischer AC, Shawker TH. The role of sonography in pediatric gynecology. *Clin Obstet Gynecol* 1987;30:735.
22. Rigsby CK, Siegel MJ. CT appearance of pediatric ovaries and uterus. *J Comput Assist Tomogr* 1994;18:72.
23. Cohen HL, Tice HM, Mandel FS. Ovarian volumes measured by US: bigger than we think. *Radiology* 1990;177:189.
24. Ivarsson SA, Nilsson KO, Persson PH. Ultrasonography of the pelvic organs in prepubertal and postpubertal girls. *Arch Dis Child* 1983;58:352.
25. Simkins CS. Development of the human ovary from birth to sexual maturity. *Am J Anat* 1932;51:465.
26. Thind CR, Carty HML, Pilling DW. The role of ultrasound in the management of ovarian masses in children. *Clin Radiol* 1989;40:180.

3

Normal Pubertal Development

Sander S. Shapiro and Joel S. Krasnow

Puberty refers to those developmental processes initiated in late childhood that culminate in adult reproductive competence. It involves a group of qualitative changes that depart from the generalized somatic growth processes that are dominant throughout childhood. Attainment of puberty is associated with profound hormonal alterations, the acquisition of secondary sexual characteristics, a short-lived increase in longitudinal growth rate, and numerous psychosocial changes (1). None of these events, however, either alone or in concert, absolutely signifies that an individual has established a reproductive capacity. Thus, puberty is a rather general term that connotes the transition period between childhood and adulthood.

The age at which the somatic changes associated with puberty occur is highly variable. A majority of North American females initiate pubertal alterations between 8 and 13 years of age. Their male counterparts initiate analogous pubertal development at 9 to 14 years of age (2). Between 1% and 2% of the population will start their transition outside of this range and thereby invite evaluation for either precocious or delayed puberty (3).

The first somatic change that occurs in females is either the beginning of breast (thelarche) or pubic hair (pubarche) development. The onset of both thelarche and pubarche are variable, with a mean of 10.9 and 11.2 years, respectively, for North American females. Tanner described five stages of breast and pubic hair development, as outlined in Figs. 3.1 and 3.2. An even earlier, but seldom documented, change is the onset of the "adolescent

growth spurt." This change in growth velocity has a mean onset of 9.6 years (4). The peak height velocity (PHV) occurs almost 2.5 years later and precedes the onset of menses (mean age 12.7 years). The interval between onset of breast development and menarche is 2.3 ± 1.0 years and is independent of the age at which thelarche occurs. However, a wider temporal range exists for the onset, duration, and completion of these transforming events. Within the spectrum of normal pubertal development, it is possible to see physical changes as much as 5 years before menarche. It also is possible for the sequence of physical changes to vary considerably from the order discussed. Such variability can lead to expressions of concern on the part of adolescents and their parents. Therefore, it is helpful for medical practitioners to have a firm sense of the wide temporal range of pubertal events and an understanding of when to initiate an evaluation for those who present outside popularly perceived norms.

The average age of pubertal onset, as well as the age of first menses (menarche), has declined steadily over the last century in this country and throughout the industrialized world. Most recently, however, this trend has leveled off and may even be going in the opposite direction (5). At present, the average age of menarche is about 12.7 years (6). This has been attributed to improved nutritional and general health conditions, as well as to altered lifestyles. In isolated nomadic tribes, where living conditions and socialization practices have not changed significantly during recent times, the trend toward earlier

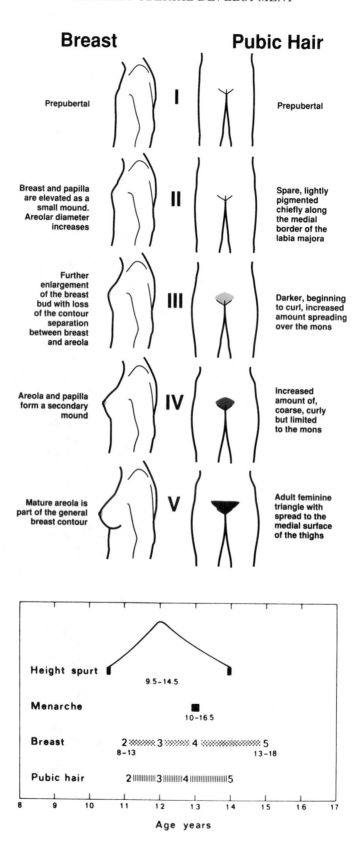

FIG. 3.1. Stages of female breast and pubic hair development during puberty as described by Marshall and Tanner. (From Marshall WA, Tanner JM. Variations in pattern of pubertal changes in girls. *Arch Dis Child* 1969;44:291, with permission.)

menarche is not found. In addition, strenuous physical activity, decreased body fat content, chronic disease, and malnutrition are all associated with delayed puberty. Conversely, females with moderately increased fat content tend to experience menarche at an earlier age. Thus, geographic, nutritional, and sociologically determined factors may affect the time at which puberty begins and its rate of progression. Furthermore, daughters frequently experience menarche at an age that is close to their mother's menarcheal age, suggesting that genetic factors may contribute to the timing of pubertal events.

ETIOLOGY OF PUBERTY

The principal factors involved in the initiation of puberty are contained within the hypothalamic-pituitary-gonadal (HPG) axis, as represented in Fig. 3.3. The arcuate nucleus, which is located in the medial basal hypothalamus, contains a group of specialized cells that have the ability to secrete gonadotropin-releasing hormone (GnRH). This neurohormone initially is synthesized as part of a 92 amino-acid precursor that undergoes post-translational processing before release as a decapeptide (7). GnRH is released into the hypothalamic-portal circulation in a pulsatile manner, which results in a high concentration within the anterior lobe of the pituitary. This

FIG. 3.2. Relationship of breast and pubic hair development to the adolescent growth spurt and menarche. Ranges are given for the changes illustrated. (From Sorva R, Tolppanen E-M, Lankinen S, et al. Growth evaluation: parent and child specific height standards. *Arch Dis Child* 1989;64:1483–1487, with permission.)

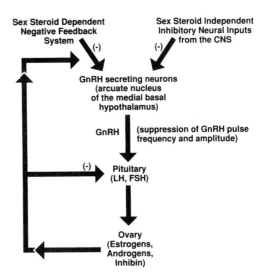

FIG. 3.3. Model of the major factors influencing the gonadotropin-releasing hormone (GnRH)-secreting neurons in the region of the medial basal hypothalamus. Before puberty, both the sex steroid-dependent and sex steroid-independent systems exert a primarily inhibitory influence on GnRH secretion. Pulsatile GnRH secretion causes the pituitary to release luteinizing hormone (LH) and follicle-stimulating hormone (FSH). The gonadotropins, in turn, stimulate ovarian activity. Ovarian secretion of sex steroids and inhibin maintain homeostasis by exerting feedback inhibition at the pituitary and hypothalamus.

stimulates the secretion of follicle-stimulating hormone (FSH) and luteinizing hormone (LH) by specific cells within that gland. These gonadotropins (FSH and LH), in turn, stimulate the production of sex steroids by the gonads. Circulating androgens, estrogens, and the gonadal peptide inhibin have inhibitory actions at the level of the pituitary and hypothalamus, which also serve to maintain homeostasis.

GnRH-producing hypothalamic cells originate in ectoderm of the nasal placode and migrate to their permanent site during embryogenesis (8). Intrinsically pulsatile, their release of hormone is thought to become synchronized through the development of synaptic communication (9). Two major systems are known to modulate GnRH secretion. The central nervous system (CNS) exerts its influence through synaptic connections terminating in the region of the medial basal hypothalamus. Summation of all neural inputs usually results in an inhibitory effect, referred to as the "intrinsic CNS inhibitory mechanism." The principal transsynaptic inhibitor of GnRH secretion is thought to be γ-aminobutyric acid (GABA) (10). The second modulating system involves the negative feedback of sex steroids at the level of the hypothalamus. Thus, the relative sensitivity of the GnRH neurons in the hypothalamus to (a) negative feedback effects of circulating sex steroids and (b) neural inputs from the CNS determine the activity of the entire HPG axis (Fig. 3.3). Puberty represents the disinhibition of these cells from the aforementioned influences and results in regular, pulsatile GnRH secretion.

DEVELOPMENT AND MATURATION OF THE HYPOTHALAMIC-PITUITARY-GONADAL AXIS

During the fourth week of embryonic development, germ cells, which have their origin in yolk sac endoderm, migrate to the genital ridge, taking up residence in the undifferentiated gonad. Organization of mesenchyme at this site progresses rapidly so that, by the seventh week of gestation, primordial testes are distinguishable. Expression of the testis-determining factor gene, which is located on the short arm of the Y chromosome, induces this differentiation (11). Absence of testis-determining factor gene expression leaves the gonad to differentiate into an ovary. Ovarian differentiation can be positively identified by 10 weeks of gestation. The germ cells then undergo multiple mitotic divisions that terminate in a single meiotic division at about 20 weeks (12). When oocytes enter the diplotene stage of prophase, they are surrounded by a single layer of granulosa cells forming a primordial follicle. The number of oocytes reaches a maximum of approximately seven million during the fifth month of gestation; from that point it declines to about two million at term (13). After approximately the fifth month of gestation, ovaries become re-

sponsive to gonadotropin stimulation resulting in follicular growth and estrogen production. Follicular development *in utero* usually proceeds to the early antral stage (1 to 2 mm in diameter) and is followed by atresia. Maintenance of a normal complement of primary oocytes depends on the presence of two normal X chromosomes. This supposition is supported by the finding that fetuses with a 45,XO karyotype have a normal complement of oocytes at midgestation but a reduced number of follicles at birth. Follicular atresia continues after birth so that few of these girls deficient in X chromosome experience menarche. On the other hand, children with 46,XX/45,XO karyotypes often have sufficient follicular development to experience menstruation and even conception. However, they usually undergo ovarian failure long before the time for normal menopause.

The HPG axis is established early in fetal development. In the human fetus, GnRH is present in the hypothalamus by 8 weeks of gestation (14), and the hypothalamic-portal system is functional by 11.5 gestational weeks. Detection of LH and FSH in the fetal pituitary is demonstrable by 12 gestational weeks. Fetal pituitary cells respond to GnRH with the synthesis and secretion of LH and FSH (14). The production of gonadotropins by the fetal pituitary appears to be necessary for normal ovarian development. Hypophysectomy of Rhesus monkey fetuses decreases the number of germ cells found in their ovaries (15). Similar changes are noted in anencephalic human fetuses. Female fetuses experience a significantly higher concentration of FSH in their serum and their pituitaries than do males (16). In the male, placental human chorionic gonadotropin (hCG) stimulates fetal Leydig cell differentiation and the secretion of testosterone. Fetal testosterone levels rise, peaking at 15 to 18 gestational weeks (17). The elevated level of testosterone in males is thought to account for the sex difference in FSH through a negative feedback effect on the male hypothalamus and pituitary. The presence of such an inhibitory effect further suggests that a functional HPG endocrine system exists *in utero*. Because this sex difference persists postnatally, a direct effect of testosterone on differentiation of the hypothalamic-pituitary unit has been postulated (18).

In utero, the fetoplacental unit is the primary estrogen-secreting organ. Thus, at delivery, FSH and LH levels are low in cord blood due to the suppressive effect brought on by high levels of circulating estrogens. Estrogen levels fall abruptly after birth. This decreases the inhibitory influence on the hypothalamic GnRH pulse generator, causing serum LH and FSH concentrations to rise gradually. As a result, gonadotropin levels remain low for the first 3 days postpartum and then increase to a peak during the third month of life (19,20). The sexual dimorphism in FSH secretion seen at midgestation is observed again after the third postpartum day. In females, plasma FSH levels rise earlier and attain higher peak values compared to males. Moreover, males experience a rapid decline in plasma FSH levels by 6 months, whereas slightly higher FSH levels may persist in the female until 4 years of age (21). FSH release after exogenous stimulation by GnRH also is greater in females in than males during this period (22). In females, ovarian production of estradiol rises in response to increasing levels of FSH during the early part of infancy (23).

In males, postpartum testosterone levels fall immediately after birth as a consequence of the loss of testicular stimulation by placental hCG. A secondary rise in testosterone that occurs several days after birth is coincident with the rise in pituitary gonadotropins. After the third postnatal month, decreasing pituitary gonadotropin secretion results in a decline in serum testosterone levels. The role of gonadotropins in testosterone secretion can be inferred from the observation that infants with panhypopituitarism do not exhibit this secondary rise. In contrast to FSH levels, the rise in plasma LH occurs earlier in males than in females during the first 2 months postpartum. In both sexes, LH levels peak in the third to fourth months and then decline, reaching low levels by 1 year of age.

As illustrated in Fig. 3.3, GnRH secretion is dependent on both sex steroid-dependent and sex steroid-independent systems. From the third trimester of pregnancy and throughout the first few months of life, fluctuations in LH and FSH can be explained largely by the negative feedback effects of circulating sex steroids. The sex steroid-independent system represents the sum of all neural inputs to the GnRH-secreting neurons. These inputs are primarily inhibitory. With continued growth and differentiation of the CNS, additional maturational changes occur, resulting in increased inhibitory input to the GnRH-secreting neurons. Evidence for the role of the "intrinsic CNS inhibitory mechanism" comes from neuroendocrine studies of the human neonate. When infants born prematurely are compared to infants born at term, both groups being of similar postnatal age and having similar sex steroid levels, the premature infants are found to have significantly higher serum LH and FSH levels. Presumably this is due to the relative immaturity of the intrinsic CNS inhibitory system (24). Similarly, premature male infants have a normal pattern of decrease in their serum testosterone levels at birth due to withdrawal of hCG. However, they have a higher and more sustained secondary rise in testosterone levels, reflecting decreased inhibition of GnRH and consequently LH secretion (24).

Agonadal patients provide a unique model for investigating the activity of the intrinsic CNS inhibitory system. These individuals secrete no gonadal steroids; therefore, the contribution of the sex steroid-dependent feedback mechanism is minimal, with hypothalamic-pituitary pulsatility inhibition being solely dependent on intrinsic CNS factors. After birth, serum gonadotropin concentrations rise to menopausal levels in agonadal infants, peaking at between 1 and 2 years of age (Fig. 3.4) (25). This suggests that, in intact infants, the governing mechanism controlling physiologic LH and FSH secretion at this time is the serum level of sex steroids.

The subsequent decline in gonadotropins to their nadir between 6 and 8 years of age sug-

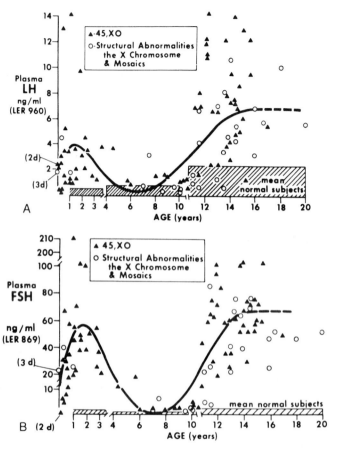

FIG. 3.4. Plasma luteinizing hormone (LH) **(A)** and follicle-stimulating hormone (FSH) **(B)** levels in patients with gonadal dysgenesis compared to normal subjects. The *curved line* represents the mean of values from females with gonadal dysgenesis; the *hatched area* represents the mean for normal females. (From Conte FA, Grumbach MM, Kaplan SS. A diphasic pattern in gonadotropin secretion in patients with the syndrome of gonadal dysgenesis. *J Clin Endocrinol Metab* 1974;40:670–675, with permission.)

gests that an intrinsic CNS inhibitory mechanism is almost exclusively responsible for restraining the GnRH pulse generator during this period (26). In midchildhood, LH and FSH begin to rise again, suggesting reversibility of this intrinsic CNS inhibitory mechanism. Here again, the higher levels of gonadotropins seen among agonadal children demonstrates the reemergence of a dominant influence by sex steroid hormones.

The principal central inhibitor of GnRH pulsatile activity during childhood is thought to be GABA. High levels of this agent are present in the median eminence of prepubertal monkeys (Fig. 3.5), and its concentration changes reciprocally with that of GnRH during puberty. Blockade of its type A receptor induces a rise in GnRH release during prepuberty, but not afterward (27). Furthermore, inhibition of glutamic acid decarboxylase production (the enzyme involved in GABA synthesis) causes a rise in GnRH release by prepubertal animals (28).

In the late juvenile period, inhibitory CNS influences on the hypothalamic pulse generator wane, initiating a rise in GnRH secretion. This results in increased secretion of sex steroids by the gonads, which is referred to as

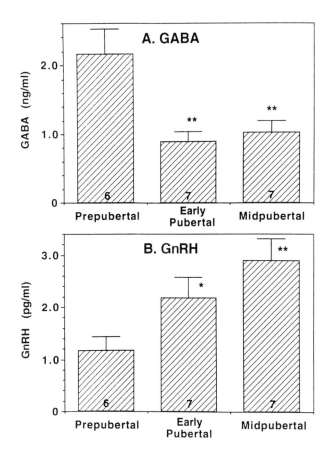

FIG. 3.5. Developmental changes in γ-aminobutyric acid (GABA) release **(A)** and gonadotropin-releasing hormone (GnRH) **(B)** measured in aliquots of the same 10-minute perfusate samples from the stalk-median eminence of female Rhesus monkeys.

"gonadarche." Dickerman et al. (29) were the first to postulate the role of increased GnRH pulse frequency in the initiation of puberty. They demonstrated that administering a bolus of GnRH resulted in the release of pituitary FSH and LH in prepubertal children. Subsequently, Wildt et al. (30) eloquently demonstrated the central role of GnRH in pubertal development. They administered GnRH in a regular pulsatile manner to prepubertal Rhesus monkeys (Fig. 3.6). Initially FSH and LH were not detectable. After 15 days of regular GnRH pulses, FSH rose to detectable levels. At 30 days, serum estradiol increased, followed by an LH surge that was not large enough to induce ovulation. Subsequently, estrogen levels declined and menses occurred. Continued GnRH administration resulted in a second rise of estradiol sufficient to produce an LH surge that resulted in ovulation. Adequate proges-

terone secretion demonstrated the presence of a functional corpus luteum. Continuation of GnRH administration produced regular 28-day menstrual cycles. When GnRH therapy was discontinued, the animals reverted to their prepubertal state. Subsequently, these animals experience menarche at the expected age. Thus, their studies in the monkey support the hypothesis that reactivation of GnRH pulsatility leads to puberty. Studies of pulse generator activity in prepubertal children further support this notion (31). What remains unexplained is the mechanism that instigates a diminution in central inhibitory influences on GnRH pulsatility and the manner in which body weight relates to this CNS governor.

The first identifiable endocrinologic sign of puberty is the release of GnRH only at night and coincident with onset of sleep (Fig. 3.7). Subsequently, LH pulses become more

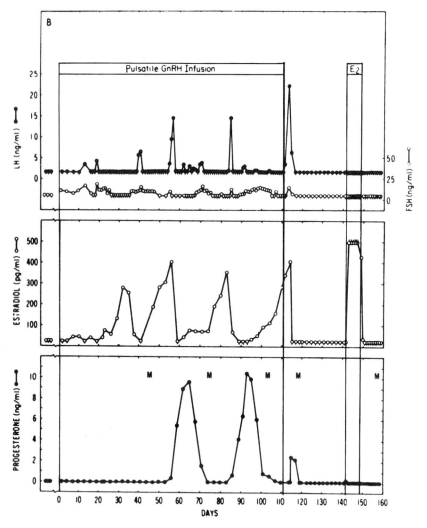

FIG. 3.6. Effect of an unvarying hourly pulsatile dose of gonadotropin-releasing hormone (GnRH) in a prepubertal Rhesus monkey. Gonadotropin and estradiol levels were undetectable before initiating stimulation with GnRH. At time 0, pulsatile GnRH was begun. This was followed by small, yet physiologically significant increases in gonadotropins. This resulted in elevated estradiol levels reflecting advancing ovarian folliculogenesis. The first rise in estradiol was ineffective in eliciting a gonadotropin surge. Nevertheless, menstruation (M) occurred as a consequence of estrogen withdrawal. The next rise in estradiol elicited a luteinizing hormone (LH) surge resulting in ovulation and progesterone secretion by the corpus luteum. Continued stimulation resulted in another ovulatory cycle 28 days later. Two days after discontinuation of GnRH infusion, a gonadotropin surge occurred in response to rising estradiol levels. Progesterone secretion was only transient due to the absence of continued hypophysiotropic stimulation. The area labeled *E2* indicates implantation of estradiol containing Silastic capsules. In the absence of hypophysiotropic stimulation, rising estradiol levels failed to induce a gonadotropin surge. (From Wildt L, Marshall G, Knobil E. Experimental induction of puberty in the infantile rhesus monkey. *Science* 1980;207:1373–1375, with permission.)

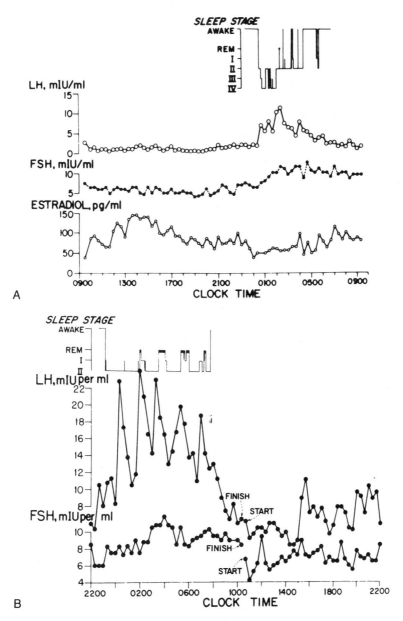

FIG. 3.7. Relationship between the onset of sleep and gonadotropin secretion in early **(A)** and mid puberty **(B)**. Gonadotropins are released in association with the onset of sleep. A sleep histogram indicating the subject's sleep stage is superimposed. The sleep stages are rapid eye movement (REM), sleep, and stages I to IV. Advancing puberty **(B)** is associated with increased gonadotropin pulse frequency and amplitude. (From Boyar R, Finkelstein J, Roffwarg H, et al. Synchronization of augmented luteinizing hormone secretion with sleep during puberty. *N Engl J Med* 1972;287:582 and Boyar RM, Wu RHK, Roffwarg H, et al. Human puberty: 24-hour estradiol patterns in pubertal girls. *J Clin Endocrinol Metab* 1976;43:1418, with permission.)

frequent but continue to occur primarily during sleep (32). With further maturation, LH pulses appear during the daytime and increase in amplitude. As menarche approaches, these pulses are detected at all hours, and a diurnal variation in pulse frequency no longer is demonstrable (33). A similar change in secretory pattern is noted for FSH. Thus, puberty represents a limited disinhibition of the GnRH neurons, resulting in a progression of secretory activity that culminates in the adult form of regular, pulsatile GnRH secretion. In concert with these maturational changes, LH levels rise and the serum ratio of LH to FSH, which had been less than one, reverses (34).

The factor(s) responsible for initiation of the hypothalamic pubertal changes described here currently is unknown. Frisch and Revelle (35) proposed that a critical body weight and body fat content are required for the initiation of menarche. Their theory is supported by the finding that there is a delay in menarche in states of malnutrition and chronic disease. Individuals who participate from an early age in highly competitive athletic training and consequently have low fat/lean muscle mass also experience menarche later than their nonathletic peers (36–38). Girls with anorexia nervosa exhibit a regression to the prepubertal pattern of gonadotropin secretion as body weight declines and revert to normal secretory patterns as their weight increases (39). To test Frisch and Revelle's hypothesis that increased body weight and fat content are required for the occurrence of menarche, urinary gonadotropin and anthropometric data were obtained from healthy children. The changes in body composition in these children did not precede, but rather occurred simultaneously with, the rise in gonadotropin secretion (40). This suggests that changes in body composition are not a prerequisite to the initiation of puberty. Nevertheless, the regressive modifications in gonadotropin secretion associated with severe weight loss, noted by Boyar et al. (39), point to the possibility that a strong link exists between nutritional status and the initiation of puberty. Presumably, that link operates at a CNS level, exerting a direct influence on hypothalamic activity. Recently, leptin, an adipose-derived protein hormone, has been identified. It is thought to play a substantial role in neuroendocrine function as well as energy homeostasis. However, serum levels of this agent do not correlate strongly with the onset of early pubertal events, and as yet there is no direct evidence that it plays a role in the waning of central inhibitory influences on hypothalamic GnRH secretory patterns (41).

Menarche is a late pubertal event, appearing in North American girls at 12.7 years. It occurs when there has been sufficient gonadotropin stimulation of the ovaries to produce a rise in serum estrogen, which, in turn, stimulates proliferation of uterine endometrium. As it grows, the endometrium becomes progressively more dependent on sustaining levels of estrogen. Eventually either the uterine lining outgrows the steroid's capacity to maintain it, or there is a dip in circulating estrogen concentration. In either case, the result is hemorrhage. However, because proliferation has occurred without subsequent progesterone exposure, the length and amount of bleeding can be highly variable. Such irregular, unpredictable menstrual flow will occur as long as the individual remains anovulatory and the endometrium remains unexposed to progesterone, usually for 6 to 18 months. Ovulatory menstrual cycles require a final maturational event: the development of a hypothalamic-pituitary positive feedback mechanism. This will produce the midcycle LH surge, subsequent ovulation, and corpus luteal progesterone secretion.

In young women, the hallmark event of puberty is ovulation. It occurs late in the long cascade of events that began with embryologic migration of GnRH-producing cells into the medial-basal hypothalamus and signals the existence of an adult, integrated, hypothalamic-pituitary-ovarian axis. Ovulation confirms that central inhibition of neuronal GnRH secretory pulsatility has ceased and that both estrogen negative and estrogen positive feedback loops are operational. For the next 25 or so years, estrogen and inhibin will act to limit the secretion of pituitary go-nadotropins (through negative feedback), while intermittent high levels of estradiol will serve (through positive feedback) to induce the midcycle LH surge. Ovulatory cycling can continue until the individual's ovarian follicular population is exhausted.

INITIATION OF ADRENARCHE

Adrenarche refers to the process of adrenal gland secretion. At approximately 3 years of age, the zona reticularis begins to form. As that zone enlarges, changes in its capacity for steroid production result in increased secretion of androgens, principally dehydroepiandrosterone (DHEA) and its sulfate (DHEAS) (42). A rise in plasma DHEAS is first detectable at about 7 years and reaches adult levels at about 15 years of age. During this period, plasma DHEAS levels rise as much as 20-fold in both sexes (43). The increased production of adrenal androgens results in the development of pubic and axillary hair and contributes to the development of acne in both sexes. Adrenal androgens also contribute to advancing bone age and linear growth. Individuals who experience premature adrenarche will have a diminished adult height, because the effect of androgens on bone maturation is considerably greater than on skeletal growth (44).

The factors that regulate zona reticularis steroid output are not well established. The increase in androgen synthesis during adrenarche occurs in the absence of any detectable change in adrenocorticotropic hormone or cortisol secretion. A corticotropin androgen-stimulating hormone has been postulated as the agent responsible for adrenarche, but to date no such molecule has been positively identified. The onset of adrenarche typically precedes any rise in gonadotropins or change in growth rate. For this reason, the initiation of adrenal androgen production has been postulated as playing a role in the onset of puberty. Although the initiating factors in both adrenarche and gonadal puberty remain unknown, considerable experimental evi-dence supports a lack of association between the two processes. This evidence originates primarily from studies of patients with gonadal dysgenesis or isolated gonadotropin deficiency who almost universally experience normal adrenarche (45). Moreover, patients with true precocious puberty experience gonadal puberty before adrenarche. It also has been observed that children with chronic adrenal insufficiency, who consequently have deficient adrenal androgen secretion, will progress through puberty normally while receiving replacement doses of only glucocorticoids and mineralocorticoids.

INITIATION OF GONADARCHE

The alterations in physical characteristics that occur around puberty are largely dependent on sex steroid production by the gonads. The process of ovarian follicular growth and atresia is a continuous process initiated *in utero*. Both ultrasound and autopsy studies have documented cystic changes in the ovaries from birth to puberty (46,47). It is not uncommon to note ovarian follicular cysts, *in utero* or in the neonatal period, that regress spontaneously following chorionic gonadotropin withdrawal. Throughout childhood, follicles continue to develop and undergo atresia, resulting in a gradual increase in ovarian stromal tissue but with only minimal estrogen secretion. The initiation of follicular development is thought to occur independent of pituitary gonadotropin stimulation. Sustained progression of follicular development to the antral stage with significant estrogen production does, however, require gonadotropins (48).

After reactivation of the HPG axis at puberty, multiple (more than five) follicles develop to a size larger than 4 mm. With maturation of the neuroendocrine unit, gonadotropin pulse frequency increases and ovarian follicles develop to a progressively larger size. As follicular maturation progresses, steroidogenic competency develops. There is a direct relationship between follicular size and steroid-synthesizing capacity (48). Follicular development to 16 mm in diameter may be expected to provide sufficient estrogen for endometrial proliferation. The earliest follicles to attain this degree of maturation usually fail to induce an LH surge and, therefore, undergo atresia without effecting ovulation. This, in turn, causes estrogen withdrawal followed by endometrial involution and menstrual bleeding. Thus, menarche follows and is usually the result of nonovulatory cycling. The length of the menstrual cycle is quite variable during the first year after menarche, with only about 15% being ovulatory (49). However, should ovulation take place during the initial cycle, pregnancy would be possible without the onset of a first menses.

Even after ovulatory competence has been achieved, abnormalities of the luteal phase (short luteal phase, inadequate luteal phase) commonly occur (50). These abnormalities are thought to be the result of inadequate follicular stimulation by the pituitary and provide evidence that the HPG axis has not achieved full maturity. With complete maturation of the HPG axis, a dominant follicle develops in each cycle, becomes fully mature, and ovulates.

Both the onset and rate of progression through puberty correlate with the age of menarche and the age at which regular ovulatory menstrual cycles are established (51). Progression from Tanner stage II breast and pubic hair to menarche occurred in 1.4 ± 0.1 years and 1.1 ± 0.2 years, respectively, in Finnish girls experiencing menarche prior to age 13 years. The majority of menstrual cycles were ovulatory within 18 months of menarche. In contrast, those girls experiencing menarche after age 13 years progressed through these same developmental stages in 2.1 ± 0.2 years and 2.0 ± 0.2 years, respectively. In this group, only 50% of all menstrual cycles were ovulatory by the fifth year after menarche (52). Other investigators have found a trend in essentially the opposite direction, with those girls undergoing early onset of puberty experiencing a longer pubertal interval (53). This observation is thought to reflect the variable velocity at which integration of the HPG axis occurs (54).

PHYSICAL EVENTS OF PUBERTY

In utero, the fetus is exposed to high estrogen levels. Acute withdrawal of estrogen at birth can result in endometrial shedding, which manifests clinically as vaginal bleeding. In infant girls between 1 and 6 months of age, the uterus decreases in size, achieving an average length of 32 mm. The ratio of corpus to cervix in the prepubertal uterus is 1:2. When GnRH pulse frequency increases sufficiently to cause multiple follicular development and estradiol production, uterine growth begins. The first change is a lengthening of the corpus, followed by an increase in the width and thickness of both corpus and cervix. This process is initiated between 7 and 9 years of age. A uterine cross-sectional area of 4×2 cm usually is achieved by 12 years of age. Before initiation of puberty, the endometrium consists of a single layer of cuboidal cells. As estradiol levels increase, the endometrium begins to proliferate. A rapid increase in endometrial thickness immediately preceding menarche can be visualized by ultrasound evaluation.

Like the uterus, the vagina is an estrogen-responsive tissue. During puberty, newly elevated estrogen levels stimulate overall growth as well as epithelial proliferation. Under the influence of estrogen, the vaginal epithelium increases in thickness, with cornification of its superficial cell layers. This change has been quantified and the karyopyknotic index used as a sign of estrogenic status. Multiple metabolic alterations of the epithelium also result from estrogen exposure. These bring about a change in vaginal secretions and pH, providing greater resistance to local infection.

Both the labia minora and majora respond to estrogen by increasing in size and thickness. Concomitantly, the hymen thickens and its orifice enlarges to about 1 cm in diameter. At the same time, the vestibular glands begin active secretion and the clitoris undergoes general enlargement. The relative contribution of estrogen and androgens to this latter change remains ill defined.

Breast development is often the first visible change of puberty, although it may follow pubarche by many months (Fig. 3.2). Before thelarche, male and female breast tissue is histologically indistinguishable. Breast development at puberty requires the presence of multiple hormones including prolactin, glucocorticoids, and insulin (55). However, it is gonadarche with its production of estrogens that induces thelarche. It is the direct estrogen stimulation of mammary epithelium that causes ductal proliferation and the site-specific adipose deposition that accounts for the majority of female breast development. Males fail to produce significant breast mass, primarily because they lack optimal levels of circulating estrogen. The extent to which testosterone inhibits breast development (during embryogenesis and/or puberty) remains uncertain. In complete testicular feminization, substantial breast tissue usually is present despite only minimal increases in estrogen compared to the testosterone-sensitive, normal male, suggesting the potential importance of androgens in limiting male breast development. Once thelarche begins, the duration of time at each Tanner stage is variable. Overall, breast development usually proceeds smoothly to maturity in about 3 years (4).

Temporally associated with the development of secondary sexual characteristics is a marked increase in growth referred to as the "adolescent growth spurt." This growth spurt, which is measured by a change in skeletal growth rate, actually represents a more global process involving an increase in muscle mass and growth of almost all internal organs. These processes are dependent on both growth hormone and sex steroids, predominantly estrogen in both sexes (56). Adrenal, as well as gonadal hormones, are thought to contribute to this change in growth rate (57). In addition to their direct anabolic effects, sex steroids have been demonstrated to increase the secretion of growth hormone and consequently insulin-like growth factor (58). The rise in serum sex steroid levels initiates a change in growth velocity that often antedates pubarche and thelarche (Fig. 3.2). A sudden increase in shoe size frequently is observed coincident with onset of the linear growth

spurt. Peak growth velocity usually is attained midway in the course of pubertal maturation in females, which is 2 years earlier than in males. Prior to the adolescent growth spurt, growth velocity averages 3 to 6 cm per year. PHV in males averages 8.8 cm, with a standard deviation of 1.05 cm per year. In females, PHV is 8.13 cm, with a standard deviation of 0.78 cm per year. By the time PHV is reached, approximately 90% of the final adult height has been achieved. On completion of the adolescent growth spurt, very little additional height is gained. The average increase in height from the onset of the growth spurt to the cessation of growth is 25 cm in females and 28 cm in males. Thus, the greater final height achieved in males is a function of both the delay in onset of the growth spurt and a greater gain in height during the growth spurt. Children who progress through puberty earlier tend to attain a greater PHV but ultimately have a shorter final adult height than their peers.

There are several common variations in normal pubertal development. For example, one breast may begin to develop up to 6 months before the other. This may lead to an asymmetry that persists into adult life. Premature development of the breast bud is referred to as premature thelarche. When this occurs in early infancy, it may represent a delay in either establishment of negative estrogen feedback on the hypothalamus or inhibition of the intrinsic pulsatile activity of the hypothalamus by higher centers. In the older child, it may be an attenuated form of sexual precocity. In both instances, endocrinologic findings may reveal increased gonadotropins or increased gonadotropin response to GnRH. Total or free estradiol level may be elevated in plasma. Radiologic evaluation usually reveals some ovarian follicular activity. Follow-up is necessary to distinguish premature thelarche from true precocious puberty. In premature thelarche, breast development ceases and may even regress, bone age is not advanced, and there are no further signs of pubertal development (59). In contrast, during premature puberty, bone age will advance significantly and

other signs of continued pubertal development, such as the appearance of pubic hair,
will occur.

Premature development of sexual hair is referred to as premature pubarche. The majority
of children with premature pubarche have
early activation of adrenal androgen secretion.
Adrenocorticotropic hormone stimulation of
these individuals will reveal responses between those of adults and prepubertal children

(60). Levels of DHEAS usually are elevated.
Because puberty and adrenarche are independent events, there are no other signs of sexual
precocity and bone age is not significantly advanced in these children.

In assessing children for suspected disorders of growth and development, charts displaying normative data provide valuable information. North American children grow
faster and on average are taller than British

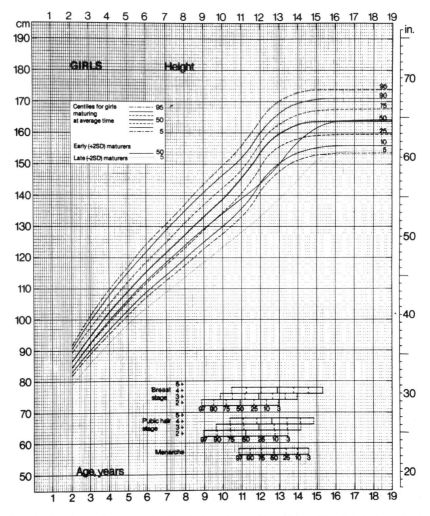

FIG. 3.8. Longitudinal growth curves for North American girls adjusted for the timing of pubertal development: the 50th and 95th centile for girls with accelerated maturation *(symbol)* and the 50th and
5th centile for girls with later maturation. Percentiles for Tanner stages and menarche are given for
North American girls. (From Tanner JW, Davies PWS. Clinical longitudinal standards for height and
height velocity for North American children. *J Pediatr* 1985;107:317, with permission.)

children; therefore, appropriate standards for the population being studied should be used. The onset of gonadarche is associated with increased growth velocity. Because the time of initiation of gonadarche is quite variable, the range of heights in pubertal aged children will be greater than the range for prepubertal children. Therefore, the use of cross-sectional population curves to follow the growth of an individual child, once puberty has begun, is invalid (61). The use of the growth curves for North American children published by Tanner in 1985 take into account the variability in pubertal progression (Figs. 3.8–3.9). For example, take two girls both destined for an adult height of 164 cm (50th percentile). At age 12 years, an "early maturer" (+2 SD) will have completed her growth spurt and measure 160 cm. The "late maturer" (−2 SD) will measure 144 cm. Because these curves are derived by

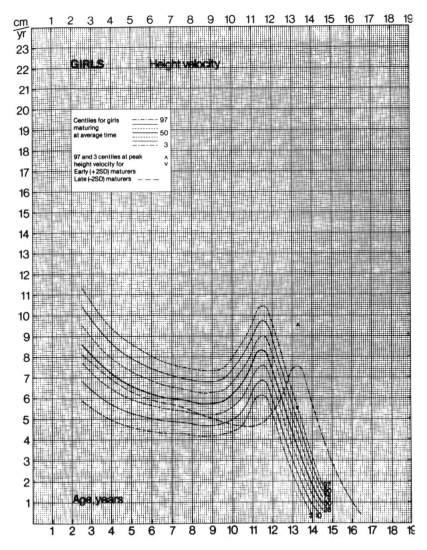

FIG. 3.9. Height velocity in North American girls adjusted for the timing of pubertal development. (From Tanner JW, Davies PWS. Clinical longitudinal standards for height and height velocity for North American children. *J Pediatr* 1985;107:317, with permission.)

averaging data from a large population, no single individual should be expected to follow the curve precisely. These graphs are particularly useful in evaluating girls with primary amenorrhea. When height and breast and pubic hair development are all progressing in accordance with the norms and an intact reproductive tract is present, the patient can be assured that menarche is imminent.

A distinction must be made between the late maturer who makes slow but steady progress and the individual exhibiting an arrest of pubertal development. Individuals who have initiated breast and pubic hair growth usually also will have noticed an increase in the size of their hands and feet. As indicated earlier, increasing shoe size is an indicator of normal pubertal development. Arrest of pubertal development is relatively rare, but when detected it may indicate hypothalamic, pituitary, gonadal, or systemic disease. Because the interval from thelarche to menarche is 2.3 ± 1.0 years (62), the absence of advancement in breast and pubic hair development and the absence of growth in the hands and feet over a 2- to 3-year period deserves further evaluation.

Girls who are late to initiate signs of pubertal development will usually also be late to experience menarche. It is not unusual for an individual initiating breast development at age 14 years to not experience first menses until age 17 or 18 years (51,53). As a general rule, one should expect healthy girls of 14 years to have begun to demonstrate the physical changes of puberty. Those that have not require special attention. When a young woman demonstrates substantial pubertal development yet has not experienced menarche by age 18 years, she too deserves thorough evaluation.

One of the more commonly seen variations from normal puberty is the failure to develop secondary sexual characteristics by age 14 years. These individuals usually are smaller than their peers due to the lack of initiation of a growth spurt. Commonly, their mothers also exhibited a delay in the onset of puberty. Bone age is useful in evaluating such patients, because it is more closely correlated with pubertal events than chronologic age. Clinical signs of pubertal development are present in approximately 95% of individuals when their bone age reaches 12.5 years (63). Constitutional delay in growth and pubertal development occurs as a result of a delay in maturation of the HPG axis. Most cases of delayed development are constitutional, but other causes of delayed puberty, as discussed in Chapter 13, need to be considered (64). In individuals with constitutional delay of pubertal development, endocrinologic findings should be consistent with the stage of development and may indicate impending onset of clinical signs (65).

In addition to changes in linear growth, the skeleton also undergoes a series of characteristic alterations in its osseous composition. These patterns define a bone age that, during adolescence, more closely correlates with the individual's state of pubertal development than with their chronologic age. A radiographically defined bone age of 11 years usually is associated with the onset of either pubarche, thelarche, or both (66).

In conjunction with the physical changes described earlier, the appearance of acne, axillary hair growth, and phenotypical alterations in adipose distribution are part of the pubertal process. Each of these can be directly associated with the newly integrated hormonal changes that underpin puberty. On the other hand, there is little current evidence to support a direct relationship between adolescent patterns of social behavior and the chemical alterations that are an integral part of the pubertal process. This concept may change as a more thorough understanding of the effects that pubertal hormone changes have on neurobiochemical processes evolves.

Growth and development throughout childhood usually progresses in an orderly fashion (67). Any deviation from the perceived norm usually results in the child being brought to medical attention. Precocious, delayed, and aberrant development can cause alarm to parents, school officials, and medical personnel. Wide variation in the onset of developmental milestones evokes concern, as comparisons usually are made between children of similar chronologic age. The physician faced with such concerns must thoroughly evaluate the child's current and past developmental status and utilize compilations of normative data including height, weight, skeletal age, and time of onset of individual pubertal events to determine the presence or absence of pathologic processes. For those children who deviate significantly from these established norms, a more thorough evaluation will be necessary. This can involve further radiologic as well as endocrinologic testing as described in Chapters 11 and 13.

REFERENCES

1. Sizonenko PC. Physiology of puberty. *J Endocrinol Invest* 1989;12[Suppl 3]:59–63.
2. Tanner JW, Davies PWS. Clinical longitudinal standards for height and height velocity for North American children. *J Pediatr* 1985;107:317.
3. Grumbach MM, Kaplan SL. Recent advances in the diagnosis and management of sexual precocity. *Acta Paediatr Jpn* 1988;30[Suppl]:155–175.
4. Largo RH, Prader A. Pubertal development in girls. *Pediatrician* 1987;14:212–218.
5. Dann TC, Roberts DF. Menarcheal age in University of Warwick young women. *Biosoc Sci* 1993;25:531–538.
6. Tanner JM. Trend toward earlier menarche in Long, Oslo, Copenhagen, the Netherlands and Hungary. *Nature* 1973;243:95.
7. Adelman JP, Mason AJ, Hayflick JS, et al. Isolation of the gene and hypothalamic cDNA for the common precursor of gonadotropic-releasing hormone and prolactin release-inhibiting factor in human and rat. *Proc Natl Acad Sci U S A* 1986;83:179–183.
8. Schwanjel-Fukuda M, Plaff DW, Crossin KL, et al. Migration of luteinizing hormone-releasing hormone neurons in early human embryos. *Soc Neurosci Abstr* 1994; 20:1491.
9. Mellon PL, Windle JJ, Goldsmith PC, et al. Immortalization of hypothalamic GnRH neurons by genetically targeted tumorogenesis. *Neuroendocrinology* 1990;5: 1–10.
10. Terasawa E. Mechanisms controlling the onset of puberty in primate: the role of GABAergic neurons. In: Plan TM, Lee PA, eds. *The neurobiology of puberty:* Society for Endocrinology, Almondbury, U.K. 1995:139–154.
11. Page DC. Sex reversal: deletion mapping the male-determining function of the human Y chromosome. *Cold Spring Harbor Symp Quant Biol* 1986;51:229.
12. Peters H. Migration of gonocytes in the mammalian gonad and their differentiation. *Phil Trans R Soc Lond B* 1970;259:91.
13. Baker TG. A quantitative and cytological study of germ cells in human ovaries. *Proc Roy Soc B* 1963;158:417.
14. Gluckman PD, Grumbach MM, Kaplan SL. The human

fetal hypothalamus and pituitary gland: the maturation of neuroendocrine mechanisms controlling the secretion of fetal pituitary growth hormone, prolactin, gonadotropin, and adrenocorticotropin-related peptides. In: Tulchinsky D, Ryan KJ, eds. *Maternal-fetal endocrinology.* Philadelphia: WB Saunders, 1980: 196–232.
15. Gulyas BJ, Hodgen GD, Tullner WW, et al. Effects of fetal or maternal hypophysectomy on endocrine organs and body weight in infant rhesus monkeys (*Macaca mulatta*): with particular emphasis on oogenesis. *Biol Reprod* 1977;16:216.
16. Kaplan SL, Grumbach MM. The ontogenesis of human foetal hormones. II. Luteinizing hormone (LH) and follicle stimulating hormone (FSH). *Acta Endocrinol* 1976;81:808–829.
17. Kaplan SL, Grumbach MM. Pituitary and placental gonadotropins in sex steroids in the human and subhuman primate fetus. *Clin in Endocrinol Metab* 1978;7:487–511.
18. Gorski RA, Gordon JH, Shryne JE, et al. Evidence for a morphological sex difference within the medial preoptic area of the rat brain. *Brain Res* 1978;148:333.
19. Winter JSD, Hughes IA, Reyes FI, et al. Pituitary-gonadal relations in infancy: 2. Patterns of serum gonadal steroid concentrations in man from birth to two years of age. *J Clin Endocrinol Metab* 1976;42:679.
20. Winter JSD, Faiman C. Pituitary-gonadal relations in female children and adolescents. *Pediatr Res* 1973;7:948.
21. Winter JSD, Faiman C, Hobson WC, et al. Pituitary-gonadal relations in infancy. I. Patterns of serum gonadotropin concentrations from birth to four years of age in man and chimpanzee. *J Clin Endocrinol Metab* 1975;40:545.
22. Plauchu H, Claustart B, Betend B, et al. Le test a l'hormone hypothalamique synthetique LHRH chez infant normal de la naissance a l'age adulte. *Pediatrie* 1980; 35:119–131.
23. Bidlingmaier F, Knorr D. Oestrogens: physiological and clinical aspects. *Pediatr Adolesc Endocrinol* 1978;4:43.
24. Tapanainen J, Koivisto M, Vihko R, et al. Enhanced activity of the pituitary-gonadal axis in premature human infants. *J Clin Endocrinol Metab* 1981;52:235–238.
25. Conte FA, Grumbach MM, Kaplan SS. A diphasic pattern in gonadotropin secretion in patients with the syndrome of gonadal dysgenesis. *J Clin Endocrinol Metab* 1974;40:670–675.
26. Ropelaton MG, Escobar ME, Gottlieb S, et al. Gonadotropin secretion in prepubertal normal and agonadal children evaluated by ultrasensitive time-resolved immunofluorometric assays. *Horm Res* 1997;48: 164–172.
27. Mitsushima D, Hei DL, Terasawa E. γ-Aminobutyric acid is an inhibitory neurotransmitter restricting release of luteinizing hormone-releasing hormone before the onset of puberty. *Proc Natl Acad Sci U S A* 1994;91: 395–399.
28. Mitsushima D, Marzban F, Luchansky LL, et al. Role of glutamic acid decarboxylase in the prepubertal inhibition of the luteinizing hormone releasing hormone release in female rhesus monkeys. *J Neurosci* 1996;16: 2563–2573.
29. Dickerman Z, Prager-Lewin R, Laron Z. Response of plasma LH and FSH to synthetic LH-RH in children at various pubertal stages. *Am J Dis Child* 1974;130:634.
30. Wildt L, Marshall G, Knobil E. Experimental induction

of puberty in the infantile rhesus monkey. *Science* 1980; 207:1373–1375.

31. Apter D, Butzow TL, Laughlin GA, et al. Gonadotropin-releasing hormone pulse generator activity during pubertal transition in girls: pulsatile and diurnal patterns of circulating gonadotropins. *J Clin Endocrinol Metab* 1993;76:940–949.

32. Boyar R, Finkelstein J, Roffwarg H, et al. Synchronization of augmented luteinizing hormone secretion with sleep during puberty. *N Engl J Med* 1972;287:582.

33. Boyar RM, Wu RHK, Roffwarg H, et al. Human puberty: 24-hour estradiol patterns in pubertal girls. *J Clin Endocrinol Metab* 1976;43:1418.

34. Kulin HE, Reiter EO. Gonadotropins during children and adolescence: a review. *Pediatrics* 1973;51:260.

35. Frisch RE, Revelle R. Height and weight at menarche and a hypothesis of critical body weights and adolescent events. *Science* 1970;169:397.

36. Frisch RE, Wyshak G, Vincent L. Delayed menarche and amenorrhea in ballet dancers. *N Engl J Med* 1980; 303:17.

37. Frisch RE, Gotz-Welbergen AV, McArthur JW, et al. Delayed menarche and amenorrhea of college athletes in relation to age of onset of training. *JAMA* 1981;246:1559.

38. Warren MP. The effects of exercise on pubertal progression and reproductive function in girls. *J Clin Endocrinol Metab* 1980;50:1150.

39. Boyar RM, Katz J, Finkelstein JW, et al. Anorexia nervosa. Immaturity of the 24-hour luteinizing hormone secretory pattern. *N Engl J Med* 1974;291:861–865.

40. Penny R, Goldstein IP, Frasier SD. Gonadotropin secretion and body composition. *Pediatrics* 1978;61:294.

41. Flier JS. What's in a name? In search of leptin's physiologic role. *J Clin Endocrinol Metab* 1998;83:1407–1413.

42. Schiebinger RK, Albertson FG, Cassorla FG, et al. The developmental changes in plasma adrenal androgens during infancy and adrenarche are associated with changing activities of adrenal microsomal 17-hydroxylase and 17,20 desmolase. *J Clin Invest* 1981;67:1177.

43. Hopper BR, Yen SSC. Circulating concentrations of dehydroepiandrosterone and dehydroepiandrosterone sulfate during puberty. *J Clin Endocrinol Metab* 1975;40:458.

44. Sizonenko PE, Paunier L. Hormonal changes in puberty. III. Correlation of plasma dehydroepiandrosterone, testosterone, FSH, and LH with stages of puberty and bone age in normal boys and girls and in patients with Addison's disease or hypogonadism or with premature or late adrenarche. *J Clin Endocrinol Metab* 1975;41:894.

45. Layman LC, Lee E, Peak DB, et al. Delayed puberty and hypogonadism caused by mutations in the follicle-stimulating hormone β-subunit gene. *N Engl J Med* 1997;337:607–610.

46. Peters H, Byskov A, Grinsted J. Follicular growth in fetal and prepubertal ovaries in humans and other primates. *Clin Endocrinol Metab* 1978;7:469.

47. Stanhope R, Adams J, Jacobs HS, et al. Ovarian ultrasound assessment in normal children, idiopathic precocious puberty, and during low dose pulsatile gonadotropin releasing hormone treatment of hypogonadotropic hypogonadism. *Arch Dis Child* 1985;60:116.

48. Ross GT. Gonadotropins and preantral follicular maturation in women. *Fertil Steril* 1974;25:522.

49. Apter D. Development of the hypothalamic-pituitary-ovarian axis. *Ann NY Acad Sci* 1997;816:9–22.

50. Knobil E. The neuroendocrine control of the menstrual cycle. *Recent Prog Horm Res* 1980;36:53.

51. Apter D, Vihko R. Premenarcheal endocrine changes in relation to age at menarche. *Clin Endocrinol* 1985;22:753–760.

52. Apter D, Vihko R. Early menarche, a risk factor for breast cancer, indicates early onset of ovulatory cycles. *J Clin Endocrinol Metab* 1983;57:82–86.

53. Marti-Henneberg C, Vizmanos B. The duration of puberty in girls related to the timing of its onset. *J Pediatr* 1997;131:618–621.

54. Vihko R, Apter D. Endocrine characteristics of adolescent menstrual cycles: impact of early menarche. *J Steroid Biochem* 1984;20:231–236.

55. Rosen JM, Paget P, Goodman H, et al. Mechanisms by which prolactin and glucocorticoids regulate casein gene expression. *Biochem Soc Symp* 1989;55:115–123.

56. Smith EP, Boyd J, Frank GR, et al. Estrogen resistance caused by a mutation in the estrogen-receptor gene in a man. *N Engl J Med* 1994;331:1056–1061.

57. Wierman ME, Beardsworth DE, Crawford JD, et al. Adrenarche and skeletal maturation during luteinizing hormone releasing hormone analogue suppression of gonadarche. *J Clin Invest* 1986;77:121–126.

58. Cara JF, Rosenfeld RL, Furlanetto RW. A longitudinal study of the relationship of plasma somatomedin-C concentration to the pubertal growth spurt. *Am J Dis Child* 1987;41:562–564.

59. Pescovity OH, Hench KD, Barnes KM, et al. Premature thelarche and central precocious puberty: the relationship between response of luteinizing hormone-releasing hormone. *J Clin Endocrinol Metab* 1988;67:474.

60. Rich BH, Rosenfield RL, Lucky AW, et al. Adrenarche: changing adrenal response to ACTH. *J Clin Endocrinol* 1981;52:1129.

61. Sorva R, Tolppanen E-M, Lankinen S, et al. Growth evaluation: parent and child specific height standards. *Arch Dis Child* 1989;64:1483–1487.

62. Marshall WA, Tanner JM. Variations in pattern of pubertal changes in girls. *Arch Dis Child* 1969;44:291.

63. Rosenfeld RL. The ovary and female sexual maturation. In: Kaplan SA, ed. *Clinical pediatric endocrinology*, 2nd ed. Philadelphia: WB Saunders, 1989:259–323.

64. Rosenfeld RL. Clinical review 6. Diagnosis and management of delayed puberty. *J Clin Endocrinol Metab* 1990;70:559–562.

65. Ehrmann DA, Rosenfield RL, Cuttler L, et al. A new test of combined pituitary-testicular function using the gonadotropin-releasing hormone agonist nafarelin in the differentiation of gonadotropin deficiency from delayed puberty: pilot studies. *J Clin Endocrinol Metab* 1989;69:963–967.

66. Porcu E, Venturoli S, Fabbri R, et al. Skeletal maturation and hormone levels after menarche. *Arch Gynecol Obstet* 1994;255:43–46.

67. Nottelmann ED, Susman EJ, Dorn LD, et al. Developmental processes in early adolescence. *J Adolesc Health Care* 1987;8:246–260.

4

Gynecologic Examination of the Adolescent

Sandra Ann Carson

Adolescence transforms a girl into a woman and often introduces the gynecologist. At this introduction, long-lasting impressions may be initiated that influence the patient's lifelong gynecologic health care habits. These patients must be approached in a kind, gentle, knowledgeable manner that assures a confidential doctor-patient relationship without alienation of their parents.

This chapter discusses specific problems that may present in the examination of the adolescent to the physician not used to dealing with this age group. Discussion is limited to problems and examination only as they differ from evaluation in the adult.

INTERVIEW

Manner

The discomfort and apprehensive feelings that a gynecologic consultation poses to most women are even more intense in teenagers. Adolescents' most frequent source of information regarding pelvic examination is their peers (1). Horror stories from adolescent peers are more likely believed by the patient than any realistic communications from adults. Therefore, the most important part of the gynecologic interview may be the time spent by the physician to dispel the patient's untoward expectations and gain her confidence.

Most visits by the adolescent to a gynecologist are prompted by a specific problem and are rarely a routine visit. Most of the time, the adolescent's anxiety stems from worry that a significant health problem will be discovered

(1). They also are afraid the examination will be painful, and many are embarrassed about undressing and personal hygiene (1).

Beginning the interview by an explanation of pelvic anatomy often is useful in putting the adolescent at ease. Most adolescents have a burning desire to learn the facts of life and facts about their body. The physician also is afforded an opportunity to demonstrate a knowledgeable and gentle manner. By directing the discussion to the adolescent, the parent (who usually is present during the interview) will be put into the background. Direct questioning of the adolescent herself may follow, encouraging her to provide useful information. The conversation can thus be comfortably geared to identify the adolescent as the patient without alienating the parent. In general, adolescents relish the opportunity to assume adult roles and in return become more cooperative and trusting.

Both the patient and her parent should be reassured that a gynecologic examination will not damage the patient's hymen and the examination will not change her virginity. A diagrammatic explanation of the pelvic examination will help the patient understand exactly what is to be done.

Parental Presence

The propriety of parental presence in the interview is a point of debate. Usually, the parent is necessary to complete the medical history for the patient; however, this may inhibit the patient from relating important facts unknown to her parents, such as sexual habits and previous venereal disease. Parental presence also impinges on developing a trusting doctor-patient relationship.

Perhaps the best compromise is to begin the interview with the parent present. Just before the examination, the parent may be dismissed, allowing the patient confidential time with her doctor. At this time, the patient can be assured that you will tell her parent only that which she allows you to tell, and it is for this reason that the parent will not be invited into the examination room. Some patients may protest, but most patients will cooperate better without a parent in the room.

Attire

A large proportion of physicians strongly believe that their attire affects the doctor-patient relationship but do not agree on the style, i.e., formal or casual, white coat or none (2). Studies document that college-age women expect their physicians to wear a white coat (3). Adolescents, however, seem less affected by their physician's dress (4), although most parents prefer the physician to wear a white coat and formal (e.g., coat and tie) rather than casual dress (1). Perhaps the best compromise is to begin with a white coat and remove it if the patient seems intimidated or uncomfortable.

MEDICAL HISTORY

Gynecologists are accustomed to interviewing adults who have a complete examination only by integration of a few consultants: internist, gynecologist, ophthalmologist. It is useful to remember that the adolescent may not have seen her pediatrician in years. The history should include all the essentials of a detailed medical history, as well as age of adrenarche, thelarche, and menarche. A thorough review of systems should be followed by interrogation of each positive symptom specifically as to frequency, relationship to menstrual cycle, and provocative events. The patient's performance in school is a tactful way to introduce questions on the patient's

temperament, social history, and boyfriends. Behavioral problems, school failure, or medical symptoms are often the presenting complaint in adolescent depression (5).

Adolescent patients have difficulty knowing what symptoms are important and require direct questioning in a specific manner. Open-ended questions allow the adolescent to express herself and become comfortable, but they are less beneficial in eliciting valuable information. Thus, more specific questions should be interspersed to obtain the necessary information.

Menstrual History

The patient's menstrual history, especially if precocious or delayed, may be explained by her mother's age of menarche. Similarly, maternal drug ingestion during a patient's gestation may be relevant to the patient's complaint.

Specific questions regarding the amount, length, and frequency of menstrual flow should be used to gain the history. Adolescents are very concerned about the regularity of their menses. The first year's menstrual cycles often have intervals as long as 6 months and continue to be irregular for the first 15 cycles (6). Such abnormalities occurred in 43% of more than 5,000 adolescents surveyed by Kantero and Widholm (7) and 68% of 1,533 adolescents surveyed by Batrinos et al. (8).

Patients who have experienced only a few menstrual periods may be unaware of what is normal, light, or heavy, and they may provide incorrect information to questions such as, "Are your menses light or heavy?" Questions regarding bleeding should identify amount by actions required to contain it. For example, is bleeding so heavy it requires both a pad and a tampon, or must the patient awaken at night to change? The number of pads or tampons used also may lead to an inaccurate assessment of menstrual pattern; some patients will change as soon as the pad is soiled, whereas others only when the pad is soaked. Heavy uterine bleeding or menses more frequent than every 21 days is abnormal. Although this often is attributed to anovulation, such bleeding has occurred with proliferative, secretory, or atrophic endometrium (9). Amenorrhea as well as abnormal uterine bleeding requires investigation in a manner discussed in Chapters 13 and 14.

Dysmenorrhea usually does not occur until after the patient begins to ovulate. Because over 80% of the first year's menses are anovulatory (10), dysmenorrhea does not usually occur in early cycles (11). Severe pain with menses requiring absence from school must be investigated. No matter what the actual pathogenesis, dysmenorrhea is "real" pain and should not be attributed to hysteria or emotional problems. Although young ladies with psychological problems may, of course, have dysmenorrhea, they do not have a higher incidence of dysmenorrhea than psychologically well-adjusted females (12). Historical inquiry about concomitant symptoms, such as diarrhea, nausea, vomiting, and irritability, suggests prostaglandin association. Gentle questions should be used to determine if the patient is trying to use dysmenorrhea as an excuse for school absence to avoid undesirable situations. During the history, the physician also may explain symptoms such as molimina and dysmenorrhea to reassure the patient experiencing them that nothing is seriously wrong.

The adolescent also may be asked if her mother experiences menstrual pain. Kantero and Widholm (7) noted dysmenorrhea in 30% of patients whose mothers had dysmenorrhea compared to only 7% of the daughters of mothers without pain. One interpretation suggests a family's perception of menstrual pain influences the patient's reaction to her menses. However, the results also may reflect a genetic predisposition to factors leading to dysmenorrhea: prostaglandin synthesis or receptors may be regulated by an autosomal dominant gene with variable expressivity. A detailed evaluation and treatment plan for dysmenorrhea is given in Chapter 15.

Urologic History

Particular attention should be given to the urologic history. Frequent urinary tract infec-

tions or previous urologic surgery may be related to a gynecologic problem. It may be difficult for some patients to distinguish between hematuria and intermenstrual spotting. Usually, all patients have difficulty distinguishing hematuria and menstrual blood in the urine.

Sexual and Contraceptive History

Parental presence during the sexual history almost always is prerequisite to incomplete information. Even the most open parental-offspring relationship limits physician access to important details of these intimate times.

The gynecologist is accustomed to hearing a variety of sexual techniques and preferences from adults without passing judgment. This should also be the rule for listening to the sexual habits of adolescents. During this time, the gynecologist has an opportunity to educate the adolescent about intercourse, venereal disease, and contraception in a way that does not frighten the patient away from sex but rather educates her. She also should be informed that females require more time for sexual arousal than males. If sex is to be pleasurable for her, she must demand her partner take the time for foreplay (13). This is also a good time to inform her that her young man undergoes no physical trauma by waiting and being considerate. A boy mature enough to have intercourse should be a man mature enough to understand the needs of his partner. Most adolescents are thankful for honest information provided in a sincere, nonjudgmental manner.

EXAMINATION

The adolescent gynecologic examination can be performed successfully only if enough time is allotted for the patient. Physicians desiring to provide care for adolescents should be willing to allot 1 full hour for the medical interview and examination of the adolescent.

Chaperone

Although, at first glance, it may seem reasonable that adolescents would feel more comfortable with a female chaperone than being alone with a male or female doctor, surveys of adolescents' preference do not attest to this. Of 100 adolescents surveyed, 60% of those 13 to 14 years old preferred being alone with a male physician known to them and 80% preferred being alone if the physician was female and known to them. Of those 15 to 17 years, 73% preferred to be alone with a male physician and 79% preferred to be without a chaperone if the physician was female. Of patients older than 19 years, 79% preferred no chaperone regardless of the physician's gender (14). Interestingly, of 292 male physicians surveyed, 37% did not routinely use a chaperone when examining an adolescent, citing patient preference as the most frequent necessity for examination with a chaperone present (15). Compelling reasons for using a chaperone included medicolegal issues, a seductive patient, and a history of rape or sexual abuse.

General Examination

The patient should be instructed to empty her bladder and then disrobe completely. A hospital gown will make the patient feel much more comfortable than a sheet alone. Her height, weight, arm span, and vital signs should be recorded. The blood pressure should be taken with a properly fitting cuff. Congenital abnormalities, hair distribution, and skin lesions may suggest systemic disease, as will lymphadenopathy, mucosal changes, or scleral icterus found during examination of the head and neck.

A heart and lung examination should be performed. Auscultation of the patient's abdomen before palpation will prevent falsely heightened bowel sounds. Abdominal contour and scars will uncover previous surgery, hernias, and masses. Palpation of the liver edge, spleen, and kidney should be attempted; and abdominal tenderness, rebound, or guarding should be noted. The presence of ascites should be ruled out.

Breast Examination

The breast examination should search for masses and elicit any nipple secretion present. Breast development should be staged according to the Tanner classification. However, the classification is a morphologic classification and may not always reflect the glandular and ductal development of the breast during adolescence, which itself reflects a myriad of hormones and growth factors acting in concert. In a patient with precocious or delayed puberty or a patient with abnormal breast development, ultrasound examination of the breast seems more reproducible and documentable. In addition, serial ultrasound examinations over time probably will prove a more reliable reflection of pubertal progression and therapeutic efficacy than Tanner staging (Fig. 4.1) (16). This is an opportune time to instruct the adolescent in

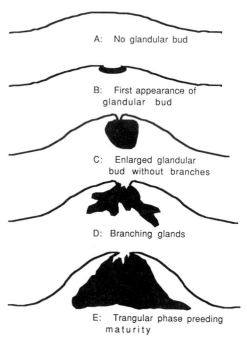

A: No glandular bud

B: First appearance of
     glandular   bud

C: Enlarged glandular
     bud without branches

D: Branching glands

E: Trangular phase preeding
     maturity

FIG. 4.1. Schematic diagram of the ultrasound stages of the breast. (Adapted from Bruni V, Dei M, Deligeoroglou E, et al. Breast development in adolescent girls. *Adolesc Pediatr Gynecol* 1990; 3:201.)

self-examination of her breasts. Although 93% of surveyed physicians thought this important, only 60% taught it (17).

Pelvic Examination

The best position for a pelvic examination in an adolescent patient depends on the comfort of the patient and maximal visualization for the physician. Although Huffman et al. (9) reported that the knee-chest position frightens children, this position may be necessary to obtain full view of the vagina as well as demonstrate abnormalities of the hymen. In a questionnaire survey, adolescents at their first pelvic examination seemed more comfortable when examined in a semisitting position (18). One method is to begin the examination in the position most comfortable to the patient and then change it as necessary for visualization once she is more relaxed.

The patient must be informed of what is to happen before each step. "This is not going to hurt" is just as unwise as "This is going to hurt." Explaining each step before gently performing it and allowing the patient to decide how painful it is or is not paves the way for patient trust and better cooperation.

Vulva

The external genitalia should be staged according to the Tanner classification. The clitoris should be measured with a small ruler. The clitoris should not be larger than the average adult clitoris: 5.4 × 4.4 mm (9).

Hymen

The hymen should be examined for patency as well as caruncles. The normal hymen will change as the patient changes position. In the knee-chest position, gravity causes the lower edge to roll outward. Examining the hymen in this position allows confirmation of hymenal abnormalities and may confirm suspected child abuse. In addition, labial traction will allow gaping of the hymen and sizing of the hymeneal opening (19). An infected urethral meatus, at the superior aspect of the hymen, often will elicit tenderness or thickness on palpation.

Vaginal Discharge

In early puberty, an adolescent may present with a thick, white, cloudy discharge that she or her parent may interpret as an infection. Usually, this is a physiologic leukorrhea resulting from the unopposed estrogen production that occurs before menarche and stimulates vaginal and cervical secretions. Microscopic examination reveals voluminous squamous cells without white blood cells or organisms. The patient should be reassured that no pathology is present and instructed in proper perineal hygiene. Indeed, improper perineal hygiene is the most common cause of adolescent vulvovaginitis resulting from *Escherichia coli* colonization (9). Daily bathing, cotton panties, dresses, and panty hose with cotton crotches will help keep the perineum dry and prevent local pruritis, itching, and odor. These instructions will be much more beneficial than attempting to change the patient's direction of tissue wiping after a bowel movement from "back to front" to "front to back." "Minipads" or "panty liners" may be recommended rather than talcum powder to maintain dryness during the day.

Although usually physiologic, all discharge should be examined for yeast, trichomonas, and bacterial vaginosis *(Gardnerella vaginalis)*. Vulvovaginal infection is treated with the same medicines in the adolescent as in the adult, except application is adjusted for the size of the vagina and inexperience of the patient (20).

Vagina and Cervix

Pelvic examination will rule out most congenital anomalies of the vagina. Visual examination of the vagina and cervix is best performed with a Huffman adolescent speculum (Fig. 4.2). The introitus of an ado-

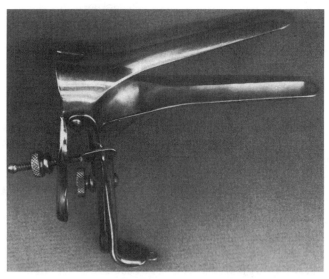

FIG. 4.2. The Huffman vaginal speculum is specially designed to fit the adolescent vagina. Its blades are 1.5 cm wide. (From Carson SA. Gynecologic problems of adolescence and puberty. In: Sciarra JJ, ed. *Gynecology and obstetrics, vol. 1.* Philadelphia: JB Lippincott, 1992:1–8, with permission.)

lescent who uses tampons or is having intercourse will easily admit the speculum. The speculum blades are 1.5 cm wide and 11 cm long. However, if the introitus is too narrow, a limited examination can be performed with a Peterson speculum or a pediatric vaginoscope (Fig. 4.3). Although the pediatric vaginoscope is useful for removal of a foreign body, it rarely allows enough visualization for an adequate cervical examination. In most cases, this instrument causes so much discomfort that the patient is less compliant for the succeeding bimanual examination; it usually is preferable to perform an examination under anesthesia in cases where cervical examination is mandated but the Huffman speculum is too large.

The speculum used should be *warm* and *lubricated.* If a cytologic smear is to be taken, then lubrication with warm water is substituted for jelly. The patient may be asked to perform a valsalva maneuver to relax the muscles of the pelvic diaphragm while inserting the speculum. The instrument should be inserted *slowly* with posterior pressure exerted on the perineal body to avoid the more tender urethra. Insertion should proceed with the blades close and pointed posteriorly toward the coccyx.

The cervix should be examined for lesions, infections, or congenital abnormalities. Although it is unlikely that anyone born after 1970 will have been exposed *in utero* to diethylstilbesterol (DES), vaginal adenosis and clear cell carcinoma do occur *de novo.* The knee-chest position will help position an eccentrically placed cervix into view.

An annual Pap smear is warranted in all sexually active adolescents. If adolescents have an easily identifiable cervix, a Pap smear may be obtained at the time of examination but, if normal, not repeated annually until she becomes sexually active.

Uterus

One lubricated finger usually can be inserted in the vagina for a bimanual examination. If the introitus is too small, the digital examination must be rectal. After entry, it is advisable to stop and allow the patient to re-

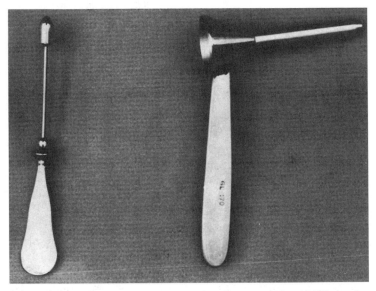

FIG. 4.3. A pediatric vaginoscope limits exposure and causes considerable discomfort, but it may be useful for removal of a foreign body. (From Carson SA. Gynecologic problems of adolescence and puberty. In: Sciarra JJ, ed. *Gynecology and obstetrics, vol. 1.* Philadelphia: JB Lippincott, 1992:1–8, with permission.)

gain composure and become accustomed to the finger in her vagina or rectum before proceeding with actual palpation. Ectopic gestation, endometriosis, and inflammation often will elicit cervical tenderness to palpation. The uterine fundus can be palpated and its position, size, shape, and consistency noted (Table 4.1). During adolescence, the uterine length enlarges from approximately 3 cm at 7 to 8 years to almost 7 cm at 15 to 16 years (21). This increase in length is accompanied by a change in proportion of a relatively larger uterine fundus compared to cervix (21). Normal tubes cannot be palpated.

Ovaries

Normal ovaries usually can be palpated in thin patients. An ultrasound survey of 75 peripubertal girls with no ovarian pathology revealed a symmetric increase in ovarian size during puberty that parallels the increase in uterine length. Most girls had multiple, bilateral, 3- to 10-mm ovarian cysts. Occasionally, a 3- to 5-cm follicular cyst was found and resolved without incident (Table 4.1) (21). Thus, enlarged ovaries in the presence of an infantile uterus or a unilateral ovarian enlargement that does not resolve is suspect of neoplasia.

TABLE 4.1. *Ovarian volume and uterine length increase during normal adolescence as viewed in 75 peripubertal girls undergoing ultrasonographic measurements*

Age	Mean uterine length (cm)	Corpus-to-cervix ratio	Mean ovarian volume (cm^2)
7–8 yr	3.28 ± 1.3	1.1:1	1.91 ± 0.7
15–18 yr	6.98 ± 1.0	1.3:1	3.52 ± 0.4
Commonly accepted adult values	8	3	12

From Winer-Muram HT, Emerson DE, Muram D, et al. The sonographic features of the peripubertal ovaries. *Adolesc Pediatr Gynecol* 1989;2:160, with permission.

Rectovaginal Examination

A rectovaginal examination with one finger in each orifice is too painful for the adolescent; thus, this examination should be avoided. A rectal examination alone will suffice.

INFORMATION AND THERAPY

Findings of the examination should be discussed with the patient immediately on completion of the examination. A brief description while the patient is still on the examining table may be followed by a more detailed discussion after she is dressed. It is a nice gesture to ask her permission to explain the findings to her parent and have the more detailed discussion along with therapeutic plans in a consultation room with both patient and parent present. Patients should be reassured repeatedly of normal findings.

At some point in the discussion, the adolescent should be informed that intercourse does not feel the same as a pelvic examination. The physician should stress that foreplay will increase vaginal compliance and lubrication allowing pleasurable lovemaking. This is, of course, a good time to inform the patient of her contraceptive choices.

Contraception

A teenager who consults a physician for contraception should be applauded, not given a lecture on being too young to have sex. Such lectures are not contraceptive and may result in teenage pregnancy. A physician willing to give contraception to a teenager only after she has demonstrated a previous pregnancy should not be taking care of adolescents. The adolescent who has decided to have intercourse will not change her mind if not given contraception. In fact, most of these young women have already had intercourse before seeking contraception (22).

Contraception does not increase adolescent promiscuity—it decreases adolescent pregnancy. Of course, it is difficult to make parents understand that withholding contracep-

tion will not decrease the sexual activity of their daughter or son. Nonetheless, sex education courses do reduce adolescent pregnancy rates (23). The laws governing prescription of contraceptives to minors vary from state to state, even though the U.S. Supreme Court ruled that minors have a constitutional right to nonprescription contraceptives (24). The physician should take the time to describe the risks and benefits of each contraceptive method available (see Chapter 22) and allow the patient a choice. When afforded the opportunity, adolescents make surprisingly wise decisions for themselves. The physician should offer guidance and stress the importance of follow-up visits.

Prescribing for Minors

Patients younger than 18 years of age are considered minors and require parental consent for surgery and treatment of nonvenereal disease. In all 50 states, physicians can treat minors for venereal disease without parental consent (25).

An emancipated minor is an individual younger than 18 years who is married, has parental consent, is self-supporting, is living apart from her parents, has parents who failed their legal responsibilities, or who has a judicial decree deeming her of the majority. These individuals can legally consent to medical or surgical therapy. However, a "legal" adult at any age may not be emotionally or physically mature. Thus, the medical approach to an emancipated minor should be with the identical cautious attitude and demeanor given to all adolescent patients. Prudent physicians are wise to consult their legal counsel regarding laws governing prescriptions for minors in their state.

Summary

Before dismissing the patient, it is wise to briefly summarize all findings and therapy plans. Asking the patient to repeat her understanding of the instructions may be the best way to confirm communication. In addition, giving the patient, and not her parent, a card with the physician's name and number along with instructions to call before prematurely stopping any medication or experiencing any side effect will identify the patient as the responsible person and codify the doctor-patient rather than doctor-parent relationship.

CONCLUSION

The care of the adolescent patient requires patience and time. Besides the initial visit, the adolescent also requires more vigilant attention to phone calls, as frequently she may be calling between classes or from a pay phone. Confidentiality may prevent return calls at a time more convenient for the physician.

REFERENCES

1. Millstein SG, Adler NE, Irwin CE Jr. Sources of anxiety about pelvic examinations among adolescent females. *J Adolesc Health Care* 1984;5:105.
2. Muram D, Gold JJ. Physician dress style and the examination of young children. *Adolesc Pediatr Gynecol* 1990;3:158.
3. Dunn JJ, Lee TH, Percelay JM, et al. Patient and house officer attitudes on physician attire and etiquette. *JAMA* 1987;257:65.
4. Neinstein LS, Stewart D, Gordon N. Effect of physician dress style on patient-physician relationship. *J Adolesc Health Care* 1985;6:456.
5. Rapp CE Jr. The adolescent patient. *Ann Intern Med* 1983;99:52.
6. Dewhurst CJ, Cowell CA, Barrie LC. The regularity of early menstrual cycles. *J Obstet Gynaecol Br Common* 1971;78:1093.
7. Kantero R, Widholm O. Correlation of menstrual traits between adolescent girls and their mothers. *Acta Obstet Gynecol Scand Suppl* 1971;14:30.
8. Batrinos ML, Panitsa-Faflia C, Courcoutsakis N, et al. Incidence, type and etiology of menstrual disorders in the age group 12–19 years. *Adolesc Pediatr Gynecol* 1990;3:149.
9. Huffman JW, Dewhurst CJ, Capraro VJ. *The gynecology of childhood and adolescence,* 2nd ed. Philadelphia: WB Saunders, 1981:85–87.
10. Apter D, Vihko R. Hormonal patterns of the first menstrual cycles. In: Flamigni C, Venturoli S, Givens JR, eds. *Adolescence in females.* Chicago: Year Book Medical Publishers, 1985;182.
11. Wilson L, Kurzrok R. Studies on the motility of the human uterus in vivo. A functional myometrial cycle. *Endocrinology* 1983;23:79.
12. Bichers W. Dysmenorrhea and menstrual disability. *Clin Obstet Gynecol* 1960;3:233.
13. Masters WH, Johnson VE. *Human sexual response.* Boston: Little Brown, 1966.
14. Buchta RM. Adolescent females' preferences regarding use of a chaperone during a pelvic examination. Observations from a private-practice setting. *J Adolesc Health Care* 1986;7:409.
15. Buchta RM. Use of chaperones during pelvic examinations of female adolescents. Results of a survey. *Am J Dis Child* 1987;141:666.
16. Bruni V, Dei M, Deligeoroglou E, et al. Breast development in adolescent girls. *Adolesc Pediatr Gynecol* 1990; 3:201.
17. Nussbaum MP, Shenker IR, Feldman JG. Attitudes versus performance in providing gynecologic care to adolescents by pediatricians. *J Adolesc Health Care* 1989;10:203.
18. Seymore C, DuRant RH, Jay MS, et al. Influence of position during examination, and sex of examiner on patient anxiety during pelvic examination. *J Pediatr* 1986; 108:312.
19. Bays J, Chewning M, Keltner L, et al. Changes in hymenal anatomy during examination of prepubertal girls for possible sexual abuse. *Adolesc Pediatr Gynecol* 1990;3:42.
20. Carson SA. Gynecologic problems of adolescence and puberty. In: Sciarra JJ, ed. *Gynecology and obstetrics, vol. 1.* Philadelphia: JB Lippincott, 1992:1–8.
21. Winer-Muram HT, Emerson DE, Muram D, et al. The sonographic features of the peripubertal ovaries. *Adolesc Pediatr Gynecol* 1989;2:160.
22. Kanter JF, Zelnik M. Contraception and pregnancy: experience of young unmarried women in the United States. *Fam Plan Perspect* 1973;5:21.
23. Mecklenburg F. Pregnancy: an adolescent crisis. *Minn Med* 1973;56:101.
24. 431. US678, 1977 (United States Supreme Court Decision).
25. Annas GJ, Glantz LH, Katz BF. *Informed consent to human experimentation: the subject's dilemma.* Cambridge: Ballinger Publisher Company, 1977.

5

Congenital Defects of the External Genitalia in the Newborn and Prepubertal Child

Claude J. Migeon and Gary D. Berkovitz

In this section, we discuss mainly the problem of ambiguous genitalia observed at delivery, as this is usually the time at which the problem becomes apparent.

At every birth, two major events take place: the first cry of the baby at the perception of the harshness of the outside world, and the first glance by the world at the external genitalia of the baby. The first cry is, of course, vitally important. But the first glance at the baby also is significant, as it establishes the sex of the individual for a lifetime. In the vast majority of cases, that casual glance is adequate in establishing sex. However, we strongly advise careful palpation of the scrotum to confirm the presence of testes before declaring the maleness of an infant.

The presence of ambiguous genitalia is always troubling to those witnessing the abnormality. At that point, it is of great importance to consult the pediatric endocrinologist, helped by the gynecologist, urologist, and psychologist experienced in problems of sex differentiation. In particular, the problem must be considered as an urgency. The first step to be taken is to explain to the parents that it is not possible to establish the sex of the infant by simple examination. Even the presence of palpable gonads does not necessarily indicate that one is dealing with testes (they can be ovotestes) or that they have a normal function. Furthermore, the parents must be told that various examinations will be needed before a decision can be made, that the labo-

ratory tests may take a few days, and that the rest of the family and friends are to be told that the baby has an abnormality in the formation of the sex organs and that it will take 1 to 2 weeks for doctors to determine the sex of the baby.

Ideally, the infant should be kept in the hospital until a decision is made about the sex of rearing. The mother, after her discharge, should be encouraged to stay with the baby to establish the appropriate bonding as well as breastfeeding and general care. Unfortunately, it is not always possible to do so.

The role of the pediatric endocrinologist will be important, not only in determining the etiology of the ambiguous genitalia but also in helping the parents to make a decision for the sex of rearing. The guiding of the family will include support and reassurance but also teaching about sexual differentiation. This will permit the physician to identify later the specific step responsible for the abnormality.

In the early stages of discussion with parents, physicians should keep an open mind about the sex of rearing of the infant. At that time, it is preferable to use neutral terms such as the baby (rather than girl or boy), the gonads (rather than testes or ovaries), and phallus (rather than penis or clitoris).

After the decision about gender has been made, then it is appropriate to emphasize the elected choice and to give a first name that is unambiguously male or female.

PHYSIOLOGY OF SEXUAL DIFFERENTIATION

The first step in sex differentiation is the determination of genetic sex (XX or XY) at the time of conception. Nonetheless, the external genitalia of the male and female fetus appear to be identical at 6 weeks of gestation. This neutral genitalia includes the genital tubercle, the labioscrotal folds, the urethral folds, and a urogenital sinus. Simultaneously, a variety of bipotential structures develop (1). The first among these are the gonads, which become apparent as a genital ridge at about 5 weeks. These structures are populated by germ cells, which migrate from the wall of the yolk sac. The fate of these germ cells (whether they develop as oocytes or spermatozoa) will be under the control of the ovary or testis that subsequently will develop from the bipotential gonad. Two sets of ducts appear at about the sixth week of fetal life: the male, wolffian ducts, and the female, müllerian ducts. These structures will give rise later to the internal accessory sex organs.

Gonadal Differentiation

The primary event in specific male sex determination is the commitment of the bipotential gonad to testicular development at about the sixth week of gestation (1). The trigger for this process is a Y chromosomal gene, termed the "testis-determining factor" (TDF). A gene termed the "sex-determining region of the Y chromosome" (SRY) was isolated from the distal segment of the short arm of the Y chromosome near the pseudoautosomal boundary and is indeed the testis-determining gene (2–6). However, other genes also appear to be necessary for testicular determination. Several genes play a role in the formation of the bipotential gonadal ridge and in differentiation of the gonads after sex determination. One example is the Wilms' tumor suppressor gene (WT1), which is involved in the formation of both the gonadal ridge and the testis. This gene also is necessary for kidney development (7). The steroidogenic factor (SF-1) gene appears to play a role in formation of the gonadal ridge as well as in Sertoli cell differentiation after the expression of SRY (8,9). By contrast, a gene termed LIM1 appears to be necessary for differentiation of the gonadal ridge before testis determination (10).

Some information is available regarding genes that play a specific role in testis or ovarian determination. The gene termed SOX9 is involved in testis differentiation and in the expression of a gene(s) necessary of chondrogenesis (11). Although little is known about the genetic mechanisms regulating ovarian determination, a gene termed DAX-1 appears to have a role as an antagonist of the SRY gene or as a direct inducer of ovarian differentiation (12). The first histologic sign of testicular determination is the appearance of Sertoli cells, which then proliferate and aggregate about germs cells to form testicular tubules (13,14). Three weeks after the appearance of Sertoli cells, Leydig cells also appear within the developing testis (1).

In the absence of TDF, the bipotential gonad undergoes ovarian determination (15). The primordial cells, which gave rise to Sertoli cells in the testis, differentiate as granulosa cells in the developing ovary and surround germ cells to form primordial follicles.

Differentiation of Accessory Sex Organs

Differentiation of accessory sex organs (wolffian ducts or müllerian ducts) occurs between 8 and 11 weeks of gestation. In the developing testis, Sertoli cells produce müllerian-inhibiting substance (MIS), which promotes the regression of female internal ducts (16). At about the same time, fetal Leydig cells begin to produce testosterone under the stimulus of maternal human chorionic gonadotropin (hCG). Biosynthesis of testosterone from cholesterol involves the action of four enzymes (17), including side chain cleavage, 3β-hydroxysteroid dehydrogenase, 17α-hydroxylase/17,20-desmolase, and 17-ketoreductase (Fig. 5.1). In the presence of high local concentrations of testos-

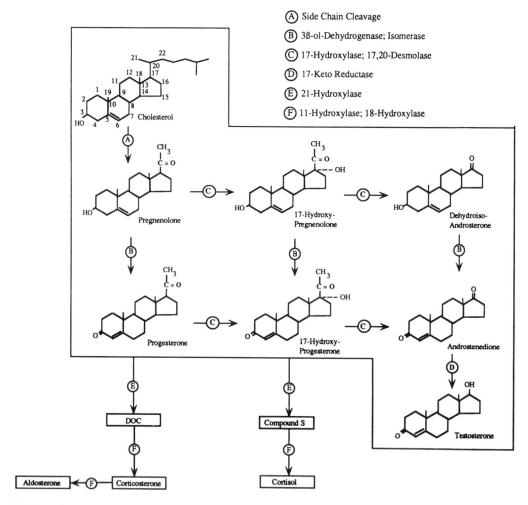

FIG. 5.1. Pathway for the biosynthesis of testosterone from cholesterol. Also shown is the pathway for the biosynthesis of glucocorticoids (cortisol, corticosterone) and mineralocorticoids (aldosterone, 11-deoxycorticosterone).

terone, wolffian ducts proliferate, giving rise to the epididymis, vas deferens, and seminal vesicles (16).

MIS also is produced in the female fetus, probably by the granulosa/theca cells, but it is not secreted until a later stage of development (18). The delay in MIS production beyond a critical commitment period permits the proliferation of müllerian ducts and the formation of the fallopian tubes, uterus, and the upper two thirds of the vagina. In the absence of fe-

tal testosterone, wolffian ducts in the female fetus regress (16).

Differentiation of External Genitalia

Masculinization of the external genitalia in the male fetus begins at around 8 weeks of gestation. This process begins with the lengthening of the anogenital distance. It results in fusion of the labioscrotal folds to form the scrotum, growth of the genital tubercle to form the penis, fusion of urethral folds to form the urethra, and regression of the utriculovaginal pouch to form the prostatic utricle (1).

Development of male external genitalia requires the conversion of testosterone to the more biologically active metabolite dihydrotestosterone (19) by the 5α-reductase pathway. Dihydrotestosterone then must bind to specific protein receptors within target tissues to permit the expression of its androgenic effects (20). These androgen receptors are part of a family of steroid hormone receptors. They consist of three major structural and functional domains: a transcriptional activation domain, a DNA-binding domain, and a ligand-binding domain (Fig. 5.2) (21). The amount of androgen receptor protein is the same in the target tissue of men and women, with the difference in androgenic effects regulated principally by the amount of androgen available to the cells (22). The gene encoding the human androgen receptor has been mapped to the long arm of the X chromosome near the centromere (Xq12) (23). Subsequently, the complete human androgen receptor cDNA has been isolated, thus facilitating a variety of studies of androgen receptors in health and disease (24,25).

Recent studies have indicated a role for coactivators of androgen receptors (26,27) and have suggested that other steroid hormone receptors may interact in the control of androgen-responsive genes (28).

In the absence of androgenic effects, the external genitalia develop along female lines. The labioscrotal folds become the labia majora, the urethral folds become the labia minora, the genital tubercle becomes the clitoris, and the urogenital sinus differentiates to form a separate urethral and vaginal opening (1).

WORKUP OF NEWBORNS WITH AMBIGUOUS EXTERNAL GENITALIA

As already stated, it is an emergency to determine the etiology of the ambiguous genitalia because it will help in the decision making as far as the sex of rearing is concerned. It also can be a medical emergency as, in some cases, the mutation responsible for the abnormal genitalia results in life-threatening symptoms. Following is an example of a schedule for tests that need to be ordered: day 1, karyotype (fluorescent Y chromosome); day 2, plasma testosterone, dihydrotestosterone, and androstenedione; day 3, plasma progesterone, 17-hydroxyprogesterone, 17-hydroxypregnenolone, and androstenedione; day 4, sonogram (gonads-uterus), genitogram with or without intravenous pyelogram; and day 6, repeat plasma 17-hydroxyprogesterone and androstenedione.

At least once a day, it is necessary to check the levels of serum electrolytes and blood glucose (dextro-stick). The infant also must be weighed carefully every day.

The results of these tests will help in determining the etiology of the ambiguous genitalia. The importance of the karyotype is self-evident. Although the search for a fluorescent Y chromosome is of interest, it is important to remember that the locus of the fluorescence is on the long arm of that chromosome, whereas the gene that initiates testicular formation (SRY) is located on the short arm. A buccal smear is not sufficient as a technique for de-

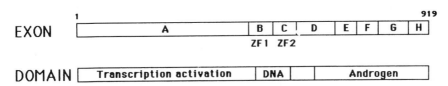

FIG. 5.2. Structural and functional domains of the human androgen receptor gene. This gene has been mapped to the long arm of the X chromosome (Xq12).

termining the sex chromosome complement and should not be used.

The study of androgens (androstenedione, testosterone, and dihydrotestosterone) must be done on a single blood sample to permit determination of the ratios of androstenedione to testosterone and of testosterone to dihydrotestosterone. Abnormally elevated ratios would be evidence of a deficiency in 17-ketosteroid reductase and 5α-steroid reductase, respectively. This investigation is timed for day 2 of life, because testicular androgen levels tend to decrease on days 3 to 8, before returning later to values of 150 to 250 ng/dL for testosterone (29).

The concentrations of 17-hydroxyprogesterone and progesterone normally are elevated in cord blood and shortly after birth (30). However, by day 3 of life they have reached levels that make possible the differentiation of normal values from those observed in patients with congenital adrenal hyperplasia due to 21-hydroxylase deficiency (31). This pattern also applies to the levels of androstenedione. On occasion, it is appropriate to repeat the assays of various steroids if the original results are not conclusive.

Sonogram and genitogram permit determination of the nature and localization of the internal ducts and their relationship to the urethra. In a markedly masculinized female, the vagina may open in the urethra via a narrow canal. In undermasculinized males, a utricular-vaginal pouch can be observed, opening in the urethra but ending blindly, without cervix or uterus.

Deficiency of some of the enzymes necessary for the biosynthesis of cortisol and aldosterone (21-hydroxylase, 3β-hydroxysteroid dehydrogenase isomerase, side chain cleavage) (Fig. 5.1) results in abnormalities of the external genitalia. In such cases, an acute adrenal crisis with hyponatremic, hyperkalemic acidosis, and hypoglycemia can develop, usually between days 2 and 6 of life. Hence, adequate monitoring of serum electrolytes and glucose are of great importance. Dehydration and marked weight loss also are symptoms of the adrenal crisis. A lack of adequate therapy may have catastrophic results (31).

WORKUP OF PREPUBERTAL CHILDREN WITH AMBIGUOUS GENITALIA

The workup of ambiguous external genitalia described in the previous section was devised for newborn infants. It is extremely important to establish early in life the etiology of the ambiguous genitalia and the preferred sex of rearing. Experience has shown that it is hazardous to make a change in sex after 1 or 2 years of age. The optimal time is in the first month of life.

On occasion, one is obliged to deal with a prepubertal child. Although the workup of the prepubertal child with abnormal external genitalia is directed to ask the same questions as those raised in infancy, the gonadal physiology has changed in certain aspects. In particular, Leydig cell function that was quite active during the first 3 months of life remains quiescent throughout childhood until puberty. To determine the potential of the gonads for androgen secretion, it is necessary to stimulate the Leydig cells by intramuscular administration of gonadotropins, usually hCG. The daily dose of hCG is adjusted for body size (3,000 IU per M^2 of body surface area). One injection is given every day for 5 consecutive days. A blood sample is obtained before the injections and on the morning of the sixth day (32).

Interpretation of the values of the various androgens is similar whether after hCG stimulation in childhood or without exogenous stimulation in infancy. An hCG stimulation test also can be helpful in the rare infants with ambiguous genitalia and suspected hypopituitarism.

In some children, the adequacy of penile response to androgen stimulation may be questioned. On such occasions, the hCG stimulation is prolonged to 6 weeks, giving two or three injections weekly. This sustained stimulation results normally in increased penile size. This diagnostic test also is used for therapeutic purposes in male children with small phallus.

DETERMINATION OF ETIOLOGY OF AMBIGUOUS GENITALIA

· The first step in determining the etiology is the karyotype (Fig. 5.3). If it is 46,XY, one is dealing with an undermasculinized infant with a "male" karyotype. If testicular determination is normal, the condition is termed male pseudohermaphroditism, but if gonadal differentiation is abnormal, then it is a partial gonadal dysgenesis. On occasion, the abnormal gonadal differentiation can lead to true hermaphroditism, defined as the presence of well-characterized ovarian and testicular elements in the same individual. Often, the two tissues are combined to form an ovotestis.

If the karyotype is 46,XX and if the ovaries developed normally, the subject is a masculinized infant with a "female" karyotype and the condition is called female pseudohermaphro-

ditism. A few subjects with XX sex chromosome complement will be true hermaphrodites.

Finally, in rare instances, an abnormality of sex chromosomes is found. This situation will be discussed separately, even though some cases may have an etiology similar to that of certain of the conditions mentioned earlier.

For etiologic classification, determination of the karyotype permits the distinction of three groups of patients: 46,XY infants with ambiguous external genitalia, 46,XX infants with ambiguous genitalia, and infants with abnormal karyotype.

46,XY Infants with Ambiguous External Genitalia

Results of the study of the concentration of androgens will permit another practical and important consideration, namely to distinguish whether the function of the Leydig cells is normal or diminished; in other words, whether testosterone levels are normal or abnormally low (Fig. 5.4).

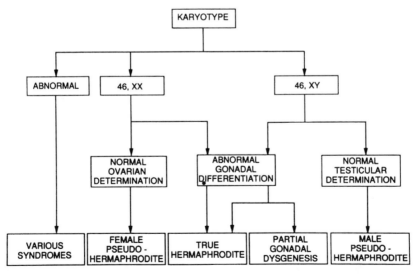

FIG. 5.3. Scheme for the determination of the pathology related to ambiguous genitalia based on the karyotype. In 46,XY infants with normal testicular formation, the condition is termed male pseudohermaphroditism. In 46,XX infants with normal ovarian formation, the condition is termed female pseudohermaphroditism. In 46,XX or 46,XY infants with abnormal gonadal differentiation, the condition may be true hermaphroditism or partial gonadal dysgenesis.

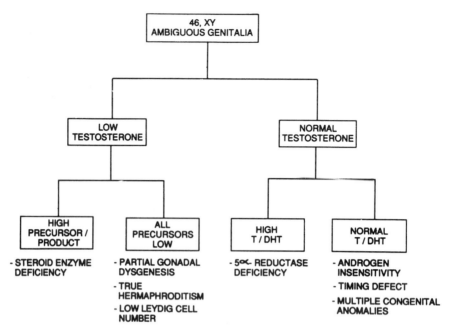

FIG. 5.4. Scheme for the determination of the pathophysiology related to ambiguous genitalia in 46,XY infants.

If testosterone is normal, a high testosterone-to-dihydrotesterone ratio (greater than 12:1 in the newborn period) will be indicative of 5α-reductase deficiency (33). This syndrome is characterized by poor masculinization of the external genitalia but normal development of the epididymis, vas deferens, and seminal vesicles (Table 5.1). This has permitted the conclusion that 5α-reduction of testosterone to dihydrotestosterone is necessary for masculinization of the external genitalia but not for proliferation of wolffian structures. Individuals with 5α-reductase deficiency who are raised as males may have normal sperm production in adult life. There is virilization at puberty with improvement in phallic length, increased muscle mass, and deepening of the voice. However, there usually is poor development of facial and body hair, and little or no hairline recession (34,35).

A normal testosterone-to-dihydrotestosterone ratio will be characteristic of androgen insensitivity, a syndrome related to abnormal androgen receptor activity resulting in an inability to express androgen effects (33). In the complete form of androgen insensitivity, patients have normal female external genitalia but lack müllerian as well as wolffian structures (Fig. 5.5). Often, diagnosis is delayed until later in childhood when subjects present with bilateral inguinal hernia, or at puberty when they present with primary amenorrhea despite normal breast development. Partial androgen insensitivity is characterized at birth by ambiguous genitalia and at puberty by poor development of secondary sexual characteristics, particularly with lack of growth of the phallus (Fig. 5.6). The diagnosis of androgen insensitivity is made by the detection of a mutation in the androgen receptor gene and if the mutation transferred in an expression vector shows decreased androgen receptor activity (36). Hence, the recent isolation of the androgen receptor gene makes it possible to evaluate defects at the molecular level (24,25).

In the "timing-defect" syndrome, androgen secretion and expression of androgen effects are normal, but they started too late in embryonic life to permit complete masculinization

TABLE 5.1. *Effects of various steroid enzyme deficiencies on the development of the external genitalia*

Enzyme deficiency	Genitalia in		Other symptoms	Congenital adrenal hyperplasia
	Males	Females		
SCC/STAR				
Partial	Ambiguous	Female	—	+
Complete	Female	Female	Salt loss	+
3βol				
Partial	Ambiguous	Ambiguous	—	+
Complete	Female	Female	Salt loss	+
17-OH				
Partial	Ambiguous	Female	Hypertension	+
Complete	Female	Female	Hypertension	+
11-Hydroxylase	Male	Ambiguous	Hypertension	+
21-OH				
Partial	Male	Ambiguous	—	+
Complete	Male	Ambiguous	Salt loss	+
17-Keto-reductase	Ambiguous	Female	—	0
5α-Reductase	Ambiguous	Female	—	0

SCC/STAR; side chain cleavage and steroid acute regulatory protein; 3β-ol, 3β-hydroxyteroid dehydrogenase; 17-OH, 17 hydroxylase; 21-OH, 21 hydroxylase.

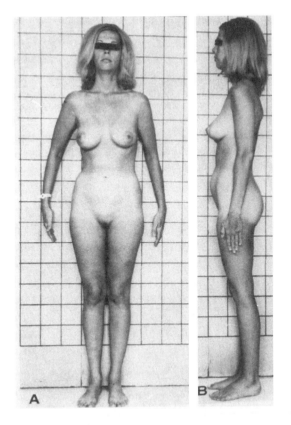

FIG. 5.5. Complete form of androgen insensitivity syndrome in a 46,XY adult subject. A mutation of the androgen receptor gene (deletion or point mutation) results in an inability to express androgen effects.

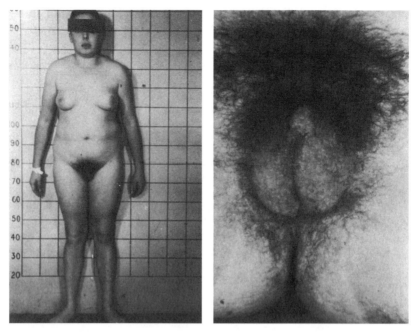

FIG. 5.6. Partial form of androgen insensitivity syndrome in a 46,XY young adult raised as a male. The mutation of the androgen receptor gene results in a partial inability to express androgen effects.

of the external genitalia (37,38). Patients with the timing defect cannot be distinguished from those with partial androgen insensitivity on the basis of hormone profile alone. Furthermore, androgen receptor-binding studies in cultured cells may be equivocal. Because patients with the timing defect develop normally at puberty whereas those with partial androgen insensitivity develop less well, it is important to differentiate between the two at the time of gender assignment. It now is possible to use molecular techniques for the study of androgen receptors, which permit detection of mutations of the receptor gene in the newborn period (39,40).

A normal testosterone-to-dihydrotestosterone ratio can be observed in infants with congenital malformations involving the genitourinary/gastrointestinal tracts. For example, a male infant with imperforate anus also can have an unusual external genitalia. This also can be seen in prune-belly syndrome (absence of abdominal wall) and in exstrophy of the bladder.

When testosterone concentrations are low, an increase in one of its precursors suggests an enzyme deficiency at the level of the abnormal precursor-to-product ratio. For example, an increase in androstenedione-to-testosterone ratio is indicative of a 17-ketosteroid reductase abnormality (41). The other enzymes (Table 5.1) involved in the formation of testosterone from cholesterol include steroid acute regulatory protein, side chain cleavage enzyme (20-hydroxylase/22-hydroxylase/20,22-desmolase), 3β-hydroxysteroid dehydrogenase, and 17-hydroxylase/17,20-desmolase. A deficiency of either the side chain cleavage enzyme (42) or 3β-hydroxysteroid dehydrogenase (43) is rare but results in a salt-losing form of congenital adrenal hyperplasia. These two conditions often are lethal in infancy. However, mild deficiencies without salt loss have been reported in children. By contrast, 17-hydroxylase deficiency results in an hypertensive form of congenital adrenal hyperplasia. It is associated with an absence of androgen secretion in the complete form, resulting in female-appearing genitalia in the affected infants. In the partial form, the genitalia are ambiguous (31).

If the levels of testosterone and its precursors are all low, then the problem might be related to 46,XY gonadal dysgenesis involving both tubules and Leydig cells. In the complete form of the disorder (pure gonadal dysgenesis), subjects develop bilateral streak gonads, normal müllerian structures, and female external genitalia. Such subjects usually are diagnosed at 12 to 15 years of age when they present with hypergonadotrophic hypogonadism (44). The 46,XY partial gonadal dysgenesis is characterized by incomplete testicular differentiation. The gonads consist of poorly formed testicular tubules mixed with ovarian stroma. The external genitalia are ambiguous, and there is frequently a mix of müllerian and wolffian structures. The degree of Leydig cell function determines the extent of the masculinization of the external genitalia (44,45). Early diagnosis of 46,XY partial gonadal dysgenesis is important, because patients with this disorder are at increased risk for developing gonadal malignancy (46). The syndrome of 46XY true hermaphroditism might be considered a form of gonadal dysgenesis. Finally, in rare cases of diminished testosterone production, the tubules appear to have normal Sertoli cells and germ cells, but the number of Leydig cells is decreased. This sometimes is referred to as Leydig cell hypoplasia.

46,XX Infants with Ambiguous External Genitalia

In female pseudohermaphroditism, the source of excessive androgen can be either the fetus or the mother (Table 5.2). Excessive production of fetal androgens is related to congenital adrenal hyperplasia (Table 5.1). Although there are several forms of this disorder, they all have a common etiology: a deficiency of one of the enzymes needed for the formation of cortisol from cholesterol (Fig. 5.1). In turn, the decreased cortisol secretion results in a compensatory increase in corticotropin-releasing hormone/adrenocorticotropic hormone output, which produces adrenal hyperplasia and hypersecretion of

TABLE 5.2. *Classification of female pseudohermaphroditism*

Excess fetal androgen
  21-Hydroxylase deficiency
    Partial (simple virilizing form)
    More complete (salt-losing form)
  11-Hydroxylase deficiency (hypertensive form)
  3β-Hydroxysteroid dehydrogenase deficiency
Excess maternal androgen
  Iatrogenic
  Virilizing tumor of ovary or adrenal
Congenital abnormalities
  Structural or teratogenic factors

adrenal androgens (except in side chain cleavage enzyme deficiency).

The most frequent form is 21-hydroxylase deficiency. The overproduced C_{19}-steroid is androstenedione, an androgen with little or no biologic activity. However, 10% of it is metabolized to testosterone, which will masculinize the female fetus (Fig. 5.7). Two of the cortisol precursors that also are hypersecreted are 17-hydroxyprogesterone and progesterone. They produce a salt-losing tendency that is compensated by an increased aldosterone secretion in the partial form of 21-hydroxylase deficiency (simple virilizing form). In the more complete form, aldosterone secretion cannot be increased, resulting in a salt-losing crisis (salt-losing form) with low Na, Cl, and CO_2, and elevated K (31).

In the 11-hydroxylase deficiency (hypertensive form), the mechanism responsible for masculinization of the female fetus is similar to that of 21-hydroxylase deficiency. However, the hypersecreted precursors of cortisol are different. They are 11-deoxycortisol that has low glucocorticoid activity and 11-deoxycorticosterone that produces hypertension (31).

Deficiency in 3β-hydroxysteroid dehydrogenase/isomerase (31,43) is extremely rare, and so is that of cytochrome P450 side chain cleavage enzyme (31,42), which permits 20-hydroxylation, 22-hydroxylation, and 20,22 desmolase. The complete deficiency of both of these enzymes results in a total lack of biologically active adrenal steroids. In such cases, there is salt loss and a lack of androgen biosyn-

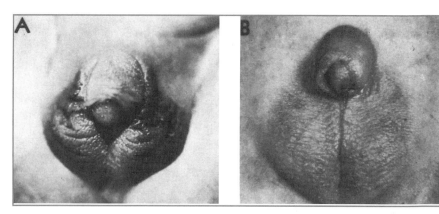

FIG. 5.7. Masculinization of the external genitalia of two 46,XX infants with congenital adrenal hyperplasia caused by 21-hydroxylase deficiency (salt-losing form). **A:** Typical abnormality including enlargement of the clitoris and scrotalization of the labia and urogenital sinus. **B:** Marked masculinization resulting in penile urethra.

thesis. Hence, female fetuses are not virilized and male fetuses present a female genitalia. When the deficiency of 3β-hydroxysteroid dehydrogenase is only partial, some androgens are secreted, and there is a mild degree of masculinization in female fetuses and an almost complete feminization in male fetuses.

A deficiency of 17-hydroxylase, also rare, leads to feminization of the male fetus with no masculinization of female fetuses, if the deficiency is complete (31,47,48). In partial forms, both males and females present ambiguous genitalia.

On rare occasions, the source of androgens is the testicular component of the gonads of a subject with 46,XX true hermaphroditism.

Excessive androgens arising in the mother can cross the placenta and masculinize the external genitalia of a female fetus. The source of abnormal amounts of maternal androgens can be related to a virilizing tumor of the ovary (hilar cell tumor, adrenal-rest tumor, Krukenberg's tumor) or adrenal gland (49). Such tumors usually arise after fecundation as excess androgens prevent ovulation and therefore pregnancy. Some of the synthetic progestins have a mild androgenic activity. Given in large amounts shortly after the start of pregnancy (as done sometimes in habitual abortion), they can masculinize the female fetus (50).

Congenital abnormalities can, on occasion, mimic abnormalities of the external female genitalia. For example, moles or hemangioma located on the hood of the clitoris may suggest an hypertrophic phallus.

Abnormal Karyotype

As shown in Table 5.3, abnormal sex chromosome complements can result in various syndromes, some of them with unquestionably male or female external genitalia, others with ambiguous genitalia.

In cases of triploidy (69 chromosomes), the XXY sex chromosome complement results in

TABLE 5.3. *Various syndromes with abnormal sex chromosome complement*

Ambiguous genitalia
  X/XY
  XX/XY
  XX/XXY
  Triploidy 69,XXY
  Rare syndromes: Opitz, Opitz-Frias
Male genitalia
  47,XXY and variants (Klinefelter's syndrome)
  47,XYY and variants (XYY syndrome)
  46,XX males
Female genitalia
  45,X and variants (Turner's syndrome)
  47,XXX and variants (super female syndrome)
  Pure gonadal dysgenesis (SRY gene deletion or
    mutation): 46,XY females; 46,X,i(Yq); 46,X,Yp-

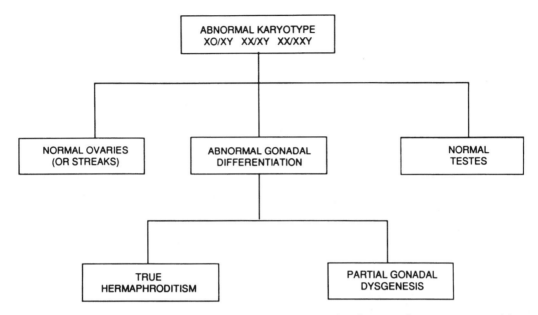

FIG. 5.8. Gonadal differentiation in subjects with karyotype showing sex chromosome mosaicism and including a Y chromosome.

ambiguous genitalia in about 50% of subjects (51). However, triploidy is quite lethal. Most triploidy cases are detected in abortuses; if pregnancy is carried to term, the baby dies early in infancy.

Rare syndromes like those described by Opitz often are accompanied by various degrees of hypospadias (51). A few individuals with 47,XXY and 47,XYY also may present ambiguous genitalia (51).

In sex chromosome mosaicisms such as 45,X/46,XY or 46,XX/46,XY or 46,XX/47,XXY, the appearance of the external genitalia will vary in relation to the amount of testicular tissue present (52). The spectrum ranges from normal male genitalia with normal testes to normal female genitalia with ovaries (46,XX/46,XY) or streak gonads (45,X/46,XY) (Fig. 5.8). Ambiguous genitalia will be observed with abnormal gonadal differentiation of the partial gonadal dysgenesis type. Some of the patients with 45,X/46,XY present a streak gonad on one side and a dysgenetic testis on the other, whereas others are true hermaphrodites. The reason for the diversity of phenotypes seems to be related to the

cloning of 45,X or 46,XX or 46,XY cells in the gonads.

GENDER ASSIGNMENT

Gender assignment is a complex issue, yet decisions need to be made as quickly as possible after the birth of an intersex child concerning male or female sex of rearing. Gender assignment is best guided by an experienced medical team including a pediatric endocrinologist/urologist/gynecologist and medical psychologist so that parents can make a well-informed decision. The team should be organized as a standing committee with its own self-imposed rules. One rule is to use only the neutral terms in early discussions with the parents (e.g., phallus rather than penis or clitoris, gonad rather than testis or ovary). This rule should be imposed on all hospital personnel in contact with the family. One other important rule is that, after appropriate discussion, the members of the team should come up with a unanimous decision as to advice for gender to be presented to the parents. Although the team members would be expected to inform the parents of the value of their advice, the parents should make the final decision. The team should make it clear that whatever the parental decision, support will be given to the family in the future. In general, decisions about gender assignment depend on the results of studies performed as part of the etiologic evaluation of the child. In particular, informed decisions will require detailed information from the physical examination, karyotype, genitourethrogram and/or sonogram, studies of androgen production, including 5α-reductase activity, and, if possible, studies of androgen receptor function.

Decisions regarding gender assignment in infants with an XX karyotype tend to be less complicated. A 46,XX individual who has been virilized by the hyperandrogenism associated with adrenal hyperplasia, or by maternal androgens, has a normal uterus, fallopian tubes, and ovaries. Hence, the potential for normal reproductive function in these patients makes a female gender assignment the reasonable choice. However, in some cultures, parents put greater value in being a man than a woman. In these cases, the medical team must explain fully the consequences of such decisions to the parents but, again, the team must respect parental decisions.

Infants with an abnormal karyotype, such as 45,X/46,XY, present a somewhat special situation. Infertility, the potential for gonadal malignancy, and the likelihood of short stature (52) suggest that female gender assignment is the better choice in the majority of these patients. The exception is in cases with well-masculinized external genitalia and with testes that are located or can be brought into the scrotum so the development of a gonadal tumor can be monitored.

Gender assignment in individuals with a 46,XY karyotype can be particularly complex. A variety of criteria regarding anatomy of the genitalia and the potential for future function need to be examined:

1. Phallic length should be determined by measuring the "stretched length" from the tip of the glans to the base of the phallus at the pubic symphysis. This can be easily accomplished in the newborn by applying slight pressure with the second and third fingers at the base of the phallus to cause erection of phallic tissue. In considering the potential for normal function if the child is raised male, one needs to question whether the penile length will be adequate for sexual function later in life. A phallic length of 1.9 cm is 2.5 SD below the mean for a normal newborn male (53) and may be considered a lower limit in assessing future function. However, the multiple surgeries necessary for gender reassignment may also be problematic.

2. The position of the urethral meatus is important, as it determines, in part, the number and complexity of the surgical procedures necessary to reconstruct the child as a male. In general, recent advances in surgical technique have greatly improved the outlook for repair of severe perineal hypospadias.

3. The presence of a vaginal pouch may strongly influence the decision regarding gender assignment. Removal of a large utriculovaginal pouch often is necessary if the child is raised as a male, as it can otherwise become the site of urinary stasis and recurrent infection. However, removal of a utriculovaginal pouch in a male invariably damages the vas deferens and results in infertility. By contrast, the absence of a vaginal pouch may argue against a female gender assignment as construction of a vaginal pouch *de novo* may be a difficult procedure.

4. The presence of normal müllerian structures is important, as their presence raises the possibility of menses or even a future pregnancy with a donor egg (54).

5. The adequacy of testosterone production can be assessed by determining blood levels in the first 3 months of life or later, after hCG stimulation. This information is useful in judging the potential for normal testosterone production at puberty and in adult life.

6. Evidence of androgen insensitivity in an infant with ambiguous genitalia creates a special case. As mentioned earlier, male subjects with partial androgen insensitivity virilize poorly at puberty despite high levels of androgens, usually develop gynecomastia, and invariably are infertile (55). On the other hand, female subjects of partial androgen insensitivity also can experience difficulties related to their feminizing surgery. For these reasons, we recommend gender assignment for infants with partial androgen insensitivity on a case-by-case basis.

Advances in medical diagnosis and surgical technique have had a significant impact on our approach to gender assignment over the past 20 years. Long-term follow-up of patients born with ambiguous genitalia will ultimately provide information on the soundness of these decisions.

MANAGEMENT

One of the major steps in the management of infants and children with ambiguous genitalia is the decision on the sex of rearing. This was discussed in the previous section. The other steps include consideration of the medical, surgical, and psychological needs of the patient.

Medical Therapy

Adrenal Steroid Replacement Therapy

As shown in Table 5.1, deficiency of enzymes required for cortisol steroidogenesis may result in undermasculinized males (partial deficiency of side chain cleavage enzymes, 3β-hydroxysteroid dehydrogenase, 17-hydroxylase) or overmasculinized females (partial or complete deficiency of 21-hydroxylase, 11-hydroxylase, or 3β-dehydrogenase). Concomitantly, there is adrenal hyperplasia. If the abnormality is quite marked, there can be hypertension in 11-hydroxylase deficiency or salt loss in the others.

Classically, the treatment includes replacement cortisol therapy (cortisol, cortisone, prednisone, dexamethasone), along with aldosterone replacement therapy (9α-fluorocortisol) if there is salt loss. Such treatment is required in both male and female patients, and it must be continued for life (31).

A deficiency of 17-ketosteroid reductase or 5α-reductase does not affect adrenocortical function (Table 5.1) and results in incomplete masculinization of male fetuses.

Sex Steroid Replacement Therapy at Puberty

Sex steroid therapy usually is not needed until pubertal age. Then, male patients with ambiguous genitalia and steroid enzyme deficiencies often will require supplemental androgen administration (testosterone enanthate 200 to 300 mg intramuscularly, once a month). Female patients with deficiency of side chain cleavage enzyme, 3β-hydroxysteroid dehydrogenase, and 17-hydroxylase require estrogen administration at puberty (Premarin 0.3 to 0.6 mg p.o., daily for 1 year, then a contraceptive pill, the first 21 days of each month).

Patients raised as males who present with partial gonadal dysgenesis, low Leydig cell number, and true hermaphroditism usually will require androgen supplement, whereas those with a timing defect do not.

Patients raised as females who have 46,XY partial gonadal dysgenesis, true hermaphroditism, or male pseudohermaphroditism will require estrogen supplementation at puberty.

Surgical Therapy

Details of the technical aspects of the reconstruction of ambiguous genitalia will be described in Chapter 6.

Patients Raised as Females

In these subjects, surgery to feminize the external genitalia is needed early in life (3 to 6 months of age). This is extremely important, as it helps the family to establish the female gender in their mind and, later, in the child. Specifically, it involves appropriate size reduction of the phallus so that it becomes inconspicuous and looks like a clitoris.

Often a second surgery will be needed to correct the shape or size of the vagina. We believe that this plastic surgery will give better results if carried out at the time the individual is ready to start her sex life.

Patients Raised as Males

The correction of ambiguous genitalia along male lines involves several steps, including release of chordee, construction of a perineal urethra, and prolongation of the urethra to the tip of the penis.

Gonads

In patients raised as males, the gonads that cannot be brought down in the scrotum must be removed because of the high risk of tumors. In patients raised as females, gonads (including streak gonads) must be removed if the karyotype is 46,XY.

Psychological Therapy

This most important part of treatment will be discussed in Chapter 7. We will only mention that psychological therapy is needed not only at the time of the choice of gender, but throughout the various stages of development of the child.

Ethical Considerations

Parents should be made aware that there is presently a major ethical debate concerning sex assignment of infants born with congenital malformations of the sex organs. One view is that patients themselves should be permitted to decide their ultimate sex of rearing when they reach the "age of reason." Proponents of this view believe that no surgical correction of the external genitalia should take place until the patient chooses a gender. Such a view, however, does not take into consideration the unrealistic situation in which parents are placed until their child reaches this "age of reason" and chooses a gender. It is of inter-

est that, in our experience with 60 adults treated for various intersex conditions, only two indicated doubt concerning their gender assignment. Furthermore, most of the 60 patients felt that parents should assign gender to their intersex child and surgical correction should be made early in life (work in progress).

REFERENCES

1. Langman J. *Medical embryology,* 2nd ed. Baltimore: Williams & Wilkins, 1969.
2. Palmer MS, Sinclair AH, Berta P, et al. Genetic evidence that ZFY is not the testis-determining factor. *Nature* 1989;342:937–939.
3. Sinclair AH, Berta P, Palmer MD, et al. A gene from the human sex determination region encodes a protein with homology to a conserved DNA-binding motif. *Nature* 1990;346:240–244.
4. Berta P, Hawkins JR, Sinclair AH, et al. Genetic evidence equating SRY and the testis-determining factor. *Nature* 1990;348:448–450.
5. Jager RJ, Anvret M, Hall K, et al. A human XY female with a frame shift mutation in the candidate testis-determining gene SRY. *Nature* 1990;348:452–454.
6. Koopman P, Gubbay J, Vivian N, et al. Male development of chromosomally female mice transgenic for Sry. *Nature* 1991;351:117–121.
7. Little MH, Wells C. A clinical overview of WT 1 gene mutations. *Human Mutations* 1997;9:209–225.
8. Luo X, Ikeda Y, Parker KL. A cell specific nuclear receptor is essential for adrenal and gonadal development and sexual differentiation. *Cell* 1994;77:481–490.
9. Shen WH, Moore CC, Ikeda Y, et al. Nuclear receptor steroidogenic factor, regulates with mullerian inhibiting substance gene: a link to the sex determination cascade cell. *Cell* 1994;77:651–661.
10. Shawlot W, Behringer. Requirement for Lim in head organizer function. *Nature* 1995;374:425–430.
11. Foster JW, Dominguez-Steglich MA, Guioli S, et al. Camptomelic dysplasia and autosomal sex reversal caused by mutations in an SRY-related gene. *Nature* 1994;372:525–530.
12. Swain A, Narraez V, Burgoyne P, et al. Dayl antogoners SRY action in mammalian sex determination. *Nature* 1998;391:761–767.
13. Magre S, Jost A. The initial phases to testicular organogenesis in the rat: an electron microscopy study. *Arch Anat Microsc Morphol Exp* 1980;69:297–318.
14. Magre S, Jost A. Dissociation between testicular organogenesis and endocrine cytodifferentiation of Sertoli cells. *Proc Natl Acad Sci U S A* 1984;81:7831–7834.
15. Swain A, Lovell-Badge R. Mammalian sex determination: a molecular drama. *Genes Dev* 1999;13:755–767.
16. Rey R, Picard J-Y. Embryology and endocrinology of genital development. In: Huges IA, ed. *Bailliere's clinical endocrinology and metabolism.* London: Bailliere Tindall, 1998:17–33.
17. Miller WL. Molecular biology of steroid hormone synthesis. *Endocr Rev* 1988;9:295–318.
18. Josso N, Picard JY. Antimullerian hormone. *Physiol Rev* 1986;66:1038–1090.

19. Wilson JD, Griffin JE, Russell DW. Steroid 5α reductase 2 deficiency. *Endocr Rev* 1993;14:577–593.

20. Brown TR. Androgen receptor dysfunction in human androgen insensitivity. *Trends Endocrinol Metab* 1995; 6:170–175.

21. O'Maley B. The steroid receptor superfamily: more excitement predicted for the future. *Mol Endocrinol* 1990; 4:363–369.

22. Keenan BS, Meyer WJ III, Hadjian AJ, et al. Androgen receptor in human skin fibroblasts: characterization of specific 17-beta-hydroxy-5-alpha-androstan—3-one-protein complex in cell sonicates and nuclei. *Steroids* 1975;25:535–552.

23. Migeon BR, Brown TR, Axelman J, et al. Studies of the locus for androgen receptor: localization on the human X chromosome and evidence for homology with the Tfm locus in the mouse. *Proc Natl Acad Sci U S A* 1981;78:6339–6343.

24. Lubahn DB, Joseph DR, Sar M, et al. The human androgen receptor: complementary deoxyribonucleic acid cloning, sequence analysis and gene expression in prostate. *Mol Endocrinol* 1988;2:1265–1275.

25. Quigley CA, DeBellio A, Marschke KB. Androgen receptor defects: historical, clinical and molecular perspectives. *Endocr Rev* 1995;16:271–321.

26. Onate SA, Tsai SY, Tsai MJ, et al. Sequence and characterization of a coactivator for the steroid hormone receptor superfamily. *Science* 1995;270:1354–1357.

27. Yeh SJ, Change C. Cloning and characterization of a specific coactivator, ARA$_{70}$, for the androgen receptor in human prostate cells. *Proc Natl Acad Sci U S A* 1996; 93:5517–5521.

28. Yen PM, Liu Y, Palvimo JJ, et al. Mutant and wild-type androgen receptors exhibit cross-talk on androgen-, glucocorticoid-, and progesterone-mediated transcription. *Mol Endocrinol* 1997;11:162–171.

29. Forest MG, Sizoneniko PC, Cathiard AM, et al. Hypophyso-gonadal function in humans during the first year of life. I. Evidence for testicular activity in early infancy. *J Clin Invest* 1974;53:818–828.

30. Forest MG, Ducharme JR. Hormones gonado tropes et gonadiques. In: Bertrand S, Rappaport R, Sizonenko PC, eds. *Endocrinologie pediatique.* Paris: Payot Lausanne, 1982:91–112.

31. Donohaue PA, Parker K, Migeon CJ. Congenital adrenal hyperplasia. In: Scriver CR, Beauolet AL, Sly WS, et al, eds. *The metabolic and molecular bases of inherited disease,* 8th ed. New York: McGraw-Hill *(in press).*

32. Berkovitz GB, Lee PA, Brown TR, et al. Etiologic evaluation of male pseudohermaphroditism in infancy and childhood. *Am J Dis Child* 1984;138:755–759.

33. Pang S, Levine LS, Chow D, et al. Dihydrotestosterone and its relationship to testosterone in infancy and childhood. *J Clin Endocrinol Metab* 1979;48:821–826.

34. Imperato-McGinley J, Guerrero L, Gautier T, et al. Steroid 5α-reductase deficiency in man: an inherited form of male pseudohermaphroditism. *Science* 1974; 186:1213–1215.

35. Walsh PC, Madden JD, Harrod MJ, et al. Familial incomplete male pseudohermaphroditism, type 2. Decreased dihydrotestosterone formation in pseudovaginal perineoscrotal hypospadias. *N Engl J Med* 1974;219:944–949.

36. Migeon CJ, Wisniewski AB, Brown TR. Androgen insensitivity syndrome in hormone resistance. In: Chrousos GP, Olefsky JM, Samuels E, eds. Philadel-

37. Meyer WJ III, Keenan BS, De Lacerda L, et al. Familial male pseudohermaphroditism with normal Leydig cell function at puberty. *J Clin Endocrinol Metab* 1978; 46:593–603.

38. Walsh PC, Migeon CJ. The phenotypic expression of selective disorders of male sexual differentiation. *J Urol* 1978;119:627–629.

39. Brown TR, Lubahn DB, Wilson EM, et al. Deletion of the steroid-binding domain of the human androgen receptor gene in one family with complete androgen insensitivity syndrome: evidence for further genetic heterogeneity in this syndrome. *Proc Natl Acad Sci U S A* 1988;85:8151–8155.

40. Lubahn DB, Brown TR, Simental JA, et al. Sequence of the intron/exon junctions of the coding region of the human androgen receptor gene and identification of a point mutation in a family with complete androgen insensitivity. *Proc Natl Acad Sci U S A* 1989;86:9534–9538.

41. Bertrand J. Familial male pseudohermaphroditism with gynecomastia due to testicular 17-ketosteroid reductase defect: in vivo studies. *J Clin Endocrinol Metab* 1971; 32:604–610.

42. Forest MG. Inborn errors of testosterone biosynthesis. In: Josso N, ed. *The intersex child.* Basel: Karger, 1981: 133–155.

43. Bongiovanni AM. The adrenogenital syndrome with deficiency of 3β-hydroxysteroid dehydrogenase. *J Clin Invest* 1962;41:2086–2092.

44. Berkovitz GD, Fechner PY, Zacur HW, et al. Clinical and pathologic spectrum of 46 XY gonadal dysgenesis: its relevance to the understanding of sex differentiation. *Medicine* 1991;70:375–383.

45. Raifer J, Walsh PC. Mixed gonadal dysgenesis-dysgenetic male pseudohermaphroditism. In: Josso N, ed. *The intersex child.* Basel: Karger, 1981:105–115.

46. Scully RE. Neoplasia associated with anomalous sexual development and abnormal sex chromosomes. In: Josso N, ed. *The intersex child.* Basel: Karger, 1981:203–217.

47. Biglieri EG, Herron MA, Brust N. 17-Hydroxylation deficiency in man. *J Clin Invest* 1966;45:1946–1954.

48. New M. Male pseudohermaphroditism due to 17α-hydroxylase deficiency. *J Clin Invest* 1970;49:1930–1940.

49. Jones HW Jr. Nonadrenal female pseudohermaphroditism. In: Josso N, ed. *The intersex child.* Basel: Karger, 1981:65–79.

50. Wilkins L, Jones HW Jr, Holman GH, et al. Masculinization of the female fetus associated with administration of oral and intramuscular progestins during gestation: nonadrenal female, pseudohermaphroditism. *J Clin Endocrinol Metab* 1958;18:559–585.

51. Jones KL. *Smith's recognizable patterns of human malformations,* 5th ed. Philadelphia: WB Saunders, 1997.

52. Forest MG. Diagnosis and treatment of disorders of sexual development. In: DeGroot LJ, ed. *Endocrinology.* Philadelphia: WB Saunders, 1995:1901–1937.

53. Lee PA, Mazur T, Danish R, et al. Micropenis I criteria, etiologies and classification. *Johns Hopkins Med J* 1980;146:156–163.

54. Sauer MV, Lobo RA, Paulson RJ. Successful twin pregnancy after embryo donation to a patient with XY gonadal dysgenesis. *Am J Obstet Gynecol* 1989;161:380–381.

55. Amrhein JA, Klingensmith G, Walsh PC, et al. Partial androgen insensitivity: the Reifenstein syndrome revisited. *N Engl J Med* 1977;297:350–356.

phia: Lippincott Williams & Wilkins *(in press).*

6

Surgical Management of Genital Ambiguity

Mark R. Feneley and John P. Gearhart

Management of the infant with ambiguous genitalia demands great care and skill. Gender assignment requires careful clinical evaluation and full understanding of its implications for future sexual and psychological development as well as fertility. The surgeon must be sensitive to concerns of the parents and the future development of the individual patient. This may pose great dilemmas, even for the infant with a normal 46,XX or 46,XY karyotype.

Ambiguous genitalia represents a spectrum of deviations of *in utero* sexual development, where the abnormal external genitalia range from predominantly male to predominantly female. These are manifestations of female pseudohermaphroditism, male pseudohermaphroditism, true pseudohermaphroditism, and mixed gonadal dysgenesis. Evaluation includes history, physical examination, and special investigations to define the phenotypic, gonadal, and chromosomal sex.

Maternal hormone therapy or intake of androgenic substances, medications that interfere with steroid metabolism, and excess steroid production secondary to maternal illness during pregnancy are etiologically important. The unexpected death of a sibling during the first weeks of life may alert the physician to the likelihood of adrenogenital syndrome with salt wasting. Family history of genital anomalies may indicate the possibility of 5α-reductase deficiency or androgen receptor insensitivity. Sterility, amenorrhea, and hernia containing a gonad also may be relevant.

On physical examination, the genitalia are ambiguous by definition and thus are neither clearly male nor female. Any of the following abnormalities may be present: (a) small phallus in the genetic male or enlarged clitoris in the genetic female, (b) inappropriately fused labioscrotal folds, (c) bifid scrotum, (d) labial rugae, (e) hypospadias, (f) chordee, (g) gonads above or below the inguinal ring, (h) palpable epididymis on the gonad, or (i) midline uterus on rectal examination. Recognizing the presence of vaginal epithelial cells in the smear of the perineal discharge obtained by milking the vagina during the rectal examination may be informative. Major anomalies involving other organ systems may be present and should be evaluated.

Blood draw for both biochemical studies and karyotyping are mandatory in all cases of genital ambiguity. Biochemical studies may reveal an underlying enzymatic defect and should include serum electrolyte analysis, 17-hydroxyprogesterone, pregnenolone, gonadotrophins, testosterone, and dihydrotestosterone, and quantification of urinary ketosteroids and pregnanetriol. Congenital adrenal hyperplasia, due to enzymatic defect that results in mineralocorticoid and glucocorticoid deficiency, leads to overproduction of adrenal androgens and masculinized genitalia in a genetic female. In the newborn, this may present as a medical emergency and early diagnosis will be life saving. Karyotype may distinguish mixed gonadal dysgenesis from true hermaphroditism. Laparotomy or laparoscopy and gonadal biopsy may be necessary in some cases to definitively diagnose mixed gonadal dysgenesis, male pseudohermaphroditism, or true hermaphroditism.

Initial evaluation of the internal genitalia includes retrograde genitogram and pelvic ultrasound examination. The genitogram will confirm the presence of müllerian structures and define the "takeoff" position of the vagina from the urogenital sinus (Fig. 6.1). These findings have significant implications for surgical reconstruction, and the surgeon will appreciate the need to be present at the time of these examinations. Müllerian duct structures may be identified by ultrasound or their absence confirmed. Magnetic resonance imaging may provide additional information. In cases where internal genital anatomy and gonadal sex remain undetermined, gonadal biopsy may be necessary.

Decisions on sex of rearing for an infant should be based on anatomy and potential for sexual function and not chromosomal karyotype or fertility potential alone. Genetic females almost invariably can be reconstructed and raised as female, whereas males with an inadequate phallus may be assigned the female sex. It is not difficult to create a vagina if one is absent, but it may be difficult to create a satisfactory penis. For genetic males with an adequate phallus, male sex assignment should be considered, but in general only patients with a stretched penile length of at least 2.5 cm who have responded to testosterone should be considered. When the phallus is particularly diminutive or rudimentary, female sex should be assigned regardless of gonadal or ductal sex of the infant. Despite major technical advances in penile reconstruction, it continues to appear that infants with a major intersex abnormality fare better psychologically and anatomically as females than as males. A contemporary long-term study recently completed at our institution has demonstrated highly favorable psychosexual and surgical outcomes in male pseudohermaphrodites following female reconstructive surgery, particularly when vaginoplasty is delayed until adolescence (1A).

NON-NEWBORN SURGICAL OPTIONS

Intersex patients who require feminine reconstruction of the perineum can be divided into two groups: (i) females with extreme masculinization of the external genitalia (the adrenogenital syndrome and female pseudohermaphroditism), and (ii) others with incomplete masculinization of the sexual structure (male pseudohermaphrodites, mixed gonadal dysgenesis, and some forms of true hermaphroditism) (1B).

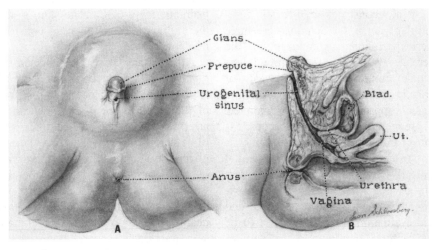

FIG. 6.1. Ambiguous genitalia with urethral takeoff from urogenital sinus. **A:** External genitalia (perineal view). **B:** Internal genitalia (sagittal view).

Surgical repair of these infants who are to be reared as females includes phallic reduction (clitoroplasty), creation of labia majora and minora (labioplasty), and exteriorization of the vagina, if present, or complete reconstruction, if not present (vaginoplasty). Gonads that are inappropriate for gender assignment and gonadal tissue with high potential for malignant transformation will require removal. Formerly, the enlarged clitoris or diminutive penis was managed by clitorectomy, and the entire structure was excised (2). This approach was superseded by more conservative procedures that included excision of the corporeal bodies without removal of the glans and symmetric wedge resection of the tunica albuginea to shorten the corpora (3,4). More recently, methods that preserve innervation to the glans with resection of the entire corporeal body have been developed (5–7). A modified approach to phallic reconstruction described by Kogan and Smey (8) has been popularized by other groups (9). Feasibility of one-stage surgical correction of the high vaginal takeoff has since been demonstrated (10). Using a modification of the sagittal transanorectal approach of Pena and Devries (11), accurate positioning of the vaginal introitus and good cosmetic results can be achieved (12).

OPERATIVE TECHNIQUE

The surgical reconstruction of female genitalia is similar whether the diagnosis is female pseudohermaphroditism secondary to the adrenogenital syndrome, male pseudohermaphroditism, mixed gonadal dysgenesis, or true hermaphroditism. Genital reconstruction and surgical approach should be planned, based on preoperative studies. Endoscopic examination of the lower genitourinary tract is mandatory to supplement preoperative genital radiographs. If a vagina is present that enters the urethra or urogenital sinus distal to the external urinary sphincter and endoscopic and radiologic evaluation show the vagina to be reachable from the perineum, a flap vaginoplasty is performed. If the vagina is too high for a simple perineal flap but is distal to the

bladder neck and urinary sphincter, a perineal approach is used, but the vagina must be detached from the urogenital sinus and brought to the perineum, often with the aid of perineal flaps. If construction of a neovagina is to be deferred, as in some patients whose vaginal entry is proximal to the external sphincter or those who have no vagina, phallic reduction and recession are the initial procedures of the perineal reconstruction.

Phallic reduction and recession usually is performed when the child is metabolically stable, as confirmed by the pediatric endocrinologist. The operation is begun by making a circumferential incision at the phallus at the coronal level, sparing the ventral mucosal groove. The perineal flap is outlined and dissected carefully from the underlying tissues to ensure an adequate blood supply (Fig. 6.2). The dorsal skin of the prepuce is dissected from the penile shaft, starting at the glans and continuing to the base of the phallus. Any inappropriate gonads can be removed easily through this incision at this time.

The suspensory ligaments are taken down (Fig. 6.3A). Because no vagina exists in some patients, the urethra in the male or urogenital sinus in the female, which may be of variable length, is opened ventrally from the meatus to the posterior bulbar area (Fig. 6.3B). The perineal flap is then brought into the bulbar urethra/urogenital sinus to provide a feminine appearance (Fig. 6.3C). The skin is divided in the midline in preparation for construction of the labia minora (Fig. 6.3C).

After taking down the suspensory ligaments, a 2-0 polyglycolic acid suture ligature is placed in each corporal body near the base of the penis to occlude the central corporal artery and to reduce blood flow into the erectile tissue (Fig. 6.4A). This maneuver minimizes the amount of bleeding during subsequent manipulation of the corporal tissues. Care is taken to avoid the neurovascular bundles. Reduction of the phallus to a normal appearance is accomplished by making an incision into each corporal body as lateral as possible to avoid injury to the neurovascular bundles (Fig. 6.4B). Enough erectile tissue is

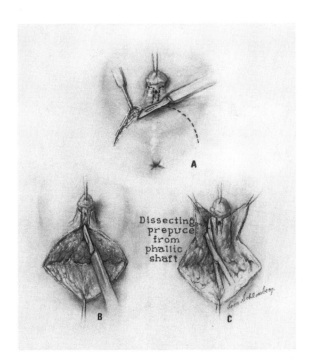

FIG. 6.2. Skin incisions for feminizing genitoplasty. **A:** Incisions for phallic dissection and perineal flap. **B:** Sparing of ventral mucosal groove and creation of perineal skin flap. **C:** Dissection of dorsal skin of prepuce from penile shaft for creation of labia minora.

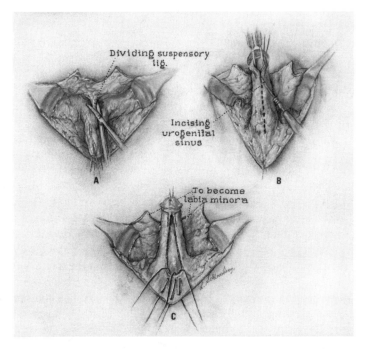

FIG. 6.3. Reconstruction of female external genitalia by flap vaginoplasty. **A:** Division of phallic suspensory ligament. **B:** Incision of urogenital sinus. **C:** Apposition of perineal skin flap into proximal urogenital sinus.

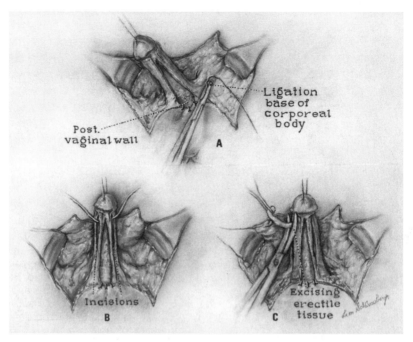

FIG. 6.4. Phallic reduction for clitoroplasty. **A:** Ligation of base of corporeal body taking care to avoid the neurovascular bundles. **B:** Bilateral incisions of corporal tissues. **C:** Excision of erectile tissues.

removed to create a clitoris of appropriate size via these two incisions (Fig. 6.4C). After excision of the erectile tissue, if the clitoris still appears to be too large, it can be reduced easily before recession by excising a ventral wedge of tissue from the glans. In this manner, the phallic structure can be reduced markedly without excising the tunica albuginea or manipulating the neurovascular bundles supplying the glans.

An often neglected part of the surgical reconstruction is fixation of the glans to the pubic bone. The glans must be fixed with at least two sutures to the base of the pubic bone. The author usually uses two sutures of 3-0 silk and sews the base of the glans to the periosteum of the pubic bone near its inferior edge, just cephalad to where the suspensory ligaments were previously cut (Fig. 6.5A–B). Care must be taken when sewing the glans to the pubis so that the dorsal neurovascular bundle is not constricted in any way. Also, for cosmetic appearances, the glans should be sewn as far cephalad as possible so that the ventral mu-

cosal strip is stretched out and does not appear redundant. Also, the glans must be well fixed to the pubis so that it will remain in a normal recessed and concealed position near the mons pubis. In this manner, a midline scar over the mons is avoided.

The two flaps that were created by dividing the phallic skin are draped around the side of the clitoris to create the labia minora. The medial edge of these flaps is sutured to the trimmed glans and to the edges of the ventral phallic urethral strip (Fig. 6.5C). The lateral aspect of the same dorsal skin flap is sutured to the labioscrotal folds. The labioscrotal flap is extended into the angle formed by the perineal flap and the labia minora (labioscrotal Y-V plasty) to advance the labia majora (Fig. 6.6). Some of the labioscrotal skin may have to be excised before the Y-V plasty is completed to prevent this tissue from having a rugated appearance.

The proper type of vaginal exteriorization procedure performed depends on the level of vaginal takeoff from the urogenital sinus. Al-

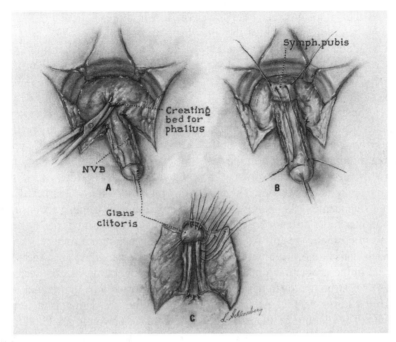

FIG. 6.5. Anchoring of recessed clitoris to symphysis pubis and reconstruction of labia minora. **A:** Creating bed for phallus. **B:** Anchoring glans to symphysis pubis. **C:** Creation of labia minora.

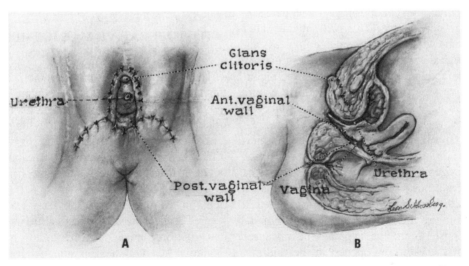

FIG. 6.6. Y-V advancement of labia majora and completion of feminizing genitoplasty. **A:** Reconstructed female external genitalia (perineal view). **B:** Separated urethra and genital tract (sagittal view).

though reported, the author has seen very few patients in whom a simple cutback of the introitus would be adequate. A preoperative retrograde genitogram and cystoscopy along with vaginoscopy at the time of genital reconstructive surgery helps in proper planning of this procedure. The crucial determination that must be made at cystoscopy is whether a sufficiently large cavity lies behind the posteriorly fused labia minora. Most often in the infant coming to reconstructive surgery, a flap-type vaginoplasty is carried out. The use of this perineal advancement flap along with a clitoroplasty allows most infants to have a very satisfactory cosmetic result from this unified approach. This author usually places a no. 12-14 sound in the urogenital sinus opening and opens this structure over the sound, placing marking sutures as the incision advances cephalad. The placing of these marking sutures allows the walls of the urogenital sinus to be well controlled when it is time to advance the perineal flap into the urogenital sinus and vagina. It is extremely important that the perineal flap be advanced well into the vagina so that an introitus of adequate size will be constructed. This will obviate later problems with stenosis, hematocolpos associated with the menarche, and recurrent urinary tract infections. Cystoscopy during the reconstructive procedure may be helpful to ensure that the flap is in good position and that it allows the vagina to be well drained.

A flap vaginoplasty is performed with incisions similar to those described previously. The urogenital sinus is opened in the midline until the posterior wall of the vagina is reached. Care must be taken at this juncture not to injure the rectum, which lies immediately posterior to the vagina. The posterior flap of the vagina is opened in the midline, and the perineal flap is advanced to exteriorize the vagina. The labioscrotal folds are sutured to the lateral borders of the urogenital sinus and the vagina using the dorsal phallic skin, which was divided previously in the midline. Although some recommend routine dilatation of this newly constructed vaginal

orifice, in our experience this usually has not been necessary.

If the vaginal entry into the urogenital sinus is proximal to the external urinary sphincter and adequate drainage of the müllerian system is evident, the vaginoplasty is deferred to avoid injury to the sphincter and subsequent stress incontinence. In these cases, a pullthrough procedure or a posterior sagittal approach is performed when the child is 18 months to 3 years of age (11,13,14). However, if the müllerian tract on either side is obstructed or serves as a diverticulum for urine, a reconstructive procedure may need to be performed before 18 months. Clean intermittent vaginal catheterization may be necessary in some patients until a definitive operation can be performed. For an individual in whom the vagina is absent, creation of the neovagina is deferred until late adolescence or young adulthood. At that time, the person will be mature, and regular dilatation of the vagina can be accomplished. This delay also allows time for the pelvis and perineal tissues to develop fully before reconstruction is performed.

POSTOPERATIVE MANAGEMENT AND COMPLICATIONS

The cosmetic and functional outcomes with this technique have been excellent. In all patients, the clitoris has normal sensation to pinprick. No episodes of glans sloughing, flap necrosis, urinary tract infections, or wound infections have been reported. It should be noted that no patient had stress incontinence as a result of this reconstruction. Of all patients in whom a flap vaginoplasty was performed at the time of the original perineal reconstruction, none has required regular dilatation to maintain an adequately sized vaginal orifice.

Most patients have experienced few immediate postoperative complications. A cross-shaped perineal pressure dressing is made from an adhesive elastic dressing and left in place for 48 hours. A Foley catheter is placed at the time of surgery and left in the bladder until the dressing is removed and the wound is examined. After 5 days, the child is given sitz baths twice daily, and a blow dryer is used to dry the perineal wound after bathing. If all is well, the Foley catheter is removed, and the parent cleans the suture lines daily with hydrogen peroxide solution.

SUMMARY

This approach to surgical reconstruction of the perineum can be used, regardless of the diagnosis, in all patients with ambiguous genitalia who are to be reared as females. The only aspect of the reconstruction that varies among patients is the timing of the vaginoplasty. However, in all cases the phallic reduction creation of the labia minora and majora and gonadectomy (if indicated) are performed when the child is approximately 3 to 6 months old. Early genitoplasty ensures that the appearance of the external genitalia is consistent with the female sex of rearing and relieves the parents' anxiety about the child with regard to the concerns of relatives and friends (15).

In this procedure, phallic reduction with phallic recession is described and incorporated. The erectile tissue is removed using two lateral corporal incisions without manipulation of the neurovascular bundles. The newly constructed, appropriately size clitoris is placed beneath the mons pubis without an overlying scar. The phallic foreskin is used to create the labia minora. A labioscrotal Y-V plasty reduces the enlarged labioscrotal folds to produce normal-appearing labia majora. A posterior perineal flap provides access to the vagina when present and to the urethra when absent. This unified approach is applicable to a variety of patients with different types of intersexual abnormalities. However, continuous core-team follow-up of the patient is needed endocrinologically, psychologically, and surgically to attain success.

REFERENCES

1A. Wisniewski AB, Migeon CJ, Meyer-Bahlburg HF, et al. Complete androgen insensitivity syndrome: medical, surgical, and psychosexual outcome. (Submitted for publication, 2000.)

1B. Donahoe PK, Hendren WH III. Perineal reconstruction in ambiguous genitalia in infants raised as females. *Ann Surg* 1984;200:363.

2. Gross RE, Randolf J, Kriggler JF Jr. Clitorectomy for sexual abnormalities: indications and technique. *Surgery* 1966;59:300.

3. Spence HM, Allen TD. Genital reconstruction in the female with adrenogenital syndrome. *Br J Urol* 1973;45:126.

4. Glassberg KI, Laungani G. Reduction clitoroplasty. *J Urol* 1981;17:604.

5. Barrett TM, Gonzalez ET Jr. Reconstruction of the female external genitalia. *Urol Clin North Am* 1980;7:455.

6. Snyder HMC III, Retik AB, Bauer SB, et al. Feminizing genitoplasty. *J Urol* 1983;129:1024.

7. Gearhart JP, Burnett A, Owen JH. Measurement of pudendal evoked potentials during feminizing genitoplasty: technique and applications. *J Urol* 1995;153:486.

8. Kogan SJ, Smey PLSB. Subtunical total reduction clitoroplasty: a safe modification of existing techniques. *J Urol* 1983;130:746.

9. Oesterling JE, Gearhart JP, Jeffs RD. A unified approach to early reconstructive surgery of the child with ambiguous genitalia. *J Urol* 1987;130:1079.

10. Passerini-Glazel G. A new 1-stage procedure for clitorovaginoplasty in severely masculinized female pseudohermaphrodites. *J Urol* 1989;142:565.

11. Pena P, Devries P. Posterior sagittal anorectoplasty: important technical considerations and new applications. *J Pediatr Surg* 1982;17:796.

12. Benedetto VD, Gioviale M, Bagnara V, et al. The anterior sagittal transanorectal approach: a modified approach to 1-stage clitoral vaginoplasty in severely masculinized female pseudohermaphrodites—preliminary results. *J Urol* 1997;157:330.

13. Hendren WH. Reconstructive problems of the vagina and the female urethra. *Clin Plast Surg* 1980;7:207.

14. Hendren WH, Donahoe PK. Correction of congenital anomalies of the vagina and perineum. *J Pediatr Surg* 1980;15:751.

15. Snyder HMC III. Clitoroplasty (part II). *Dial Pediatr Urol* 1985;8:2.

7

Psychological Aspects of
Sexual Differentiation Disorders

Sarah E. Herbert

How a child or adolescent understands and copes with a disorder of sexual differentiation depends in part on where he or she is developmentally and how the specific disorder impacts the child or adolescent's life. Other important factors are how the family handles the disorder and what the societal and cultural biases around gender and sexuality are. This chapter will look at general developmental issues pertaining to individuals with sexual differentiation disorders and then explore what is known about the psychological, social, and sexual aspects of specific disorders of sexual differentiation.

DEFINITIONS

Before describing the psychological impact of sexual differentiation disorders, it would be helpful to define some of the terms that will be used, that is, biologic sex, gender identity, gender role behaviors, and sexual orientation. Biologic sex is made up of a number of different components: chromosomes, gonads, internal genitalia, external genitalia, sex hormones, and secondary sex characteristics (1). In children and adolescents with disorders of sexual differentiation, these components are not consistently associated with one biologic sex or the other. Gender identity is the individual's self-designation as male or female, the self-image of his or her biologic sex (2). Gender role behaviors are those behaviors, attitudes, and personality traits that a society in a given culture and historical period desig-

nates as masculine or feminine (2). These include nonsexual attributes and behaviors that are considered characteristic of one gender or the other, such as physical appearance, dress, mannerisms, speech, emotional responsiveness, and aggressiveness. Gender role identity is the individual's self-perception as feminine or masculine. Sexual orientation is the person's erotic preference for persons of the same, opposite, or either sex. Components of sexual orientation include emotional attachments, sexual fantasies, and sexual behavior (3). Traditionally these have been referred to in our culture as homosexual, heterosexual, or bisexual. An alternative manner of noting sexual orientation that is more easily applicable to individuals with sexual differentiation disorders is to refer to the gender of the person they desire sexually; that is, they are described as androphilic, gynecophilic, or ambiphilic.

DEVELOPMENTAL ISSUES IN
SEXUAL DIFFERENTIATION
DISORDERS

The impact that disorders of sexual differentiation have on individuals will depend in part on the age of that person at diagnosis. The developmental stage of the child or adolescent will affect his or her ability to understand and cope with such a diagnosis. Likewise, the ability to cooperate with medical care and comply with treatment regimens will depend in part on the level of maturity. In the following sections, the impact of sexual differentiation disorders will be viewed from the vantage point of developmental phases.

ISSUES AT BIRTH AND THE NEONATAL PERIOD

Significant issues in the neonatal period are the diagnosis and assignment of gender to the child with ambiguous genitalia at birth. This is generally a very stressful time for the parents and extended family. It has been considered vitally important to provide support to parents at this time. Time is devoted to educating the parents about normal sexual differentiation of the fetus to help them understand better what has gone wrong in their child's development. It has been feared that parents who do not get a clear early message about the child's gender will pass this confusion on to their child or, worse, that the parents will reject their child. At the time of birth, it has been suggested that physicians address the issue with parents by telling them that their baby's genitals are not fully developed, and further testing will be necessary to determine the baby's sex (4). Telling parents that the baby is half-male and half-female is only likely to increase their anxiety and confusion (4). At this stage, it often is helpful to allow parents the opportunity to voice their feelings about having a sexually atypical baby. Feelings of humiliation, shame, or self-blame may be present. It may come as a shock to the parents, because the technical advances associated with ultrasound and amniocentesis have allowed many parents to know the sex of their child before delivery or to feel reassured that there were no major birth defects. If parents have informed other family members and friends of the child's sex ahead of time, they may need assistance in knowing what to say or how to disclose information about the infant's gender under these circumstances.

The speed with which medical professionals are advised to assign a gender to the child no doubt heightens anxiety in the immediate postnatal period. Medical textbooks traditionally have informed medical professionals that it is vitally important to quickly assign a gender to the child born with ambiguous genitalia (5). Therefore, multiple tests are performed in the immediate postnatal period to determine what the child's gender assignment should be, and parents must await these results before announcing to which gender the child has been assigned. Many surgical and pediatric textbooks recommend early surgical correction of the genitalia, thereby increasing the pressure on medical professionals to make an early and appropriate decision and likewise increasing the anxiety experienced by parents. Thus, the parents may experience pressure to give permission for surgical procedures early in the infant's life, without much time to consider alternatives for a condition that may not be life threatening. The rationale for early surgery apparently is to help the child look normal and thus avoid rejection by parents and other caretakers. There is not much documentation, however, to support the claim of parental rejection of infants whose genitals remained ambiguous and without early surgical intervention. In the past few years, there have been newer recommendations suggesting less surgical intervention or deferring surgical procedures until the child is older (6–8). If early surgical intervention does not take place and the genitals remain ambiguous, then parents may need counseling about what to say to others who provide care for their child, such as grandparents or day care workers.

ISSUES IN CHILDHOOD

Advice on clinical management of these conditions in early childhood has stressed that not only should gender be assigned shortly after birth, but the child should be consistently and unambiguously reared in this gender (1,4,9). There is little controversy about consistently rearing a child in one gender or the other. Flexibility may be needed, however, in the area of gender role behaviors. Children born with ambiguous genitalia may have undergone atypical hormonal exposure *in utero,* and their gender role behaviors may not fit the stereotypic picture for a child of that gender.

Although ridicule and subsequent shame and embarrassment may occur for young children with genital anomalies, it is possible that much more has been made of this than is warranted (10). Children can label themselves as male or female early in the preschool years, but it takes longer to develop gender constancy. Gender constancy is the concept that being male or female is a biologic characteristic and cannot be changed by changing superficial attributes such as clothing or hairstyle. It takes much longer to develop, often not until middle childhood (11,12). Thus, it is not likely that preschool or early school-age children will attribute great significance to some degree of genital ambiguity. Given the sexual modesty taught to children in our culture and the fact that children spend most of their time clothed, it is unlikely that even school-age children will spend a great deal of time comparing genitals. If there are occasions when the child is unclothed and the genitals are exposed, children with these anomalies can be coached about how to deal with unkind remarks or intrusive questions in the same way that children with various other congenital anomalies are taught to handle this issue. It is helpful to prepare some simple explanations that children can be prepared to use in response to questions from peers or siblings.

A major issue that arises in the childhood years is the decision about when and how the child should be told about her condition. It has been recommended that children learn about their condition in gradual steps and in developmentally appropriate ways. Simple explanations can be used and knowledge built up incrementally over time. Because school-age children think in concrete ways, it is best to tailor explanations to fit this way of thinking. John Money illustrated one way to do this in the explanation he gave a 46,XY girl about her chromosomal status. He told her that her Y chromosome was like an X with an arm broken off, totally incapable of doing Y work (13), a concrete image that any prepubertal child could relate to. Pictures and diagrams, rather than just words, can be effective in educating children about their condition.

The intrusiveness of genital examinations, often performed by multiple medical professionals at teaching institutions, and nude medical photography have been noted to be problematic for some children. It has been likened to childhood sexual abuse in its impact on some individuals (14). Consequences have included a phobic response to hospitals and genital procedures during childhood and avoidance of medical care in the adult years (14,15).

ISSUES AT PUBERTY AND THE ADOLESCENT YEARS

Certain sexual differentiation disorders do not manifest themselves until puberty or the adolescent years. Girls with complete androgen insensitivity (CAI) generally present in the adolescent years with amenorrhea and a lack of adrenarche. Children with 5α-reductase deficiency who have been raised as girls since birth will begin to experience growth of the phallus, descent of the testes, and production of testosterone leading to increased hirsutism and muscle development. Likewise, true hermaphrodites being reared as girls might experience masculinization at puberty if there is one testis producing testosterone.

A major developmental task of puberty and early adolescence is accepting and adjusting to the multitude of bodily changes that take place at this age (16). Girls expect to develop breasts and start menses; they do not expect to develop facial and body hair or to become increasingly muscular at puberty. Adolescence is a time of heightened sensitivity to others' perceptions and a desire to be accepted by one's peers. A lack of the anticipated pubertal physical changes or growth in ways that are the opposite of what is expected have the potential to lead to confusion, increased anxiety, a negative self-image, and alienation from peers.

Identity issues are also quite significant for adolescents. This is the age at which some intersex individuals begin to articulate questions about their identities as male or female based on physical changes, as well as internal feelings. It also may be the time when some intersex adolescents begin to consider a change of gender (17,18).

Adolescence is a time for becoming aware of sexual feelings, developing romantic relationships, becoming aware of one's sexual orientation, and, for a sizable percentage of teens, becoming sexually active. Sexual orientation for children born with genital ambiguity may not be what they, or their parents, expected, based on the assigned gender and the assumption of heterosexuality. These feelings can be confusing and upsetting for adolescents born without any genital ambiguity, so one can imagine how confusing it might be for adolescents with genital ambiguity. Both adolescents and their parents may need help in understanding and accepting an atypical sexual orientation. Given that over 50% of adolescents in the 15- to 19-year-old age group are sexually active (19), one would expect that this would be a particularly problematic time for individuals with genital anomalies or conflicts around sexual activity. There are very limited data on the sexual functioning of adults with disorders of sexual differentiation and almost none about teens with these disorders. This is a particularly important time to be available to provide appropriate sex education for the patient and to assist her parents in this endeavor. In addition to making sure the young woman has adequate sex education, discussion of her sexual history in a matter of fact and nonjudgmental way is important at this time.

The adolescent years are the time when cognitive development may reach the level of formal thinking, thus allowing the individual to have more ability to abstract and imagine the future (16). Therefore, it is a better time for patients to receive more complex explanations about their particular disorder from their physicians, particularly with regard to issues around infertility and reproductive technologies that might potentially help with fertility. Girls born without a vagina become candidates for vaginoplasty at this time. Because compliance with dilatation is such an impor-

tant issue in keeping the neovagina functional, it has been recommended that this surgical procedure take place when the girl or young woman can understand the importance of the regular dilatation regimen required after vaginoplasty and that she is motivated to comply with it.

Adolescence is a time of increasing desire for autonomy. Data on adolescent decision making suggest that by the age of 15 years, most individuals have a decision-making capacity similar to adults (20–22). If further surgical procedures are recommended, this would be a better time to consider them. Adolescence is an appropriate time to allow the girl or young woman opportunities to participate in her medical care and in decisions made about her body.

FAMILY ISSUES IN SEXUAL DIFFERENTIATION DISORDERS

Our culture's discomfort regarding sexual matters makes it likely that the family of a child born with ambiguous genitalia will be anxious about disclosure of this information. The anomaly often becomes a family secret, and parents may have difficulty sharing information with the child, close relatives, or others. Individuals born with ambiguous genitals have recently begun to speak out about their experiences with these issues during childhood and adolescence (15,23,24). Many have described feelings of betrayal and alienation from their family because of not being told, or because they found out in unexpected or unsupportive ways. The secrecy surrounding their status at birth and the difficulty obtaining this information from parents or physicians has been most troublesome to adults who attempt to gain information about their earliest years.

Families have been placed in a bind regarding their child's genital anomaly. Professionals tell parents that they must consistently reinforce a particular gender identity so their child will feel no ambiguity about their assigned male or female gender. In trying to carry out the physicians' advice regarding consistent reinforcement of gender, parents may not be as open as they might otherwise have been about the circumstances surrounding their child's genital abnormality. Parents and physicians alike have often thought they were acting in the child or adolescent's best interest in not disclosing information, not realizing the detrimental impact this secrecy eventually might have.

CULTURAL ASPECTS OF SEXUAL DIFFERENTIATION DISORDERS

In western European culture, only two genders—male and female—have been recognized. There has been an implicit assumption that an individual had to have normal-looking and sexually functional genitals to be considered a member of that gender (10). These concepts have been particularly salient for males in western European culture. When male infants sustained traumatic injuries to their genitals or were born with a micropenis or ambiguous genitalia, such that they would never look "normal" and would not be able to perform urinary or genital functions in a typical way, recommendations were made to reassign them as girls. Girls born with an enlarged clitoris or otherwise masculinized genitals often in the past had early genital surgery to repair what had been considered defective genitals.

In cultures more patriarchal than our own, where significant advantages accrue to being male, parents or adolescents may still choose assignment to the male gender for boys who have ambiguous genitals or who may never function sexually in typical ways (21). In some more primitive cultures, intersex individuals have been given a label, possibly indicating a third sex or intersex identity. For example, in the Dominican Republic, the label guevodoces ("balls at 12") or *machihembra* ("macho missy") was given to boys who masculinized at puberty but initially were reared as females (13). Among the Sambia of Papua, New Guinea, a boy with the same disorder was called "turnim-man" (25).

SPECIFIC DISORDERS OF SEXUAL DIFFERENTIATION

The impact of sexual differentiation disorders will vary not only according to the age at diagnosis but also according to the nature of the disorder. What is known about the psychological, social, and sexual aspects of selected disorders will be summarized in this section. Disorders most likely to come to the attention of the gynecologist treating the pediatric and adolescent population are congenital adrenal hyperplasia (CAH), 5α-reductase deficiency, Turner's syndrome, androgen insensitivity syndrome, and Mayer-Rokitansky-Küster-Hauser syndrome.

Congenital Adrenal Hyperplasia

CAH is one of the most common types of sexual differentiation disorders. Due to a recessive genetic disorder that involves a defect in the biosynthesis of cortisol, it leads to overproduction of adrenal androgens and results in a type of female pseudohermaphroditism when the fetus is a 46,XX female. At birth, masculinized or indeterminate external genitalia are present; typically there is enlargement of the clitoris, partial fusion and rugation of the labioscrotal folds, and a urogenital sinus. Internally there are ovaries and normal müllerian duct structures (26).

Today these children are raised according to their chromosomal sex, although in the past some were mistakenly reared as males. Girls with this disorder have atypical gender role behaviors, showing more evidence of tomboyism than their female siblings. They prefer rough-and-tumble play and have an interest in boys' toys, but gender identity has been consistent with the sex of rearing (27). This does not preclude, however, some concerns that adolescent girls with CAH express about their body image. There is some controversy about whether there is actually a higher prevalence of atypical sexual orientation in this group compared to the general population (27,28). There does appear to be a higher prevalence of homosexual and bisexual fantasies in the studies that have been done, but the data regarding actual sexual behavior are equivocal. Some studies show a higher prevalence of homosexual behavior than one would expect, but some do not (26,27,29). Adolescents with CAH showed evidence of delays in dating and sexual relations compared to a control group of girls with chronic illness (28). Several different authors evaluated the sexual functioning of adult women with this disorder. They usually defined sexual functioning as the ability to have comfortable vaginal intercourse. Research regarding orgasmic capability in CAH women who had surgical correction has rarely been undertaken. One small study that included nine patients who had the surgery as infants found that eight of the nine patients were orgasmic (30). CAH women appear to be less sexually active, with a substantial number not attempting intercourse. Of the ones who have attempted coitus, only 62% in one study were able to have comfortable intercourse (31). When studied as adults, CAH women more often were single and had fewer children than controls. The salt-wasting form of CAH, which leads to more significant virilization compared to the simple virilizing form of CAH, has been associated in some studies with more difficulties establishing intimate relationships and more unhappiness with regard to sex (28). Thus, the major issue of psychological importance to this group of patients appears to be the impact of masculinization on their body image and the effect of the disorder on their sexual functioning as adolescents and adults.

Traditionally, surgical correction of the enlarged clitoris was done early in the child's life, and corrective surgery on the vagina or dilatation to enlarge an inadequately sized vagina was undertaken in the adolescent years. The practice of surgically altering the clitoris, particularly through clitorectomy or excision of sensitive clitoral tissue, has been criticized by intersex adults (24), individuals in the fields of gender studies and ethics (10,32,33), as well as individuals within the medical and surgical community (6–8,30). The impetus for this is related to impairment

of sensitivity and orgasmic ability in women who have surgical correction of the clitoris. As noted, there is a significant lack of data on sexual functioning of these women as adults, yet recommendations for early surgical correction of the enlarged clitoris persist.

Intellectual impairment has not been associated with this condition when affected girls are compared to controls. In fact, prenatal exposure to androgens in these patients may be associated with enhancement in spatial relationships when they are compared to controls (26,34).

Androgen Insensitivity Syndrome

Androgen insensitivity syndrome, or testicular feminizing syndrome as it also is named, is a type of male pseudohermaphroditism due to peripheral unresponsiveness to androgen. The karyotype is 46,XY, testes are present but generally undescended, and there are no müllerian duct structures. These children have female-appearing genitalia if there is CAI; ambiguous genitalia may indicate only partial androgen insensitivity. The initial diagnosis may not be made until they present with amenorrhea in the adolescent years. There is breast development, but pubic and axillary hair is minimal (26).

Research suggests that these young women have a female gender identity and typically feminine gender role behaviors (1,26). Their sexual orientation has been found to be heterosexual for the gender of rearing. This apparently has been true for girls with only partial androgen insensitivity who have some degree of masculinization of their external genitalia.

Increased psychiatric, psychosocial, or cognitive problems have not been reported to be associated with this sexual differentiation disorder (26). This is remarkable in that the issues of prime importance are potentially quite upsetting to an adolescent girl's identity and image of her body. An adolescent girl diagnosed with CAI would learn that she is not only behind her peers in physical development, but she will never have periods, nor will she be able to conceive a child. She also would learn at this time that surgery will be required to remove her potentially carcinogenic gonads, and she will require vaginal dilatation or surgery to have comfortable sexual intercourse. A recent article on long-term psychological evaluation of intersex children did, however, find more evidence of psychiatric problems than had been previously thought (35). Approximately half of the girls who looked completely female at birth (12 of 14 had CAI) exhibited some type of psychopathology, including depression, anxiety disorders, sexual problems, oppositional defiant disorder, and mental retardation (35). One of the eight individuals with partial androgen insensitivity not only had depression and sexual problems, but also showed evidence of a gender identity disorder (35).

Mayer-Rokitansky-Küster-Hauser Syndrome

Congenital absence or abnormal development of the vagina, uterus, and fallopian tubes characterizes this syndrome. Ovaries are present, and the karyotype is 46,XX. The psychological issues faced by girls with this syndrome are much like those noted for girls with androgen insensitivity syndrome: amenorrhea, sterility, and the need for creation of an adequate vagina for sexual intercourse. Major differences, however, are that these girls do not have to come to terms with information regarding a 46,XY karyotype and the presence of testes. They can be expected to have their genetic offspring with oocyte harvest and gestational carriers.

A search of the literature reveals little, if any, information regarding psychopathology in these young women. Surgical correction to create a vagina that can comfortably permit sexual intercourse is the focus of most articles. There are many more articles on techniques of surgery than on long-term follow-up to determine sexual functioning. What information exists about sexual functioning in these young women shows that some are sexually active and have comfortable vaginal in-

tercourse, but a significant percentage are not sexually active. The reasons for the lack of sexual activity are not clear. Many of the women surveyed have required, or will require, repeat surgical procedures to correct stenotic vaginas. Whether physical discomfort or psychological reasons account for the lack of sexual activity is not clear from the existing data.

True Hermaphroditism

True hermaphroditism is a rare condition, defined by the presence of both ovarian and testicular tissue in the same person (13). A combination of ovary, testis, or ovotestis may be present; thus, the physical effects may vary. It may be diagnosed at birth or not until later. Due to the rarity of this condition, most of the information on psychosocial and sexual functioning is in the form of case studies, many of which were reported by Money et al. (36–38).

The majority of psychological issues that have been explored for this group of patients are related to assignment of sex and subsequent gender identity, gender role, and sexual orientation. The numbers are too small to draw any significant conclusions. Reference to the discussion of pseudohermaphroditic syndromes with similar manifestations should help in understanding the psychological impact of this particular disorder.

Turner's Syndrome and Pure Gonadal Dysgenesis

Girls with Turner's syndrome are phenotypically female at birth and generally have a 45,X or 45,X/46,XX mosaic karyotype. It is a syndrome characterized by a failure of gonadal development; in place of ovaries these girls have gonadal streaks. Like the girls with androgen insensitivity syndrome and Mayer-Rokitansky-Küster-Hauser syndrome, they may present with amenorrhea. However, the associated physical features of short stature, webbed neck, digital defects, and cardiac or renal anomalies may lead to diagnosis before puberty. Congenital primary gonadal insufficiency in patients with the physical characteristics of Turner's syndrome but without the chromosomal abnormality has been defined as "pure" gonadal dysgenesis. These girls will need replacement hormone therapy to make up for the lack of estrogen and progesterone normally produced by the ovaries. However, because they have a uterus, treatment with the hormones will permit menstruation to begin. Androgen may be added to enhance sexual desire (13). Hormone therapy, however, may be deferred until later in adolescence in an effort to maximize adult height using growth hormone or a growth-promoting synthetic anabolic steroidal hormone (13). Newer reproductive technologies may permit pregnancy using a donor egg and *in vitro* fertilization.

The issues faced by girls with Turner's syndrome are in some respects similar to, but also different from, those described previously. They have a more lengthy delay in the onset of pubertal development, including menses and breast development. Because girls with this disorder have always looked younger due to their short stature, this is likely to enhance the perception of them as much younger through the important adolescent years. However, they do not have to deal with the prospect of amenorrhea or certain sterility, or the knowledge of a karyotype and gonads associated with the opposite sex.

Systematic research on the psychological, social, and sexual impact of this disorder has been much more extensive than for the other disorders of sexual differentiation discussed. Standardized instruments have been used for assessment, and control groups have been used. Self-image, psychological distress, and social functioning have been evaluated in adolescent girls. Educational, vocational, social, and sexual functioning have been investigated in adult women with gonadal dysgenesis.

Gender identity development and gender role development have been described as typically feminine for children, adolescents, and adults with Turner's syndrome. During childhood and adolescence, the differences between girls with Turner's syndrome and girls with constitutional short stature were all in the direction of more feminine gender role behaviors for the Turner's syndrome girls (39). They had more interest in girls' toys and playing with dolls in a nurturing way. They were less frequently labeled a tomboy and reported less rough-and-tumble play in childhood, along with less physical strength and athletic ability as adolescents. They reported fewer overt expressions of anger in childhood and adolescence. As adults, they continued to report more traditionally feminine behaviors and interests (39).

Girls with Turner's syndrome have repeatedly been shown to have more difficulties with social relationships than their peers. In one recently published study, they had fewer friends, engaged in fewer social activities, and had more behavior problems of the internalizing type compared to normative data (40). Even when compared to controls who also had short stature, girls with Turner's syndrome reported fewer friends and more negative interactions with peers. Peer teasing about general appearance was found to be the most significant factor with regard to self-image and depression in a group of adolescent girls with Turner's syndrome, more significant than dissatisfaction with their height and image of their body in general (41).

Adult women with Turner's syndrome likewise have been reported to have a lower self-concept compared to a normative sample (39,42,43). Research has given somewhat equivocal results concerning psychiatric status and psychopathology among women with Turner's syndrome. Initially these patients were described as emotionally well adjusted, with a personality style characterized by low arousal and high stress tolerance (43). More recent research data using standardized tests and diagnostic criteria from the *Diagnostic and Statistical Manual of Mental Disorders, Fourth Edition (DSM-IV)* found a significant subgroup of women who reported psychiatric problems (predominantly depression) and low self-esteem (43).

Adult psychosocial and sexual functioning of individuals with Turner's syndrome suggest only a fair adjustment. Their social functioning has been reported as adequate in relationship to female friends, but heterosexual contact has been reported to be more limited (43). These women began dating later than their peers and had their first experience with intercourse at a later age. A smaller percentage of women with gonadal dysgenesis have married (1,40) compared to rates for women of similar age. Lower sex drive, reduced orgasmic capacity, and less sexual activity have been described for women with gonadal dysgenesis compared to an age-matched control group (43,44). However, the 24 women in one study who were in a stable partnership at the time they were interviewed were not significantly different from controls on one of the three instruments used to evaluate sexual functioning (44).

ETHICAL ISSUES IN SEXUAL DIFFERENTIATION DISORDERS

There are a number of important ethical issues that confront medical professionals and parents of children with ambiguous genitalia. Conflict may arise regarding the most beneficent or nonmaleficent course of action. Physicians often have advised parents that early surgical intervention is the most beneficent course of action. In their opinion, it would be most harmful to have the parents reject the child because of atypical genitals or to have the child endure potential ridicule and embarrassment in the early childhood years. Impairment of adult sexual functioning, however, has been attributed to this early surgical intervention by a number of intersex individuals who are speaking out about their condition as adults. In their opinion, the surgical intervention to make them look "normal" was not worth the sexual dysfunction they experience as adults. Cheryl Chase, founder of the Intersex Society of North America (ISNA), states, "Nonconsensual surgery cannot erase intersexuality and produce whole males and females; it produces emotionally abused and sexually dysfunctional intersexuals" (24, p. 214).

Surrogate decision making is another ethical issue being considered. Decisions about sex assignment at birth and surgical intervention in infancy do not allow the child or adolescent to have a role in the decision-making process. If surgery were to be postponed until the teenage years, the affected individuals would be able to make the decision themselves about this important issue, thus taking a course that respects the person and permits more autonomy.

Ethical conflicts have arisen for parents and medical professionals when telling the truth about the anomaly has come into conflict with secrecy that is believed to be in the best interest of the child or adolescent. Some adult patients have described feeling so betrayed because of lies by parents or medical specialists that they became alienated from their families and avoided medical care for many years. The diagnosis of androgen insensitivity syndrome in an adolescent girl illustrates the complexity of ethical issues. Because this diagnosis often is made in the adolescent years, there has been a good deal of debate about when and how she should be told about her chromosomal status and the presence of testes (15,23,45,46). Some professionals do not recommend telling patients about this information, at least until they are more mature and in their adult years, because identity and sexuality are such important issues in adolescence (47). Other physicians recommend partial truths, reassuring these patients and their parents that they are genetically female, but just have some "male chromosomal material, and gonads that will need to be removed" (29). Other health professionals and patients have recommended a more open approach to disclosing information. They suggest that it is better to learn the truth in circumstances where physicians and parents are available to provide education and support, rather than risk unplanned disclosure that leaves the individual feeling alienated and betrayed by those she trusted.

Major conflicts have arisen when parents and physicians disagree about the advisability of surgical correction of genital ambiguity.

There has been consideration of whether parental refusal of surgery is grounds for declaring medical neglect or abuse and overriding the parents' decision. This has not come about, because a child has to be in imminent danger of dying for the legal system to consider removing parental rights as surrogate decision makers for their child (48).

RECOMMENDATIONS FOR MANAGEMENT: PSYCHOSOCIAL AND SEXUAL ISSUES

Practical suggestions for management of intersex patients have been made by a number of different authors (7–9,13,29,49,50). The following suggestions are grouped according to the developmental phase of the child's life.

Birth

Because it is not common to have the diagnosis of genital ambiguity made before delivery, supportive interventions should begin with the parents at birth of the child. Parents will need to understand the diagnosis, prognosis, and treatment plan. The rationale for recommendations regarding sex assignment should be carefully explained. Medical professionals will need to be understanding and respectful of parental attitudes, values, and cultural beliefs.

Preschool Age

Parents will likely need continuing education and counseling regarding gender identity and gender role issues for their child. They should be helped to understand what it means to reinforce a consistent gender identity. If their children exhibit atypical gender role behaviors, they may need help in understanding that it does not mean they have failed. Concrete suggestions about what to say to others caring for the child will be needed by parents. Likewise, they will need suggestions about how to prepare their child to be around other children.

School Age

School-age children will need education regarding their condition and supportive counseling. They will need advice on how to manage issues that arise in day-to-day life with peers or siblings. Gender identity and gender role behaviors can be monitored. Medical professionals should be sensitive to the fact that genital examinations may lead to increased anxiety or phobic responses.

Puberty

Children with disorders of sexual differentiation will need preparation for the body changes that occur at puberty, just as their more typical peers do. They will need to know what type of development to expect and whether this will occur naturally or with the use of exogenous hormones. Issues addressed by the medical professional should include the pubertal child's body image, gender identity, and relationships with peers and siblings. Individual counseling or therapy should be offered if it would be of benefit to the child.

Adolescence

The progress of pubertal changes and the individual's adjustment to these changes should be monitored during the adolescent years. Social adjustment, acceptance by the peer group, and interest in dating are all important issues in the adolescent's development. Sex education should help prepare the young person for developing sexuality. Assessment of sexual feelings, attachments, and behaviors will shed light on the individual's sexual orientation. In preparation for sexual relationships, youths may need help in knowing how to inform their sexual partners about the genital anomaly if this is a relevant issue.

Assessment of readiness for vaginoplasty and preparation for the procedure generally take place in the adolescent years. Informed consent should be obtained from the adolescent as well as her parents. Compliance with hormonal therapy and dilatation procedures should be monitored after surgery. If there is noncompliance, the reasons for this should be sought from the adolescent. This is the phase in which parenting, infertility, and newer reproductive technologies can best be discussed with the patient.

CONCLUSION

Children born with sexual differentiation disorders have always presented medical professionals with difficult decisions, particularly at the time of diagnosis. Optimal management requires a team effort, which includes appropriate medical and mental health specialists. Parents require education and support, not just in the neonatal period but throughout the child's early years and adolescence. Likewise, the children need developmentally appropriate ongoing support and counseling from the medical professionals treating them and their parents. Problems may arise in the child's or adolescent's self-image, relationships with peers, and sexual relationships. More research needs to done to determine if children with sexual differentiation disorders have a higher rate of mental health problems than other children with chronic medical problems or other children in general. Mental health intervention is appropriate to monitor the child's and family's adjustment.

Management of children with sexual differentiation disorders has become controversial in recent years. There has been criticism about early surgical intervention and the cultural assumptions about gender that underlie some of the decisions regarding sex assignment. Recommendations have been to assign gender early but to defer surgical intervention when possible until the child or adolescent is older. Parents and medical professionals have the opportunity to see if gender assignment has been appropriate, and the child or adolescent is old enough to participate actively in her care and give assent or consent for treatment.

Much more systematic long-term follow-up needs to be undertaken for children born with sexual differentiation disorders. Outcome should be viewed in terms of appropriateness of gender assignment, social and psychological adaptation during middle childhood and adolescence, and adjustment to adult social and sexual roles.

REFERENCES

1. Money J, Ehrhardt AA. *Man and woman, boy and girl: the differentiation and dimorphism of gender identity from conception to maturity.* Baltimore: The Johns Hopkins Press, 1972.
2. Zucker KJ, Bradley SJ. *Gender identity disorder and psychosexual problems in children and adolescents.* New York: Guilford Press, 1995.
3. Coleman E. Assessment of sexual orientation. In: Coleman E, ed. *Integrated identity for gay men and lesbians.* New York: Harrington Park Press, 1987:9.
4. Meyers-Seifer CH, Charest NJ. Diagnosis and management of patients with ambiguous genitalia. *Semin Perinatol* 1992;16:332.
5. Migeon CJ, Berkovitz GD, Brown TR. Sexual differentiation and ambiguity. In: Kappy MS, Blizzard RM, Migeon CJ, eds. *Diagnosis and treatment of endocrine disorders in childhood and adolescence,* 4th ed. Springfield: Charles C. Thomas Publisher, 1994:573.
6. Schober JM. Early feminizing genitoplasty or watchful waiting. *J Pediatr Adolesc Gynecol* 1998;11:154.
7. Reiner WG. Sex assignment in the neonate with intersex or inadequate genitalia. *Arch Pediatr Adolesc Med* 1997;151:1044.
8. Diamond M, Sigmundson HK. Management of intersexuality. Guidelines for dealing with persons with ambiguous genitalia. *Arch Pediatr Adolesc Med* 1997;151:1046.
9. Meyer-Bahlburg HFL. Gender identity development in intersex patients. *Child Adolesc Psychiatr Clin North Am* 1993;2:501.
10. Kessler SJ. *Lessons from the intersexed.* New Brunswick, NJ: Rutgers University Press, 1998.
11. Marcus DE, Overton WF. The development of cognitive gender constancy and sex role preferences. *Child Dev* 1978;49:434.
12. Goldman R, Goldman J. *Children's sexual thinking.* London, UK: Routledge and Kegan Paul, 1982.
13. Money J. *Sex errors of the body and related syndromes,* 2nd ed. Baltimore: Paul H. Brookes Publishing, 1994.
14. Money J, Lamacz M. Genital examination and exposure experienced as nosocomial sexual abuse in childhood. *J Nerv Ment Dis* 1987;175:713.
15. Groveman S. Letter to editor. *Can Med Assoc J* 1996; 154:1829.
16. Gemelli R. *Normal child and adolescent development.* Washington, DC: American Psychiatric Press, 1996.
17. Elsayed SM, Al-Maghraby M, Hafeiz HB, et al. Psychological aspects of intersex in Saudi patients. *Acta Psychiatr Scand* 1988;77:297.
18. Imperato-McGinley J, Paterson RE, Gautier T. Androgens and the evolution of male gender identity among male pseudohermaphrodites with 5 alpha-reductase defiency. *N Eng J Med* 1979;300:1233–1237.
19. Leigh BC, Morrison DM, Trocki K, et al. Sexual behavior of American adolescents. *J Adolesc Health* 1994; 15:117–125.

20. Grisso T, Vierling L. Minors' consent to treatment: a developmental perspective. *Profess Psychol* 1978;9: 412–427.

21. Weithorn LA. Children's capacities for participation in treatment decision-making. In: Schetky DH, Benedek EP, eds. *Emerging issues in child psychiatry and the law.* New York: Brunner/Mazel, 1985:22–35.

22. Mann L, Harmoni R, Power C. Adolescent decision-making: the development of competence. *J Adolesc* 1989;12:265–278.

23. Kemp BD. Letter to editor. *Can Med Assoc J* 1996;154: 1829.

24. Chase C. Affronting reason. In: Atkins D, ed. *Looking queer: body image and identity in lesbian, bisexual, gay, and transgender communities.* New York: Harrington Park Press, 1998:205.

25. Herdt GH, Davidson J. The Sambia "turnim-man": sociocultural and clinical aspects of gender formation in male pseudohermaphrodites with 5-alpha-reductase deficiency in Papua New Guinea. *Arch Sex Behav* 1988;17:33.

26. McCauley E. Disorders of sexual differentiation and development. Psychological aspects. *Pediatr Clin North Am* 1990;37:1405.

27. Zucker KJ, Bradley SJ, Oliver G, et al. Psychosexual development of women with congenital adrenal hyperplasia. *Hormones Behav* 1996;30:300.

28. Kuhnle U, Bullinger M, Schwarz HP. The quality of life in adult female patients with congenital adrenal hyperplasia: a comprehensive study of the impact of genital malformations and chronic disease on female patients' life. *Eur J Pediatr* 1995;154:708.

29. Money J, Schwartz M, Lewis VG. Adult erotosexual status and fetal hormonal masculinization and demasculinization: 46,XX congenital virilizing adrenal hyperplasia and 46,XY androgen insensitivity syndrome compared. *Psychoneuroendocrinology* 1984;9:405.

30. Newman K, Randolph J, Parson S. Functional results in young women having clitoral reconstruction as infants. *J Pediatr Surg* 1992;27:180.

31. Azziz R, Mulaikal RM, Migeon CJ, et al. Congenital adrenal hyperplasia: long-term results following vaginal reconstruction. *Fertil Steril* 1986;46:1011.

32. Dreger AD. "Ambiguous sex" or ambivalent medicine? Ethical issues in the treatment of intersexuality. *Hastings Center Rep* 1998;28:24.

33. Kessler SJ. The medical construction of gender: case management of intersexed infants. *Signs J Women Cult Soc* 1990;16.

34. Hurtig AL. The psychosocial effects of ambiguous genitalia. *Comp Ther* 1992;18:22.

35. Slijper FME, Drop SLS, Molenaar JC, et al. Long-term psychological evaluation of intersex children. *Arch Sex Behav* 1998;27:125.

36. Money J, Devore H, Norman BF. Gender identity and gender transposition: longitudinal outcome study of 32 male hermaphrodites assigned as girls. *J Sex Marital Ther* 1986;12:165.

37. Money J, Lobato C. Matched pair of siblings concordant for 46,XY hermaphroditism with female sex assignment and discordant for erotosexual outcome. *Psychiatry* 1988;51:65.

38. Money J, Norman BF. Gender identity and gender transposition: longitudinal outcome study of 24 male hermaphrodites assigned as boys. *J Sex Marital Ther* 1987; 13:75.

39. Downey J, Ehrhardt AA, Morishima A, et al. Gender role development in two clinical syndromes: Turner syndrome versus constitutional short stature. *J Am Acad Child Adolesc Psychiatr* 1987;26:566.

40. Siegel PT, Clopper R, Stabler B. The psychological consequences of Turner syndrome and review of the National Cooperative Growth Study psychological substudy. *Pediatrics* 1998;488:102–491.

41. Rickert VI, Hassed SJ, Hendon AE, et al. The effects of peer ridicule on depression and self image among adolescent females with Turner syndrome. *J Adolesc Health* 1996;19:34.

42. Pavlidis K, McCauley E, Sybert VP. Psychosocial and sexual functioning in women with Turner syndrome. *Clin Genet* 1995;47:85.

43. McCauley E, Sybert VP, Ehrhardt AA. Psychosocial adjustment of adult women with Turner syndrome. *Clin Genet* 1986;29:284–290.

44. Raboch J, Kobilkova J, Horejsi J, et al. Sexual development and life of women with gonadal dysgenesis. *J Sex Marital Ther* 1987;13:117.

45. Minogue BP, Taraszewski R. The whole truth and nothing but the truth? *Hastings Center Rep* 1988;Oct/Nov:34.

46. Goodall J. Helping a child to understand her own testicular feminisation. *Lancet* 1991;337:33.

47. Natarajan A. Medical ethics and truth telling in the case of androgen insensitivity syndrome. *Can Med Assoc J* 1996;154:568.

48. Catlin AJ. Ethical commentary of gender reassignment: a complex and provocative modern issue. *Pediatr Nurs* 1998;24:63.

49. Money J. Psychological aspects of disorders of sexual differentiation. In: Carpenter SE, Rock JA, eds. *Pediatric and adolescent gynecology.* New York, Raven Press, 1992:103–116.

50. Money J. Hormones, hormonal anomalies, and psychologic health care. In: Kappy MS, Blizzard RM, Migeon CJ, eds. *Diagnosis and treatment of endocrine disorders in childhood and adolescence,* 4th ed. Springfield: Charles C Thomas Publisher, 1994:1141.

8

Trauma to the Female Perineum

David L. Dudgeon and Enrique R. Grisoni

Accidental trauma to the pediatric female perineum is relatively common and occurs most often in the 4- to 12-year-old age group. Fortunately, most female pediatric external genitalia injuries are superficial and have a relatively low morbidity. However, because of differences in the anatomy of children and adults, relatively innocuous-appearing pediatric perineal trauma can result in significant injury (1). A study of 22 children over a 10-year period demonstrated that these differences make blunt injury, penetrating wounds, and superficial lacerations potentially catastrophic injuries characterized by major hemorrhage, intraperitoneal urinary injury, intestinal viscus injury, or possible rectovaginal fistula (2).

ANATOMY OF THE FEMALE PERINEUM

The female perineum is a diamond-shaped area bounded anteriorly by the symphysis pubis, posteriorly by the coccyx, and laterally by the ischial tuberosities. The perineal region can be divided into two triangular-shaped areas, urogenital and anal, by drawing an imaginary line between the two ischial tuberosities and passing the line anterior to the anus (Fig. 8.1). The urogenital or anterior triangle contains the labia majora, labia minora, the body and glans of the clitoris, and the vaginal orifice (3). The urethral orifice, which also is included, is found in the superior portion of the urogenital triangle. The anal or posterior tri-

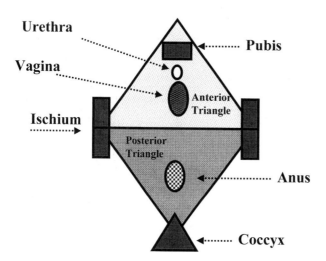

FIG. 8.1. Diagram of the female perineum.

Adult Perineum Pelvis

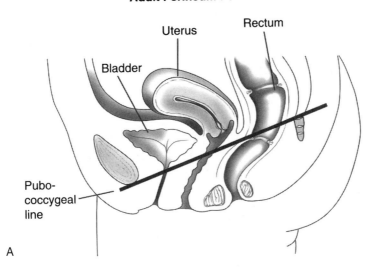

Pediatric Perineum Pelvis

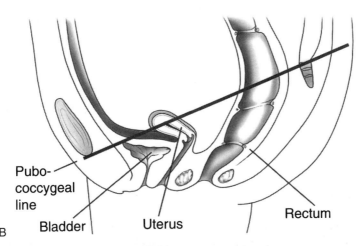

FIG. 8.2. A: Adult perineum pelvis. The bladder, uterus, and rectum are more separated, in an extrapelvic location above the pubococcygeal line, and are less vulnerable to superficial perineal penetrating trauma. **B:** Pediatric perineum pelvis. The bladder, uterus, and rectum are in close proximity, in an intrapelvic location below the pubococcygeal line, and are more vulnerable to superficial penetrating perineal injuries.

angle contains the anal canal and the surrounding area. This area is also termed the ischiorectal fossa. It is important to note that children have a relatively shorter distance between the perineal body and a very thin rectovaginal septum.

Blood supply to the perineum is provided primarily by the internal pudendal artery, which traverses the ischiorectal fossa in the pudendal canal and enters the anterior urogenital triangle. The levator ani and coccygeus muscles surround the terminal portions of the urethra, vagina, and anus and form the pelvic diaphragm. The urogenital diaphragm, spanning the pelvic outlet anteriorly, is formed by the sphincter muscle of the urethra. This region is superficial in children. An understanding of this anatomic structure, their unique differences in children, and the presence and characteristics of perineal trauma will guide management decisions (Fig. 8.2) (4).

ETIOLOGY OF PERINEAL TRAUMA

Injuries to the perineum and lower genital tract occur more commonly than do those of the upper genital organs. Blunt trauma is the most common cause of perineal injury. In the pediatric patient, there are five common mechanisms of injury. They are "straddle" injuries, accidental penetration (including foreign bodies), sexual abuse, tearing or tissue lacerations due to sudden abduction of the lower extremities, and lacerations as a result of a pelvic fracture. Missed or improperly treated female genital injuries can result in hemorrhage, sepsis, and loss of endocrine and reproductive function.

Straddle Injuries

Straddle injuries, described as a forced compression of soft tissues within the perineal region by a hard surface or object, account for approximately 75% of all genital injuries in young girls (5). These injuries often are sports related and can occur as a result of straddling sports or gymnastic equipment, the center bar of a boy's bicycle, or waterskiing equipment. Generally, injuries are minor and include lacerations, hematomas, and abrasions to the highly vascularized perineal region. These lesions may involve the mons, clitoris, urethra, and/or anterior portions of both the labia minora and labia majora.

Hymeneal and vaginal injuries resulting from this form of trauma are extremely rare and more commonly are associated with penetrating mechanisms either unintentional or by sexual assault (5). The resultant trauma can

appear as a small perineal ecchymotic area or a more significant hematoma with painful swelling over the labial area. However, hematuria, urethral trauma, and/or bloody staining of diapers or undergarments may be noted even with an apparently nonpainful periurethral lesion.

Accidental Penetration

Accidental penetration usually is the result of falling on a relatively sharp object. It occurs most frequently in the 2- to 4-year-old age group. Curiosity and self-manipulation with the use of foreign bodies such as pens and pencils are the usual culprits. These lesions can vary in appearance from a punctiform ecchymotic area to an obvious puncture wound with or without associated hemorrhage. The actual site of injury may not be obvious, and the child may present with hematuria, vaginal discharge, or bleeding. Vaginal bleeding in association with consensual sexual intercourse has been reported among adolescents. Bhagat (6) described such a case in which a posterior vaginal wall laceration and hemoperitoneum were found in a 13-year-old presenting with a 4-day history of increasing abdominal pain and rigidity after consensual intercourse.

If microscopic hematuria is present, very careful urethral catheterization is indicated, because forceful insertion efforts against resistance can result in complete disruption of a partial urethral tear. Resistance to the attempted passage of a catheter is an indication for cessation of the catheterization effort and utilization of a voiding cystourethrogram. Gross hematuria requires immediate cystourethrogram without a preceding catheterization effort. A perineal injury also may occur in the child who presents not with a visible puncture site or genitourinary symptom, but with rectal pain or bleeding. As previously noted, the differences in anatomy make an intraperitoneal injury in this situation much more likely in a child (7). Therefore, a thorough abdominal examination, including abdominal roentgenographs, anoscopy, and sigmoidoscopy, must be performed.

Lesions caused by impalement injury, a form of accidental penetrating trauma, can be surgically challenging and potentially life threatening. The extent of injury is dependent on the dimensions of the penetrating object, the patient's weight, the force and direction of the impaled object, and the object's final resting place. Lesions may be simple and require only minimal intervention. However, complex injuries, such as diaphragmatic, lung parenchymal, and duodenal trauma, have been reported with perineal impalement (8). Peritoneal penetration and associated abdominal injuries also have been described with accidental anorectal impalement (9). Patient prognosis is influenced by a variety of factors, including the amount of manipulation of the impaled object before and during transport to a treatment facility, presence and extent of associated lesions, degree of bacterial contamination, and patient's age and physical condition (10). Complex lesions are associated with a high mortality rate, reported between 50% and 75% (11).

Retained vaginal foreign bodies occur most frequently in the 2- to 4-year-old age group. Vaginal discharge, occasionally purulent but usually bloody, is the most common symptom. The patient may have genital pruritus, low-grade fever, abdominal pain, or even symptoms of generalized sepsis (12). Regardless of the apparent paucity of accompanying symptoms or suggestive history, the presence of a persistent vaginal discharge in a toddler or young girl requires a vaginal examination under general anesthesia. Vaginal foreign bodies can vary from a firm wad of toilet paper to small hard objects such as buttons, coins, and toys. An undetected vaginal foreign body can result in peritonitis due to ascent of the purulent secretions proximally into the fallopian tubes (13). Because of their insidious course and, thus, late diagnosis, even a spherical foreign body may be embedded in the vaginal wall and be very difficult to extirpate. Therefore, a careful examination is required after removing the foreign body to detect any residual defect in the vaginal wall.

Sexual Abuse

Recognition of sexual abuse as the source of genital or perineal trauma, except in the case of an unstable physiologic status, demands a modified diagnostic and therapeutic approach and complete documentation of the examiner's diagnostic impression. This is imperative to meet the emotional needs of the patient as well as the legal requirements for successful future prosecution of the perpetrator. Wissow discusses this difficult diagnostic and therapeutic problem in detail in Chapter 28. Unfortunately, sexual abuse is common, with an incidence of approximately 90% in all pediatric female perineal injures reported in one series (14).

Abduction Injuries

Vaginal orifice lacerations can occur as a result of sudden forceful abduction of the legs. The lesion can be produced during gymnastic exercises, while waterskiing, or as a result of major motor vehicular trauma. Pain and bloody vaginal discharge are the most prominent findings. This accidental injury, which frequently can extend posteriorly into the vaginal fornix in a manner very similar to the lesion produced by sexual abuse, usually can be differentiated from forced penetration by the presence or absence of associated injuries and/or a suspicious patient history. The extent of these lesions should be determined by a complete examination under general anesthesia, because severe complications can result from undetected or underestimated injury with incomplete repair. This is more significant if the lesion has rectovaginal septum involvement and/or extension of the laceration into the peritoneal cavity.

Fractures/Perineal Injury

Genitourinary injuries are common with complex pelvic fractures; however, vaginal lacerations are less common and more often reported in adult females. Nevertheless, high-speed, high-impact vehicular injuries, with massive pelvic fractures resulting in bony spicules or hip joint disruption, can produce severe vaginal or combined urogenital lacerations (15). Additionally, fractures of the pubic arch pose a considerable risk for urethral injury (16). These lesions occur in the severely injured patient and must not be overlooked as a source of significant intraabdominal symptoms or signs, including severe hemorrhage (17).

Perineal Trauma/Other Etiologies

An unusual form of accidental penetration is related to a high-pressure liquid injection into the vagina. A vaginal vault laceration due to this injury has been reported in a young girl held over a swimming pool fountain (18). Similar trauma induced by high pressure occurred with a waterslide-related injury (19). Although more commonly associated with straddle injuries, waterskiing cannot be ruled out as a cause in this mechanism of injury. Forceful entry of water into the lower genital tract in this case may contribute to cervical injury, perineal lacerations, tuboovarian abscess, and salpingitis (13).

Clitoral strangulation or ischemia is a rare traumatic lesion reported in infants. It usually is the result of a hair, from a caretaker, accidentally wrapped circumferentially about the base of the organ (7). This is a difficult diagnosis, resulting in symptoms of irritability in association with engorgement and/or cellulitis of the area. Clinical outcome, including possible auto amputation, depends on the degree of ischemia and further emphasizes the need for an early complete perineal examination in all females, regardless of age, who present with symptoms of genital irritation or trauma.

EVALUATION AND MEDICAL MANAGEMENT

Initial resuscitation in any pediatric trauma should begin with the primary survey: stabilization of airway, breathing, circulation, neurologic status, and gross bleeding. A secondary survey should complete the assessment in a head-to-toe fashion, including a complete perineal examination. Performance of the initial resuscitation and assessment must be documented in writing.

Evaluation of blunt perineal injuries must commence with a thorough examination of the perineal area (Fig. 8.3). An examination may be difficult to perform in the young patient, especially if she is in pain. If the patient is neurologically and hemodynamically stable, sedation should always be used to evaluate the perineum. First, attempt to assess the origin of any bleeding site. This can be done by gently retracting the labia and looking for hematomas, gross blood, and feces. The vulvar area must be inspected carefully for external hematoma and lacerations. Similarly, the urethral meatus should be examined. The American Association for the Surgery of Trauma (AAST), Organ Injury Scaling Committee, classified vulva, vaginal, urethral, bladder, and anal-rectal injuries on an ascending scale from I to V (Tables 8.1–8.3) (25–27). Most minor perineal hematomas require conservative management. Specifically, observation and the use of cold compresses during the acute phase (the first 6 hours), with warm sitz baths for symptomatic relief of tenderness during the recovery period. Expanding hematomas of the vulva must be opened and thus require general anesthesia for ligation of bleeding points under direct vision. Fewer complications and a reduced need for transfusions and antibiotics have been reported with this management approach (20).

Superficial vaginal or vulva lacerations, AAST grades I or II, should be debrided and closed using absorbable sutures in either single or multiple layers. However, deep vaginal lacerations, grades III to V, involve the surrounding muscle and fat and often are associated with injuries extending to the anus, rectum, urethra, or bladder. These perforations, evaluated by a complete perineal examination, are managed with preoperative antibiotics, proximal diverting colostomy, presacral drainage, washout of the defunctionalized bowel, and closure of the laceration. Postoperative complications include abscess, os-

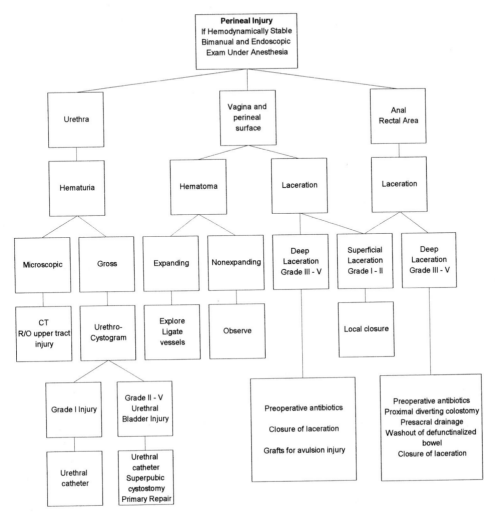

FIG. 8.3. Approach to the patient with perineal trauma.

TABLE 8.1. *AAST organ injury scaling of vulva and vagina*

Grade	Injury description
Vulva injury	
I	Contusion/hematoma
II	Superficial laceration (skin only)
III	Deep laceration (into fat/muscle)
IV	Avulsion (skin/fat/muscle)
V	Injury into adjacent organs (anus, rectum, urethra, bladder)
Vagina injury	
I	Contusion/hematoma
II	Superficial laceration (skin only)
III	Deep laceration (into adjacent fat/muscle)
IV	Laceration-complex into cervix
V	Injury into adjacent organs (anus, rectum, urethra, bladder)

From Moore EF, Jurjovich GJ, Knudson MM, et al. Organ injury scaling. VI: extrahepatic biliary, esophagus, stomach, vulva, vagina, uterus (nonpregnant), uterus (pregnant), fallopian tube, and ovary. *J Trauma* 1995;39:1069, with permission (25).

TABLE 8.2. *AAST organ injury scaling of urologic injury*

Grade	Injury description
Bladder injury	
I Hematoma	Contusion, intramural hematoma
Laceration	Partial thickness
II Laceration	Extraperitoneal bladder wall laceration <2 cm
III Laceration	Extraperitoneal (>2 cm) or intraperitoneal (<2 cm) bladder wall lacerations
IV Laceration	Intraperitoneal bladder wall laceration >2 cm
V Laceration	Intraperitoneal or extraperitoneal bladder wall laceration extending into the bladder neck or ureteral orifice (trigone)
Urethral injury	
I Contusion	Blood at urethral meatus; urethrography normal
II Stretch injury	Elongation of urethra without extravasation on urethrography
III Partial disruption	Extravasation of urethrographic contrast medium at injury site, with contrast visualized in the bladder
IV Complete disruption	Extravasation of urethrographic contrast medium at injury site, without visualization in the bladder; <2 cm of urethral separation
V Complete disruption	Complete transection with >2 cm of urethral separation or extension into the prostate or vagina

From Moore EE, Cogbill TH, Jurjovich GJ, et al. Organ injury scaling. III: chest wall, abdominal vascular, ureter, bladder, and urethra. *J Trauma* 1992;33:337, with permission (26).

teomyelitis, urethral strictures, and vaginal-rectal fistulas (21). Grafts may be required for complete closure of avulsion-type injuries. An injury involving the urogenital diaphragm lends a high index of suspicion for associated pelvic and/or intraabdominal organ injury.

An intravaginal foreign body may be difficult to detect in the small child, especially if it has been present for a prolonged time. The use of sonography and vaginography are useful diagnostic tools (22,23).

Microscopic hematuria in association with vaginal or vulva trauma should be evaluated with a computed tomographic scan. Gross hematuria requires a voiding cystourethrogram and a possible computed tomographic scan.

In the evaluation of perineal trauma, it is important to perform a bimanual examination. In the prepubital female, this can be a rectal/abdominal examination. A complete perineal examination under general anesthesia for a young female includes a vaginal inspection using appropriately sized instruments, such as a small nasal speculum or vaginoscope for visualization in an infant or young girl; cystoscopic examination for suspected bladder perforation; and an anorectoscopic examination for suspected anorectal trauma. A significant penetrating wound with involvement of intraperitoneal organs requires, as noted, an exploratory laparotomy (24). Enteric injury with gross contamination and/or generalized peritonitis will require

TABLE 8.3. *AAST organ injury scaling of rectal injury*

Grade	Injury description
Rectal injury	
I Hematoma	Contusion, or hematoma without devascularization
Laceration	Partial thickness laceration
II Laceration	Laceration <50% of circumference
III Laceration	Laceration ≥50% of circumference
IV Laceration	Full-thickness laceration with extension into the perineum
V Laceration	Devascularized segment

From Moore EE, Cogbill TH, Malangoni MA, et al. Organ injury scaling. II: pancreas, duodenum, small bowel, colon and rectum. *J Trauma* 1990;30:1427, with permission (27).

temporary intestinal bypass stomas. Repair of a bladder perforation, grades III to V, requires either a suprapubic cystostomy or urethral catheter, depending on the location of the bladder injury. Significant urethral injuries determined by voiding cystourethrogram should be primarily repaired and a urethral and/or suprapubic catheter placed for postoperative decompression. A urethral catheter as both a stent and decompressing mechanism can treat less severe urethral injuries or those without disruption.

SUMMARY

In summary, a high index of suspicion is necessary when evaluating trauma to the vulva and vagina in the pediatric age group. Straddle injuries, accidental penetration, sexual abuse, tearing from forced abduction, and lacerations due to pelvic fractures are the five most common mechanisms. Differences in the child's anatomy make more significant injury a distinct possibility. Management should begin with a primary and secondary survey. A decision then should be made about sedation or usually general anesthesia to evaluate the perineum. Finally, the complete evaluation should include assessment of the urethra and rectum, as well as the vagina.

ACKNOWLEDGMENTS

The authors wish to thank Teresa A. Volsko, BS, RRT, Research Coordinator for the Rainbow Pediatric Trauma Center, for assistance with this chapter.

REFERENCES

1. Okur H, Kucikaydin M, Kazez A, et al. Genitourinary tract injuries in girls. *Br J Urol* 1996;78:446.
2. Reinberg O, Yazbeck S. Major perineal trauma in children. *J Pediatr Surg* 1989;24:982.
3. Thotak P. *Anatomy in surgery,* 2nd ed. Philadelphia: JB Lippincott, 1962:544.
4. Propst AM, Thorp JM. Traumatic vulvar hematomas: conservative versus surgical management. *South Med J* 1998;91:144.
5. Dowd MD, Fitamaurice L, Knapp JF, et al. The interpretation of urogenital findings in children with straddle injuries. *J Pediatr Surg* 1994;29:7.
6. Bhagat M. Coital injury presenting in a 13 year old as abdominal pain and vaginal bleeding. *Pediatr Emerg Care* 1996;12:354.
7. Sterioff S Jr, Izant RJ, Persky L. Perineal injuries in children. *J Trauma* 1969;9:56.
8. Grindlinger GA, Vester SR. Transvaginal injury to the duodenum, diaphragm and lung. *J Trauma* 1987;27:575.
9. Jona JZ. Accidental anorectal impalement in children. *Pediatr Emerg Care* 1997;13:40.
10. Kelly IP, Attwood SE, Quilan W, et al. The management of impalement injury. *Injury* 1995;26:191.
11. DeRosa G, Peppas C, Vincenti B, et al. Impalement injuries. A clinical case. *Minerva Chir* 1997;52:143.
12. Pierce EH. Retained vaginal tampon: a unique cause of acute abdomen. *South Med J* 1973;66:640.
13. Grey JJ. A risk of waterskiing for women. *West J Med* 1982;136:169.
14. Herman-Giddens ME, Frothingham TE. Prepubertal female genitalia: examination for evidence of sexual abuse. *Pediatrics* 1987;80:203.
15. Thambi Dorai CR, Boucaut HA, Dewan PA. Urethral injuries in girls with pelvic trauma. *Eur Urol* 1993;24:371.
16. Koraitim MM, Marzouk ME, Atta MA, et al. Risk factors and mechanism of injury in pelvic fractures. *Br J Urol* 1996;77:876.
17. Beck W, Weckbach A. Necrotizing fasciitis after closed pelvic ring fracture. Case report and review of the literature. *Unfallchirurgie* 1993;19:234.
18. Holloway GA. Vaginal vault tear following a high pressure douche. *S Afr Med J* 1987;71:886.
19. Kunkel NC. Vaginal injury from a water slide in a premenarcheal patient. *Pediatr Emerg Care* 1998;14:201.
20. Benrubi G, Newman C, Nuss RC. Vulvar and vaginal hematomas: a retrospective study of conservative verses operative management. *South Med J* 1987;80:991.
21. Maull KI, Sachatello CR, Ernst CB. Deep perineal laceration—an injury frequently associated with open pelvic fractures: a need for aggressive surgical management. *J Trauma* 1977;17:685.
22. Caspi B, Zalel Y, Katz Z, et al. The role of sonography in the detection of vaginal foreign bodies in young girls: the bladder indentation sign. *Pediatr Radiol* 1995;25(1):S60.
23. Wu MH, Huang SC, Lin YS, et al. Intravaginal foreign body retained for a long duration. *Int J Gynaecol Obstet* 1995;50(2):193.
24. Reinburg O, Uazbeck S. Major perineal trauma in children. *J Pediatr Surg* 1989;24:982.
25. Moore EE, Jurjovich GJ, Knudson MM, et al. Organ injury scaling. VI: extrahepatic biliary, esophagus, stomach, vulva, vagina, uterus (nonpregnant), uterus (pregnant), fallopian tube, and ovary. *J Trauma* 1995;39:1069.
26. Moore EE, Cogbill TH, Jurjovich GJ, et al. Organ injury scaling. III: chest wall, abdominal vascular, ureter, bladder, and urethra. *J Trauma* 1992;33:337.
27. Moore EE, Cogbill TH, Malangoni MA, et al. Organ injury scaling. II: pancreas, duodenum, small bowel, colon and rectum. *J Trauma* 1990;30:1427.

9

Vulvar Disease in the Prepubertal Girl

Wilberto Nieves-Neira, Bhagirath Majmudar, and Ira R. Horowitz

During childhood, the vulva is one of the most important anatomic areas examined. Genetic and mutation anomalies as well as tumors frequently are diagnosed after examining the vulvar and urogenital tract. Vulvovaginitis is a common disease during childhood and adolescence, representing more than half of the gynecologic problems seen during these age periods (1).

SEXUALLY TRANSMITTED DISEASES

Vulvovaginal manifestations of sexually transmitted diseases (STDs) are important to recognize in the prepubertal child. These infections may result from sexual abuse or from maternal transmission (2,3). Maternal transmission of STDs is responsible for significant morbidity and mortality in the newborn. In contrast, prepubertal children are more likely to contract the diseases through sexual contact (4,5). Although there has been a decrease in the number of reported cases of gonorrhea and syphilis in the general population and among children ages 10 to 14 years, STDs continue to be a significant public health problem (6). Nonsexual transmission of infections such as gonorrhea, chlamydia trachomatis, herpes genitalis, trichomonas vaginalis, syphilis, chancroid, and granuloma inguinale is an infrequent occurrence (7). In addition to identification of manifestations of the disease, evidence of trauma must be investigated. Attempted intercourse often results in lacerations of the perineum or the anal orifice. As is the case with an adult, if one STD is identified, the patient should be evaluated for coexistent infections. The American Academy of Pediatrics (AAP) Committee on Child Abuse and Neglect has suggested guidelines for STD screening in children being evaluated for suspected sexual abuse (8). Using specific criteria for evaluating children suspected of sexual abuse supports limited STD testing in prepubertal girls (9,10). The psychological impact of STDs and sexual abuse in the child cannot be underestimated and should be handled through a multidisciplinary approach. Several conditions have manifestations that may be mistaken for trauma associated with sexual abuse (11). An awareness of such clinical features is essential to properly guide police and child protection worker intervention.

Gonorrhea

The vulva is covered by stratified squamous epithelium, which is not directly infected by the gonococcus, because the latter primarily invades nonsquamous mucus membrane. The thin premenarchal vaginal epithelium is cuboidal and, therefore, infected by the gonococcus. The associated vaginal discharge commonly results in vulvar skin irritation. Generalized vulvar skin erythema and vaginal discharge are the most common findings (12). Gonorrhea infection may be the result of sexual abuse, but nonvenereal transmission also has been reported (13,14). A positive gram stain is helpful but not diagnostic, as other *Neisseria* species may be present in the vagina. It is important to obtain cultures and sensitivity results for gonococcus before the patient is treated with penicillin. Because of the increased prevalence of resistance to penicillin, the use of a third-generation cephalosporin is recommended. A single intramuscular dose of 125 mg of ceftriaxone is adequate treatment (15). This treatment also may be effective for syphilis, but not for chlamydia trachomatis. A single intramuscular dose of spectinomycin (40 mg/kg for children weighing less than 45 kg, otherwise 2 g) is a safe and efficacious regimen for uncomplicated gonococcal infection in prepubertal children who are penicillin allergic (16). One approach used in the past was the use of intravaginal estrogen suppositories to induce squamous change in the vaginal mucosa. It was observed that gonorrhea can resolve spontaneously at the time of menarche. Thickening of the vaginal epithelium may eliminate the infection and thus the resulting dermatitis. However, it is recommended that a gonorrheal infection, even when silent, should be completely treated with antibiotics because of its potential for pelvic and distant spread. Local vulvar irritation may be treated by cool sitz baths with or without aluminum acetate (Domeboro) powders. The Domeboro powder reduces swelling associated with the infection. The urethra may be irritated. It may be infected directly or through the infection of the urethral mucus glands. In either case, the patient will complain of pain on voiding. The gonococcus rarely produces cystitis and conjunctivitis (Fig. 9.1). Local treatments usually are effective in relieving the discomfort. Distant organ involvement of PID (pelvic inflammatory disease), arthritis, endocarditis, and septicemia should be considered.

Syphilis

Manifestations of syphilis in the vulva of the child may be confusing. In the primary stage, instead of the classic chancre, the lesions frequently are superficial ulcerations, often with striking edema (Fig. 9.2). As in the adult, they are asymptomatic, although for some patients they may cause irritation. In secondary syphilis, condyloma lata can be confused with condyloma acuminata, particularly in the perirectal area where the lesions may be raised and convoluted rather than flat grayish-white coalescing papules (17,18) (Fig. 9.3). Mucous patches that are painless grayish-white erosions occur most commonly in the oropharynx and perirectal area (19). Lymphadenitis usually is present and asymptomatic. Evaluation of preschool children with syphilis is confounded by several factors, including the possibility of congenital disease and problems with recognition of clinical disease (20). Household nonsexual transmission of syphilis from parents with secondary syphilis has been reported (18,21). Diagnosis is based on visualization of treponemas by dark-field microscopy of samples from genital or skin lesions in the primary stage and Warthin-Starry silver stain in condy-

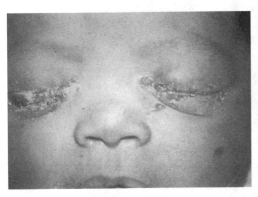

FIG. 9.1. Bilateral purulent conjunctivitis secondary to gonorrheal infection.

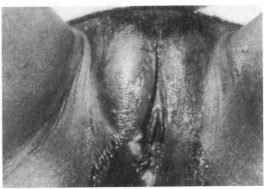

FIG. 9.2. Syphilis in a 14-year-old girl. Vulva and anal orifice. Multiple ulceration with marked edema.

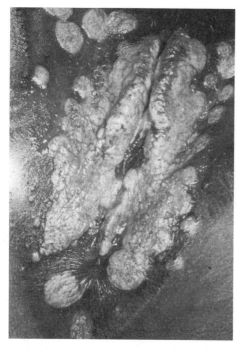

FIG. 9.3. Raised, convoluted, confluent labial and perianal lesions of condyloma lata.

loma lata (Fig. 9.4). Screening by serology is more helpful in the secondary stage and accomplished by nontreponemal tests, which include the Venereal Disease Research Laboratory (VDRL) and the rapid plasma reagin (RPR) tests. Higher titers are indicative of active disease. Specific antitreponemal tests should be performed when necessary. The most commonly used tests are the microhemagglutination assay for antibodies to treponema pallidum (MHA-TP) and the fluorescent treponemal antibody-absorption (FTA-ABS) test (22). Penicillin remains the drug of choice for treatment of syphilis. Benzathine penicillin G in a single intramuscular dose is the treatment for primary and secondary syphilis. The dose is 50,000 U/kg, up to an adult dose of 2.4 million units (23). For latent syphilis of more than 1-year duration, three weekly doses are recommended. In the penicillin-allergic child, erythromycin is an adequate substitute for penicillin.

Congenital syphilis resulting from vertical transmission of *Treponema pallidum* to the newborn is more serious because up to 66% of neonates will have no gross external manifestations of the disease (22). Diagnosis of congenital syphilis often is difficult, and new guidelines were established by the Centers for Disease Control and Prevention in 1989 (24,25). The signs of congenital syphilis are the result of an inflammatory response against *T. pallidum* in multiple organs or tissues. Erythematous maculopapular rash and hepatosplenomegaly are characteristic. Diagno-

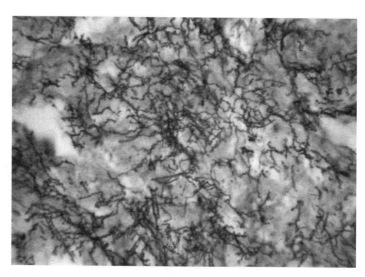

FIG. 9.4. Warthin-Starry stain from a biopsy of condyloma lata showing numerous spirochetes.

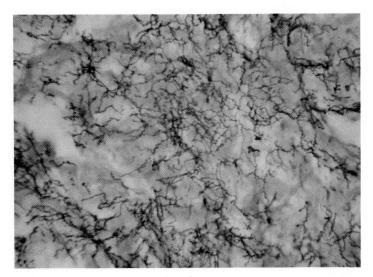

COLOR PLATE 1. Warthin-Starry stain from a biopsy of condyloma lata showing numerous spirochetes.

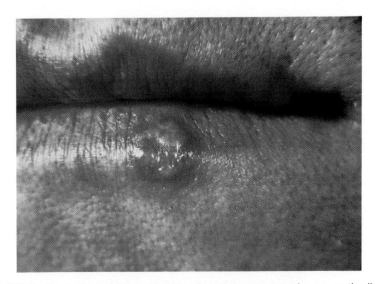

COLOR PLATE 2. Centrally umbilicated lesion of molluscum contagiosum on the lip of a child.

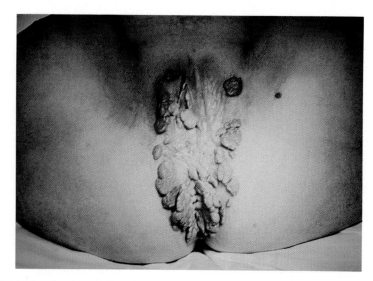

COLOR PLATE 3. Confluent, velvety, verrucous lesions of vulva and anal canal due to condyloma acuminata.

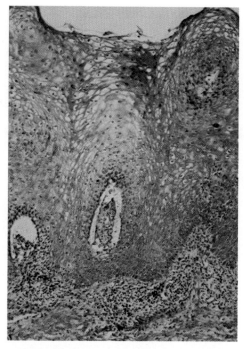

COLOR PLATE 4. Microscopic section of condyloma acuminata showing papillomatosis of the epidermis. Intense inflammation is seen in the upper dermis.

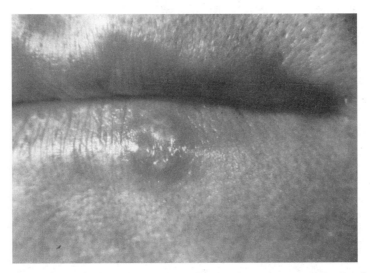

FIG. 9.5. Centrally umbilicated lesion of molluscum contagiosum on the lip of a child.

sis is established by visualization of spirochetes in suspicious lesions, body fluids, or
tissues. As with adults, the RPR or the VDRL
test can be used for diagnostic purposes. Detection of FTA-ABS-[19]S-IgM antibody in the
newborn serum is evidence of congenital infection (22).

Molluscum Contagiosum

Molluscum contagiosum is seen most frequently in children, usually on the face, trunk,
and extremities (Fig. 9.5). Vulvar lesions can
result from autoinoculation from other parts
of the body or from close contact (sexual
or nonsexual) with an affected individual
(26,27). In the child, molluscum produces the
classic, slightly elevated, waxy, 2- to 5-mm diameter nodules with a central umbilication
(Fig. 9.6). The umbilication contains a pulpy
core that can be removed (28). The lesions are
asymptomatic and can be recognized by either
the child or the mother. The diagnosis is confirmed by cytology or biopsy as prominent viral inclusions (molluscum bodies) (Fig. 9.7)
are visualized. The biopsy can be performed

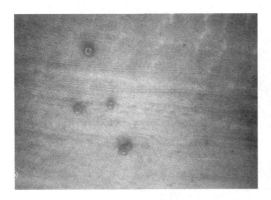

FIG. 9.6. Multiple lesions of molluscum contagiosum with central umbilication. Multiplicity often is secondary to self-inoculation.

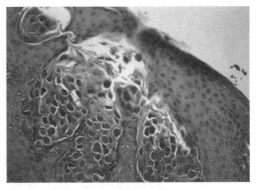

FIG. 9.7. Prominent viral inclusions (molluscum
bodies) seen in the epidermis of a skin biopsy
from molluscum contagiosum.

using a small Keys punch biopsy device with the patient under local anesthesia. Many molluscum infections will resolve spontaneously over a 6- to 12-month period. Cryotherapy with application of liquid nitrogen using a cotton applicator can be performed every 3 weeks until the lesions resolve (27). Curettage of the central core of each lesion with the patient under local anesthesia is effective and provides a surgical pathology specimen. Scratching of the lesions is an important mode of spreading the disease by autoinoculation.

Herpes

Vulvar herpes simplex in the newborn may have been transmitted through the vaginal canal. The appearance of lesions during the first week of life suggests this possibility even if no lesions were demonstrated in the mother (29,30). Herpes seen during childhood strongly suggests transmission by sexual contact (31,32). Vulvar herpes vulvitis may be caused by herpes simplex either type 1 or type 2 (31–34). Sexual abuse seems to be less frequent in children with concomitant oral lesions, but an index of suspicion should always be maintained (34). Herpes simplex infection should be considered in the presence of any vesicular or ulcerative lesion of the genitalia, conjunctiva, or generalized skin (Figs. 9.8–9.9). Infection begins as a cluster of painful vesicles with an erythematous base. The vesicles rupture easily and may leave erosions or ulcerations that may be covered with a yellowish crust (Fig. 9.10). Careful inspection is important in any child complaining of vulvar pain, as sometimes the vesicles may be small. During primary outbreaks, inguinal adenopathy, malaise, fever, and myalgias may be present.

Diagnosis is made on the basis of serology, cultures, or visualization of giant cells on a Tzanck smear (Fig. 9.11). It should be kept in mind that the Tzanck smear is not specific for herpes simplex, as varicella zoster will result in the same cellular changes (35). Topical acyclovir reduces the duration of the outbreak but not the pain (36). For children over 40 kg, an adult dosage of 200 mg four to five times a day has been used with no adverse effects. For primary outbreaks, acyclovir is administered intravenously or orally to a maximum of 80 mg/kg/day in two to five divided doses. Acyclovir, famciclovir, and valacyclovir treatments for recurrence are clinically equivalent; however, only acyclovir is approved by the Food and Drug Administration for use in children (37).

Erythema multiforme is a common childhood consequence of herpes infection (38,39). Reported cases of erythema multi-

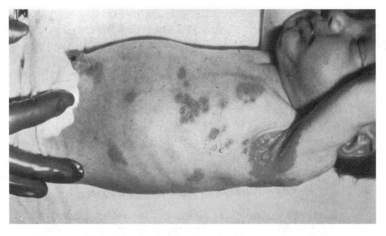

FIG. 9.8. Generalized rash of herpes in a child.

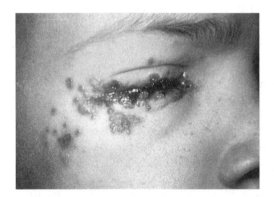

FIG. 9.9. Herpetic conjunctivitis.

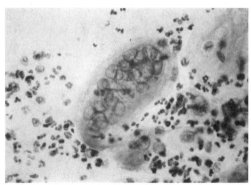

FIG. 9.11. Cytology of herpetic lesion showing a multinucleated giant cell containing molded, ground-glass nuclei.

forme have been associated with herpes labialis or facialis, but not genitalis (40). Recurrences of erythema multiforme could be abrogated by prophylactic acyclovir (40). Vulvar involvement of varicella zoster is a rare condition even in the adult (41). Varicella zoster is seen more frequently in immunocompromised children. Involvement of the third sacral dermatome can cause vulvar lesions. As in the adult, the lesions occur more frequently around the girdle area. Four cases of genital herpes zoster have been reported (35,42). Direct fluorescent antibody testing is a sensitive and specific diagnostic test to differentiate the vesicular rash from herpes simplex 1 or 2 (42). Treatment with acyclovir 1,000 mg/day in divided doses or famciclovir 500 mg/day three times a day is recommended for children who weigh at least 40 kg. Smaller children are treated with acyclovir 20 mg/kg four times a day (37). Chickenpox may produce dramatic manifestations in the vulva

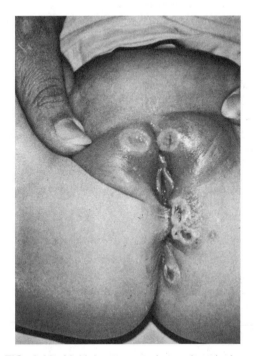

FIG. 9.10. Multiple encrusted, purulent lesions of genital herpes.

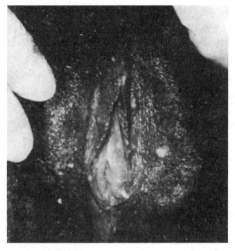

FIG. 9.12. Chickenpox on vulva.

and vagina (Fig. 9.12) (43). Generally vulvar chickenpox is associated with evidence of systemic disease. Antibiotic cream can be applied to avoid superinfection.

Condyloma Acuminata

Human papilloma virus (HPV) causes condyloma acuminatum. Approximately 75 types of HPV have been identified. Anogenital condylomata most often are caused by HPV types 6 and 11, but other types, including 16, 18, 31, 33, 35, 45, and 56, have been identified (44). HPV viral types recovered from genital papillomas in children are the same as those found in the lesions of adults (45,46). HPV type 2, which is associated with cutaneous warts, may result in vulvar lesions typical of condyloma acuminatum (47). The epidemiology of anogenital HPV infection in childhood and the associated condyloma acuminata is not well known. There has been a steady increase in the incidence of childhood condyloma acuminata (48). Between 1940 and 1980, only 19 documented cases of prepubertal condyloma acuminata had been reported in the English literature (49,50). The increasing number of HPV-infected children parallels the adult HPV epidemic that began in the mid-1960s (51). Condylomata can be acquired through sexual contact, vertical transmission at birth, autoinoculation, or nonsexual heteroinoculation (52–55). HPV DNA amplification in amniotic fluid of pregnant patients with cervical HPV has been reported (56). To date there has been one report of congenital condylomata identified in a male neonate (57). Pakarian et al. (58) reported a 55% transmission rate of HPV types 16 and 18 in 31 infants born to mothers with proven HPV 16 and 18 infection before delivery. They also reported a persistence rate of 26% at 6 weeks from delivery (58). Nevertheless, other studies on the presence of HPV DNA in children born to infected mothers reported transmission rates between 1% and 73% (59–62). Using more sensitive techniques,

Rice et al. (63) reported vertical transmission from at least 30% of HPV-infected mothers to their infants and persistence of the virus throughout childhood. In a study of 18 girls with external genital warts, Gutman et al. (64) detected HPV types 6, 11, and 16 DNA in 17 biopsy specimens. Sexual abuse was confirmed in seven of nine girls over 3 years of age (64). On the other hand, subclinical HPV infection has been found to be uncommon in children victims of sexual abuse (65). Rapid progression of condyloma lesions after chickenpox infection has been observed (66). Neonatal HPV infection has been associated with laryngeal papillomatosis seen in prepubescent children (67).

Lesions typically present as multiple 2- to 3-mm papules that resemble flat warts. Even in the presence of larger verrucae, small papules can be visualized after application of acetic acid. The perianal area alone is the most common site of manifestation, followed by the labia (55). The flesh-colored lesions can be difficult to visualize in the hypoestrogenized mucosa. In the vaginal and anal areas, the lesions may be confluent and form a velvety mat around the orifice (Fig. 9.13). Diagnosis can be established by cytology and biopsy done under local anesthesia (Fig. 9.14). HPV DNA testing of clinical samples, including biopsies, vaginal washings, or perineal swabs, is the most sensitive and specific test, but it usually is applied as a research tool. Use of caustic agents including podophyllotoxin is not advocated in children due to poor tolerance of the pain associated with this method. In the past, excision by electrocautery was commonly used and effective. Carbon dioxide laser ablation is one of the more effective treatments for condyloma, with response rates up to 95% (68). Ablation of condylomata with the ultrasonic surgical aspirator provides a sample for pathologic evaluation and is associated with minimal discomfort, rapid healing, and no scarring (69). Because of its oncogenic potential, all patients with HPV infection should be followed on a long-term basis.

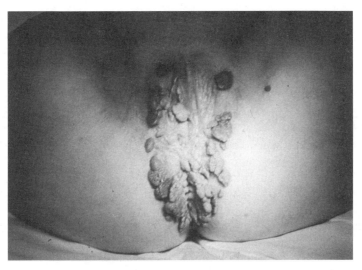

FIG. 9.13. Confluent, velvety, verrucous lesions of vulva and anal canal due to condyloma acuminata.

VULVITIS

Vulvitis is the most common pediatric gynecologic problem and frequently manifests as vulvovaginitis. Prepubertal girls are prone to vulvitis because the anus is physically closer to the vestibule, and the labia lack the fat pads and pubic hair that provide protection after puberty. Poor hygiene habits as well as bizarre genital care practices may contribute to this condition (70). Most cases of vulvitis have no specific identifiable etiology. Bacteriologic studies of the vaginal flora in asymptomatic children and children evaluated for vulvovaginitis found a similar microbiologic pattern (71). Anaerobes such as *Peptococci, Peptostreptococci,* and *Bacteroides* species have been found to be part of the vaginal flora in asymptomatic girls (72), but these organisms as well as yeasts such as *Candida albicans* are significantly more frequent in symptomatic children (71). When evaluating laboratory culture reports, it is important to obtain a colony count of all organisms identified. A pathophysiologic response to an organism commonly is related to inoculum size, particularly in the case of enteric organisms (73). A laboratory report of "normal vaginal

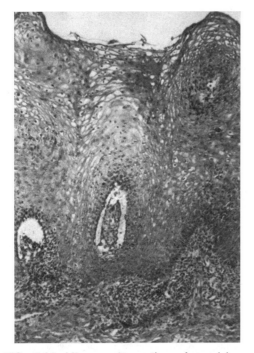

FIG. 9.14. Microscopic section of condyloma acuminata showing papillomatosis of the epidermis. Intense inflammation is seen in the upper dermis.

flora" is inadequate, because it has not been determined what is normal for the prepubertal girl.

Bacterial Vulvitis

Bacterial vulvitis (and vulvovaginitis) is caused most commonly by group A β-hemolytic streptococcus. Vulvar infection can result from autoinoculation from pharyngitis, cutaneous infections, or the gastrointestinal tract, although no recent association with upper respiratory tract infections, tonsillitis, or nasopharyngitis is common (74). Presentation is acute in most cases, with an evolution of several days only. The most common symptoms are dysuria, vaginal discharge, and vulvar pain. On examination, erythema of the vulva or a fiery-red rash resembling cellulitis and vaginal discharge are the most frequent findings. The vaginal discharge is serosanguinous in about half the patients presenting with this finding (75). Other findings include edema, local excoriation, and tenderness. Final diagnosis is made by cultures, which should include proper medium to support the growth of hemolytic streptococcus (5% sheep blood agar with a bacitracin disk) (74). Treatment with penicillin, a cephalosporin, or erythromycin is effective and a response usually is obtained within 24 hours (75).

Group A β-hemolytic streptococcal vulvovaginitis is a well-recognized complication of scarlet fever (76,77). Nowadays scarlet fever is sporadic in nature. A case of coexisting group A streptococcal proctitis and vulvovaginitis, which required 21 days of erythromycin for treatment, was reported (78). Other streptococcal infections may result in significant vulvar disease. *Streptococcus pneumoniae* has been associated with vulvar and intragluteal abscesses (79). Pneumococcus may be isolated from the pharynx and the vagina simultaneously in symptomatic as well as asymptomatic girls (80). Impetigo is a common childhood skin condition caused by staphylococcal or streptococcal organisms. Sources include the mother, other children, or a nosocomial infection. Lesions develop as 1- to 2-mm vesicles that, after eroding, develop a crust and then form vesicles and bullae on the face, extremities, and "diaper area." Treatment includes systemic antibiotics to cover streptococcal and staphylococcal organisms (81).

Other bacterial pathogens have manifested symptoms of vulvovaginitis. Shigella vaginitis may occur alone or may be associated with shigella gastroenteritis (82). The most common presentation is a bloody vaginal discharge and vulvar irritation with inflammation and/or erosion. Chronic vulvovaginitis has been associated with *Shigella flexneri* (83). In areas where shigellosis is endemic, 6% of girls presenting with vulvovaginitis have positive cultures for *S. flexneri*. Interestingly, a low prevalence of shigella in the rectum of patients with shigella vulvovaginitis was found (84). Ampicillin and trimethoprim-sulfamethoxazole are effective antibiotics. Patients with resistant isolates to these antibiotics respond well to nalidixic acid 50 mg/kg/day for 7 days (85). A case of *Yersinia enterocolitica* vulvovaginitis that responded well to trimethoprim-sulfamethoxazole was reported (86). A labial abscess associated with Yersinia infection in household dogs also was reported (86). *Escherichia coli* may be a frequent isolate in girls with vulvovaginitis, suggesting that hygiene and contamination with bowel flora are important factors in the development of the condition (77,87). It usually presents with a purulent vaginal discharge.

Haemophilus influenzae type B has been associated with purulent vulvovaginitis (77, 88). In some populations, *H. influenzae* is the second most common organism identified in girls with vulvovaginitis (89). Autoinoculation is probably an important mode of transmission. Amoxicillin is adequate treatment, with few recurrences. *Mycoplasma* sp have been found to be a cause of vulvovaginitis in children (90). In 1897, Williams (91) reported a case of diphtheria of the vulva, although in his own discussion he acknowledged that the "diphtheritic membrane" was not a justifiable reason to believe that the infection was true diphtheria (91). In the last 30 years, two cases of vulvar diphtheria have been reported (92,93).

Virus-Induced Vulvitis or Ulcerations

Epstein-Barr virus (EBV) may be shed from the genital tract of both males and females (94,95). The uterine cervix is recognized as a site of active viral shedding even in asymptomatic adult females or adolescents (96–98). EBV also has been identified in acetowhite lesions of the vulva (99). The virus has been isolated from genital ulcers (100). Although uncommon, genital ulceration and vulvitis may be a primary manifestation of infectious mononucleosis in children (101,102). This entity was first described by Lipschutz (103). The genital ulceration usually precedes the systemic symptoms of fever, pharyngitis, oral lesions, and cervical adenopathy (104). The ulcerations have a characteristic dark edge, and edema of the vulva is common. A case of necrotizing labial ulcerations was reported in a prepubertal girl (105). The mechanism of acute genital ulceration during EBV infection is unclear.

Vaccinia of the vulva has been reported and is shown in Figs. 9.15–9.16 (106,107). Most cases occur in children and seem to be related to smallpox vaccination, with transmission of the virus by autoinoculation or heteroinocula-

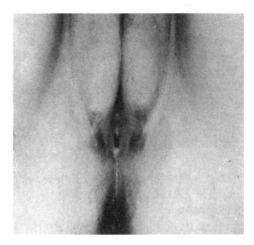

FIG. 9.16. Healing lesions after vaccination.

tion. The most common presentation is vulvar erythema and edema with the presence of characteristic umbilicated vesicles. The last case report of vulvar vaccinia was published in 1980 (108). That same year, the World Health Organization declared the eradication of smallpox throughout the world.

The vulvar manifestations of herpes viruses were addressed earlier in this section.

Pinworms

Enterobius vermicularis (pinworm) should be suspected in girls who present with vulvar and/or perianal itching as the main symptom. Nocturnal exacerbation of the pruritus increases the degree of suspicion. This occurs as the female worm emerges from the anus to deposit the eggs on the external skin. As many as 20% of girls infested with pinworms develop an associated vulvitis (80). Rarely, a female worm may become trapped in the vagina and cause primary vaginitis. Pinworms are a cause of persistent or recurrent vulvovaginitis. Pinworm infestation has been associated with increased incidence of *E. coli* cultures from the introitus and recurrent urinary tract infections (109). Usually there is perianal and vulvar erythema. Because the patient often scratches, vulvar skin abrasions are likely to be present. Diagnosis is based on the direct

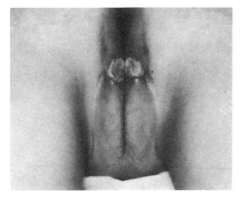

FIG. 9.15. Postvaccination ulcerations on vulva in an 8-year-old girl.

observation of the worm or more commonly its eggs. The Scotch tape test usually is effective in establishing the diagnosis. Stool samples for ova and parasites usually do not detect pinworm ova. The most common treatment is mebendazole as a single 100-mg tablet (80). For patients with vulvovaginitis, a second course of treatment may be advisable to cover any possible eggs in the vaginal introitus. Other regimens include pyrantel pamoate 11 mg/kg up to 1 g or pyrvinium pamoate 5 mg/kg up to 350 mg. Vulvar granulomas secondary to *E. vermicularis* eggs have been reported (110).

Candidiasis and Fungal Infections

Candidiasis is frequent in children but much less than in adults. Contrary to adults, it is most frequently a vulvar disease rather than a vulvovaginitis. *Candida* grow well in the estrogenized mucosa of adults that has a higher content of glycogen. Up to 25% of girls with vulvovaginitis grow *C. albicans* in cultures (71). Candida vulvitis presents as a spectrum of severity, from mild erythema and edema with pruritus to an intense red, macerated, eczematoid dermatitis with pustules. Chronic candidiasis presents with thickened, reddish-brown skin and areas of excoriation (80). Underlying skin disorders, such as atrophy and atopic and seborrheic dermatitis, are likely to present initially as Candida infection. Secondary infection with Candida is common in diaper rash, which is a contact dermatitis. Antecedent use of antibiotics or diabetes mellitus is more common than in adults. Recurrent Candida infections occur in immunocompromised children. Diagnosis can be established by visualization of pseudohyphae in a saline or potassium hydroxide wet smear or by cultures. Treatment involves decreasing the inflammation with local measures such as sitz baths for a day or two. Antifungal agents such as miconazole or clotrimazole creams then are applied for 1 week. In the case of seborrheic dermatitis with secondary candidiasis, hydrocortisone cream can be applied and allowed to dry, followed by nystatin powder.

Pityriasis versicolor is rare before puberty and in the genital area (111). The *Pityrosporum orbiculare* has been reported in the genital area in Afro-Caribbeans (112). Skin scrapings show the mycelia and spora. Topical agents such as clotrimazole are effective treatment.

Vaginal Foreign Bodies

Foreign bodies in the vagina usually produce a purulent or sanguinous discharge that causes significant vulvar irritation. Foreign objects should be considered in cases of persistent or recurrent vulvitis. Frequently the child denies this possibility. In these cases, a crusty erythematous or hyperpigmented line develops along the dependent part of the labia majora (Fig. 9.17). The most common foreign object recovered in prepubertal girls is wads of toilet paper (113). These can appear as gray masses at the vaginal introitus. A case of a vaginal foreign body retained for 20 years since childhood was reported (114). Rectal examination, ultrasonography, and radiographic studies fail to detect most foreign bodies. Initial efforts for removal of a foreign object include vaginal lavage using a 10 to 12 red rubber catheter. Vaginoscopy should be per-

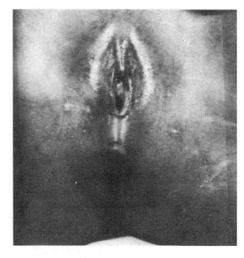

FIG. 9.17. Dermatitis due to a foreign body in vagina and resultant discharge.

formed. Foreign objects have a tendency to become embedded into the vaginal walls as inflammation produces a papillary growth of the mucosa (73).

Local Care of the Vulva in Patients with Vulvitis

In addition to the specific agents mentioned for particular infections, local care of the vulva is important and necessary in the treatment of vulvitis. Bland compresses or sitz baths are usually the initial treatment for vulvitis. Tap water and Burow's (borate) or Domeboro powder solutions are adequate and soothing. For specific cleansing of the vulva, a cotton ball with bland oil can be used. Otherwise, gentle cleansing of the vulva with a mild, nonmedicated, nonperfumed soap should be done two or three times a day. Adequate hygiene after bowel movements is important, and the child should be taught to wipe front to back. Cotton underwear should be used and tight clothing avoided (26).

DERMATOLOGIC CONDITIONS

It is important to recognize the difference between atrophic vulvar mucosa and other dermatologic problems. Atrophic mucosa has a "road map" appearance due to the pattern of capillaries coursing the vulva with an increased density in the vestibular sulcus. Erythema due to inflammation has a uniform redness that occurs most intensely at the medial aspects of the labia majora. The capillaries are not visible due to edema. A hyperpigmented line of demarcation along the medial aspect of the labia majora may be present in chronic vulvitis (73).

Dermatitis

The terms dermatitis and eczema often are used synonymously. There are two main types of dermatitis (115). Exogenous dermatitis (irritant dermatitis, allergic contact dermatitis) is caused by outside agents. Irritant dermatitis is acute in onset. Allergic contact dermatitis is

a delayed cell-mediated reaction and requires preexposure to the offending agent. Endogenous dermatitis (atopic and seborrheic dermatitis) is a skin reaction without environmental stimulus.

Irritant dermatitis is characterized by acute burning on contact with the substance. There is erythema and edema that may last from minutes to hours. Affected skin may appear dry and parched, and fissures may occur. Common irritants include soaps, bubble baths, alcohol, propylene glycol, topical medications, rubber, deodorants, and bromide in swimming pools. The irritant effect of fluorinated hydrocarbon propellants used in deodorants is well known (116). Diaper rash is a type of contact irritant dermatitis of the convex surfaces with the skin creases spared (Fig. 9.18). It is caused by friction, continuous wetness, and continuous exposure to stool and ammonia produced from urine by fecal bacteria. The condition usually begins around 3 months of age and presents as a parchment-like erythema with erosion and vesiculation (117). In cases of severe edema, 1% hydrocortisone cream or, alternatively, cool Domeboro compresses can be applied. A mixture of

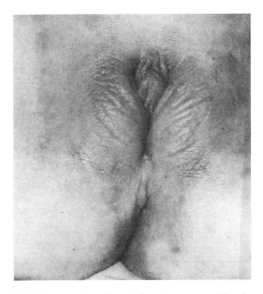

FIG. 9.18. Dermatitis with edema, possibly diaper rash.

cornstarch and zinc oxide usually is very effective treatment. Secondary candidiasis is common with superficial pustules and red satellite papules (118). Miliaria (prickly heat) results from obstruction of the eccrine sweat glands and is the direct result of the hot and humid environment produced by the diaper. In the newborn, miliaria presents as clear, superficial vesicles without inflammation (miliaria crystallina). Small, erythematous papules and pustules are characteristic in older infants (miliaria rubra) (118).

Allergic contact dermatitis usually develops 48 hours after exposure to the offending agent. Lesions are well circumscribed to the area of exposure. Itching, burning, and discomfort are the most common symptoms (115). Mild reactions cause erythematous macules and papules; severe or chronic reactions may cause edema and vesicle or bulla formation (Fig. 9.19). Sometimes it is possible to elicit a history indicating the introduction of the environmental agent. In some cases, an acute irritant vulvitis may be followed by contact dermatitis on reexposure to the specific agent. Lesions may last up to 3 weeks. Definitive treatment is avoidance of the etiologic agent. Multiple allergens have been implicated in vulvar dermatitis, including ethylenediamine, neomycin, clobetasol

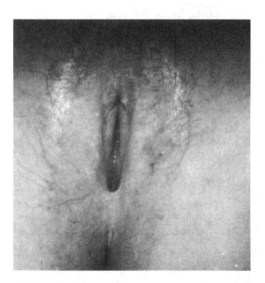

FIG. 9.19. Chronic eczematoid dermatitis.

propionate, local anesthetic preparations used for hemorrhoids, nickel, and rubber (115,119). In the acute phase, local care measures will decrease the inflammation. Topical corticosteroids such as 1% hydrocortisone or 0.05% desonide may accelerate resolution of the condition.

Atopic dermatitis is a hereditary condition with a chronic fluctuating course. Patients characteristically have a history of asthma, allergic rhinitis, or family members with atopic dermatitis. The vulva may be affected in children with a generalized eruption. Vulvar itching is prominent. Examination reveals erythema with dry, papular, scaly skin patches. Similar lesions may be present in the face, neck, trunk, and extremities. Antihistamines are useful in controlling itching, which is important in treating this condition. Pruritus is exacerbated by heat or cold, so baths should be lukewarm. Short-term topical corticosteroids are effective (26).

Seborrheic dermatitis affects 2% to 5% of the population. Vulvar manifestations of seborrhea include erythematous patches, fissures, or simply secondary infection. Usually patients are asymptomatic unless labial fissuring occurs. Fissures characteristically run between the labia majora and minora, extend anterior to the clitoris, and join in the midline (117). Scaling may be present anterior to the clitoris. Diagnosis is aided by identifying erythematous lesions with oily scales and indistinct borders on the scalp, face, and intertriginous areas (120). Candidal or bacterial secondary infections are common. Exacerbating factors include tight clothing, low humidity, and cold temperatures. Treatment with sitz baths or Burow's solution compresses is adequate in combination with an intermittent low-potency topical corticosteroid. Secondary infections are treated with systemic antibiotics or topical antifungals.

INFLAMMATORY DERMATOSES

Lichen Sclerosus

Perhaps the most striking prepubertal vulvar skin disorder is lichen sclerosus. This is a destructive inflammatory condition involving the vulvar, perineal, and/or perianal skin (hourglass or figure-of-eight pattern) in prepubertal and postmenopausal females. Only 6% of patients with lichen sclerosus do not have a genital localization (121). Children constitute 10% to 15% of all cases of lichen sclerosus. Vulvar itching is the most prominent symptom. Intractable itching or burning can occur with minimal findings on examination. Conversely, extensive tissue changes may exist with minimal symptoms. Early lichen sclerosus may be difficult to diagnose due to subtle physical findings. Common presenting symptoms are vulvar itching, bleeding, dysuria, and painful bowel movements (122). Lesions usually begin as white, polygonal macules and papules that coalesce into hypopigmented plaques or opalescent patches (123). A presentation of bleeding may be due to vesicles or bullae that become hemorrhagic (Fig. 9.20). The lesions occur in the genitocrural areas with no involvement of the vagina. In children, cracking of the skin is more extensive. Erosions, bleeding, bruising of the labia, and anal fissures are findings that occur more often than in adults. These presentations may be confused with sexual abuse

(11,124–126). Later changes include atrophy of the labia minora, scarring of the clitoris, narrowing of the introitus, and labial adhesions (Fig. 9.21). Treatment of lichen sclerosus consists of the application of high-potency corticosteroids such as clobetasol propionate. The safety and superior efficacy of clobetasol propionate has been demonstrated (127). In children, the use of betamethasone dipropionate 0.05% ointment for 4 months resulted in complete resolution of vulvar findings in nine of eleven girls who were not responsive to other therapies (128). More recently, other series involving ten girls treated with several ultrapotent topical corticosteroids (0.05% clobetasol, 0.05% betamethasone dipropionate, 0.05% diflorasone diacetate) reported significant symptomatic and clinical improvement after 6 to 8 weeks of treatment. Recurrences in six girls were described as mild and responded to short courses of the topical steroids. No skin atrophy changes were noted on follow-up (129).

The natural history of childhood lichen sclerosus has not been well studied. Ridley (130) reported the persistence for up to 14 years of unequivocal vulvar changes of lichen sclerosus in 36 of 37 girls; however, many of the patients were asymptomatic. Wallace indi-

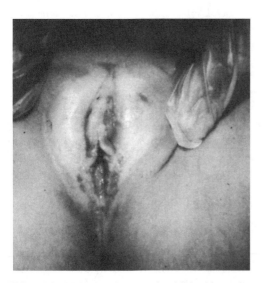

FIG. 9.20. Lichen sclerosus in child with ecchymoses.

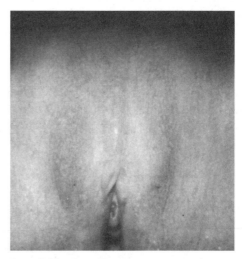

FIG. 9.21. Lichen sclerosus with agglutination of minor folds producing paraphimosis.

cated resolution or marked improvement of symptoms at or around the time of menarche, although subjective improvement was not always accompanied by lessening of objective changes (121). Retrospective studies indicate that 4% of women with lichen sclerosus develop squamous cell carcinoma of the vulva (131). Lichen sclerosus has been found in up to 61% of vulvar squamous cell carcinoma specimens (132). Vulvar squamous carcinoma has been observed in a few adolescents and young adults who had lichen sclerosus during childhood (121,133–134).

Lichen Planus

Lichen planus is rare in children. It can affect the mucous membranes of the mouth and vagina with white patches or erosions and the flexor surfaces of the extremities with shiny pruritic papules. The classic definition of lichen planus includes "five Ps": purplish, pruritic, polygonal papules, and plaques (120). Scaling is faint with surface streaking (Wickham's striae). These are grayish-white, hyperkeratotic striae with a lacy or reticular pattern (26). Extensive desquamation of the vagina may occur in severe cases. Diagnosis is based on biopsy. The course of the disease is unpredictable, with exacerbations and recurrences. Occasionally the condition is self-limited. Topical steroids are the treatment of choice for lichen planus. Vulvitis and erosive vaginitis may be controlled with potent steroid creams (clobetasol propionate) for 1 to 2 weeks followed by gradual tapering of the dosage and then switching to hydrocortisone (120). Antihistamines are indicated to control pruritus.

Lichen Simplex Chronicus

Lichen simplex chronicus (neurodermatitis) is rare in children. It results from constant scratching and rubbing of the skin. Chronic inflammation leads to pruritus and, therefore, an itch-scratch cycle that is difficult to break. The result is lichenified plaques. Excoriations

and fissures are common and may dominate the clinical picture. In the labia, whitening or altered pigmentation as well as hypertrophy and edema are common (115). Treatment consists of topical steroids. Potent corticosteroids (desoximetasone or fluocinonide) are followed by mild ones to decrease inflammation and gradually reduce the hyperkeratosis. It is important to break the itch-scratch cycle with antihistamines, topical lidocaine (Xylocaine), and ice packs (135). Hydrocortisone 1% is excellent maintenance therapy. Localized plaques of the vulva respond well to injected triamcinolone acetonide (120).

Psoriasis

Psoriasis is a hereditary (autosomal dominant) chronic inflammatory skin condition. It affects 1% to 3% of the population (136). A large series showed that around 10% of patients develop psoriasis before the age of 10 years (137). The most common pattern of the disease (psoriasis vulgaris) consists of red plaques with thick silvery-white scales on the scalp, knees, elbows, sacrum, and anogenital areas. Pinpoint sites of bleeding (Auspitz's sign) are seen when adherent scales are removed. Vulvar lesions tend to be less demarcated. The lateral aspects of the labia majora are involved in most cases, usually bilaterally (138). Appearance varies from moist grayish plaques on the labia majora to glossy red plaques without scales in the skin folds (120). Maceration and fissures are common. Psoriasis in infants and toddlers usually presents in the diaper area as the primary manifestation of the disease (118). The plaque's scaling may be absent in the diaper area and in infants is not as thick. Diagnosis may be delayed until the appearance of the more classic lesions in other areas of the body and the occurrence of nail dystrophy and pitting, which may be congenital (139). Genital lesions usually respond well to topical hydrocortisone, which can be used for a long time. When skin changes are severe with fissuring and maceration, short-term use of fluorinated steroid creams is effective and enhances healing.

VESICOBULLOUS DISEASES

Vesicles and bullae are the characteristic lesions for this group of dermatologic conditions. Erosions of mucous membranes and the vulva also are common. Immunobullous diseases are caused by autoimmune reactions to antigens in the epidermis and basal membrane leading to acantholysis and blistering. These are rare in childhood and often are misdiagnosed (140). Diagnosis is based on skin biopsies and direct immunofluorescence (136).

Aphthous ulcers of the oral and genital mucosa are shallow erosions with a grayish-yellow base that vary in size from 1 to 10 mm. The lesions usually are painful. Recurrence of the ulcers is common, followed by resolution within 7 to 10 days (135). Vulvar and oral erosions may be treated with topical steroids. Clobetasol 0.05% cream is effective for vulvar lesions in adults.

Chronic bullous disease of childhood (linear IgA disease) is characterized by linear IgA deposition at the basement membrane zone (141). The condition usually presents by age 10 with bullae on the groin, perineum, and buttocks. Mucosal involvement of the eyes, nose, and vulva occurs in 80% of patients. Clusters of bullae are the most common presentation in the genital area and may be confused with herpes infection or sexual abuse (142). Skin bullae may resemble traumatic burns. Oral sulfapyridine over a period of 1 to 2 years produces remission in over 60% of children (143). Resistant cases require the use of systemic antibiotics.

Childhood cicatricial pemphigoid may be considered a more severe form of linear IgA disease because it has the same immunofluorescence findings (143). The mucosal involvement is extensive. Lesions begin as blisters in the mouth, eyes, nose, and genital area with rapid erosion. Vulvar and ocular scarring are prominent. Anterior fusion of the labia or stenosis of the introitus may occur (142). Treatment is similar to that for linear IgA disease, but remission is rare. Therefore, persistence into adult life is common.

Bullous pemphigoid is a rare occurrence in children but several cases have been reported (144). Childhood bullous pemphigoid is characterized by linear deposition of IgG and C3 at the basement membrane. Pruritus may be a presenting feature, but mucosal lesions may be asymptomatic. Initially the lesions are plaque-like but progress to widespread, tense bullae (141). The spectrum of disease ranges from localized lesions to extensive vulvar scarring (145). Treatment starts with oral prednisone. Dapsone or sulfapyridine can be added. Most children achieve remission within 1 year (141). Vulvar involvement may be the only manifestation of the condition (146,147). Response to topical steroids is good in patients with isolated vulvar lesions (145). More recently, IgG autoantibodies targeting the C-terminus of collagen XVII/BP180 have been described. This finding suggests that localized vulvar pemphigoid of childhood is a variant of bullous pemphigoid (148). However, differentiation between the scarring and the nonscarring course of the disease is not possible with the present diagnostic markers. Cicatricial pemphigoid is another rare condition in children. Scarring of the vulva may be prominent. The condition may be confused with lichen sclerosus (149). Some authors have proposed that cicatricial pemphigoid is a severe form of chronic bullous disease of childhood (143).

Pemphigus vulgaris is extremely rare in childhood. Adult females with pemphigus vulgaris have vulvar involvement (142). Rare cases of pemphigus vulgaris manifesting with oral mucosa and vulvar erosion have been reported in adolescence in association with angiofollicular lymph node hyperplasia (Castleman's disease) (150).

VULVAR MANIFESTATIONS OF SYSTEMIC DISEASE

Behçet's disease is a chronic, recurrent, inflammatory disease of unknown etiology that involves multiple systems and mucous membranes. Diagnosis is based on the presence of oral and genital ulcers and at least two of the following clinical findings: uveitis, cutaneous vasculitis, arthritis, meningoencephalitis, or cutaneous hyperreactivity to minor trauma. Recurrences and exacerbations characterize the disease. Ulcerations usually are painful and often occur on the labia minora. The ulcers usually are less than 1 cm in diameter and have a yellow, necrotic center with peripheral edema (151). Genital ulcerations tend to be less painful than the oral ones. In Behçet's disease with childhood onset, the average time interval between the onset of oral ulcerations and the appearance of genital ulcers is around 9 years (152). Perianal aphthosis appears to be a specific feature of childhood Behçet's disease (153). Manifestations of Behçet's disease are similar in adults and children, but the course of the condition seems to be less severe in children (153,154). Systemic corticosteroids often are needed. Ulcers generally resolve in 1 to 2 weeks but may heal with scar formation. Thalidomide 100 mg/day has been shown to be effective for treating the oral and genital ulcers as well as follicular lesions of Behçet's disease in adults (155). An infant with features of Behçet's disease who did not respond to corticosteroids and cytotoxic agents had marked improvement and resolution of symptoms when treated with thalidomide (156). Sucralfate suspension application to the oral and genital ulcers has been shown to significantly decrease frequency, healing time, and pain (157).

Crohn's disease is a chronic granulomatous disease that primarily affects the terminal ileum and can involve the entire gastrointestinal tract. The skin is the most common site of extraintestinal manifestation. Common genital features of Crohn's disease in women include abscesses, fistulas, ulcers, fissures, and infections of the internal pelvic organs as well as the vulva, vagina, and perineum (158,159). A vulvar lesion may be an extension of an anal lesion or can arise separately (metastatic). Children and adolescents may present vulvar lesions several months before the development of gastrointestinal symptoms (160,161). Initial lesions may present as labial hypertrophy or vulvar swelling (162,163).

Metastatic lesions may present as vulvar swelling or ulcerations (164,165). Perianal manifestation of Crohn's disease is associated with severe, mutilating tissue destruction and is refractory to treatment (166). When the manifestations are limited to the vulva, treatment is oral metronidazole with local symptomatic relieve measures. Topical or systemic corticosteroids may be needed.

HYPOPIGMENTED AND HYPERPIGMENTED LESIONS

Vitiligo is a patchy but complete loss of skin pigmentation due to the absence of melanocytes. Microscopically there is no specific alteration, and on examination the texture of the skin is normal. Pinkish-white to ivory patches are sharply demarcated and may spread and coalesce (Fig. 9.22) (26). The patches of depigmented skin may occur anywhere in the body and are asymptomatic. Vulvar involvement should be assessed carefully. Trauma or irritation may lead to loss of pigmentation in the vulva. Likewise, it should not be confused with lichen sclerosus. There

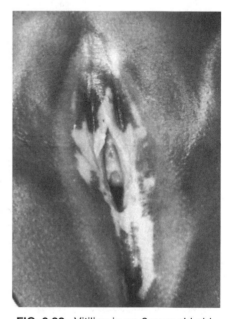

FIG. 9.22. Vitiligo in an 8-year-old girl.

is no specific treatment. Reassurance to the patient and mother should make them aware that no serious problems are associated with vitiligo.

Melanocytic nevi (common moles) occur anywhere on the body, including the vulva. Nevi are caused by nests of melanocytes within the dermis and epidermis. They present as 2- to 5-mm, flat, well-circumscribed, brown or black macules. Compound melanocytic nevi are raised, dome-shaped, brown or skin-colored papules. Lentigenes are flat areas of hyperpigmentation caused by increased numbers of melanocytes in the basalis. Lesions are 1- to 2-mm, brown or brown-black macules on the skin and mucous membranes (135).

An epidermal nevus is a congenital cutaneous anomaly that can occur at any skin site, including the anogenital region. The lesion is characterized by a linear and whorled pattern with a midline demarcation (Blashcko's lines). Epidermal nevi usually are present at birth, but they may not become apparent until childhood. The initial appearance is a smooth, hyperpigmented patch or a rough, skin-colored plaque. With time, epidermal nevi become verrucous and thus may be confused with condylomata. An inflammatory variant may be pruritic and present with unilateral, linear vulvar erosions (167).

OTHER CONGENITAL DISEASES

Hailey-Hailey disease (benign familial pemphigus) is a rare autosomal dominant dermatosis. The disease is characterized by a chronic, recurrent, erosive papular eruption of skin folds, including the groin. Disease severity varies among patients, but typically it waxes and wanes. Darier's disease (keratosis follicularis) is another rare autosomal dominant disorder. Despite the clinical and histologic overlap of both diseases, mutations of different genes are associated with each disorder (168). Darier's disease is seen more commonly in the adult, although it is an inherited condition. Lesions usually are symmetric, keratotic, reddish-brown papules in the seborrheic areas of the body. A localized, unilateral variant has been identified (169). Pruritus is a common symptom. Childhood vulvar lesions associated with Darier's disease are extremely rare (Fig. 9.23) (170). Lesions present as verrucous papules coalescing into plaques in the labia majora and may be confused with genital warts (171). Warty dyskeratoma is a noninherited, isolated, single keratotic nodule typically confined to the head and neck. Histologically, warty dyskeratoma is indistinguishable from Darier's disease. Isolated warty dyskeratoma of the vulva has been observed in the absence of any other skin lesions (172).

Biopsy is needed to establish the diagnosis. Both conditions are extremely difficult to treat. The conventional treatment of both disorders consists of topical or oral corticosteroids and antibiotics to control secondary infection. Long-term remission is difficult to achieve (173). Ablation of lesions with carbon dioxide laser is a useful modality (174). Erbium:YAG laser treatment, which produces

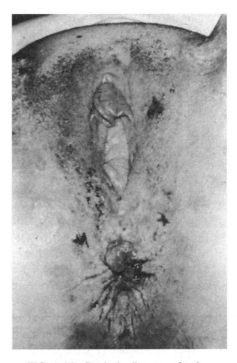

FIG. 9.23. Darier's disease of vulva.

less thermal damage than the CO_2 laser, has been reported to achieve complete remissions (175). Oral and topical use of retinoids has been reported to be a useful modality capable of achieving remission (176–178).

LABIAL ADHESIONS

Agglutination of the labia is a common condition in prepubertal girls. Severe cases of agglutination may be confused with an imperforate hymen or ambiguous genitalia. Agglutination is an acquired condition. A fine line of demarcation between the clitoral hood (prepuce) and the labia minora that runs to the midline under the clitoris is always present (73). In ambiguous genitalia, a normal urethral meatus is identifiable on the floor of the vestibule just anterior to the imperforate hymen. Ambiguous genitalia is discussed in Chapters 5 and 6.

The etiology of labial adhesions is unknown but appears to be the result of a combination of vulvitis and the hypoestrogenic state of the prepubertal girl (179). Most children with agglutination of the labia are asymptomatic and require no treatment. Over 80% of cases of agglutination resolve spontaneously within 1 year. Most patients present between 2 months and 2 years of age, with 90% of cases presenting before age 6 years (180,181). Partial adhesions are common (182).

Patients presenting with urinary tract symptoms such as obstruction or urinary tract infections require therapy. Treatment should be offered if there is marked parental anxiety. Usually parents require considerable reassurance. The treatment of choice is topical estrogen cream applied at bedtime. It is effective in 90% of cases in 2 to 8 weeks (182,183). Separation may be maintained by application of a bland emollient twice a day for 1 to 2 months. Recurrences may be treated in the same way. Conditions responsible for irritation or vulvitis should be addressed. Thin adhesions could be teased apart using a moistened swab after application of

lidocaine gel. Mechanical rupture of the adhesions by applying traction to the labia with the thumbs is not recommended. The resulting raw surfaces may cause reagglutination. Surgery rarely is necessary.

Adhesions may develop between the glans of the clitoris and the prepuce. Patients usually present with this condition until the age of 7 or 8 years. Patients are asymptomatic unless smegma accumulates under the prepuce or inflammation occurs. Spontaneous separation is common and will occur at the time of menarche; therefore, treatment is seldom necessary. When chronic inflammation is a problem, application of estrogen cream at bedtime for several weeks induces separation of the adhesions (26).

TUMOR-LIKE LESIONS

Hemangiomas

Hemangiomas are the result of anomalous development of blood vessels. They are congenital malformations consisting of dilated blood vessels that may cause tumors in the dermis or subcutaneous tissues. Hemangiomas are the most common soft-tissue tumors of infancy, occurring in approximately 5% to 10% of 1-year-old children (184). The female-to-male ratio is 3:1. Hemangiomas may be visible at birth or become apparent in the first few weeks of life. Normally they go through a phase of growth followed by stabilization and even regression over the course of several years. In general, hemangiomas regress at the time of menarche and rarely leave any distortion of the normal architecture. A case of capillary-venous malformation worsening after puberty has been reported (185). Lesions vary from small hemangiomas commonly adjacent to the clitoris (Fig. 9.24) to large vascular dilatations that may develop in the prepuce (Fig. 9.25). Ulceration is the most common complication of hemangiomas. Ulcerations may be extremely painful and are associated with secondary infection, bleeding, and scarring (186). This presentation of vulvar hemangiomas may be confused with

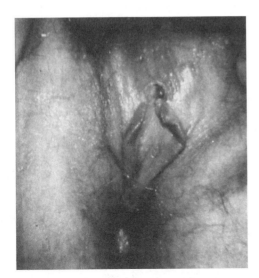

FIG. 9.24. Small periclitorial hemangioma in a 5-year-old girl.

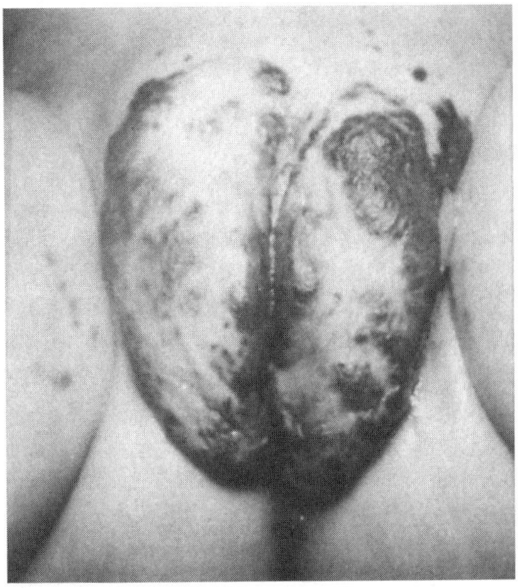

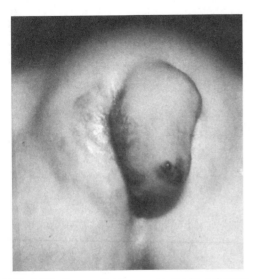

FIG. 9.25. Congenital hemangioma in a 3-year-old girl.

FIG. 9.26. Congenital hemangioma at age 3 years (resolved spontaneously at menarche).

sexual abuse (186). Expectant management should be followed in most cases. Cool sitz baths and Domeboro compresses often relieve local discomfort and edema of larger lesions (Fig. 9.26). Local control measures are sufficient to stop bleeding from capillary heman- giomas. Systemic corticosteroids have become a mainstay in the treatment of hemangiomas (prednisone or prenisolone 2 to 3 mg/kg/day) (184). Approximately one third of hemangiomas exhibit dramatic shrinkage with this therapy. Surgical excision or ablation may treat small hemangiomas that do not regress spontaneously using an argon or Nd:YAG laser (135,187). Cavernous hemangiomas are composed of larger vessels and may result in profuse bleeding if injured. Consumptive coagulopathy may occur, and radiographic embolization may be needed before definitive treatment. Unilateral varices with recurrent bleeding may require ligation of vessels in the inguinal canal as most of the blood supply to the upper external genitalia comes from the pampiniform plexus (170). It should be recognized that the area below the clitoris is supplied by the pudendal vessels.

Cysts

Cysts of the vulva may develop at any age and are of mucinous or mesonephric type. Common inclusion cysts (sebaceous) are rare because secretion of the sebaceous gland in

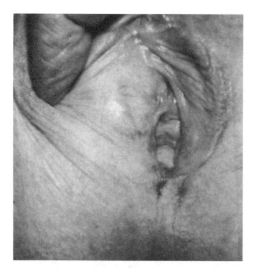

FIG. 9.27. Cyst of minor vestibular gland.

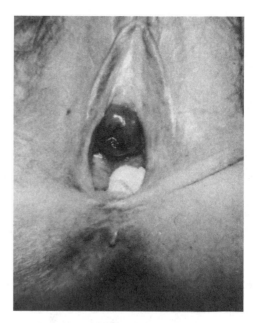

FIG. 9.28. Prolapsed urethral mucosa.

the hair shaft is not occluded. Rarely hair grows before puberty. On rare occasions, the vestibular glands are active and cysts develop (Fig. 9.27). Treatment with simple incision is indicated in symptomatic children or if infection develops (170). Epidermoid cysts are benign inclusion cysts that present as a firm, nodular mass. They usually are asymptomatic and rare in children. Infection or rupture may cause tenderness. Treatment is simple excision with pathologic confirmation (26). These cysts have been associated with ritual female circumcision (188,189).

Periurethral cysts of the newborn frequently are confused with hydromucocolpos or bulging imperforate hymen. Careful probing with a feeding tube reveals patency of the vagina. The cysts are 2 to 4 cm and are a yellowish color. Suburethral cysts may stretch the hymen. Most cysts resolve spontaneously over the first month of life. Excision or drainage is not necessary unless the cysts become symptomatic or infected (73).

Urethral Prolapse

Prolapse of the urethra is a circular eversion of the urethral mucosa protruding through the meatus. It presents as a friable, red-blue annular mass (Fig. 9.28). The mass may be ulcerated, infected, or even gangrenous. Careful examination will reveal the urethral meatus in the center of the mass and the vaginal introitus posterior to it. Visualization of voiding, catheterization, or cystourethroscopic examination may be required for diagnosis (190). The average age of presentation is 5 years. Most patients are African-Americans (191). Onset usually is sudden, and most patients present with painless vaginal bleeding (190,192). Dysuria, urinary frequency, or vulvar pain are other presenting features.

A history of genital trauma or increased abdominal pressure produced by crying, temper tantrums, coughing, or constipation has been associated with the onset of the prolapse. The etiology and pathophysiology remain obscure. Proposed etiologies include neuromuscular disorders, fascial defects, increased width of the urethra, urethral malposition, submucosal weakness, and elastic tissue deficiency (190).

Conservative measures include sitz baths, local care, and systemic antibiotics if infection coexists (193). Topical estrogens and antibiotics have been used. These measures are simple and effective, but the rate of recurrence is as high as 66% (194). Excision of the prolapsed mucosa with approximation of the mucosal edges is the most common approach and has the lowest complication rate (195). Cauterization and cryosurgery are other options for treating urethral prolapse in children (195).

Urethral polyps are a well-known entity in boys. Few cases of urethral polyps in girls have been reported (196). The polyp presents as an interlabial mass and usually arises in the posterior urethra. They may be asymptomatic or present with spotting. Urethral polyps are effectively treated by simple excision and fulguration of the base. No recurrences after excision have been reported.

Urethral caruncles are the most common benign tumors of the female urethra; most occur in postmenopausal women. Several cases of urethral caruncles in prepubertal girls have been reported, including one present at birth (197,198). The most common location for the growth is the posterior lip of the urethral meatus, but other locations have been reported. Urethral caruncles frequently are asymptomatic, but bleeding may be a presenting feature (199). Local care with sitz baths and topical estrogen cream are effective measures (11). Simple surgical resection provides a specimen for pathologic confirmation.

Cervical Prolapse

Cervical prolapse is rare in childhood. The most common presentation is a mass protruding from the vulva in the first few days of life (200,201). Most reported cases are associated with meningomyelocele or other central nervous system anomalies (202). Genital prolapse has been described in preterm infants with no nervous system anomalies (203). Prompt reduction is important. The two most successful management approaches are digital replacements and the use of small pessaries (204). Digital replacement requires multiple reductions (200). A nipple inserted in the vagina can be used as a pessary, or it can be made with a rolled Penrose drain attached to a silk guide string (205,206).

Hymenal Tags

Hymenal tags are seen in 6% to 13% of female neonates (207,208). The tags are smooth, firm, pink nodules protruding from the margin of the hymen. The most common location is the dorsal margin of the hymen near the fourchette. Sometimes, more than one tag is present. Most hymenal tags resolve spontaneously during the first few weeks of life as the maternal estrogen effect wanes (207). By age 3 years, up to 68% of tags have resolved spontaneously but new ones may develop (209,210). No specific treatment is necessary. Persistence should be evaluated by biopsy.

DISORDERS OF SWEAT GLANDS

Eccrine miliaria has been described previously.

Hidradenitis affects the apocrine glands and the primary lesion may be in the follicular epithelium. Onset generally is considered to occur after puberty. Hidradenitis is more prevalent in women. Active genitofemoral lesions are more common in females than in males (211). The breasts and axillae often are involved. Keratinous plugging of the apocrine sweat gland leads to duct dilatation, inflammation, and bacterial infection. Deep inflammation develops with sinuses and bridged scars leading to edema and induration (111). Epithelium-lined sinuses, tracts, and skin contractures favor chronic infections and may lead to significant tissue destruction. Treatment with long-term antibiotics may result in transitory improvements. Recurrences are characteristic. The use of isotretinoin has yielded contradictory results ranging from no response to significant improvements (212, 213). Surgery is reserved for chronic relapsing cases with significant scarring. A case of vulvar hidradenitis suppurativa was described in a 7.8-year-old premenarchal girl who had premature adrenarche (214). Another case of vulvar hidradenitis suppurativa with onset at age 10 years and requiring radical excision and grafting by age 13 years has been described (215).

MISCELLANEOUS PROBLEMS

Vulvar Edema

Edema may develop without an apparent cause. Edema may be transitory and related to constriction of the prepuce. Occasionally, paraphimosis may be associated (Figs. 9.29–9.30) (136). Lymphatic obstruction, temporary or permanent, may produce such a problem. Careful examination should be undertaken to evaluate any possible lymphatic blockage of the inguinal or pelvic area and its underlying cause. Treatment consists of local care with cool Domeboro soaks.

Clitoris Tourniquet Syndrome

Clitoris tourniquet syndrome is produced by clitoral strangulation by hair. Few cases of this condition have been reported in prepubertal girls (216,217). Patients present with an

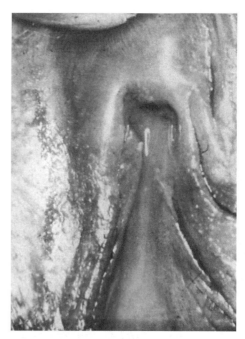

FIG. 9.30. Phimosis and edema of labia minora.

enlarged, erythematous, and extremely tender clitoris. Bleeding and ulceration may occur as the obstruction progresses. The strands of hair may be difficult to visualize because they become embedded in the edematous tissue (218). Therefore, a high index of suspicion is required. Conservative management consists of removing the hair wrapped around the clitoris and local care to reduce the edema.

Female Circumcision

Female circumcision is a traditional or ritual practice that is still widespread in Africa, the Middle East, and southeast Asia. Female circumcision is significantly associated with poverty, illiteracy, and low status of women. In societies that practice female circumcision, the woman who is not circumcised is stigmatized, ostracized, and not sought in marriage (219). Several national and international organizations have opposed all forms of medically unnecessary surgical modification of the female genitalia. Nevertheless, the eradication of a practice based on cultural and traditional patterns that can be traced back for more than

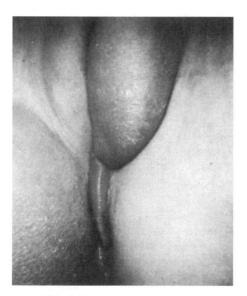

FIG. 9.29. Prepubertal edema.

2,000 years is a difficult and delicate task that requires promoting awareness and education.

Female circumcision usually is performed before adolescence between the ages of 1 week and 14 years. There are several forms of female genital mutilation. The most common procedures performed are (1) removal of the clitoral prepuce, (2) excision of the clitoris, and (3) removal of the clitoris and labia minora. Occasionally, much of the labia majora is removed and the two sides are sutured together to occlude the vagina (infibulation) (220,221). Immediate complications include infection, tetanus, shock due to the violent pain or hemorrhage, and even death. Long-term sequelae include chronic pelvic infections, vulvar abscesses, keloids, sterility, incontinence, obstetric complications, sexual dysfunction, and depression.

REFERENCES

1. Koumantais EE, Hassan EA, Deligeoroglou EK, et al. Vulvovaginitis during childhood and adolescence. *J Pediatr Adolesc Gynecol* 1997;10:39–43.
2. De Jong AR. Sexually transmitted diseases in sexually abused children. *Sex Transm Dis* 1986;13:123–126.
3. Hadlich SF, Kohl PK. Sexually transmitted diseases in children. A practical approach. *Dermatol Clin* 1998; 16:859–861.
4. DeJong AR. Sexually transmitted diseases in children. *Am Fam Physician* 1984;30:185–193.
5. Anderson C. Childhood sexually transmitted diseases: one consequence of sexual abuse. *Public Health Nurs* 195;12:41–46.
6. Waldman HB. Sexually transmitted diseases and children: there is good news, but.... *ASDC J Dent Child* 1998;65:60–64.
7. Neinstein LS, Goldenring J, Carpenter S. Nonsexual transmission of sexually transmitted diseases: an infrequent occurrence. *Pediatrics* 1984;74:67–76.
8. American Academy of Pediatrics Committee on Child Abuse and Neglect. Guidelines for the evaluation of sexual abuse of children. *Pediatrics* 1991;87:254–260.
9. Siegel RM, Schubert CJ, Myers PA, et al. The prevalence of sexually transmitted diseases in children and adolescents evaluated for sexual abuse in Cincinnati: rationale for limited STD testing in prepubertal girls. *Pediatrics* 1995;96:1090–1094.
10. Ingram DL, Everett VD, Flick LAR, et al. Vaginal gonococcal cultures in sexual abuse evaluations: evaluation of selective criteria for preteenaged girls. *Pediatrics* 1997;99:8–16.
11. Bays J, Jenny C. Genital and anal conditions confused with child sexual abuse trauma. *Am J Dis Child* 1990; 144:1319–1322.
12. Frewen TC, Bannatyne RM. Gonococcal vulvovaginitis in prepubertal girls. *Clin Pediatr* 1979;18:491–493.
13. Folland DS, Burke RE, Hinman AR, et al. Gonorrhea in preadolescent children: an inquiry into source of infection and mode of transmission. *Pediatrics* 1977;60: 153.
14. Shore WB, Winkelstein JA. Nonvenereal transmission of gonococcal infections to children. *J Pediatr* 1971; 79:661.
15. Estabrook M. Gonococcal infections. In: Nelson WE, Behrman RE, Kliegman RM, et al., eds. *Nelson's textbook of pediatrics*, 15th ed. Philadelphia: WB Saunders, 1996:771–775.
16. Rettig PJ, Nelson JD, Kusmiesz H. Spectinomycin therapy for gonorrhea in prepubertal children. *Am J Dis Child* 1980;134:354–363.
17. Goldering JM. Secondary syphilis in a prepubertal child. Differentiating condyloma lata from condyloma acuminata. *N Y State J Med* 1989;89:180–181.
18. Ozturk F, Gurses N, Sancak R, et al. Acquired secondary syphilis in a 6-year-old girl with no history of sexual abuse. *Cutis* 1998;62:150–151.
19. Ginsburg CM. Acquired syphilis in prepubertal children. *Pediatr Infect Dis* 1983;2:232–234.
20. Christian CW, Lavele J, Bell LM. Preschoolers with syphilis. *Pediatrics* 1999;103:E4.
21. Rubins S, Janniger CK, Schwartz RA. Congenital and acquired early childhood syphilis. *Cutis* 1995;56: 132–136.
22. Hollier LM, Cox SM. Syphilis. *Semin Perinatol* 1998; 22:323–331.
23. Centers for Disease Control and Prevention. Guidelines for treatment of sexually transmitted diseases. *MMWR Morb Mortal Wkly Rep* 1998;47(RR-1): 1–118.
24. Centers for Disease Control. Congenital syphilis: New York, NY, 1986–1988. *MMWR Morb Mortal Wkly Rep* 1989;38:825–829.
25. Glaser JH. Centers for Disease Control and Prevention guidelines for congenital syphilis. *J Pediatr* 1996;129: 488–490.
26. Williams TS, Callen JP, Owen LG. Vulvar disorders in the prepubertal female. *Pediatr Ann* 1986;15:588–589, 592–601, 604–605.
27. Felman YM, Phil M, Nikitas JA. Genital molluscum contagiosum. *Cutis* 1980;26:28–32.
28. Janniger CK, Schwartz RA. Molluscum contagiosum in children. *Cutis* 1993;52:194–196.
29. Arvin AM, Hensleigh PA, Prober CG. Failure of antepartum maternal cultures to predict the infant's risk of exposure to herpes simplex virus at delivery. *N Engl J Med* 1986;315:796–800.
30. Brown ZA, Vontver LA, Benedetti J, et al. Genital herpes in pregnancy: risk factors associated with recurrences and asymptomatic viral shedding. *Am J Obstet Gynecol* 1985;153:24–30.
31. Kaplan KM, Fleisher GR, Paradise JE, et al. Social relevance of genital herpes simplex in children. *Am J Dis Child* 1984;138:872–874.
32. Gushurst CA. The problem of genital herpes in prepubertal children. *Am J Dis Child* 1985;139:542–544.
33. Hare MJ, Mowla A. Genital herpes virus infection in a prepubertal girl. *Br J Obstet Gynaecol* 1977;84: 141–142.
34. Nahmias AJ, Dowdle WR, Naib ZM, et al. Genital infection with herpes virus hominis types 1 and 2 in children. *Pediatrics* 1968;42:659–666.

35. Boyd M, Jordan S. Unusual presentation of varicella suggestive of child abuse. *Am J Dis Child* 1987;141: 940.

36. Corey L, Nahmias AJ, Guinan ME, et al. A trial of topical acyclovir in genital herpes simplex infection. *N Engl J Med* 1982;306:1313–1319.

37. Grose C, Wiederman J. Generic acyclovir vs famciclovir and valacyclovir. *Pediatr Infect Dis J* 1997;16:838–841.

38. Weston WL. What is erythema multiforme? *Pediatr Ann* 1996;25:106–109.

39. Weston WL, Brice SL, Jester JD, et al. Herpes simplex virus in childhood erythema multiforme. *Pediatrics* 1992;89:32–34.

40. Weston WL, Morelli JG. Herpes simplex virus-associated erythema multiforme in prepubertal children. *Arch Pediatr Adolesc Med* 1997;151:1014–1016.

41. Brown D. Herpes zoster of the vulva. *Clin Obstet Gynecol* 1972;15:1010–1014.

42. Simon HK, Steele DW. Varicella: pediatric genital/rectal vesicular lesions of unclear origin. *Ann Emerg Med* 1995;25:111–114.

43. Paryani SG, Arvin AM. Intrauterine infection with varicella-zoster virus after maternal varicella. *N Engl J Med* 1987;316:1366–1370.

44. Bauer HM, Ting YI, Greer CE, et al. Genital human papillomavirus infection in female university students as determined by a PCR-based method. *JAMA* 1991; 265:472–477.

45. Rock B, Naghashfar Z, Barnett N, et al. Genital tract papillomavirus infection in children. *Arch Dermatol* 1986;122:1129–1124.

46. Gibson PE, Gardner SD, Best SJ. Human papillomaviruses in anogenital warts in children. *J Med Virol* 1990;30:142–145.

47. Obalek S, Misiewicz J, Jablonska S, et al. Childhood condyloma acuminatum: association with genital and cutaneous human papillomaviruses. *Pediatr Dermatol* 1993;10:101–106.

48. Boyd AS. Condyloma acuminata in the pediatric population. *Am J Dis Child* 1990;14:817–824.

49. Grace DA, Ochsner JA, McLain CR, et al. Vulvar condylomata acuminata in prepubertal females. *JAMA* 1967;201:137–138.

50. Stumpf PG. Increasing occurrence of condyloma acuminata in premenarchal children. *Obstet Gynecol* 1980;56:262–264.

51. Frasier LD. Human papillomavirus infections in children. *Pediatr Ann* 1994;23:354–360.

52. Storrs FJ. Spread of condyloma acuminata to infants and children. *Arch Dermatol* 1977;113:1294.

53. Seidel J, Zonana J, Totten E. Condyloma acuminata as a sign of sexual abuse in children. *J Pediatr* 1979;95: 553–554.

54. De Jong AR, Weiss JC, Brent RL. Condyloma acuminata in children. *Am J Dis Child* 1982;136:704–706.

55. Cohen BA, Honig P, Androphy E. Anogenital warts in children. Clinical and virologic evaluation for sexual abuse. *Arch Dermatol* 1990;126:1575–1580.

56. Armsruster-Moraes E, Ioshimoto LM, Leao E, et al. Presence of human papillomavirus in amniotic fluids of pregnant women with cervical lesions. *Gynecol Oncol* 1994;54:152–158.

57. Tang CK, Shermeta DW, Wood C. Congenital condylomata acuminata. *Am J Obstet Gynecol* 1978;131: 912–913.

58. Pakarian F, Kaye J, Cason J, et al. Cancer associated human papillomaviruses: perinatal transmission and persistence. *Br J Obstet Gynaecol* 1994;101:514–517.

59. Smith EM, Johnson SR, Cripe T, et al. Perinatal transmission and maternal risks of human papillomavirus infection. *Cancer Detect Prev* 1995;19:196–205.

60. Puranen M, Yliskoski M, Saarikoski S, et al. Vertical transmission of human papillomavirus from infected mothers to their newborn babies and persistence of the virus in childhood. *Am J Obstet Gynecol* 1996;174: 694–699.

61. Watts DH, Koustky LA, Holmes KK, et al. Low risk of perinatal transmission of human papillomavirus: results from a prospective cohort study. *Am J Obstet Gynecol* 1998;178:365–373.

62. Cason J, Jewers RJ, Kambo PK, et al. Perinatal infection and persistence of human papillomavirus types 16 and 18 in infants. *J Med Virol* 1995;47:209–213.

63. Rice PS, Cason J, Best JM, et al. High risk genital papillomavirus infections are spread vertically. *Rev Med Virol* 1999;9:15–21.

64. Gutman LT, St. Claire KK, Everett VD, et al. Cervical-vaginal and intraanal human papillomavirus infection of young girls with external genital warts. *J Infect Dis* 1994;170:339–344.

65. Siegfried E, Rasnick-Conley SE, Cook S, et al. Human papillomavirus screening in pediatric victims of sexual abuse. *Pediatrics* 1998;101:43–47.

66. Persaud DI, Squires J. Genital papillomavirus infection: clinical progression after varicella infection. *Pediatrics* 1997;100:408–412.

67. Hallden C, Majmudar B. The relationship between juvenile laryngeal papillomatosis and maternal condylomata acuminata. *J Reprod Med* 1986;31:804–807.

68. Davis AJ, Emans SJ. Human papillomavirus infection in the pediatric and adolescent patient. *J Pediatr* 1989; 115:1–9.

69. Smith YR, Isacson C, Namnoum AB. Ultrasonic surgical aspiration to treat genital condyloma acuminata in children. *J Pediatr Adolesc Gynecol* 1996;9:145–147.

70. Herman-Giddens ME, Berson NL. Harmful genital care practices in children. *JAMA* 1989;261:577–579.

71. Gerstner GJ, Grunberger W, Boschitsch E, et al. Vaginal organisms in prepubertal children with and without vulvovaginitis. A vaginoscopic study. *Arch Gynecol* 1982;231:247–252.

72. Hammerschlag MR, Alpert S, Onderdonk AB, et al. Anaerobic microflora of the vagina in children. *Am J Obstet Gynecol* 1978;131:853–856.

73. Pokorny SF. Prepubertal vulvovaginopathies. *Obstet Gynecol Clin North Am* 1992;19:39–58.

74. Schwartz RH, Wientzen RL, Barsanti RG. Vulvovaginitis in prepubertal girls: the importance of group A streptococcus. *South Med J* 1982;75:446–447.

75. Straumanis JP, Bocchini JA. Group A beta-hemolytic streptococcal vulvovaginitis in prepubertal girls: a case report and review of the past twenty years. *Pediatr Infect Dis J* 1990;9:845–848.

76. Hedlund P. Acute vulvovaginitis in streptococcal infections. *Acta Paediatr* 1953;42:388–389.

77. Heller RH, Joseph HM, Davis HJ. Vulvovaginitis in the premenarcheal child. *J Pediatr* 1969;74:370–377.

78. Figueroa-Colon R, Grunow JE, Torres-Pinedo R, et al. Group A streptococcal proctitis and vulvovaginitis in a prepubertal girl. *Pediatr Infect Dis* 1984;3:439–442.

79. Zieguer NJ, Galvano A, Comparato MR, et al. Vulvar abscesses caused by streptococcus pneumonia. *Pediatr Infect Dis J* 1992;11:335–336.

80. Altchek A. Pediatric vulvovaginitis. *J Reprod Med* 1984;29:359–375.

81. Ridley C. Vulvar disease in the pediatric population. *Semin Dermatol* 1996;86:69–75.

82. Murphy TV, Nelson JD. Shigella vaginitis: report of 38 patients and review of the literature. *Pediatrics* 1979; 63:511–516.

83. Davis TC. Chronic vulvovaginitis in children due to Shigella flexneri. *Pediatrics* 1975;56:41–44.

84. Bogaerts J, Lepage P, De Clercq A, et al. Shigella and gonococcal vulvovaginitis in prepubertal central African girls. *Pediatr Infect Dis J* 1992;11:890–892.

85. Watkins S, Quan L. Vulvovaginitis caused by Yersinia enterocolitica. *Pediatr Infect Dis* 1984;3:444–445.

86. Wilson HD, McCormick JB, Feeley BS. Yersinia enterocolitica infection in a 4 month old infant associated with infection in household dogs. *J Pediatr* 1976;89: 767–769.

87. Emans SJ, Goldstein DP. The gynecologic examination of the prepubertal child with vulvovaginitis: use of the knee-chest position. *Pediatrics* 1980;65:758–760.

88. Macfarlane DE, Sharma DP. Haemophilus influenzae and genital tract infections in children. *Acta Paediatr Scand* 1987;76:363–364.

89. Cox RA. Haemophilus influenzae: an underrated cause of vulvovaginitis in young girls. *J Clin Pathol* 1997;50:765–768.

90. Hammerschlag MR, Doraiswamy B, Cox P, et al. Colonization of sexually abused children with genital mycoplasmas. *Sex Transm Dis* 1987;14:23–25.

91. Williams JW. Diphtheria of the vulva. Paper presented at the Clinical Society of Baltimore, 1897.

92. Barabe P, Delpy P, Vedy J, et al. Primary vulvovaginal diphtheria. *Med Trop (Mars)* 1972;32:637–639.

93. Charles V, Charles SX. A case of vulvo-vaginal diphtheria in a girl of seven years. *Indian Pediatr* 1978;15: 257–258.

94. Naher H, Gissman L, Freese UK, et al. Subclinical Epstein-Barr virus infection of both the male and female genital tract—indication for sexual transmission. *J Invest Dermatol* 1992;98:791–793.

95. Sixbey JW, Lemon SM, Pagano JS. A second site for Epstein-Barr virus shedding: the uterine cervix. *Lancet* 1986;2:1122–1124.

96. Taylor Y, Melvin WT, Sewell HF, et al. Prevalence of Epstein-Barr virus in the cervix. *J Clin Pathol* 1994; 47:92–93.

97. Gradilone A, Vercillo R, Napolitano M, et al. Prevalence of human papilloma virus, cytomegalovirus and Epstein-Barr virus in the cervix of healthy women. *J Med Virol* 1996;50:1–4.

98. Andersson-Ellstrom A, Bergstrom T, Svennerholm B, et al. Epstein-Barr virus in the uterine cervix of teenage girls. *Acta Obstet Gynecol Scand* 1997;76:779–783.

99. Voog E, Ricksten A, Lowhagen GB, et al. Demonstration of Epstein-Barr virus DNA in acetowhite lesions of the vulva. *Int J STD AIDS* 1994;5:25–28.

100. Portnay J, Ahronheim GA, Ghibu F, et al. Recovery of Epstein-Barr virus from genital ulcers. *N Engl J Med* 1984;311:966–968.

101. Lampert A, Assier-Bonnet H, Chevallier B, et al. Lipschutz's genital ulceration: a manifestation of Epstein-

Barr virus primary infection. *Br J Dermatol* 1996;135: 663–665.

102. Wilson RW. Genital ulcers and mononucleosis. *Pediatr Infect Dis J* 1993;12:418.

103. Lipschutz B. Ulcus vulvae acutum. *Handbuch der Haut und Geschl* 1927;21:392.

104. Sisson BA, Glick L. Genital ulceration as a presenting manifestation of infectious mononucleosis. *J Pediatr Adolesc Gynecol* 1998;11:185–187.

105. Hudson LB, Perlman SE. Necrotizing genital ulcerations in a premenarcheal female with mononucleosis. *Obstet Gynecol* 1998;92:642–644.

106. Humphrey DC. Localized accidental vaccinia of the vulva. Report of 3 cases and a review of the world literature. *Am J Obstet Gynecol* 1963;86:460–469.

107. Weary PE, Wheeler CE, Lingamfelter CS, et al. Localized accidental vaccinia. *Arch Dermatol* 1960;82: 804–811.

108. Kanra G, Sezer VM, Gurses N, et al. Accidental vaccinia vulva vaginitis. *Cutis* 1980;26:267–268.

109. Kropp KA, Cichocki GA, Bansal NK. Enterobius vermicularis (pinworms), introital bacteriology and recurrent urinary tract infection in children. *J Urol* 1978; 120:480–482.

110. Sun T, Schwartz NS, Sewell C, et al. Enterobius egg granuloma of the vulva and peritoneum: review of the literature. *Am J Trop Med Hyg* 1991;45:249–253.

111. Ridley CM. Vulvar disease in the pediatric population. *Semin Dermatol* 1996;15:29–35.

112. Jelliffe DB, Jacobson FW. The clinical picture of tinea versicolor in negro infants. *J Trop Med Hyg* 1954;57: 290.

113. Pokorny SE. Long-term intravaginal presence of foreign bodies in children. A preliminary study. *J Reprod Med* 1994;39:931–935.

114. Caldwell J, Gastonia NC. Foreign body in the vagina for twenty years. Report of a case. *Am J Obstet Gynecol* 1953;66:899–901.

115. Marren P, Wojnaroswska F. Dermatitis of the vulva. *Semin Dermatol* 1996;15:36–41.

116. Gowdy JM. Feminine deodorant sprays. *N Engl J Med* 1972;287:203.

117. Altchek A. Vulvovaginitis, vulvar skin disease, and pelvic inflammatory disease. *Pediatr Clin North Am* 1981;28:397–432.

118. Jacobs AH. Eruptions in the diaper area. *Pediatr Clin North Am* 1978;25:209–224.

119. Marren P, Wonjnarowska F, Powell S. Allergic contact dermatitis and vulvar dermatoses. *Br J Dermatol* 1992;126:52–56.

120. McKay M. Vulvitis and vulvovaginitis: cutaneous considerations. *Am J Obstet Gynecol* 1991;165:1176–1182.

121. Wallace HJ. Lichen sclerosus et atrophicus. *Trans St John's Hosp Dermatol Soc* 1971;57:9–30.

122. Loenig-Baucke V. Lichen sclerosus et atrophicus in children. *Am J Dis Child* 1991;145:1058–1061.

123. Barclay DL, Macey HB, Reed RJ. Lichen sclerosus et atrophicus of the vulva in children. A review and report of 5 cases. *Obstet Gynecol* 1966;27:637–642.

124. Jenny C, Kirby P, Fuquay D. Genital lichen sclerosus mistaken for child sexual abuse. *Pediatrics* 1981;83: 597–599.

125. Handfield-Jones SE, Hinde FRJ, Kennedy CTC. Lichen sclerosus et atrophicus in children misdiagnosed as sexual abuse. *Br Med J* 1987;294:1404–1405.

126. Young SJ, Wells DL, Ogden EJ. Lichen sclerosus, genital trauma and child sexual abuse. *Aust Fam Phys* 1993;22:729, 732–733.

127. Bracco GL, Carli P, Sonni L. Clinical and histological effects of topical treatments of vulvar lichen sclerosus. *J Reprod Med* 1993;38:37–40.

128. Fischer G, Rogers M. Treatment of childhood vulvar lichen sclerosus with potent topical corticosteroids. *Pediatr Dermatol* 1997;14:235–238.

129. Garzon MC, Paller AS. Ultrapotent topical corticosteroid treatment of childhood genital lichen sclerosus. *Arch Dermatol* 1999;135:525–528.

130. Ridley CM. Genital lichen sclerosus (lichen sclerosus et atrophicus) in childhood and adolescence. *J R Soc Med* 1993;86:69–75.

131. Ridley CM. Lichen sclerosus: a review. *Eur J Dermatol* 1994;4:99–105.

132. Leibowitch M. Lichen sclerosus. *Semin Dermatol* 1996;15:42–46.

133. Cario GM, House MJ, Paradinas FJ. Squamous cell carcinoma of the vulva in association with mixed vulvar dystrophy in an 18-year-old girl. Case report. *Br J Obstet Gynaecol* 1984;91:87–90.

134. Pelisse M. Lichen sclereux. *Ann Dermatol Venereol* 1987;114:411–419.

135. Fivozinsky KB, Laufer MR. Vulvar disorders in prepubertal girls. A literature review. *J Reprod Med* 1998; 43:763–773.

136. Howard R, Tsuchiya A. Adult skin disease in the pediatric patient. *Dermatol Clin* 1998;16:593–608.

137. Farber EM, Nall ML. Natural history of psoriasis in 5,600 patients. *Dermatologica* 1974;148:1–18.

138. Weinrauch L, Katz M. Psoriasis vulgaris of labium majus. *Cutis* 1986;38:333–334.

139. Farber EM, Jacobs AH. Infantile psoriasis. *Am J Dis Child* 1977;131:1266–1269.

140. Weston WL, Morelli JG, Huff JC. Misdiagnosis, treatments and outcomes in the immunobullous diseases in children. *Pediatr Dermatol* 1997;14:264–272.

141. Nemeth AJ, Klein AD, Gould EW, et al. Childhood bullous pemphigoid. *Arch Dermatol* 1991;1127:378–386.

142. Marren P, Wojnarowska F, Venning V, et al. Vulvar involvement in autoimmune bullous diseases. *J Reprod Med* 1993;38:101–107.

143. Wojnarowska F, Marsden RA, Bhogal B, et al. Chronic bullous disease of childhood, childhood cicatricial pemphigoid and linear IgA disease of adults. A comparative study demonstrating clinical and immunopathologic overlap. *J Am Acad Dermatol* 1988;19:792–805.

144. Edwards S, Wakelin SH, Wojnarowska F, et al. Bullous pemphigoid and epidermolysis bullosa acquisita: presentation, prognosis, and immunopathology in 11 children. *Pediatr Dermatol* 1998;15:184–190.

145. Farrell AM, Kirstschig G, Dalziel KL, et al. Childhood vulval pemphigoid: a clinical and immunopathological study of five patients. *Br J Dermatol* 1999;140:308–312.

146. DeCastro P, Jorizzo JL, Rajaram S, et al. Localized vulvar pemphigoid in a child. *Pediatr Dermatol* 1985; 2:302–307.

147. Guenther LC, Shum D. Localized childhood vulvar pemphigoid. *J Am Acad Dermatol* 1990;22:762–764.

148. Schumann H, Amann U, Tasanen K, et al. A child with localized vulval pemphigoid and IgG autoantibodies targeting the C-terminus of collagen XVII/BP180. *Br J Dermatol* 1999;140:1133–1138.

149. Marren P, Walkden V, Mallon E, et al. Vulval cicatricial

150. Coulson IH, Cook MG, Bruton J, et al. Atypical pemphigus vulgaris associated with angio-follicular lymph node hyperplasia (Castleman's disease). *Clin Exp Dermatol* 1986;11:656–663.

pemphigoid may mimic lichen sclerosus. *Br J Dermatol* 1996;134:522–524.

151. Mundy TM, Miller JJ. Behçet's disease presenting as chronic aphthous stomatitis in a child. *Pediatrics* 1978;62:205–208.

152. Kim DK, Chang SN, Bang D, et al. Clinical analysis of 40 cases of childhood-onset Behçet's disease. *Pediatr Dermatol* 1994;11:95–101.

153. Kone-Paut I, Yurdakul S, Bahabri SA, et al. Clinical features of Behçet's disease in children: an international collaborative study of 86 cases. *J Pediatr* 1998;132:721–725.

154. Krause I, Uziel Y, Guedj D, et al. Childhood Behçet's disease: clinical features and comparison with adult-onset disease. *Rheumatology* 1999;38:457–462.

155. Hamuryudan V, Mat C, Saip S, et al. Thalidomide in the treatment of the mucocutaneous lesions of the Behçet syndrome. A randomized, double-blind, placebo-controlled trial. *Ann Intern Med* 1998;128:443–450.

156. Shjek LP, Lee YS, Lee BW, et al. Thalidomide responsiveness in an infant with Behçet's syndrome. *Pediatrics* 1999;103:1295–1297.

157. Alpsoy E, Er H, Durusoy C, et al. The use of sucralfate suspension in the treatment of oral and genital ulceration of Behçet disease: a randomized, placebo-controlled, double-blind study. *Arch Dermatol* 1999;135: 529–532.

158. Donaldson LB. Crohn's disease: "its gynecologic aspect." *Am J Obstet Gynecol* 1978;131:196–202.

159. Vettraino IM, Merritt DF. Crohn's disease of the vulva. *Am J Dermatopathol* 1995;17:410–413.

160. Lally M, Orenstein SR, Cohen BA. Crohn's disease of the vulva in an 8 year old girl. *Pediatr Dermatol* 1988; 5:103–106.

161. Wallis SM, Walker-Smith J. An unusual case of Crohn's disease in a West Indian child. *Acta Pediatr Scand* 1976;65:749–751.

162. Werlin SL, Esterly NB, Oechler H. Crohn's disease presenting as unilateral labial hypertrophy. *J Am Acad Dermatol* 1992;27:893–895.

163. Tuffnell D, Buchan PC. Crohn's disease of the vulva in childhood. *Br J Clin Pract* 1991;45:159–160.

164. Kim NI, Eom JY, Sim WY, et al. Crohn's disease of the vulva. *J Am Acad Dermatol* 1992;27:764–765.

165. Schrodt BJ, Callen JP. Metastatic Crohn's disease presenting as chronic perivulvar and perirectal ulcerations in an adolescent patient. *Pediatrics* 1999;103:500–502.

166. Tolia V. Perianal Crohn's disease in children and adolescents. *Am J Gastroenterol* 1996;91:922–926.

167. Siegfried EC, Frasier LD. Anogenital skin diseases of childhood. *Pediatr Ann* 1997;26:321–331.

168. Welsh SA, Ikeda S, Peluso AM, et al. Hailey-Hailey disease is not allelic to Darier's disease. *J Invest Dermatol* 1994;102:992–993.

169. O'Malley MP, Haake A, Goldsmith L, et al. Localized Darier disease. Implications for genetic studies. *Arch Dermatol* 1997;133:1134–1138.

170. Woodruff JD. Vulvar disease in the prepubertal child. In: Carpenter SE, Rock JA, eds. *Pediatric and adolescent gynecology*. New York: Raven Press, 1992: 127–128, 134–135.

171. Salopek TG, Krol A, Jimbow K. Case report of Darier

disease localized to the vulva in a 5-year-old girl. *Pediatr Dermatol* 1993;10:146–148.

172. Duray PH, Merino MJ, Axiotis C. Warty dyskeratoma of the vulva. *Int J Gynecol Pathol* 1983;2:286–293.

173. Burge SM, Wilkinson JD. Darier-White disease: a review of the clinical features in 163 patients. *J Am Acad Dermatol* 1992;27:40–50.

174. Touma DJ, Krauss M, Feingold DS, et al. Benign familial pemphigus (Hailey-Hailey disease). Treatment with the pulsed carbon dioxide laser. *Dermatol Surg* 1998;24:1411–1414.

175. Beier C, Kaufmann R. Efficacy of erbium:YAG laser ablation in Darier disease and Hailey-Hailey disease. *Arch Dermatol* 1999;135:423–427.

176. Hunt MJ, Salisbury EL, Painter DM, et al. Vesiculobullous Hailey-Hailey disease: successful treatment with oral retinoids. *Aust J Dermatol* 1996;37:196–198.

177. Burge S. Management of Darier's disease. *Clin Exp Dermatol* 1999;24:53–56.

178. English JC 3rd, Browne J, Halbach DP. Effective treatment of localized Darier's disease with adapalene 0.1% gel. *Cutis* 1999;63:227–230.

179. Bowles HE, Childs LS. Synechias of vulva in small children. *Am J Dis Child* 1943;66:258–263.

180. Christensen EH, Oster J. Adhesions of labia minora (synechiae vulvae) in childhood. *Acta Paediatr Scand* 1971;60:709–715.

181. Capraro VJ, Greenberg F, Greenberg H. Adhesions of the labia minora. *Obstet Gynecol* 1972;39:65–69.

182. Khanam W, Chogtu L, Mir Z, et al. Adhesions of the labia minora—a study of 75 cases. *Obstet Gynecol Surv* 1978;3:364–365.

183. Aribarg A. Topical oestrogen therapy for labial adhesions in children. *Br J Obstet Gynaecol* 1975;82:424–425.

184. Drolet BA, Esterly NB, Frieden IJ. Hemangiomas in children. *N Engl J Med* 1999;341:173–181.

185. Kempinaire A, De Raeve L, Roseeuw D, et al. Capillary-venous malformation in the labia majora in a 12-year-old girl. *Dermatology* 1997;194:405–407.

186. Levin AV, Selbst SM. Vulvar hemangioma simulating child abuse. *Clin Pediatr (Phila)* 1988;27:213–215.

187. Preeyanont P, Nimsakul N. The Nd:YAG laser treatment of hemangioma. *J Clin Laser Med Surg* 1994;12:225–229.

188. Ofodile FA, Oluwasanmi JO. Post-circumcision epidermoid inclusion cysts of the clitoris. *Plast Reconstr Surg* 1979;63:485–486.

189. Onuigbo WI. Vulval epidermoid cysts in the Igbos of Nigeria. *Arch Dermatol* 1976;112:1405–1406.

190. Richardson DA, Hajj SN, Herbst AL. Medical treatment of urethral prolapse in children. *Obstet Gynecol* 1982;59:69–74.

191. Capraro VJ, Bayonet-River NP, Magoss I. Vulvar tumor in children due to prolapse of urethral mucosa. *Am J Obstet Gynecol* 1970;108:572–575.

192. Venable DD, Markland C. Urethral prolapse in girls. *South Med J* 1982;75:951–953, 958.

193. Redman JF. Conservative management of urethral prolapse in female children. *Urology* 1982;19:505–506.

194. Jerkins GR, Verheeck K, Noe HN. Treatment of girls with urethral prolapse. *J Urol* 1984;132:732–733.

195. Adducci JE. Cryosurgical treatment of urethral prolapse. *Minn Med* 1981;64:769–770.

196. Klee LW, Rink RC, Gleason PE, et al. Urethral polyp presenting as interlabial mass in young girls. *Urology* 1993;41:132–133.

197. Kim KK, Sin DY, Park HW. Urethral caruncle occurring in a young girl. A case report. *J Korean Med Sci* 1993;8:160–161.

198. Jarvi OH, Marin S, deBoer WGRM. Further studies of intestinal heterotopia in urethral caruncle. *Acta Pathol Microbiol Immunol Scand Sect (A)* 1984;92:469–474.

199. Turkeri L, Simsek F, Akdas A. Urethral caruncle in an unusual location occurring in prepubertal girl. *Eur Urol* 1989;16:153–154.

200. Bayatpour M, McCann J, Harris T, et al. Neonatal genital prolapse. *Pediatrics* 1992;90:465–466.

201. Ellis JB, Boes EG. Genital prolapse in the neonate. A case report. *S Afr Med J* 1986;69:836.

202. Shuwarger D, Young RL. Management of neonatal genital prolapse: case reports and historic review. *Obstet Gynecol* 1985;66:61S–63S.

203. Bader D, Davidovitch M, Berger A. Genital prolapse in a preterm female infant. *J Perinatol* 1993;13:159–161.

204. Loret de Mola JR, Carpenter SE. Management of genital prolapse in neonates and young women. *Obstet Gynecol Surv* 1996;51:253–260.

205. Dixon RE, Acosta AA, Young RL. Penrose pessary management of neonatal genital prolapse. *Am J Obstet Gynecol* 1974;119:855–857.

206. Carpenter SE, Rock JA. Procedentia in the newborn. *Int J Gynecol Obstet* 1987;25:151–153.

207. Mor N, Merlob P, Reisner SH. Tags and bands of the female external genitalia in the newborn infant. *Clin Pediatr (Phila)* 1983;22:122–124.

208. Berenson A, Heger A, Andrews S. Appearance of the hymen in newborns. *Pediatrics* 1991;87:458–465.

209. Berenson AB. A longitudinal study of hymenal morphology in the first 3 years of life. *Pediatrics* 1995;95:490–496.

210. Berenson AB. Appearance of the hymen at birth and one year of age: a longitudinal study. *Pediatrics* 1993;91:820–825.

211. Jemec GB, Heidenheim M, Nielsen NH. The prevalence of hidradenitis suppurativa and its potential precursor lesions. *J Am Acad Dermatol* 1996;35:191–194.

212. Dicken CH, Powell ST, Spear KL. Evaluation of isotretinoin treatment of hidradenitis suppurativa. *J Am Acad Dermatol* 1984;11:500–502.

213. Brown CF, Gallup DG, Brown VM. Hidradenitis suppurativa of the anogenital region: response to isotretinoin. *Am J Obstet Gynecol* 1988;158:12–15.

214. Lewis F, Messenger AG, Wales JK. Hidradenitis suppurativa as a presenting feature of premature adrenarche. *Br J Dermatol* 1993;129:447–448.

215. Young AW Jr, Tovell HM, Sadri K. Erosions and ulcers of the vulva: diagnosis, incidence, and management. *Obstet Gynecol* 1977;50:35–39.

216. Press S, Schachner L, Paul P. Clitoris tourniquet syndrome. *Pediatrics* 1980;66:781–782.

217. Chapman HL. Digital strangulation by hair wrapping. *Can Med Assoc J* 1968;98:125.

218. Rich MA, Keating MA. Hair tourniquette syndrome of the clitoris. *J Urol* 1999;162:190–191.

219. WHO, FIGO. Female circumcision. *Eur J Obstet Gynecol Reprod Biol* 1992;45:153–154.

220. ACOG Committee Opinion. Female genital mutilation. Number 151. *Int J Gynaecol Obstet* 1995;49:209.

221. American Academy of Pediatrics. Committee on Bioethics. Female genital mutilation. *Pediatrics* 1998;102:153–156.

10

Vaginal Discharge and Vaginal Bleeding in Childhood

Michele D. Wilson

The genital tract of the prepubertal child is quite different from that of a woman of reproductive age. At birth, the baby's vaginal mucosa is thickened from intrauterine estrogen stimulation. After a few weeks of extrauterine life, the vaginal epithelium changes into smooth, thin, atrophic, columnar epithelium that is extremely delicate. The prepubertal vagina has a neutral pH, which provides an optimal environment for bacterial growth. Additionally, the vagina lacks antibodies that may be present later in life to help fight infection. The vagina is short, measuring 3 to 4 cm in length during infancy. In a child, the ratio of the size of the cervix to the size of the uterine fundus is 3:1, whereas the ratio of the size of the cervix to fundus is reversed to 1:3 in an adult. The labia are thin, and the vaginal and vulvar tissues are sensitive.

The normal flora of the prepubertal vagina has been investigated. Hammerschlag et al. (1) obtained vaginal samples for aerobic and facultative anaerobic bacteria cultures from girls who ranged in age from 2 months to 15 years. The following bacteria were recovered in the designated percentages of individuals: diphtheroid 78%, *Staphylococcus epidermidis* 73%, α-hemolytic streptococci 39%, lactobacilli 39%, nonhemolytic streptococci 34%, *Escherichia coli* 34%, *Klebsiella* sp 15%, *Gardnerella vaginalis* 13.5%, group D streptococcus 8.5%, *Staphylococcus aureus* 7%, *Haemophilus influenzae* 5%, *Pseudomonas aeruginosa* 5%, and *Proteus* sp 5%. Genital mycoplasma cultures showed that 6% and

27% of the girls harbored *Mycoplasma hominis* and *Ureaplasma urealyticum,* respectively. Yeast species were identified in 28% of individuals. Vaginal cultures for anaerobic bacteria were performed in a subset of the patients. *Bacteroides fragilis* and peptococci each were found in 76% of the girls; peptostreptococci and *Bacteroides melaninogenicus* each were recovered in 56% of the patients. Paradise et al. (2) conducted a study to examine vulvovaginitis in premenarcheal girls. As part of their study, they obtained vaginal cultures from healthy age-matched controls who had no genitourinary complaints. They considered lactobacilli, α-hemolytic streptococci, and diphtheroid to be normal vaginal flora. They found normal flora alone in 80.8% of the girls and normal flora with one or more additional isolate in 19.2% of the other girls. Asymptomatic individuals also were colonized with the following organisms: *Bacteroides* sp 27.5%, β-hemolytic streptococci (not group A or B) 4%, *E. coli* 8%, group B streptococcus 2%, coagulase-positive staphylococcus 2%, and yeast 4%. Both of these studies provide important information regarding normal vaginal flora in girls.

VULVOVAGINITIS

Vulvovaginitis is the most common gynecologic problem in prepubertal girls (Table 10.1). Several physiologic factors contribute to the child's increased susceptibility to vul-

TABLE 10.1. *Etiologies of vaginal discharge and vaginal bleeding in childhood*

Nonspecific vaginitis
Physiologic discharge
  Newborn
  Physiologic leukorrhea
Sexually transmitted disease organisms
  Neisseria gonorrhoea
  Chlamydia trachomatis
  Herpes simplex virus
  Genital warts
  Trichomonas vaginalis
  Gardnerella vaginalis
Other infectious causes
  Shigella
  Yersinia enterocolitica
  Staphylococcus aureus
  Haemophilus influenzae
  Group A β-hemolytic streptococci
  Streptococcus pneumoniae
  Neisseria meningitidis
  Candida
  Branhamella catarrhalis
  Pinworms (*Enterobius vermicularis*)
Congenital anomalies
  Ectopic ureter
Chemical disorders
  Bubble bath, perfumes, harsh soaps, deodorants
Skin disorders
  Seborrhea
  Eczema
  Psoriasis
  Lichen sclerosus et atrophicus
  Adhesive vulvitis
Systemic illness
  Roseola
  Varicella
  Scarlet fever
  Stevens-Johnson syndrome
  Kawasaki disease
  Pelvic abscess
Genital trauma
Foreign body
Urologic disorders
  Urethral prolapse
  Urethral polyp
  Prolapsed ureterocele
Hemangioma
Physiologic vaginal bleeding in the newborn
Precocious puberty
Iatrogenic or factitious puberty
Carcinoma (sarcoma botryoides)
Bleeding disorders

vovaginitis. A pubertal female has physical barriers that help to prevent infection. In contrast, the young girl lacks labial fat pads, she has no pubic hair, and the labia minora are relatively small. In addition, the proximity of the rectum to the vagina permits easy fecal contamination of the vagina. All of these factors combined with suboptimal hygiene, which is common among young children, result in decreased protection of the vulva and vagina.

Nonspecific Vulvovaginitis

Nonspecific vulvovaginitis is the single greatest cause of prepubertal vulvovaginitis, accounting for between 25% and 93% of all cases in various clinical series (2,3). When vaginal cultures are obtained in a patient with nonspecific vulvovaginitis, they will grow organisms considered to be part of normal vaginal flora, i.e., lactobacilli, diphtheroids, *S. epidermidis,* α-hemolytic streptococci, or gram-negative intestinal organisms, particularly *E. coli*. Despite normal flora, vulvar irritation develops for several reasons. Frequently, poor perineal hygiene associated with wiping from the rectum anteriorly toward the vagina is the key issue. Tight-fitting clothes, nylon underpants or stockings, and prolonged exposure to wet bathing suits or dance leotards may contribute to the problem. Once inflammation has begun, scratching may follow, which will predispose to bacterial superinfection. Symptoms of nonspecific vulvovaginitis include vaginal discharge, genital pain, pruritus, irritation, and dysuria.

The cornerstone of treatment as well as prevention of subsequent episodes of nonspecific vulvovaginitis is the institution of good perineal hygiene. Proper wiping technique is essential to prevent fecal contamination of the vagina and vulva. The child should wear white cotton underwear and use white toilet paper because the dyes and perfumes used in clothing and toilet paper can be irritants. The child should use a mild, nondeodorant, nonperfumed soap to bathe. After bathing, she or her parent should dry her vulva by patting gently with a towel, but without rubbing. Nylon stockings, ballet leotards, tight-fitting clothes, and prolonged exposure to wet bathing suits or wet clothes should be avoided. The goal is to keep the genital area cool and dry. It is important to discontinue using bubble baths or harsh soaps. In the acute phase of irritation, sitz baths of warm water alone or warm water mixed with baking soda, colloidal oatmeal, or cornstarch are beneficial. Wet compresses of Burow's solution may provide relief for weeping lesions. For the more recalcitrant condition, antibiotics may be indicated. A 10-day course of one of the following oral antibiotics is recommended: amoxicillin, amoxicillin combined with clavulanate, or a cephalosporin. In persistent cases, it may be necessary to prescribe a course of low-dose antibiotics for as long as 2 months. Topical estrogen cream applied to the vulva for 2 to 3 weeks is efficacious when there is inadequate recovery with improved hygienic measures. Caution must be exercised in prescribing topical estrogens because prolonged use can result in iatrogenic precocious puberty.

Physiologic Discharge

A physiologic discharge frequently occurs in the newborn female due to intrauterine exposure to maternal estrogens. The discharge is characteristically white, mucoid, and without odor. It persists for approximately 1 week. After the first few days, the discharge may become bloody, due to withdrawal of estrogen stimulation to the endometrial lining of the uterus. After the newborn period, there is no visible vaginal discharge in a healthy prepubertal female. Then, during puberty, physiologic leukorrhea begins in response to increased levels of circulating estrogens. It develops weeks to months before the onset of menarche and may persist for several years. It generally is described as a copious, clear-to-white colored vaginal discharge with a tenacious consistency and without odor. The discharge is composed of desquamated vaginal cells, vaginal transudate, and endocervical mucus. The discharge is completely normal. Reassurance of the patient and her family is the only required treatment.

Specific Etiologies for Vulvovaginitis

In an individual with a specific etiology for vulvovaginitis, vaginal cultures usually will identify the pathogen. Most of these pathogens generally are categorized as sexually transmitted disease, respiratory, or intestinal organisms.

Sexually Transmitted Pathogens

Child sexual abuse is unfortunately a frequent phenomenon. It is estimated that one in four girls has been sexually abused by age 18 years (4). A study investigated the incidence of sexually transmitted diseases in children with suspected sexual abuse. The study included 409 children (360 girls) under 13 years of age. Sexually transmitted diseases were identified in 54 (13%) children. Forty-six children had gonorrhea, six had syphilis, four had trichomonas, and three had condyloma acuminata (5).

Gonococcal Infection

In contrast to the mature woman in whom the acidic, estrogenized vagina is inhospitable to gonorrhea and the cervix is the primary site of gonococcal infection, the vagina is the site of infection in the prepubertal child. Before approximately 9 or 10 years of age, the endocervix is closed and, therefore, upper tract extension is extremely rare. Gonococcal vaginitis usually is manifested by a copious, green, purulent vaginal discharge. Severe vulvitis can occur secondary to irritation from the discharge. The child may complain of pruritus or dysuria. Proof of infection by a positive culture is essential. Furthermore, an appropriate laboratory must confirm positive culture results for *Neisseria gonorrhoeae* in a prepubertal child. False-positive results have occurred due to misidentification of nonpathogenic *Neisseria* species and may have serious negative *consequences (6)*. The recommended treatment for *N. gonorrhoeae* is a single intramuscular injection of ceftriaxone 125 mg for a child weighing less than 45 kg. Children weighing 45 kg or more should be treated with one of regimens recommended for adults.

The American Academy of Pediatrics has stated that physicians should assume that if a child has gonorrhea, she acquired it sexually and presumably abusively (7). Gonorrhea, outside the newborn period, is transmitted through sex play, sexual abuse, or sexual intercourse (8). When anogenital gonorrhea is found in a prepubertal girl, a thorough evaluation coupled with reporting to the appropriate authorities for sexual abuse must ensue. A complete search for adult contacts should be undertaken. Siblings of the index case should be examined and cultured. It is crucial to provide for the child's safety while the investigation is proceeding. Gonococcal infection has been diagnosed in 3% to 20% of sexually abused children in various series (9,10).

Chlamydial Infection

Children acquire *Chlamydia trachomatis* genital infection by either perinatal exposure or sexual abuse. *Chlamydia trachomatis* is increasingly recovered from sexually abused children in whom the reported incidence rates range from 4% to 17% (11–13).

Chlamydial infection acquired perinatally may persist for over a year. Therefore, when *C. trachomatis* is recovered from a young child, the clinician should always consider but not presume that the infection was acquired by sexual abuse. On the other hand, studies support the view that sexual abuse is more probable when *C. trachomatis* is recovered in an older child (12,14).

Because of the implications of finding a sexually transmitted disease agent in a prepubertal child, the diagnosis of *C. trachomatis* should always be made by cell culture technique.

The recommended treatment of *C. trachomatis* for a child under 8 years of age who weighs less than 45 kg is oral erythromycin base 50 mg/kg/day divided into four doses for 10 to 14 days. For children under 8 years of age who weigh 45 kg or more, the treatment is a single dose of azithromycin 1 g orally. For children 8 years of age or older, the treatment is oral azithromycin 1 g as a single dose or doxycycline 100 mg twice a day for 7 days.

Herpes Simplex Virus

Type 1 or 2 herpes simplex viruses can cause vulvovaginitis in prepubertal children. The child with an oral infection may spread it to her genital area with her hand (15). Alternatively, genital herpes simplex virus infection may be a consequence of sexual abuse. Herpes simplex virus type 1 has been most closely identified with oral infection, and herpes simplex virus type 2 has been related to genital infection. Although specific serotypes of herpes simplex virus have been associated with unique sites of infection, isolation of either distinctive serotype neither proves nor excludes the possibility of sexual contact. Thus, the possibility of abuse must be explored in any child with herpes vulvovaginitis, type 1 or 2. Diagnosis usually is suspected by detecting the typical ulcers and should be confirmed by culture. Lesions of varicella may be mistaken for genital herpes (16). It is important to recognize that recurrences of genital herpes may occur after an episode of primary infection without repeat exposure.

Genital Warts

The same types of human papillomaviruses that infect the anogenital area of adults cause genital warts. It is believed that perinatal exposure, sexual abuse, or close physical contact transmits human papillomaviruses. The length of time after birth that perinatally acquired infection can present remains uncertain. It is thought that genital warts that present within the first 1 to 2 years of life are likely to have been acquired perinatally. As the age at which the child is diagnosed with genital warts increases, the suspicion of sexual abuse also should rise. More than 50% of children with anal or genital warts have histories of sexual abuse (17,18).

Trichomonas Vaginalis

Trichomoniasis, an infection caused by a flagellated protozoan, rarely occurs in prepubertal girls outside the newborn period because the organism prefers an estrogenic environment (19). Seeing motile trichomonads on wet-mount preparation generally makes the diagnosis. Culture is a more sensitive method to diagnose trichomonas and therefore may increase the yield. Wet-mount examinations are positive in only 60% of adult cases that subsequently are found to be positive by culture technique (20). In adults, wet towels have been shown to act as fomites in the spread of trichomonas. If the organism is recovered from a child, sexual abuse is extremely likely. The treatment regimen is oral metronidazole 15 mg/kg/day divided every 8 hours for a 7- to 10-day course.

Gardnerella Vaginalis

The association between *G. vaginalis* and sexual abuse remains unclear because this organism has been recovered from girls for whom there was no suspicion of sexual abuse. In some series, *G. vaginalis* is recovered more frequently from sexually abused versus nonsexually abused girls, 14.6% versus 4.2% in one study (21). By contrast, Ingram et al. (22) found no difference in rates of *G. vaginalis* based on history of sexual abuse. Bacterial vaginosis, which is a mixed infection of *G. vaginalis* and anaerobes, has been diagnosed in sexually abused children. Hammerschlag et al. (23) examined 31 abused and 23 nonabused girls aged 2.5 to 13 years. The diagnosis of definite bacterial vaginosis was made if two criteria were met: (i) vaginal washings contained clue cells and (ii) vaginal secretions had an amine odor after addition of 10% solution of potassium hydroxide. A diagnosis of possible infection was made if only one of two characteristics was found. They found that four of 31 (13%) girls who were sexually abused had definite infection and an additional four of 31 (13%) girls who were sexually abused had possible infection. In comparison, none of the 23 control subjects had definite bacterial vaginosis and only one of 23 (4%) control subjects had possible bacterial vaginosis. These data suggest that sexual activity or abuse may have a role in transmission of bacterial vaginosis.

Other Infectious Etiologies, Not Sexually Transmitted

Shigella

Shigella is an enteric pathogen that can be spread from the gastrointestinal tract to the genital region in prepubertal girls resulting in infectious vulvovaginitis. The patient with shigella vulvovaginitis typically presents with a mucopurulent and malodorous vaginal discharge. In one series, the discharge was bloody in 47% of individuals with shigella vaginitis (24). Concomitant vulvitis has been described. Diarrhea is absent in the majority of patients. The recommended treatment is combination therapy with oral combined trimethoprim 8 mg/kg/day and sulfamethoxazole 40 mg/kg/day for 5 days for suspected organisms.

Yersinia Enterocolitica

Rare cases of *Yersinia enterocolitica* vulvovaginitis have been reported (25).

Staphylococcus Aureus

Staphylococcus aureus may be part of the normal vaginal flora in prepubertal girls. The organism is carried by 7% of asymptomatic girls (1). In the study by Paradise et al. (2), symptomatic girls were no more likely than asymptomatic girls to be colonized with coagulase-positive staphylococcus (2). When *S. aureus* is found in a symptomatic individual without another infectious agent, it usually is treated as a pathogen. The recommended approach is to administer oral antibiotics, specifically cephalexin 25 to 50 mg/kg/day for 7 to 10 days, dicloxacillin 25 mg/kg/day for 7 days, or amoxicillin-clavulanate 20 to 40 mg/kg/day for 7 to 10 days.

Haemophilus Influenzae

The significance of recovering *Haemophilus influenzae* type b in cultures of vaginal secretions remains unclear. *Haemophilus influenzae,* which is a respiratory organism, was found in 5% of normal girls (1). In the series of Paradise et al. (2), there were two patients with vulvovaginitis for whom *H. influenzae* was recovered from vaginal cultures. One patient improved without treatment and the other patient did not improve despite antibiotic treatment. If *H. influenzae* is the only pathogen recovered in a symptomatic individual, a trial of oral antibiotics is indicated. The usual regimen is oral amoxicillin 20 to 40 mg/kg/day for 7 days for susceptible organisms and either amoxicillin-clavulanate or cefixime for resistant strains.

Group A β-Hemolytic Streptococcus (Streptococcus Pyogenes)

Group A β-hemolytic streptococcus is an important specific cause of bacterial vulvovaginitis. Streptococcal infection may be manifested by vaginal bleeding or a blood-tinged vaginal discharge associated with distinctive fiery-red vulvitis and/or with perianal involvement. Group A β-hemolytic streptococcal infection typically presents 7 to 10 days after a sore throat and upper respiratory tract infection. Vaginal cultures will confirm the diagnosis. The recommended treatment regimen is oral penicillin V potassium 250 mg three times a day for a 10-day course.

Other Respiratory Pathogens

Streptococcus pneumoniae, pneumococcus, is a respiratory organism that may be spread by the oral-digital route to the perineal area, causing an infection that is often asymptomatic. Treatment is oral penicillin V potassium or erythromycin for 10 days. *Neisseria meningitidis* and *Branhamella catarrhalis* occasionally will cause vulvovaginitis.

Candida Vulvovaginitis

Candida vulvovaginitis occurs frequently in women but rarely in prepubertal girls. The child who develops Candida typically has one of the following risk factors: she is still in diapers, she is taking or has recently taken an antibiotic, she has diabetes mellitus, or she is immunocompromised. When Candida vulvovaginitis is recurrent and resistant to treatment, the clinician should consider an evaluation for diabetes mellitus or immunodeficiency. The signs and symptoms of vulvovaginal candidiasis can range from mild vulvar erythema with pruritus to severe erythema with excoriations and maceration. The discharge is white and often has the appearance of thrush. If secretions are mixed with 10% potassium hydroxide solution, hyphae and/or spores can be seen microscopically. Fungal cultures may be performed. One should treat initially with a topical antifungal agent such as nystatin, miconazole, or clotrimazole, which is applied to the external vulva. If the initial treatment is not successful, intravaginal nystatin liquid or antifungal suppositories that have been cut to size should be gently inserted with a medicine dropper or cotton-tipped swabs.

Pinworms

Pinworm infestation, caused by *Enterobius vermicularis*, is a frequent problem in young children. Most girls who have pinworms do not develop associated vulvovaginal complaints. The classic symptom is perianal and vulvar itching at night when adult female pinworms emerge from the rectum to lay eggs. The diagnosis is confirmed if the parents, who are asked to check with a flashlight at night, see the pinworms crawling around the rectum or if the characteristic eggs are recovered by clear cellophane tape applied to the perianal region. The treatment regimen is oral mebendazole, a single 100-mg tablet at the time of diagnosis and again 2 weeks later, given to all members of household over 2 years of age, excluding pregnant women.

Congenital Anomalies

An ectopic ureter may open onto the perineum or into the vagina, cervix, uterus, or urethra, resulting in a discharge of clear urine or urine mixed with purulent material when the urine is infected. Urine, which appears as a chronic watery vaginal discharge, sometimes is visualized emerging from the opening. An intravenous pyelogram often is needed to make the diagnosis.

Chemicals

Chemical substances, including bubble baths, perfumes, and harsh soaps, can act an irritants to sensitive skin of the vulva and cause vulvovaginitis. Treatment involves discontinuation of use of the offending agent and institution of good perineal hygiene as described for the management of nonspecific vulvovaginitis.

Skin Disorders

Vulvar skin may be affected by dermatologic conditions such as seborrhea, psoriasis, and eczema. These dermatologic conditions tend to affect the outer labia minora and labia majora. Seborrheic dermatitis may involve the vulva in addition to other areas of the body. Psoriasis is a less common condition in children that can involve the vulva. Typical lesions of eczema are dry, papular patches that cause severe pruritus. This common childhood condition can involve the vulva. When topical steroids are used, mild, nonfluorinated types should be selected for the genital region.

Lichen sclerosus et atrophicus is a rare dermatologic disorder affecting the region surrounding the genitals. It is manifested by itching, irritation, soreness, dysuria, vaginal discharge, or bleeding. This condition has been mistaken for child abuse (26). Physical examination reveals white, parchment-like skin, with vulvar atrophy. Because of vulvar and perianal involvement, the rash gives a figure-of-eight or hourglass appearance. Lichen sclerosus may be confused with vitiligo due to skin discoloration. Vesicles that bleed easily are characteristic of this disorder. It is recognized by either its distinctive appearance or by obtaining a skin biopsy when the clinical presentation is unclear.

Adhesive Vulvitis

Adhesive vulvitis is a condition in which the labia minora fuse together, presumably secondary to chronic irritation associated with vulvitis. The peak incidence for this condition is between 2 and 6 years of age. The usual treatment is topical estrogen cream applied directly to the adhesion twice a day for 2 to 4 weeks.

Systemic Illnesses

Systemic illnesses such as roseola, varicella, scarlet fever, Stevens-Johnson syndrome, and Kawasaki disease may involve the vulvar skin. In addition, a draining pelvic abscess from inflammatory bowel disease may present with symptoms of vulvovaginitis.

VAGINAL BLEEDING

The prepubertal girl who presents with vaginal bleeding is a cause for concern, and she requires careful evaluation (Table 10.1).

Genital Trauma

Genital trauma is a serious cause of vaginal bleeding. Sexual molestation, automobile and bicycle injuries, and being kicked in the pelvic area are frequent causes of injury. Straddle injuries often result from climbing over a fence or a similar structure. Blunt trauma results in a hematoma that may appear as a bluish-red mass. Treatment entails the use of ice packs or ice sitz baths. If the hematoma continues to expand, evacuation and ligation of the bleeding artery may be indicated. Hymenal tears strongly suggest that the vagina has been penetrated. There may be internal injuries involving the bladder, intestines, and peritoneal cavity. Most extensive lacerations will necessitate sedation or general anesthesia for adequate evaluation and repair.

Foreign Bodies

Vaginal foreign bodies account for approximately 4% of gynecologic problems in children (27). A foreign body in the vagina may present with a foul-smelling, bloody discharge. The strong odor is often the prominent concern. Foreign bodies are discovered in many girls with vaginal bleeding, and the bleeding is described as bright red in color, light in amount, and intermittent. In one series, girls with foreign bodies complained of vaginal bleeding more frequently than they complained of vaginal discharge (27). It is rare that the child will disclose the essential history of having inserted a foreign body in her vagina. Most foreign bodies are not radiopaque and, consequently, x-ray studies usually are not indicated. The most commonly found item is toilet paper. Large items usually are removed with bayonet forceps. Small items may be irrigated out using a small bladder catheter. Use of lubricant or lidocaine (Xylocaine) gel may help in the process. Sedation or general anesthesia occasionally is required.

Urologic Disorders

Urethral prolapse often presents with bleeding that generally is painless. Physical examination will reveal a friable, annular, periurethral mass that is the source of the bleeding. The average age of onset for this condition is 5 years (28). Urethral prolapse usually occurs after an episode of increased abdominal pressure. Treatment includes use of sitz baths. Topical estrogens may hasten the healing process. Topical antibiotics or oral antibiotics are indicated if infection occurs. Urethral prolapse generally resolves within 4 weeks. If the tissue becomes necrotic, surgery is indicated. Urethral polyps, caruncles, cysts, and prolapsed ureterocele may have similar clinical presentations.

Hemangiomas

Hemangiomas in the genital area may become irritated and bleed. At times, bleeding due to a hemangioma may be mistaken for bleeding due to sexual abuse (26).

Physiologic Vaginal Bleeding in the Newborn

In the neonate, withdrawal of maternal estrogen stimulation to the endometrial lining of the uterus may result in vaginal bleeding. This condition is self-limited and requires no treatment other than reassurance of the parents.

Precocious Puberty

The onset of precocious puberty with menarche may first come to medical attention because of a concern about vaginal bleeding. In the individual with precocious puberty, vaginal bleeding is associated with accelerated growth and other signs of pubertal development. A rare entity known as premature menarche without other evidence of precocious puberty has been described (29).

Iatrogenic or Factitious Precocious Puberty

Use of hormonal creams or ingestion of oral estrogens or oral contraceptives can lead to iatrogenic or factitious puberty. Treatment involves discontinuation of the offending agent.

Carcinoma

Sarcoma botryoides is a malignant tumor that can involve the vagina, uterus, bladder, or urethra. The hallmark sign of sarcoma botryoides is passage of a polypoid mass from the vagina or urethra. Other manifestations include vaginal bleeding or discharge, abdominal pain, or palpable abdominal mass on examination. The peak incidence occurs before 2 years of age; 90% of patients with sarcoma botryoides are diagnosed before age 5 years. The tumor is rapidly growing and very aggressive.

Bleeding Disorders

Children with bleeding disorders rarely present with vaginal bleeding.

Other Disorders

Some of the entities previously described that cause vulvovaginitis may present with the chief complaint of vaginal bleeding. Vaginitis caused by group A β-hemolytic streptococcus and shigella often results in bleeding. Bleeding may be a predominant feature of pinworm infection if scratching and resulting excoriations are severe. Genital warts may present with bleeding. Dermatologic disorders including lichen sclerosus et atrophicus, seborrheic dermatitis, psoriasis, and atopic dermatitis that involve the vulva may present with vaginal bleeding.

EVALUATION OF THE PREPUBERTAL GIRL WITH SYMPTOMS OF VULVOVAGINITIS OR VAGINAL BLEEDING

History

The chief complaint may include vaginal bleeding, vaginal discharge, dysuria, itching, or genital pain. The parent of a nonverbal child may state that her child scratches, rubs, or is irritable with urination and defecation. It is important to know when the problem began and if there are any associated symptoms. If a discharge is present, one should inquire about the quality, quantity, color, and odor of the discharge. Has the child previously experienced a similar problem? If so, how was it treated and did the condition respond to therapy? Inquiries regarding the child's perineal hygiene are essential. Does the child use appropriate wiping technique and has she been exposed to any chemicals or irritants including harsh soaps, bubble baths, perfumes, or deodorants? Does the child have any underlying medical conditions such as diabetes mellitus or an immunodeficiency state that could predispose the patient to Candida infection? Is there a history of any skin conditions such as eczema, seborrhea, or psoriasis that is presently affecting the vulva? Has the patient had a recent upper respiratory tract infection or sore throat to suggest group A β-hemolytic

streptococcus or other respiratory pathogens as the etiology? It is important to inquire about recent use of medications, specifically antibiotics and hormonal preparations. The possibility of sexual abuse must be explored and questions about who cares for the child should be posed. Family history of related medical problems such as allergic or skin disorders or diabetes mellitus may help focus the investigation.

Physical Examination

It is essential to start with a good general examination. Growth and development should be assessed, and one should look for indications of puberty. The skin is inspected for any pertinent dermatologic disorder. The pharynx and cervical lymph nodes should be examined. Palpating the abdomen for masses is important. The extent of the pelvic examination should be individualized, with consideration of the severity and nature of the symptoms. Inspection of the patient's underpants can provide significant information regarding any vaginal discharge or bleeding. One should inspect the perineum either in the frog-leg position, with the hips flexed and the soles of the feet meeting, or in the knee-chest position. Using these techniques, one can adequately visualize the lower segment, if not all, of the vagina. If the discharge is purulent, persistent, recurrent, or grossly bloody, a more complete initial evaluation is indicated. In these situations, one should obtain specimens for culture and microscopy. Samples can be obtained using a moistened swab. Vaginal instrumentation so as to fully visualize the vagina is required if there is bleeding, evidence of significant trauma, suspicion of foreign body, tumor, or persistence of symptoms. Depending on the child's age and level of cooperation, sedation or general anesthesia may be required to accomplish vaginal instrumentation. Rectal examination usually is indicated if there is persistent or purulent discharge, bleeding, or associated abdominal pain. During the rectal examination, one can milk the vagina for discharge, feel for the presence of hard foreign bodies in the vagina, palpate the cervix, and check for any adnexal masses. When pinworm infestation is being considered as a possible diagnosis, clear cellophane tape is applied to the anus. It is important to recall that a normal examination does not exclude the possibility of sexual abuse, because the majority of sexually abused girls have a normal examination.

Laboratory Tests

A wet mount is prepared by mixing vaginal secretions with saline to look for trichomonads. Secretions combined with 10% potassium hydroxide solution are inspected microscopically for fungal forms. Cultures are obtained for gonorrhea, chlamydia, and aerobic organisms when indicated. The clear cellophane tape from the pinworm preparation is applied to a glass slide and examined microscopically for the characteristic eggs.

Assessment

The qualities of the discharge help to direct the investigation. If the discharge is foul smelling, a foreign body is likely. When there is a bloody discharge, Shigella and group A β-hemolytic streptococci are probable causes. An odorless, bloody discharge suggests the possibility of vulvar irritation, trauma, foreign body, precocious puberty, or genital warts. A purulent discharge occurs most often with gonorrhea, chlamydia, or foreign body.

REFERENCES

1. Hammerschlag MR, Albert S, Rosner I, et al. Microbiology of the vagina in children: normal and potentially pathogenic organisms. *Pediatrics* 1978;68:57–62.
2. Paradise JE, Campos JM, Friedman HM, et al. Vulvovaginitis in premenarcheal girls: clinical features and diagnostic evaluation. *Pediatrics* 1982;70:193–198.
3. Altchek A. Pediatric vulvovaginitis. *J Reprod Med* 1984;29:359–375.
4. Finkelhor D, Hotaling G, Lewis IA, et al. Sexual abuse in a national survey of adult men and women: prevalence, characteristics, and risk factors. *Child Abuse Neg* 1990;14:19–28.
5. White ST, Loda FA, Ingram DL, et al. Sexually transmitted diseases in sexually abused children. *Pediatrics* 1983;72:16–21.
6. Whittington WL, Rice RJ, Biddle JW, et al. Incorrect identification of *Neisseria gonorrhoeae* from infants and children. *Pediatr Infect Dis J* 1988;7:3–10.
7. American Academy of Pediatrics: Committee on Child Abuse and Neglect. Gonorrhea in prepubertal children. *Pediatrics* 1998;101:134–135.
8. Neinstein LS, Goldenring J, Carpenter S. Nonsexual transmission of sexually transmitted diseases: an infrequent occurrence. *Pediatrics* 1984;74:67–76.
9. Ingram DL. *Neisseria gonorrhoeae* in children. *Pediatr Ann* 1994;20:341–345.
10. Siegel RM, Schubert CJ, Myers PA, et al. The prevalence of sexually transmitted diseases in children and adolescents evaluated for sexual abuse in Cincinnati: rationale for limited STD testing in prepubertal girls. *Pediatrics* 1995;96;1090–1094.
11. Ingram DS, Runyan DK, Collins AD, et al. Vaginal *Chlamydia trachomatis* infection in children with sexual contact. *Pediatr Infect Dis* 1984;3:97–104.
12. Ingram DL, White ST, Occhiuti AR, et al. Childhood vaginal infections: association of *Chlamydia trachomatis* with sexual contact. *Pediatr Infect Dis* 1986;5:226–229.
13. Fuster CD, Neinstein LS. Vaginal *Chlamydia trachomatis* prevalence in sexually abused prepubertal girls. *Pediatrics* 1987;79:235–238.
14. Hammerschlag MR. Chlamydia and suspected sexual abuse. *Pediatrics* 1988;81:600–601.
15. Nahmias AJ, Dowdle WR, Naib ZM, et al. Genital infection with herpes-virus hominis types 1 and 2 in children. *Pediatrics* 1968;42:659–666.
16. Boyd M, Jordan SW. Unusual presentation of varicella suggestive of sexual abuse trauma. *Am J Dis Child* 1990;144:1319–1322.
17. American Academy of Dermatology Task Force on Pediatric Dermatology. Genital warts and sexual abuse in children. *J Am Acad Dermatol* 1984;11:529–530.
18. Shelton TB, Jerkins GR, Noe HN. Condylomata acuminata in the pediatric patient. *J Urol* 1986;135:548–549.
19. Jones JG, Yamauchi T, Lambert B. *Trichomonas vaginalis* infestation in sexually abused girls. *Am J Dis Child* 1985;139:846–847.
20. Krieger JN, Tam MR, Stevens CE, et al. Diagnosis of trichomoniasis: comparison of conventional wet-mount examination with cytological studies, culture, and monoclonal antibody staining of direct specimens. *JAMA* 1988;259:1223–1227.
21. Bartley DL, Morgan L, Rimsza ME. *Gardnerella vaginalis* in prepubertal girls. *Am J Dis Child* 1987;141:1014–1017.
22. Ingram DL, White ST, Lyna PR, et al. *Gardnerella vaginalis* infection and sexual contact in female children. *Child Abuse Negl* 1992;16:847–853.
23. Hammerschlag MR, Cummings M, Doraiswamy B, et al. Nonspecific vaginitis following sexual abuse in children. *Pediatrics* 1985;75:1028–1031.
24. Murphy TV, Nelson JD. Shigella vaginitis: report of 38 patients and review of the literature. *Pediatrics* 1979;63:511–516.
25. Watkins S, Quan L. Vulvovaginitis caused by *Yersinia enterocolitica*. *Pediatr Infect Dis* 1984;3:444–445.

26. Bays J, Jenny C. Genital and anal conditions confused with child sexual abuse trauma. *Am J Dis Child* 1990; 144:1319–1322.

27. Paradise JE, Willis ED. Probability of vaginal foreign body in girls with genital complaints. *Am J Dis Child* 1985;139:472–476.

28. Capraro VJ, Bayonet-Rivera NP, Magoss I. Vulvar tumors in children due to prolapse of urethral mucosa. *Am J Obstet Gynecol* 1970;108:572–575.

29. Heller ME, Dewhurst J, Grant DB. Premature menarche without other evidence of precocious puberty. *Arch Dis Child* 1979;54:472–475.

11

Precocious Puberty

Leslie Plotnick

Puberty involves an increase in both gonadal steroid production (gonadarche) and adrenal steroid production (adrenarche). It is initiated by changes in the sensitive negative feedback that operates between the gonad and the hypothalamus and pituitary (see Chapter 3).

In the majority of girls, puberty begins between the ages of 8 and 13 years. The average time from onset to completion of puberty is 4.2 years (range 1.5 to 6 years). The time from breast buds to menarche is 2.3 ± 1.0 years. Classically, if a girl shows signs of pubertal development before age 8 years, this is considered precocious and an evaluation is warranted. Recent data indicate that 5.0% of white girls and 15.4% of African-American girls have begun breast development by 7 to 7.99 years of age and 2.8% and 17.77%, respectively, have begun pubic hair development by this age (1). These data suggest a more appropriate age for concern may be 7 years for white girls and 6 years for African-American girls. The timing of progression also is important. Pubertal changes that progress too rapidly require evaluation, as do heterosexual changes (i.e., virilization).

Puberty is initiated as the gonadostat begins to lose its sensitivity to negative feedback by sex hormones. This change allows increasing pulsatile gonadotropin-releasing hormone (GnRH) secretion from the hypothalamus. There is increased sensitivity of the pituitary to GnRH leading to increased luteinizing hormone (LH) and follicle-stimulating hormone (FSH) secretion, detectable first during sleep. The gonads also develop increased sensitivity to LH and FSH secretion,

grow in size, and produce increases in levels of sex steroids. These events are synergistic and lead to accelerated change. With further maturation, a positive feedback system develops that enables the LH surge necessary for ovulation (see Chapter 3) (2).

PRECOCIOUS SEXUAL MATURATION

Table 11.1 lists the causes of precocious or inappropriate sexual maturation (3,4).

Puberty generally has been considered classically precocious when it begins before the age of 8 years in girls, but younger ages (20) may be more appropriate.

TABLE 11.1. *Precocious or inappropriate sexual development in girls*

True (or central) precocious puberty (central gonadotropin mediated)
  Idiopathic
  CNS tumor
    Hamartomas
    Other
  Other CNS disorders
    Trauma
    Hydrocephalus
    Postinfectious
    Cranial irradiation
Independent of pituitary gonadotropins
  Exposure to exogenous estrogens
  Estrogen-secreting tumors (adrenals or ovaries)
  Ovarian cysts
  McCune-Albright syndrome
  Primary hypothyroidism
Heterosexual development
  Congenital adrenal hyperplasia
  Androgen-secreting tumors (adrenals or ovaries)
  Exposure to exogenous androgens
Variations of normal puberty
  Premature thelarche
  Premature adrenarche

It is important initially to distinguish between true or central precocious puberty, which is central gonadotropin mediated, and puberty that is independent of pituitary gonadotropins.

TRUE (OR CENTRAL) PRECOCIOUS PUBERTY

In girls, the vast majority of cases of precocious puberty are central in origin, due to early maturation of hypothalamic GnRH secretion. In many cases, this is idiopathic, i.e., no organic lesion can be found. With idiopathic central precocious puberty, the pattern of development and timing of progression are normal, although the onset is at an early age.

Central nervous system (CNS) tumors, particularly hypothalamic hamartomas, are known causes of central precocious puberty. Gliomas, neurofibromas, and others have been seen. Central precocious puberty also may occur with hydrocephalus (with or without associated meningomyelocele), after head trauma (5), or after CNS infections (encephalitis, meningitis) or CNS irradiation.

Girls with central precocious puberty have an acceleration in their linear growth velocity, advancement in skeletal age, and pubertal levels of gonadotropins (LH and FSH) and sex steroids. Because LH and FSH levels fluctuate, single samples may not be helpful in making this diagnosis. Therefore, multiple samples taken at 20-minute intervals for several hours, particularly at night, and/or an infusion of GnRH with LH and FSH levels measured at regular intervals may be important in making this diagnosis.

Once the diagnosis of central precocious puberty is made, CNS imaging with computed tomography (CT) (6) or magnetic resonance imaging (MRI) is indicated to look for an underlying CNS abnormality,

Knowledge of the importance of the frequency of GnRH pulses for pituitary LH and FSH secretion has led to development of long-acting GnRH agonists. These agonists produce downregulation of pituitary GnRH receptors, desensitize pituitary gonadotrophs, and inhibit LH and FSH release. This treatment stops progression of puberty, and secondary sex characteristics often regress. Specifically, there is reduction in breast size. On ultrasound examination, a decrease in ovarian and uterine size may be seen.

Thus, treatment with GnRH analogues produces a prepubertal hormonal state that causes cessation or slowing of growth acceleration, bone age advancement, and pubertal progression. Use of a GnRH agonist is the treatment of choice in central precocious puberty. Subcutaneous, intranasal, and depot intramuscular preparations are available (7–13).

The decision to treat central precocious puberty depends on several factors. The girl's age and her psychosocial adjustment to her degree of pubertal maturation must be considered. For example, a 2-year-old girl clearly needs treatment, whereas a 7-year-old girl may be well able to psychologically handle the changes. Rapidity of progression also must be considered. In "older" girls with precocious puberty, a major issue in decisions about treatment is the degree of bone age advancement and its speed of progression, the degree of compromise of adult stature, and calculated decreases in predicted adult height.

To assess adequate suppression in a girl being treated with a GnRH agonist, it may be useful to do a GnRH infusion test to be sure LH and FSH levels remain suppressed after this stimulus.

PRECOCIOUS PUBERTY INDEPENDENT OF PITUITARY GONADOTROPINS

Girls with precocious puberty independent of pituitary gonadotropins have an independent source of estrogen as the cause of their sexual maturation. A search must be made for an exogenous estrogen source, for example, in medications (e.g., oral contraceptives) or in certain skin creams. There have been some cases where ingestion of meat of an estrogen-treated animal, especially poultry, has been implicated in producing estrogenization in a child.

Ovarian (14) or adrenal estrogen-producing tumors also must be considered. These tumors are likely to present with rapid onset and progression of pubertal changes as well as have high levels of estradiol. Ovarian estrogen-producing tumors are uncommon. They may be palpable with careful abdominal examination. Ultrasound usually will demonstrate the ovarian mass (15,16). Adrenal estrogen-producing tumors are rare and may be associated with increased levels of adrenal androgens in addition to high estrogen levels. MRI or CT should visualize the adrenal mass. Treatment involves surgical removal of the tumor and, if it is malignant, appropriate additional treatment. Tumor excision will produce regression of sexual precocity.

Ovarian cysts associated with increased estradiol levels are another cause of gonadotropin-independent precocious puberty (17). These cysts may be recurrent. Ultrasound imaging will identify these cysts and their regression, progression, or recurrence. Because of the incidence of recurrence, surgical excision may not affect the child's long-term clinical course. These cysts may produce recurrent episodes of breast development, and vaginal bleeding may occur. Estradiol levels may be high. Testolactone, which blocks estrogen synthesis by inhibiting aromatase, may be considered.

McCune-Albright syndrome is a syndrome of irregular café-au-lait spots, polyostotic fibrous dysplasia, and GnRH-independent precocious puberty. It is caused by a mutation in the α-subunit of the stimulatory G-protein producing constitutive activation (18). In girls, breast development and vaginal bleeding, which may be periodic, are related to intermittent increases in estradiol levels in association with one or more ovarian cysts. LH and FSH levels are prepubertal. Excessive hormone production by other endocrine glands (e.g., thyroid, adrenal, parathyroid) may occur. Treatment of the sexual precocity in McCune-Albright syndrome involves use of testolactone (19). Testolactone, spironolactone, and ketoconazole may be used for treatment in gonadotropin-independent precocious puberty (20).

With these causes of gonadotropin-independent precocious puberty, prolonged or repeated estrogen exposure of the CNS may lead to central precocious puberty. In this situation, after the specific estrogen source is removed or treated, central puberty will progress. Treatment with GnRH analogues is useful in this situation.

Severe and prolonged primary hypothyroidism has been associated with sexual precocity. Also, the clinical coincidence of primary hypothyroidism and precocious puberty has been associated with pituitary enlargement of galactorrhea. In this clinical situation, bone age and growth velocity typically are subnormal. Treatment with thyroxine reverses the precocious puberty.

HETEROSEXUAL DEVELOPMENT

In girls, heterosexual development, or virilization, is caused by excess androgen production from the adrenal in congenital adrenal hyperplasia or by androgen production from adrenal or ovarian tumors.

Adrenal enzyme deficiencies (21-hydroxylase, 11-hydroxlase, and 3β-hydroxysteroid dehydrogenase) may produce genital ambiguity in a female neonate but also may present in later childhood. Plasma levels of sex steroids including androgen precursors must be measured in girls showing virilization and diagnostic imaging (ultrasound, CT, or MRI) performed to identify tumors. As with other forms of gonadotropin-independent precocious puberty, treatment or removal of the excess androgen may, if the bone age is accelerated enough, be associated with progression of central (gonadotropin-dependent) precocious puberty. If this occurs, treatment with GnRH analogues is effective.

Exposure to exogenous androgens must be considered, especially with the current abuse of anabolic steroids in the athletic community.

VARIATIONS OF NORMAL PUBERTY

Premature thelarche occurs commonly in girls, most frequently between the ages of 1 and 4 years. Breast enlargement is seen, often without development of the nipple or areolae. There is no sexual hair development and no acceleration of linear growth or bone age. Minimal or no progression occurs on follow-up. Laboratory evaluation shows prepubertal gonadotropin dynamics, prepubertal or mildly increased estradiol levels, and complete estrogenization of the vaginal mucosa.

Possible causes include ovarian cysts and transient, nonprogressive secretion of pituitary gonadotropins. No treatment is necessary. However, because the early stages of precocious puberty may be clinically identical to premature thelarche, close follow-up is important (21).

Premature adrenarche is defined as the precocious appearance of sexual hair (pubic and/or axillary). The pubic hair often begins on the labia. Premature adrenarche is due to early activation of adrenal androgen secretion. Height and bone age often are slightly greater than the mean but are usually within 2 SD. Adrenal androgen levels are in the early pubertal range, as are urinary 17-ketosteroids (androgen metabolites). It is not uncommon for children with neurologic problems to have premature adrenarche.

Late-onset adrenal hyperplasia may have a similar presentation. Measurement of 17-hydroxprogesterone (and 17-hydroxypregnenolone) is indicated, especially in girls with bone age advancement. Dynamic testing with adrenocorticotropic hormone is helpful to evaluate for these adrenal enzyme deficiencies.

REFERENCES

1. Herman-Giddens ME, Slora EJ, Wasserman RC, ct al. Secondary sexual characteristics and menses in young girls seen in office practice: a study from the pediatric research in office settings network. *Pediatrics* 1997;99: 505–512.
2. Rosenfield RL. The ovary and female sexual maturation. In: Kaplan SA, ed. *Clinical pediatric endocrinology.* Philadelphia: WB Saunders, 1990;259–323.
3. Plotnick LP. Puberty and gonadal disorders. In: Oski FA, ed. *Principles and practice of pediatrics,* 2nd ed. Philadelphia: Lippincott–Raven, 1994;1968–1972.
4. Kaplan SA, Grumbach MM. Clinical review 14. Pathophysiology and treatment of sexual precocity. *J Clin Endocrinol Metab* 1990;71:785–789.
5. Sockalosky JJ, Kriel RL, Krach LE, et al. Precocious puberty after traumatic brain injury. *J Pediatr* 1987;110: 373–377.
6. Rieth KG, Comite F, Dwyer AJ, et al. CT of cerebral abnormalities in precocious puberty. *Am J Roentgenol* 1987;148:1231–1238.
7. Beopple PA, Mansfield MJ, Wierman MF, et al. Use of a potent long acting agonist of gonadotropin-releasing hormone in the treatment of precocious puberty. *Endocrinol Rev* 1986;7:24–33.
8. Lin TH, LePage ME, Henzl M, et al. Intranasal nafarelin: an LH-RH analogue treatment of gonadotropin-dependent precocious puberty. *J Pediatr* 1986;109: 954–958.
9. Manasco PK, Pescovitz OH, Feuillan PP, et al. Resumption of puberty after long term luteinizing hormone-releasing hormone agonist treatment of central precocious puberty. *J Clin Endocrinol Metab* 1988;67:368–372.
10. Kappy M, Stuart T, Perelman A, et al. Suppression of gonadotropin secretion by a long-acting gonadotropin-releasing hormone analog (leuprolide acetate, Lupron Depot) in children with precocious puberty. *J Clin Endocrinol Metab* 1988;69:1087–1089.
11. Lee PA, Page JG. Effects of leuprolide in the treatment of central precocious puberty. *J Pediatr* 1989;114:321–324.
12. Manasco PK, Pescovitz OH, Hill SC, et al. Six year results of luteinizing hormone releasing hormone (LHRH) agonist treatment in children with LHRH-dependent precocious puberty. *J Pediatr* 1989;115:105–108.
13. Parker KL, Lee PA. Depot leuprolide acetate for treatment of precocious puberty. *J Clin Endocrinol Metab* 1989;69:689–691.
14. Biscotti CV, Hart WR. Juvenile granulosa cell tumors of the ovary. *Arch Pathol Lab Med* 1989;113:40–46.
15. Fleischer AC, Shawker TH. The role of sonography in pediatric gynecology. *Clin Obstet Gynecol* 1987;30: 735–746.
16. Salardi S, Orsina LF, Cacciari E, et al. Pelvic ultrasonography in girls with precocious puberty, congenital adrenal hyperplasia, obesity, or hirsutism. *J Pediatr* 1988;112:680–687.
17. Case records of the Massachusetts General Hospital. Weekly clinicopathological exercises. Case 47-1989. A six-year-old girl with sexual precocity. *N Engl J Med* 1989;321:1463–1471.
18. DiMeglio LA, Prescovitz OH. Disorders of puberty: inactivating & activating molecular mutations. *J Pediatr* 1997;131:S8–S12.
19. Feuillan PP, Foster CM, Pescovitz OH, et al. Treatment of precocious puberty in the McCune-Albright syndrome with the aromatase inhibitor testolactone. *N Engl J Med* 1986;315:1115–1119.
20. Wheeler MD. Update on therapy for precocious puberty. *Compr Ther* 1994;20:351–355.
21. Pescovitz OH, Hence KD, Barnes KM, et al. Premature thelarche and central precocious puberty: the relationship between clinical presentation and the gonadotropin response to luteinizing hormone-releasing hormone. *J Clin Endocrinol Metab* 1988;67:474–479.

12

The Menstrual Cycle

Eugene Katz and Uluğ Uluğ

The menstrual cycle with its periodic desquamation of the endometrium is unique to the primate. It is believed to have developed as a consequence of evolutionary changes of both the maternal tract and the embryo (1). Its occurrence is a result of a delicate interaction between the hypothalamus, pituitary gland, and ovaries. This dynamic relationship is manifested in the cyclic stimulation of the ovaries to develop and extrude an oocyte (gametogenesis) and to release into the general circulation, among other hormones, estrogen throughout the cycle and progesterone after ovulation (steroidogenesis). In addition to modulating the hypothalamic pituitary function, estrogens promote the growth of the endometrium, whereas progesterone prepares the tissue for the eventual implantation of a zygote (Fig. 12.1).

The close proximity between the gametes and the steroidogenic apparatus suggests that the two elements communicate with each other, resulting in a perfect coordination between them.

The completion of a normal ovulatory menstrual cycle is the culmination of a maturational process, which begins before the appearance of the first external signs of puberty. This process is first evident by the appearance of nocturnal pulsatile secretion of gonadotropins, a reflection of pulsatile secretion of hypothalamic gonadotropin-releasing hormone (GnRH). Gonadotropins—follicle-stimulating hormone (FSH) and luteinizing hormone (LH)—promote estrogen biosynthesis, which in turn promotes the development of secondary sexual characteristics (i.e., thelarche) and endometrial proliferation. During the first years of puberty, anovulatory cycles induce continuous endometrial proliferation with sporadic and/or irregular menses. Maturation is completed when the hypothalamus displays continuous pulsatile secretion of GnRH and all the feedback mechanisms within the hypothalamic-pituitary-ovarian axis are operational. This will result in the cyclic activity of the system made evident externally by the appearance of regular ovulatory menstrual cycles. This chapter describes how, given a mature hypothalamus and an intact pituitary, the ovary modulates the hypothalamic-pituitary-ovarian axis to maintain normal ovulatory cycles.

Ovulation divides the menstrual cycle into two phases: follicular and luteal. The follicular or proliferative phase is characterized by the development of a follicle, increasing estrogen secretion, and oocyte maturation. Proliferative refers to the estrogen effect on the endometrium. During ovulation, the follicle undergoes rupture while the oocyte resumes meiosis and is extruded. The luteal or secretory phase is characterized by the production of progesterone by the newly formed corpus luteum. Progesterone promotes endometrial glandular secretion (secretory phase) and stromal changes (decidualization) that will allow implantation of the embryo. In the absence of pregnancy, the corpus luteum ceases to function and the lack of hormonal support brings about desquamation of the endometrium or menstruation.

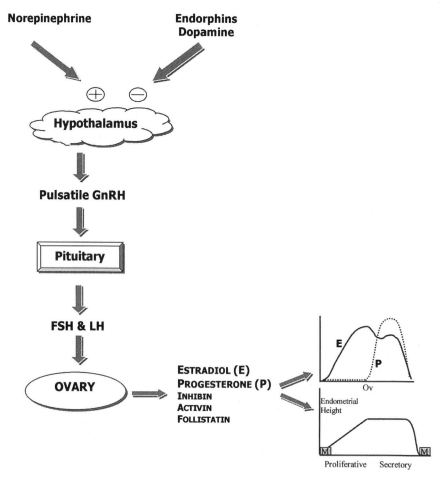

FIG. 12.1. The hypothalamic pituitary axis. Its final products, estrogen and progesterone, promote endometrial proliferation and secretory changes respectively. FSH, follicle-stimulating hormone; GnRH, gonadotropin-releasing hormone; LH, luteinizing hormone; Ov, ovulation.

FOLLICULAR PHASE

The follicular phase lasts 10 to 14 days. During this phase, a dominant follicle selected from a cohort of primordial follicles reaches final maturity (Fig. 12.2). The follicle, the functional unit of the ovary, contains a germinal cell surrounded by granulosa cells. The origin of this structure can be traced to the identification of germ cells as early as the third week of gestation. The primordial germ cells migrate from the yolk sac toward the genital ridge to induce and sustain gonadal development, reaching a maximum of 6 mil-

lion at 20 weeks of gestation. The proliferation of the local coelomic germinal epithelium provides cells that surround the germ cells giving birth to a "primordial follicle." The oocyte, arrested in the diplotene stage of prophase of the first meiotic division, is surrounded by a single layer of flattened pregranulosa cells. From that stage, the tendency of primordial follicles is toward involution or atresia. This process appears to be gonadotropin independent and occurs throughout life. The mechanism underlying this phenomenon may be apoptosis, which is an active form of programmed cell death characterized

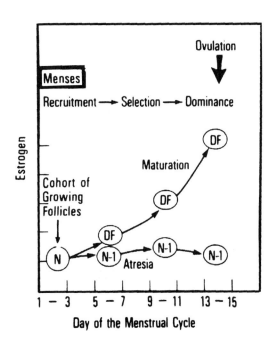

FIG. 12.2. Representation of the fate of a cohort of follicles (N) initiating growth during the follicular phase of the cycle. With the exception of the dominant follicle destined to rupture (ovulation), the remaining follicles (N-1) suffer atresia. (From Hodgen GD. Physiology of follicular maturation. In: Jones HW Jr, Jones GS, Hodgen GD, et al., eds. *In-vitro fertilization.* Baltimore: Williams & Wilkins, 1986:11, with permission.)

by a series of morphologic changes evident at the ultrastructural level (2,3). Thus, one to two million germ cells are present at birth and only 300,000 remain at puberty. Although only one follicle reaches maturity during each menstrual cycle, few germ cells remain in the ovary at menopause.

Escape from this fate is gonadotropin dependent. Thus, FSH promotes the maturation of a cohort of follicles, a process that has been termed "recruitment." It takes place not later than the first day of the cycle, and it extends to the fourth day of the cycle. The continuous stimulation by FSH transforms the primordial follicle into a primary follicle. It is characterized by a primary oocyte surrounded by a single layer of now cuboidal granulosa cells. The latter are surrounded in turn by a basement membrane that separates the granulosa cells from the theca cells of stromal origin. In addition, FSH increases the number of granulosa cells (mitogenic effect) and therefore the overall number of FSH receptors. The follicle surrounded by several layers of granulosa cells is now called the "secondary or preantral follicle" (Fig. 12.3). Meanwhile, the oocyte is

surrounded by a translucent mucopolysaccharide material called the zona pellucida.

In addition to its mitogenic action, FSH stimulates aromatase activity, which catalyzes the conversion of androgens provided by the theca cells into estrogens (Fig. 12.4). Functionally and anatomically, the follicle contains two compartments: the theca cell compartment, which produces androgens, mainly androstenedione; and the granulosa cell compartment, which produces estrogens by aromatizing the theca cell androgen precursors. This model is known as a two-cell theory. Early in the cycle, the capacity of the preantral follicles to aromatize androgens is limited. Because an environment dominated by androgens promotes atresia, further maturation depends on the capacity to acquire aromatization capabilities. Estrogens, the product of androgen aromatization, promote further increase in follicular FSH and estrogen receptors, an important paracrine effect. In addition, estrogens, the most important marker of follicular maturation, further promote mitosis of granulosa cells and amplify FSH-dependent aromatase induction. Estro-

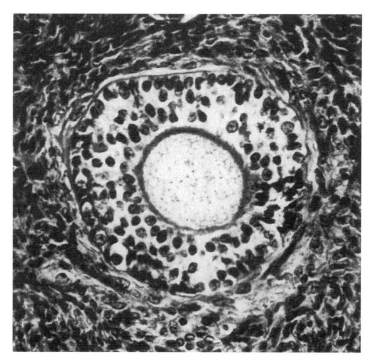

FIG. 12.3. Secondary or preantral follicle. The oocyte is surrounded by several layers of granulosa cells separated from the stroma by a basement membrane. (From Clement PB. Anatomy and histology of the ovary. In: Kurman RJ, ed. *Blaustein's pathology of the female genital tract.* New York: Springer Verlag, 1994:571, with permission.)

gens also stimulate the formation of "gap junctions" between granulosa cells. The relevance of the action of estradiol is exemplified in women unable to synthesize sex steroids due to a 17-hydroxylase deficiency in which, despite high circulating levels of gonadotropins, there is no follicular development. Likewise, in gonadotropin-stimulated immature rats, aromatase inhibitors decrease the number of healthy antral follicles (4).

During its development, the follicle secretes follicular fluid, which accumulates in a cavity or "antrum." The resultant structure becomes a "tertiary or antral follicle" (Fig. 12.5). The oocyte within the follicle remains in an eccentric position surrounded by granulosa cells in what is called the cumulus oophorus.

Recruitment is followed by "selection" (Fig. 12.2). From the initial cohort of follicles recruited, a dominant follicle is chosen, a process that takes place on day 5 to 7 of the menstrual cycle. The selection of a particular follicle depends on its intrinsic capacity to synthesize estrogen and to overcome an androgenic microenvironment. Indeed, by day 5 to 7, the ovary containing the dominant follicle can be shown to secrete more estradiol than the contralateral ovary (5). Furthermore, its follicular fluid milieu is characterized by a high estrogen-to-androgen ratio.

Estrogens in conjunction with FSH induce LH receptors. The two-cell theory assigns specific roles to the two compartments of the follicular apparatus. Thus, LH stimulates theca cells to take up cholesterol carried in the circulation in low-density lipoproteins (LDL) and to convert the precursors into androstenedione and testosterone. Meanwhile, FSH stimulates the aromatization of these androgens into estrone and estradiol, respectively. The final product, estradiol, in turn increases FSH receptors, amplifies FSH action, and as-

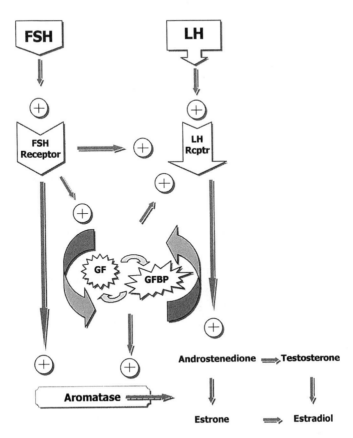

FIG. 12.4. Schematic events occurring as a result of the stimulation of the ovaries by gonadotropins. FSH, follicle-stimulating hormone; GF, growth factor; GFBP, growth factor binding protein; LH, luteinizing hormone.

sists FSH in inducing more FSH receptors not only in the theca cells but also in the granulosa cell compartment (Fig. 12.4). The lack of adequate LH receptors induced before ovulation will result in impaired steroidogenic function of the corpus luteum.

Other substances may play a role in folliculogenesis. Much attention initially was given to insulin-like growth factors (IGFs), specifically to IGF-I, formerly called somatomedin-C. Although traditionally associated with the growth-promoting effect of growth hormone, this 70-amino-acid-long peptide whose most abundant source is the liver has been found in many other tissues, including the ovary. Both the granulosa and theca cells possess receptors for IGF-I, but the IGF-I gene is expressed only in the former. Thus, intrafollicular concentrations of immunoreactive IGF-I are substantially higher in dominant follicles (6). IGF-I increases FSH-induced estrogen and progesterone synthesis as well as FSH-mediated steroid biosynthesis and acquisition of LH receptors (Fig. 12.4) (7). In addition to this autocrine effect, IGF-I may exert a paracrine effect on the theca-interstitial cell compartment by increasing ovarian androgen, which subsequently is aromatized into estrogens (8). IGF-II, a 67-amino-acid polypeptide with 62% homology with IGF-I, is present in preantral and mature follicles with receptors in theca and granulosa cells. IGF-II is the principal IGF in humans. IGF function is further modulated by several IGF-binding proteins (9).

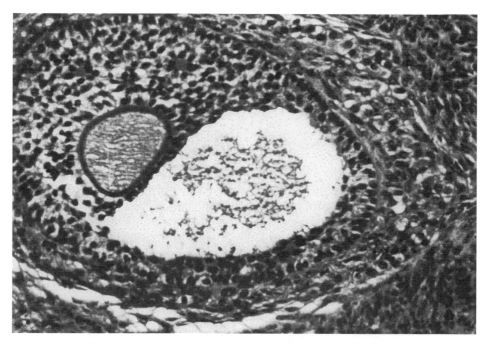

FIG. 12.5. Antral follicle. (From Clement PB. Anatomy and histology of the ovary. In: Kurman RJ, ed. *Blaustein's pathology of the female genital tract.* New York: Springer Verlag, 1994:571, with permission.)

Several growth factors other than IGF may have a role in folliculogenesis. For instance, granulosa cells of larger follicles appear to secrete endotheliotropic factors involved in microvascular remodeling that may explain the richer vascular network surrounding the dominant follicle (10–12). Such a network may further facilitate growth by increasing access to gonadotropins. Other growth factors found in human ovarian include transforming growth factor α (TGF-α), TGF-β, fibroblast growth factor, interleukin 1, and tumor necrosis factor.

As follicles mature, they secrete increasing amounts of estradiol, which inhibits gonadotropin secretion via a negative feedback mechanism. Steroid secretion in the ovary is modulated by inhibin, activin, and follistatin. These local peptides, when stimulated by pituitary gonadotropins, exert paracrine and autocrine effects (13). Inhibin also exerts classic (in distant tissues, i.e., pituitary) hormonal actions. Whereas inhibin serum levels vary widely throughout the menstrual cycle, ac-

tivin and follistatin levels remain low and stable. Inhibin is composed of two subunits, α and β. The β-subunit determines the type of inhibin. Thus, bound to the α-subunit, inhibin A includes an β_A-subunit (α-β_A) and inhibin B an β_B-subunit (α-β_B). In addition to the negative feedback of estradiol on the pituitary secretion of FSH, circulating inhibin further inhibits FSH secretion at the pituitary level. However, at the local level, inhibin enhances LH-stimulated androstenedione production, which serves as a substrate for aromatase (14). Follicular fluid also contains activin, a dimer of the β-subunit, either a homodimer β_A-β_A or a heterodimer β_A-β_B that belongs to the TGF-β superfamily. Activin displays folliculogenic activity. It stimulates FSH-induced estrogen production by rat granulosa cells, increases gonadotropins receptors, increases germinal vesicle breakdown, and decreases androgens (15). Although it stimulates FSH secretion by pituitary cell *in vitro*, it does not appear to exert any action *in vivo* given that it circulates in serum bound to proteins.

Unrelated to activin and inhibin is follistatin. It is formed by a single-chain glycosylated polypeptide that appears to inhibit activin-inhibin interaction with their receptors (13). In an environment in which circulating estradiol and inhibin decrease circulating FSH, the follicle with the highest number of gonadotropin receptors continues to thrive. The remaining follicles in the cohort initially recruited, unable to maintain an estrogenic microenvironment, become atretic.

In general, the process of selection represents a victory of a follicle over the natural tendency to become atretic. Once selection is completed on day 7 to 8 of the cycle, the dominant follicle continues to mature until ovulation. Meanwhile, lesser follicles are unable to aromatize and therefore accumulate androgens. Androgens reduce estrogen receptors and inhibit cell mitosis and aromatase activity, arresting development of the follicle and leading it to atresia. This last phenomenon culminates with the replacement of the follicles by fibroblasts and scarring. Theca cells, however, become part of the ovarian stroma, thus retaining potential function.

PREOVULATORY PERIOD

Increasing circulating levels of estradiol and inhibin reduce pituitary FSH secretion. This negative feedback mechanism is operational since childhood. At puberty, a positive feedback phenomenon between estradiol and gonadotropins becomes functional. Increasing estradiol levels elicit a positive LH response from the pituitary by increasing its sensitivity to GnRH. With the surge of LH, the follicle, having acquired LH receptors induced by estradiol and FSH, secretes 17-hydroxyprogesterone and progesterone (16,17). Progesterone appears to assist in the gonadotropin response, particularly in the midcycle FSH rise (14).

The mature follicle measuring 18 to 20 mm in diameter controls its own fate. Its steroidogenic activity produces high persistent circulating estradiol levels that trigger

the acute release of LH and FSH by the pituitary gland (18). The initiation of LH surge precedes follicular rupture by 36 to 42 hours (Fig. 12.6). Circulating LH peaks in 14 hours and lasts 48 hours. It is accompanied by a rapid fall in estradiol levels (17,19). This surge affects the oocyte, follicular wall, and granulosa cells. It triggers resumption of meiosis, formation of the first polar body, follicular rupture and extrusion of the egg (ovulation), and luteinization.

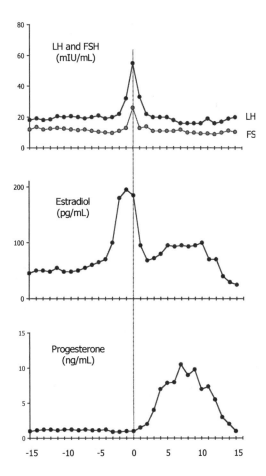

FIG. 12.6. Levels of circulating luteinizing hormone (LH), follicle-stimulating hormone (FSH), and progesterone (P) during the menstrual cycle. (Modified from Thorneycroft IH, Mishell DR Jr, Stone SC, et al. The relation of serum 17-hydroxyprogesterone and estradiol-17β levels during the human menstrual cycle. *Am J Obstet Gynecol* 1971;111:947, with permission.)

OVULATION

During ovulation, the dominant follicle protrudes from the ovarian cortex. This is followed by a gentle release of the oocyte surrounded by the cumulus granulosa cells. Several hypotheses have been formulated to explain follicular rupture.

Increased Follicular Pressure

Changes in the composition of the antral fluid, namely proteoglycans, may result in increases in the colloid-osmotic pressure and further growth of antral cavity. Although an increase in intrafollicular pressure has not been detected in the primate, drugs known to inhibit smooth muscle contraction (calcium antagonists, prostaglandin synthetase inhibitors) inhibit follicular rupture and extrusion of the oocyte (20).

Enzymatic Rupture of the Follicular Wall

Both LH and FSH stimulate the production of plasminogen activator by granulosa cells (21). This results in the conversion of plasminogen activator into plasmin. Plasmin increases fibrinolytic activity, thereby producing a breakdown of the follicular wall. LH may play an additional role by increasing prostaglandin E, which also increases plasminogen activator. Moreover, prostaglandin $F_{2\alpha}$ induces the appearance of lysosomes under the follicular wall, which may further enhance proteolytic activity.

Luteinization

After ovulation, vascular capillaries cross the basement membrane, invading the granulosa cell compartment and greatly increasing the availability of LDL-bound cholesterol. At the same time, LH stimulates the binding of LDL to its ovarian receptors. Moreover, LH increases 3α-hydroxysteroid dehydrogenase activity, thus directing the cholesterol-derived pregnenolone to production of progesterone.

Although estrogens continue to be produced, the luteal phase is characterized by the marked secretion of progesterone. Progesterone induces endometrial maturation and suppresses follicle maturation in the ipsilateral ovary (22). Clinically, the hormone displays a thermogenic activity evidenced by increased basal body temperatures, which is an effect of the steroid on the hypothalamic thermoregulatory center. In the laboratory, luteinization is assumed to have occurred when circulating progesterone levels exceed 3 ng/mL (23). Peak progesterone levels occur 7 to 8 days into the luteal phase (Fig. 12.6). The luteal phase lasts 14 days, although some variation (±2 days) may occur.

The corpus luteum is sustained by LH secretion; however, it soon loses sensitivity to gonadotropins, and luteolysis ensues. Luteolysis is inevitable unless pregnancy occurs and the trophoblast rescues the corpus luteum by secreting high amounts of human chorionic gonadotropin. The resultant decline in circulating hormones (estradiol and progesterone) brings about desquamation of the endometrium (menses). In the late luteal phase, the reduction of estrogen and progesterone allows gonadotropin to rise, which is the first stimulus for a new recruitment cycle. The regressed corpus luteum becomes the "corpus albicans," an avascular scar.

MENSTRUATION

The target of ovarian steroidogenic production and the external hallmark of the menstrual cycle is, after growth and maturation, the periodic desquamation of the endometrium. Of course, if fertilization and implantation take place, embryonic chorionic gonadotropin will further stimulate the corpus luteum to continue steroidogenesis and menstruation will not occur. Immediately before menses, the endometrium is infiltrated by leukocytes. An initial vasoconstriction causes ischemia and early desquamation, which is followed by arteriolar relaxation, bleeding, and tissue breakdown. About 20 to 60 mL of blood is lost.

THE ENDOMETRIUM

The endometrium is formed by a "zona basalis" adjacent to the myometrium and a "functionalis layer" that, although it is a continuum, is commonly divided into a "zona compacta" adjacent to the uterine cavity and a "spongiosum layer." Estrogen-induced mitotic activity in the glands and stroma during the follicular phase rapidly increases endometrial thickness from 2 to 8 mm or more from basalis to opposing basalis layer. Sonographically, the interface of basalis layers with the myometrium on both sides and the endometrial surfaces appears as a trilaminar layer (Fig. 12.7).

After ovulation and with increasing production of progesterone, mitotic activity is severely restricted. The glands produce and later secrete glycogen-rich vacuoles. There is increased stromal edema, stromal cells enlarge, and spiral arterioles develop and rapidly lengthen and coil. On ultrasound, the endometrium loses its trilaminar semblance and appears as a homogeneous layer (Fig. 12.8).

THE HYPOTHALAMIC ROLE IN THE MENSTRUAL CYCLE

Thus far, the cycle has been described in terms of the interplay between the ovary, its compartments with each other, and the pituitary. However, the pituitary function is GnRH dependent. GnRH activity is first evident at puberty. Nocturnal pulsatile activity induces a similar release of gonadotropins, which in turn initiate and maintain the secretion of estradiol. The continuous pulsatile release of GnRH induces the appearance of increased GnRH receptors in the gonadotroph (self-priming effect). Whereas small pulses display a priming effect, longer ones result in release of gonadotropins.

The pulsatile secretion of GnRH depends on the activity of a pulse generator with intrinsic rhythmicity located in the arcuate nucleus of the mediobasal hypothalamus (24). Each pulsatile episode of LH results from a corresponding hypothalamic discharge of GnRH. Experimentally, the loss of GnRH pulsatility (i.e., continuous administration of GnRH) results in downregulation of pituitary GnRH receptors and inhibition of pituitary secretion of gonadotropins (25).

The release of GnRH is modulated by external neural signals as well as by steroid hormones directly and indirectly via neurotransmitters. For instance, dopamine and β-endorphins decrease GnRH activity whereas norepinephrine stimulates GnRH release (Fig. 12.1). Progesterone and testosterone each reduces GnRH pulse frequency, a phenomenon mediated in part by the opioidergic system (26). On the other hand, estradiol increases pulse frequency and amplitude in normal preovulatory primates, but it exerts the opposite effect in castrated primates (27). During the follicular phase, GnRH pulses occur hourly. During the luteal phase, while estrogen and progesterone reduce the pulse frequency to one pulse every 90 minutes, amplitude is increased (28). Although GnRH, gonadotropins, and circulating steroids modulate GnRH release, the importance of the modulation of the "pulse generator" by these hormones has not been clearly defined. Ovulation can be induced in women with hypothalamic failure by administering GnRH in a fixed pulsatile fashion. In this respect, more important is the regulation of pituitary function by ovarian steroids.

Estrogens exert both a negative and a positive feedback action at the level of the pituitary gland. To explain this apparent paradox, the existence of two pools of gonadotropins in the pituitary gland has been postulated: a "releasable gonadotropin pool" reflecting "sensitivity" to a discrete GnRH stimulus and a "reserve" pool that becomes apparent when the pituitary is exposed to increased and more prolonged GnRH stimulation. In this scenario, the two pools are stimulated, and the resulting secretion reflects both pools or the total "capacity" of the gonadotrophs (29,30).

Estrogen appears to stimulate both pools but preferentially the reserve pool. Therefore, during the follicular phase, the negative feedback action of estrogen on the pituitary is exerted on release rather than synthesis or reserve pool. Late in the follicular phase, higher and sustained estradiol levels promote the transfer of LH from the reserve into the acute release pool, resulting in the acute discharge

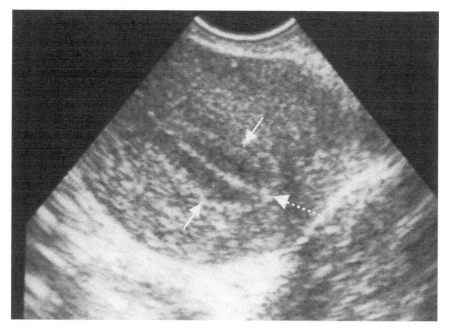

FIG. 12.7. Sonogram of the late proliferative endometrium. Echodense lines at the endometrial-myometrial border *(solid arrows)* and at the endometrial cavity *(broken arrow)* result in the typical trilaminar appearance.

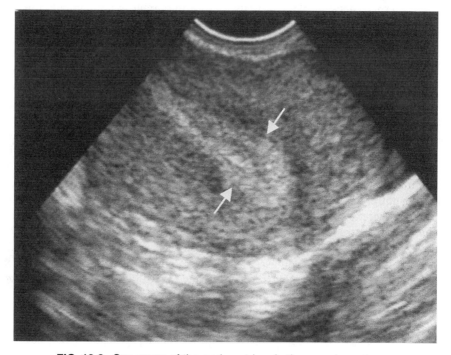

FIG. 12.8. Sonogram of the endometrium in the secretory phase.

of LH (positive feedback). This not with-standing, a steroid-induced preovulatory GnRH surge may play a role in the generation of the LH surge (31,32). The small preovulatory increase in circulating progesterone increases the LH response. In the clinical settings, some patients undergoing ovulation induction with gonadotropins display a premature LH surge induced by the high estradiol levels. Such surges can be avoided by downregulating pituitary GnRH receptors with long-acting GnRH agonists.

It is evident from the description of the events that the follicle controls the cycle directly by modulating the pituitary response and indirectly through the hypothalamus. The intraovarian regulation is complex and may include roles for vasopressin, oxytocin, relaxin, aromatase inhibitors, and other substances for which the physiologic role has not been clearly delineated. The regulatory mechanism governing the ovarian and higher centers appears optimum because it makes use of the two intraovarian signals to coordinate steroidogenesis and oogenesis locally and of extraovarian messengers to modulate gonadotropin secretion distally.

REFERENCES

1. Finn CA. Menstruation: nonadaptive consequence of uterine evolution. *Q Rev Biol* 1998;73:162.
2. DePol A, Vaccina F, Forabusco A, et al. Apoptosis of germ cells during human prenatal oogenesis. *Hum Reprod* 1997;12:2235.
3. Izawa M, Nhuyen PH, Kim HH, et al. Expression of the apoptosis related genes caspase-1, caspase-3, DNA fragmentation factor, and apoptotic protease activating factor-1, in human granulosa cells. *Fertil Steril* 1998; 70:549.
4. Selveraj N, Shetty G, Vijayolakshmi K, et al. Effect of blocking estrogen synthesis with a new generation aromatase inhibitor CGS 16949A on follicular maturation induced by pregnant mare serum gonadotropin in the immature rat. *J Endocrinol* 1994;142:563.
5. DiZerega GS, Hodgen GD. Folliculogenesis in the primate ovarian cycle. *Endocrinol Rev* 1981;2:27.
6. Eden JA, Jones J, Carter GD, et al. A comparison of follicular fluid levels of insulin-like growth factor-I in normal dominant and cohort follicles, polycystic and multicystic ovaries. *Clin Endocrinol* 1988;29:327.
7. Adashi EY, Resnick CE7, D'Ercole AJ, et al. Insulin-like growth factors as intraovarian regulators of granulosa cell growth and function. *Endocrinol Rev* 1985;6: 400.
8. Hernandez ER, Resnick CE, Svoboda ME, et al. Somatomedin-C/insulin-like growth factor I (Sm-C/IGF-I) as an enhancer of androgen bio-synthesis by cultured rat ovarian cells. *Endocrinology* 1981;122:1583.
9. Iwashita M, Kudo Y, Yoshimura Y, et al. Physiological role of insulin-like-growth-factor-binding protein-4 in human folliculogenesis. *Horm Res* 1996;46[Suppl]:31.
10. Zeleznik AJ, Schuler HM, Reichert LE. Gonadotropin-binding sites in the rhesus monkey ovary: role of the vasculature in the selective distribution of human chorionic gonadotropin to the preovulatory follicle. *Endocrinology* 1981;109:356.
11. Katz E, Rone JD, Garcia J, et al. Evidence for the production of a non-steroidal endotheliotropic factor by human granulosa cells in culture. *Fertil Steril* 1992;57: 107.
12. Ravindnanath L, Little-Ihring LL, Phillips HS, et al. Vascular endothelial growth factor messenger ribonucleic acid expression in the primate ovary. *Endocrinology* 1992;131:254.
13. Halvorson LM, DeCherney AH. Inhibin, activin, and follistatin in reproductive medicine. *Fertil Steril* 1996; 65:459.
14. Hsue AJW, Dahl KD, Vaughan J, et al. Heterodimers and homodimers of inhibin subunits have different paracrine action in the modulation of luteinizing hormone-stimulated androgen biosynthesis. *Proc Natl Acad Sci U S A* 1987;84:5082.
15. Burger HG, Findlay JK. Potential relevance of inhibin to ovarian physiology. *Semin Reprod Endocrinol* 1989; 7:69.
16. Thorneycroft IH, Mishell DR Jr, Stone SC, et al. The relation of serum 17-hydroxyprogesterone and estradiol-17β levels during the human menstrual cycle. *Am J Obstet Gynecol* 1971;111:947.
17. Thorneycroft IH, Sribyatta B, Tom WK, et al. Measurement of serum LH, FSH, progesterone, 17-hydroxyprogesterone and estradiol-17β levels at 4-hour intervals during the periovulatory phase of the menstrual cycle. *J Clin Endocrinol Metab* 1974;39:754.
18. Hackeloer J, Fleming R, Robinson HP, et al. Correlation of ultrasonic and endocrinologic assessment of human follicular development. *Am J Obstet Gynecol* 1979;135: 122.
19. World Health Organization Task Force Investigators. Temporal relationships between ovulation and defined changes in the concentration of plasma estradiol 17-β, luteinizing hormone, follicle-stimulating hormone, and progesterone. *Am J Obstet Gynecol* 1980;138:383.
20. Katz E, Dharmarajan AM, Suoka K, et al. Effects of systemic administration of indomethacin on ovulation, luteinization, and steroidogenesis in the rabbit ovary. *Am J Obstet Gynecol* 1989;161:1361.
21. Strickland S, Beers WH. Studies on the role of plasminogen activator in ovulation. *J Biol Chem* 1976;251: 5694.
22. DiZerega GS, Hodgen GD. The interovarian progesterone gradient: a spatial and temporal regulator of folliculogenesis in the primate ovarian cycle. *J Clin Endocrinol Metab* 1982;54:495.
23. Israel R, Mishell DR Jr, Stone SC, et al. Single luteal phase serum progesterone assay as an indicator of ovulation. *Am J Obstet Gynecol* 1972;112:1043.
24. Kessner JS, Kaufmann JM, Wilson RC, et al. On the short-loop feedback regulation of the hypothalamic

luteinizing hormone releasing hormone "pulse generator" in the rhesus monkey. *Neuroendocrinology* 1986;
42:109.

25. Belchetz PE, Plant TM, Nakai Y, et al. Hypophyseal responses to continuous and intermittent delivery of hypothalamic gonadotropin-releasing hormone. *Science*
1978;202:631.

26. Plan TM. Gonadal regulation of hypothalamic gonadotropin-releasing hormone release in primates. *Endocrinol Rev* 1986;7:758.

27. Djahanhakhch O, Warner P, McNeilly AS, et al. Pulsatile release of LH and estradiol during the pre-ovula-
tory period in women. *Clin Endocrinol* 1984;20:579.

28. Reame N, Sauder SE, Kelch RP, et al. Pulsatile gonadotropin secretion during the human menstrual cycle:
evidence for altered frequency of gonadotropin-releasing hormone secretion. *J Clin Endocrinol Metab* 1984;
59:328.

29. Yen SSC, Lein A. The apparent paradox of the negative

and positive feedback control system on gonadotropin
secretion. *Am J Obstet Gynecol* 1976;126:942.

30. Hoff JD, Lasley BL, Wang CF, et al. The two pools of
pituitary gonadotropins: regulation during the menstrual cycle. *J Clin Endocrinol Metab* 1977;44:302.

31. Levine JE, Normal RI, Gliessmann FR, et al. In vivo gonadotropin-releasing hormone release and serum luteinizing hormone measurements in ovariectomized estrogen-
treated rhesus monkeys. *Endocrinology* 1985;117:711.

32. Filicori M, Flamigni C, Campaniello E, et al. Evidence
for a specific role of GnRH pulse frequency in the control of the human menstrual cycle. *Am J Physiol* 1984;
257:E930.

33. Hodgen GD. Physiology of follicular maturation. In:
Jones HW Jr, Jones GS, Hodgen GD, et al, eds. *In-vitro
fertilization.* Baltimore: Williams & Wilkins, 1986:11.

34. Clement PB. Anatomy and histology of the ovary. In:
Kurman RJ, ed. *Blaustein's pathology of the female genital tract.* New York: Springer Verlag, 1994:571.

13

Adolescent Amenorrhea

Thomas M. Price and G. William Bates

Amenorrhea is the absence or cessation of menses, which may be primary or secondary. Primary amenorrhea is the lack of onset of menses by the age of 16 years in a female with secondary sexual characteristics or by the age of 14 years in an adolescent without secondary sexual development. Secondary amenorrhea is the cessation of menses for a period of 6 months in a female who previously had initiation of menses. This classification, however, gives no insight into the etiology of the amenorrhea or the prognosis for future ovulation and menstruation. In this chapter, the classification of primary and secondary amenorrhea is not absolute but is referred to as a marker for timing the onset of amenorrhea. An understanding of amenorrhea is developed that is based on the physiology of puberty and ovulation. We have found that the evaluation of patients with amenorrhea is simplified by placing patients into four diagnostic categories based on physical development. These categories are females with breast development, females without breast development, females with androgen excess,

and females with hyperprolactinemia. Each category characterizes levels of estrogen, androgens, or prolactin, which are key to the etiology of amenorrhea.

PUBERTY

Secondary Sexual Development

The process of secondary sexual maturation occurs in an orderly, predictable sequence. It reflects the secretion and action of hypothalamic peptide factors, anterior pituitary protein hormones, adrenal steroid hormones, and ovarian sex steroids. This sequence of development in girls was described by Marshall and Tanner (1) and is presented in Table 13.1.

Breast development is the first physical sign of puberty in the majority of girls and occurs at a median age of 9.8 years. The breast bud presents as a small mound beneath the nipple and is more easily palpated then visualized, especially in obese young girls. Estradiol secretion from the ovaries is requisite for

TABLE 13.1. *Sequence of sexual maturation in girls*

Event	Age (yr)	Hormones (yr)
Breast budding	10–11	Estradiol
Sexual hair growth	10.5–11.5	Androgens
Growth spurt	11–12	Growth hormone
Menarche	11.5–13	Estradiol
Adult breast development	12.5–15	Progesterone
Adult sexual hair pattern	13.5–16	Androgens

From Marshall WA, Tanner JM. Variations in the pattern of pubertal changes in girls. *Arch Dis Child* 1969;44:291, with permission.

breast development. In the absence of direct ovarian estradiol secretion, such as with gonadal dysgenesis, estrone produced by peripheral conversion of adrenal and ovarian androgens is insufficient to induce breast development. Development of the breast involves initial proliferation of the epithelial ductal system with subsequent growth of adipose and connective tissue. Ultimate breast size is determined by genetic and nutritional factors, but the molecular mechanisms regulating this phenomenon still are unknown.

The appearance of pubic hair quickly follows breast development at 10.5 years. Androgens of either adrenal or ovarian origin may be sufficient for pubic hair development, as evidenced by pubic hair in children less than 8 years old with premature adrenarche and the development of pubic hair at the time of gonadarche in children with primary adrenal insufficiency. The combination of androgens from both the ovary and adrenal probably optimizes pubic hair growth. In approximately 10% of normal girls, pubic hair development is the first sign of puberty, preceding breast development by a few months. An earlier onset of pubic hair growth, disparate from breast growth, may suggest a developing condition of androgen excess such as late-onset congenital adrenal hyperplasia (CAH).

An increase in growth velocity is actually the first clinical sign of puberty in girls, preceding breast development. Maximum growth rate correlates with Tanner III to IV stages at approximately 11.4 years. The difference in final height between males and females is primarily influenced by two factors. Females start the growth spurt at a younger age and thus with less height; the height obtained during the spurt itself is less (2). Estradiol appears to be the primary hormone responsible for epiphyseal plate closure in both women and men. The role of estrogen for bone growth and closure, even in males, was made evident by a case report of a man with an estrogen receptor abnormality, characterized by extreme height and severe osteoporosis (3). Final height in women thus correlates with the

age of onset of puberty. The earlier the onset of puberty, in general, the less the final height. At the age of menarche, a woman has completed greater than 95% of her growth with, on average, only 2.5 cm of growth remaining.

Menarche with the establishment of regular ovulatory cycles is the culmination of puberty. The median age of menarche in the United States is 12.7 years. The initial episode of uterine bleeding may not necessarily be the result of ovulation. Up to 55% of cycles may be anovulatory within the first 2 years of puberty, with this number decreasing to 20% within 5 years (4). Within 3 to 5 years of menarche, most women establish a menstrual pattern that will be characteristic of their remaining reproductive years, barring dramatic changes in weight or medical status. Thus, cycle irregularity in the late teenage years is a common predictor of ovulatory dysfunction in the subsequent reproductive years.

Hypothalamic-Pituitary-Ovarian Axis

The onset of puberty is characterized by an "awakening" of hypothalamic function, with increased gonadotropin-releasing hormone (GnRH) production compared to the quiescent childhood years. For many years, a relationship between body weight and puberty in girls has been realized. In general, a weight of 48 kg with a body fat percentage of 21% correlates with the onset of menarche (5). Improved nutrition and weight gain are primarily responsible for the decline in the age of menarche from 17 years in the mid 1800s to the present day age. Girls with modest obesity experience an earlier menarche compared to girls of normal weight. In contrast, delayed puberty is common in individuals with low body fat, such a gymnasts, ballet dancers, and sufferers of anorexia nervosa. The signal between the fat stores of the body and the brain was not realized until the recent discovery of the protein leptin. Leptin, a 16-kD protein, is the product of the obese *(ob)* gene found in mice. Although many cell types, including hematopoietic cells, trophoblasts, and breast epithelial cells, produce leptin, adipose tissue appears to be the primary source of circulating leptin in humans. Leptin levels correlate directly with body mass index. Several observations suggest that leptin is intimately related to the onset of puberty. Leptin treatment restores puberty and fertility in the *ob/ob* mouse that has a total deficiency of leptin, and in starved normal mice. Leptin treatment in normal prepubertal mice stimulates the onset of puberty (6). In humans, leptin levels rise just before puberty, and children with central precocious puberty have higher circulating leptin levels compared to weight-matched controls (7,8). In a study by Garcia-Mayor and colleagues (9), changes in leptin levels were correlated with gonadotropin and estradiol levels and the stages of puberty (Fig. 13.1). Leptin levels increase just before the rise in follicle-stimulating hormone (FSH) levels associated with early puberty. Interestingly, leptin has a diurnal pattern in humans, with higher levels during sleep as is seen with luteinizing hormone (LH) during puberty. The evidence that leptin influences the onset of puberty is strong, but the exact mechanisms by which this protein regulates the production of GnRH remain to be elucidated. Neurotransmitters such as neuropeptide Y, glutamate, and γ-aminobutyric acid may act as intermediates between leptin and the GnRH neurons (9).

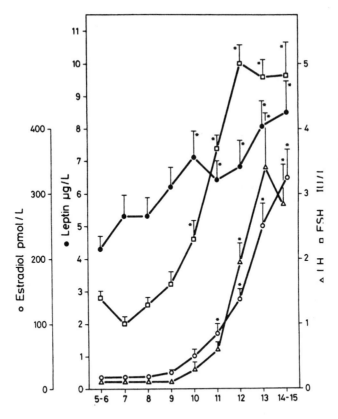

FIG. 13.1. Relationship of leptin (●), follicle-stimulating hormone (FSH; □), luteinizing hormone (LH; △), and estradiol (○) in normal girls according to age. Values are given as mean ± SEM. *Asterisks* represent values significantly different from the 5- to 6-year-old group. (From Garcia-Mayor RV, Andrade A, Rios M, et al. Serum leptin levels in normal children: relationship to age, gender, body mass index, pituitary-gonadal hormones and pubertal stage. *J Clin Endocrinol Metab* 1997;82:2849–2855, with permission.)

With increasing GnRH secretion, FSH levels initially rise followed by LH levels. LH secretion is characterized by sleep-related pulses in mid to late puberty that are not seen after puberty in adult women. These endogenous changes may be elicited by stimulation testing. Exogenous GnRH stimulation testing before puberty shows no gonadotropin response, at the time of thelarche shows an FSH-dominant response, and in late puberty and adult women shows an LH-dominant response. Women with anorexia show a reversal in the GnRH stimulation response as body fat is lost. Girls with isolated premature thelarche have an FSH-dominant GnRH response, whereas girls with central precocious puberty demonstrate an LH-dominant response.

Physiology of Ovulation

Many causes of amenorrhea are related to abnormalities of ovulation. Ovulation is an intricate process that depends on the cyclic interaction of hypothalamic GnRH, pituitary FSH and LH, and ovarian estradiol and progesterone. These hormones have positive and negative regulating effects on each other. These effects are summarized in Table 13.2.

Pulsatile release of GnRH from the arcuate nucleus of the medial basal hypothalamus controls the pituitary secretion of FSH and LH. Under normal physiologic conditions, GnRH pulses in the follicular phase occur at approximate 60-minute intervals and are of low amplitude. The pulse interval decreases as estradiol levels rise preovulatory, ultimately leading to the LH and lesser FSH surges. In the luteal phase, progesterone modulates GnRH pulses to long intervals with high amplitude. Other neurotransmitters regulate GnRH secretion, including augmentation by epinephrine and norepinephrine, whereas serotonin, opioids, and dopamine inhibit GnRH secretion.

FSH and LH secretion also are modulated by estradiol and progesterone production from the ovaries. During menses, estradiol levels are low, leading to increased FSH. FSH is primarily responsible for granulosa cell proliferation and initial recruitment of the cohort of follicles. As the follicular phase progresses, FSH levels decline due to negative feedback of rising estradiol levels. A dominant follicle emerges from the cohort and is able to progress while other follicles undergo atresia because the dominant follicle has the most granulosa cells and the most efficient estradiol production in the face of declining FSH. During the follicular phase, LH levels slowly rise. LH is responsible for the production of androgens from theca cells. Androgens, primarily androstenedione, diffuse across the avascular basement membrane into granulosa cells, where they are converted into estradiol by aromatase. Late in the follicular phase, FSH induces LH receptors in granulosa cells that are necessary for ovulation.

Ovulation is initiated by an estradiol level greater than 200 pg/mL for at least 48 to 50 hours, which triggers the LH surge. Ovulation occurs 34 to 36 hours after the initiation and 10 to 12 hours after the peak of the LH surge. The LH surge is related to many processes, including the resumption of meiosis with extrusion of the first polar body, changes in the follicle content of prostaglandins and proteolytic enzymes, and breakdown of the avascular membrane separating granulosa and theca cells with initiation of angiogenesis.

The hallmark of the luteal phase is formation of the corpus luteum, with massive pro-

TABLE 13.2. *Hormonal interrelationships*

Hormone	Effects on other reproductive hormones
FSH	Stimulates follicular maturation (estradiol production)
LH	Triggers ovulation (stimulates androgen production)
Estradiol	Stimulates LH; downregulates FSH
Progesterone	Downregulates LH and FSH

FSH, follicle-stimulating hormone; LH, luteinizing hormone.

duction of progesterone. No longer separated by an avascular membrane, granulosa lutein cells and theca lutein cells now function as a single unit in the production of estradiol and progesterone. Cholesterol derived from circulating lipoproteins now is available to the granulosa lutein cells, with progesterone as the end product due to a lack of the enzyme 17α-hydroxylase. Estradiol production continues with aromatization of theca-derived androgens. The function of progesterone is to develop an adequate secretory endometrium for implantation. The quantity of progesterone produced depends directly on the quality of the original dominant follicle. A poorly developed dominant follicle may still be capable of ovum release but forms a poor corpus luteum, resulting in low progesterone production, inadequate secretory endometrium development, and low likelihood of a successful implantation. The lifespan of the corpus luteum is fixed at 14 days unless rescued by implantation and initiation of human chorionic gonadotropin (hCG) production.

The intricacy of the ovulation process allows for many possible perturbations leading to dysfunction. Disorders may involve GnRH pulsatility, gonadotropin release, and ovarian sex steroid production. The pulse frequency of GnRH may be altered by low or excessive body weight, stress, excessive physical exercise, or use of marijuana. Hypothalamic-pituitary regulated gonadotropin secretion may be altered by abnormalities of other pituitary hormones such as prolactin, growth hormone, adrenocorticotropic hormone (ACTH), or thyroid-stimulating hormone (TSH). Inappropriate circulating levels of sex steroids, including androgens and estrogens, may lead to dysfunctional hypothalamic-pituitary regulated gonadotropin secretion. Disorders of ovulation may be chronic, leading to prolonged amenorrhea, or they may be intermittent, leading to irregular cycles (10).

CAUSES OF AMENORRHEA

The causes of amenorrhea are listed in Table 13.3.

Amenorrhea with Breast Development

Outflow Tract Obstructions

The presence of breast development confirms that, at some time, the patient had significant circulating levels of estradiol. Amenorrhea in this category suggests either that there is an outflow abnormality such as a blockage or congenital lack of development, or that estrogen has stopped being produced because of gonadal failure or lack of gonadotropin stimulation.

Imperforate hymen is the most common outflow tract abnormality, with an incidence of one in 1,000 to 10,000 (11). The cause of this condition is unknown, but it represents a failure of canalization of the junction between the caudal end of the paramesonephric ducts and the cephalad end of the urogenital sinus. The most common presentation is at the time of expected menarche, with cyclic or persistent pelvic pain, pelvic mass, and a bulging, bluish-tinged hymen. Other less common symptoms include urinary retention (12) and pain with defecation (13). Less commonly, cases may be seen in the fetal or neonatal period, with hydrocolpos and hydrometrocolpos from cervical and vaginal mucus stimulated by high circulating maternal estrogen levels. Outflow tract obstructions are second only to hydronephrosis as a cause of abdominal mass in the female neonate (11). The vast majority of cases of imperforate hymen are sporadic, with no associated abnormalities. Rarely, familial cases have been reported (14).

Transverse vaginal septum is a much less common cause of outflow obstruction (Fig. 13.2). The septum may be complete, leading to cryptomenorrhea, or it may have a pinpoint opening, leading to prolonged scant bleeding (15). Symptoms of pelvic pain, or more rarely, urinary retention or painful defecation usually present. Unlike an imperforate hymen, a bulging vaginal mass is not noted. In a review of 26 cases by Rock and colleagues (13), a high vaginal septum found just distal to the cervix accounted for 46% of the cases. These septums usually were thicker than lower septums. A midvaginal septum was

TABLE 13.3. *Causes of amenorrhea*

Amenorrhea with breast development	Ovarian Tumors
Outflow obstruction	Sertoli-Leydig cell
Imperforate hymen	Lipoid cell
Transverse vaginal septum	Hilar cell
Asherman's syndrome	Granulosa-theca cell
Müllerian agenesis	Thecoma
Androgen insensitivity syndrome	Brenner tumor
Hypothalamic/pituitary (without hyperprolactinemia)	Cystadenoma/adenoca
Low body weight	Adrenal Disease
Anorexia/bulemia	Cushing's disease
Malnutrition/malabsorption	Ectopic adrenocorticotropic hormone source
Strenuous exercise	Adrenocortical tumor
Cancer/chronic disease	Amenorrhea with hyperprolactinemia
Immunodeficiency syndrome	Drugs
Premature Ovarian Failure	Estrogen-containing compounds
Idiopathic	Dopamine-depleting agents
Autoimmune with Addison's	Methyldopa
Autoimmune without Addison's	Reserpine
Resistant ovary (Savage syndrome)	Monoamine oxidose inhibitors
Injury	Dopamine-receptor blocker
Infectious	Haloperidol
Chemotherapy	Phenothiazines
Radiation therapy	Metoclopramide
Galactosemia	Sulpiride
Amenorrhea without breast development	Pimozide
Gonadal dysgenesis	Domperidone
Turner's syndrome	Anesthesia
Mosaic Turner's	Opiates
Deletion of long arm of X chromosome	Amphetamines, hallucinogens
Triple X syndrome	Cimetadine
Pure gonadal dysgenesis	Tumors
XX karyotype	Prolactinoma
XY karyotype (Swyer syndrome)	Acromegaly
Gonadal agenesis	Nonhormone adenoma
Vanishing testes syndrome	Craniopharyngioma
Enzyme deficiencies	Cushing's disease
17-OH/17,20 lyase deficiency	Glioma
5α-Reductase deficiency	Dermoid
17β-Hydroxylase deficiency	Bronchogenic cancer
Aromatase deficiency	Infiltrating diseases
GnRH deficiency	Sarcoidosis, tuberculosis
Kallmann's syndrome	Histiocytosis
Idiopathic hypogonadotropic hypogonadism	Hemochromatosis
Hypothalamic disorders	Trauma/infection
Amenorrhea with androgen excess	Encephalitis, meningitis
Polycystic ovarian syndrome	Radiation
Hyperthecosis	Stalk transection, shunt placement
Congenital adrenal hyperplasia	Renal failure
21α-hydroxylase deficiency	Hypothyroidism
11β-hydroxylase deficiency	Chest wall trauma, surgery

found in 35% of cases; the lower vaginal septum was the least common at 19% of cases. Pelvic endometriosis more commonly is associated with transverse vaginal septum than with imperforate hymen. This may be due to a longer time to diagnosis or possibly to a greater amount of retrograde flow with a septum because the distensible vaginal reservoir is absent. Endometriosis also may play a part in the lower pregnancy rate seen in women with transverse septums (13). Similar to imperforate hymen, associated abnormalities with transverse vaginal septum are uncommon. In the same series by Rock et al., 8% of

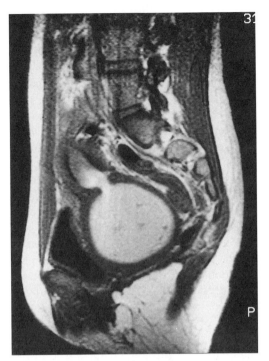

FIG. 13.2. Pelvic magnetic resonance imaging in an adolescent with primary amenorrhea due to a high vaginal septum showing hematometria and hematocolpos.

women with transverse septum had a congenital renal abnormality including hypoplasia of the kidney and duplication of the ureter.

Vaginal Absence Syndromes

Müllerian agenesis or Mayer-Rokitansky-Küster-Hauser syndrome is the most common cause of primary amenorrhea in women with normal breast development, with an incidence of one in 5,000 (Fig. 13.3). This syndrome originally was described by Mayer in 1829 and then redescribed by Rokitansky in 1838 (16). Typically, the vagina that is proximal to the hymen and the uterus fail to develop. Visual inspection of the pelvis often shows bilateral small muscular swellings at the proximal end of each fallopian tube. The uterine anlagen usually are rudimentary, with functional endometrium found in less than 10% of cases (17). The ovaries are normal; thus, all

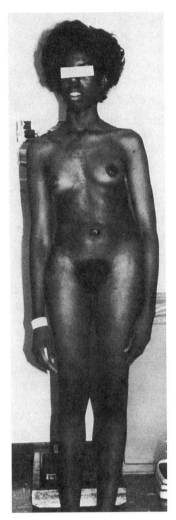

FIG. 13.3. A 16-year-old girl with primary amenorrhea due to müllerian agenesis. Note the full secondary sexual maturation. Scoliosis occurs in approximately 15% of cases.

other aspects of puberty, including breast development, pubic hair development, and growth spurt, occur as expected. The etiology of müllerian agenesis remains unknown. The discovery of homeobox genes responsible for segmental development in lower animals may provide a clue to the cause of this syndrome. Occasionally, young women with müllerian agenesis will complain of cyclic pelvic pain. In this situation, a functional uterine anlagen needs to be excluded, but the transient discomfort more often is due to periovulatory pain. Typically, Rokitansky syndrome is sporadic. In 40% to 50% of cases, associated renal abnormalities, including renal agenesis, ectopic kidney, horseshoe kidney, and duplication of the collecting system, are found (18). Bony abnormalities in 10% to 15% of cases typically are found in the axial skeleton, including hemivertebra leading to scoliosis, missing and abnormal ribs, and pelvic bone abnormalities. Other syndromes involving müllerian agenesis have been described. MURCS association includes müllerian agenesis, renal aplasia, and cervicothoracic spinal deformities. Other cases of vaginal agenesis have been associated with congenital deafness due to developmental abnormalities of the malleus, stapes, and incus bones. Finally, cases of müllerian agenesis have been associated with abnormalities of the distal extremities, instead of the axial skeleton, such as missing and abnormal digits. These cases, characterized by hand-foot-uterus syndrome, usually are inherited in an autosomal dominant manner (19,20).

Androgen insensitivity syndrome (AIS), also called testicular feminization syndrome, is a less common cause of primary amenorrhea with breast development. This X-linked disorder is caused by an abnormality of the gene for the androgen receptor located on the long arm of the X chromosome (21). More than 100 different gene defects, including deletions and point mutations, have been described. Most mutations result in complete inactivity of the receptor. The presentation is of a genetic male appearing as a phenotypical female lacking signs of androgen expression (Fig. 13.4). Testes usually are intraabdominal, but they also may be herniated into the labia. The normal secretion of müllerian inhibitory factor (MIF) results in lack of development of the upper vagina, uterus, and fallopian tubes. In addition, the lack of a functional androgen receptor results in absence of male internal structures such as vas deferens, seminal vesicles, and prostate. Affected persons appear as normal females at birth. With puberty, breast development ensues due to peripheral conversion of circulating androgens to estrogen. Breast development often is abundant due to the lack of any opposing androgen effect. Pubic and axillary hair is scant to absent and is the main distinguishing characteristic of this syndrome. The vagina is shortened but often not to the extent as seen with müllerian agenesis. Circulating testosterone levels are in the high-normal range for a male. This is due to higher than normal levels of LH because of lack of appropriate negative feedback to the pituitary. Unlike müllerian agenesis, concomitant renal or skeletal abnormalities are not found with AIS. Less commonly, muta-

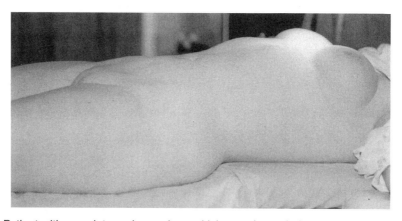

FIG. 13.4. Patient with complete androgen insensitivity syndrome being prepared for gonadectomy. Note the characteristic lack of pubic hair.

tions of the androgen receptor lead to a partially active receptor with androgen expression. The presentation includes ambiguous genitalia at birth, with clitoral enlargement and fusion of labioscrotal folds. Virilization occurs at puberty to a degree that depends on the activity of the receptor (22).

Central Disorders

Disorders of hypothalamic-pituitary function may lead to amenorrhea. Many of these disorders result in hyperprolactinemia with galactorrhea and will be discussed in a later section. The most common functional disorder affecting hypothalamic-pituitary function of the adolescent female is low body fat composition. Low body weight is very common in adolescent females and may be associated with eating disorders, such as anorexia and bulimia, or strenuous physical exercise, such as is common with ballet dancers, long-distance runners, and gymnasts. Malnutrition and chronic disease states, such as malabsorption, cancer, and acquired immunodeficiency syndrome, may lead to hypothalamic-pituitary dysfunction. The presentation is characterized by a delay in pubertal events with inadequate breast development. The underlying endocrine abnormality associated with low body weight is insufficient GnRH production. Multiple contributing factors lead to this decrease in GnRH, including increased levels of corticotropin-releasing hormone, dopamine, and β-endorphin. As discussed earlier, inappropriately low leptin levels may be a key factor in decreased GnRH.

End-Organ Failure

In contrast to a central lack of gonadotropins, premature ovarian failure (POF) may lead to amenorrhea. Most commonly, POF results in secondary loss of menses, but it can occur in the peripubertal time period and result in limited breast development with lack of menses. The causes of POF are varied, with a large number of cases remaining idiopathic. Known causes include autoimmune disease, infectious disorders, metabolic diseases, and ovarian destruction secondary to cancer therapy. POF due to autoantibodies has been an area of significant confusion. These patients usually fall into two categories: those with preexisting autoimmune polyglandular syndromes, and those with POF as the presenting symptom. The typical autoimmune polyglandular syndromes include Addison's disease in association with mucocutaneous candidiasis and hypoparathyroidism (type 1) (23) or Addison's disease in conjunction with hypothyroidism (type 2) (24). POF is found in 60% of the former and in 10% of the latter. POF associated with adrenal disease is of a classic autoimmune nature, with histochemical evidence of oophoritis and the presence of antiadrenal antibodies, most commonly to the 21α-hydroxylase enzyme (25). Of all POF cases, only 2% to 10% are associated with adrenal autoimmune disease.

In cases in which POF is the presenting problem without adrenal disease, the evidence for an immune etiology is not as strong. The ovarian histology varies significantly. Approximately 60% will appear fibrotic and lacking any follicles, whereas 40% will have recognizable primordial follicles. The presence of ovarian follicles in the face of POF was first described by Jones and de Moraes-Ruehsen (26) in 1969 and named the "Savage syndrome" after their first patient. The ovarian histology rarely shows oophoritis in POF without adrenal disease. Autoimmune antibodies have been identified in POF without adrenal disease, but they are not nearly as common. Antibodies are found to the thyroid in 14%, to the parietal cells of the stomach in 4%, to the pancreas in 2%, and to acetylcholine receptors in 2% (24,27). Although not all patients with antibodies have the corresponding diseases, higher incidences of hypothyroidism and diabetes are seen. In one study of 119 cases, 27% had hypothyroidism, 2.6% had diabetes, and 2.5% had Addison's disease (28). Other less common diseases associated with POF include pernicious anemia, myasthenia gravis (29), sicca syndrome (30), systemic lupus erythematosus, vitiligo, and rheumatoid arthritis (24). The presence and significance of antibodies to the ovary in POF without adrenal disease remains an area of debate (31,32). Possibilities include blocking antibodies to the FSH and LH receptors and antibodies to the zona pellucida. At this time, the data on antiovarian antibodies remain controversial, and it is unclear if these antibodies are the cause or the consequence of ovarian failure.

The only well-recognized metabolic disease leading to POF in young women is galactosemia. This rare autosomal recessive disease has an incidence of about one in 55,000 live births and is due to a deficiency of the enzyme galactose-1-phosphate-uridyl-transferase. The resulting buildup of galactose-1-phosphate leads to multiorgan dysfunction that includes the liver, kidneys, brain, eyes, and gonads (33,34). Unlike other organs, the ovarian damage does not correlate with the severity or age at diagnosis of the disease. The suggested explanation for this observation is that the ovarian damage primarily occurs during fetal life.

Direct ovarian damage to the ovary is uncommonly caused by infectious agents such as mumps oophoritis (35), but more commonly it is due to treatment of childhood cancers with radiation or chemotherapy. The presentation after childhood cancer treatment depends on the age at treatment and may result in lack of puberty, or puberty with primary or secondary amenorrhea. With both radiation and chemotherapy, the age at treatment correlates with the odds of irreversible POF. The radiation dose to the ovary is dependent on the area of radiation and the total dosage. The dosage directly to the ovary necessary for failure is approximately 4 to 8 Gy (Gy = 100 rad) (36). For example, in a study of Hodgkin's disease treated with only radiation, the total dose to mantle and paraaortic fields was 40 to 44 Gy, but the calculated scattered dose to the ovaries was only 3.2 Gy. Thus, only 2.7% of patients experienced POF (37). In contrast, 37 of 38 children and adolescents receiving 20 to 30 Gy of whole abdominal radiation for treatment of

Wilms' tumor or neuroblastoma had irreversible ovarian failure. Similar doses of flank radiation rarely led to POF (38). The chance of POF with chemotherapy depends on the type of drug, total dosage, and age of the patient. Alkylating agents such as cyclophosphamide appear to have the highest risk, whereas antimetabolites, such as methotrexate and fluorouracil, rarely cause ovarian damage. Hodgkin's disease is the most common malignancy in adolescents requiring chemotherapy. Several different drug combinations have been used to maximize treatment while decreasing side effects. Although some variation can be found between drug combinations, the general incidence of POF is 50% to 60% (39,40). The odds of permanent versus transient POF is dependent on the age at treatment, with women less than 25 years having a significantly higher chance of regaining ovarian function than women over 35 years.

Diagnosis and Treatment

The diagnosis in this category is reached by history and physical examination and confirmed by appropriate laboratory testing (Fig. 13.5). Physical examination confirms the finding of imperforate hymen or vaginal septum. Concomitant pelvic mass due to hematocolpos almost always is present. With vaginal septums, pelvic magnetic resonance imaging (MRI) is often of great value in determining the exact thickness and distance from the septum to the cervix. This information is very helpful in planning a surgical repair. The incidence of significant renal abnormalities with septums is low and probably does not warrant evaluation. Surgical correction of these abnormalities should be performed as promptly as prudent after the diagnosis. Correction of an imperforate hymen is straightforward, with a cruciate incision into the bulging hymen. Aggressive resection of the hymenal tags should be avoided due to an increased possibility of scarring. Surgical correction of a vaginal septum is much more prone to complications, with the difficulty of the operation corresponding to the height of the septum.

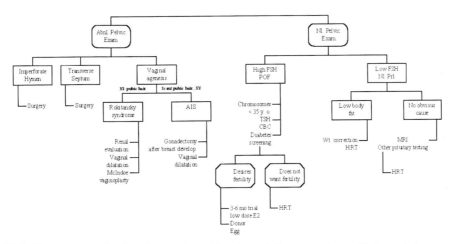

FIG. 13.5. Flow diagram for the diagnosis and treatment of amenorrhea with breast development.

Mid to high vaginal septum repairs require significant expertise and are well described in other chapters of this book.

The conditions of müllerian agenesis and complete AIS usually are easily differentiated by the scant or absent pubic and axillary hair in the latter. The diagnosis is confirmed by karyotype or measuring a serum testosterone level. Cases of müllerian agenesis need renal evaluation. Renal ultrasound will detect major abnormalities, whereas an intravenous pyelogram would be necessary to screen for ureteral duplications. Because the medical significance of ureteral abnormalities is low, a renal ultrasound is adequate and much more easily tolerated. Skeletal problems should be screened for by physical examination and radiographs taken to confirm abnormalities.

With a diagnosis of AIS, removal of the gonads is necessary due to the possibility of neoplastic formation. The odds of neoplastic formation are low, being less than 4% by age 30 years and 33% after age 50 years (41). For this reason, removal of the gonads should be delayed until breast development has been achieved. In both müllerian agenesis and AIS, creation of a neovagina often is necessary for sexual function. Vaginal creation procedures include nonsurgical dilatation and surgical in-

terventions. In the 1930s, Frank described the use of increasing sizes of vaginal dilators applied with pressure three times a day. Ingram modified the technique in 1981, such that patients would sit on a bicycle seat to apply pressure with specially designed lucite dilators. Vaginal dilatation works best with patients who already have a small vaginal dimple in which to begin the dilatation. Care should be taken in women who lack a vaginal dimple so that the urethral meatus is not unintentionally dilated. In highly motivated patients, approximately 75% are able to achieve satisfactory intercourse (42). The most common surgical vaginal creation is the McIndoe vaginoplasty. A mold constructed from Styrofoam or foam rubber is covered with a skin graft and placed into a space created in the soft tissue between the bladder and rectum. The skin graft usually is obtained from the buttock for the best cosmetic effect. After a week of total bed rest, the mold is removed and replaced with a removable mold suitable for daily cleansing. Intercourse is permitted after 3 months of healing. Substitutes for skin, such as peritoneum or amnion, have been considered but each has significant problems, such as the invasiveness necessary for obtaining peritoneum and the possible infectious disease risk of amnion. Other techniques for vaginoplasty have used segments of bowel, which has the problem of chronic mucus secretion, and by swinging in myocutaneous flaps, which requires more invasive surgery. The Vecchietti operation is a unique procedure more commonly used in Europe for vaginal creation. Traction sutures attached to an acrylic olive are brought from the potential neovaginal space through the abdominal cavity to the anterior abdominal wall. Traction on the olive creates the vaginal space, which negates the need for a skin graft. Disadvantages of this procedure include the necessity for an intraabdominal procedure and the possibility of bladder and rectal injury (42).

There are significant psychological and reproductive concerns that need to be discussed with patients who have müllerian agenesis and AIS. Patients with müllerian agenesis should be counseled that having children is possible with the use of gestational carriers and that normal sexual function will be obtained after vaginal creation. Discussion of the diagnosis of the AIS patient is a very delicate process, which must take into consideration the education level of the subject. In most patients, we have informed them that they were born with a genetic problem that caused lack of development of the uterus and abnormal gonads, which have to be removed due to the chance of tumor formation. Under most circumstances, discussion concerning a Y chromosome or reference to testes is counterproductive.

The differential diagnosis between hypothalamic-pituitary dysfunction and POF is determined by analyzing levels of FSH and LH. Gonadotropin levels less than 2 IU/L are suggestive of hypothalamic-pituitary dysfunction; an FSH level greater than 20 IU/L is diagnostic of POF. In the case of hypogonadotropic hypogonadism, other anterior pituitary hormones should be evaluated, including prolactin, TSH, insulin-like growth factor I (indirect assay of growth hormone), and a.m. and p.m. cortisol levels (indirect assay of ACTH function). Unless the cause of

the dysfunction is readily apparent, such as low body weight, MRI of the pituitary should be obtained to evaluate for a tumor. Treatment for hypothalamic-pituitary dysfunction includes hormone replacement therapy until the underlying disorder is corrected. Further evaluation for POF should include a karyotype in women less than 35 years, thyroid function testing, and screening for diabetes and anemia. Screening for other conditions associated with POF probably is not cost effective unless directed by the history or physical examination. Although most cases of gonadal dysgenesis present without breast development, a mosaic or presence of a gonadal tumor may result in initiation of puberty followed by amenorrhea. Treatment recommendations for POF depend on the fertility desires of the patient and may be difficult due to the unpredictability of the condition. Often cases of POF may be transient with intermittent episodes of ovarian function. Also, the initiation of low-dose estrogen therapy occasionally will result in renewed ovulation, possibly due to altering gonadotropin receptor levels in the ovary (43). Patients wishing to avoid pregnancy should use birth control for the first 6 months of hormone replacement therapy, until the permanency of the situation is more assured. In contrast, infertility patients may wish to consider a brief attempt at conservative therapy. The chance of renewed ovulation with estrogen therapy may inversely correlate with the level of FSH. Treatment with low-dose estradiol, such as with a 0.05 Climara patch, may be considered for up to 6 months in patients comfortable with the low probability of success. The treatment of choice for fertility in POF remains donor egg *in vitro* fertilization. Future treatment possibilities for this condition include *in vitro* maturation of immature oocytes, because 40% of patients with POF retain oocytes in the inactive ovaries.

Preservation of ovarian function is the main consideration in young women requiring treatment with radiation or chemotherapy. Lateral transposition of the ovaries should be performed in women needing pelvic radiation. This procedure can be performed laparoscopically by swinging the ovary into the colonic gutter and suturing to the lateral peritoneum. The ovarian pedicle may need to be incised, and a surgical clip should be left adjacent to the ovary to enable localization on x-ray film (44). With regard to chemotherapy, pretreatment ovarian suppression remains an area of future possibility and investigation. That ovarian failure after chemotherapy is lower in prepubescent compared to postpubertal females suggests that ovarian suppression may be of benefit. Use of GnRH agonists has been shown effective in decreasing the risk of chemotherapy-associated POF in Rhesus monkeys. One study showed that pretreatment with GnRH agonists significantly decreased the risk of POF in women undergoing chemotherapy for lymphoma. Other studies showed a lack of effect. Treatment with oral contraceptives does not appear to have the same benefit. At this time, this area of treatment needs further investigation (45).

Amenorrhea without Breast Development

Genetic Abnormalities

The lack of breast development is the most sensitive indicator that the ovaries never secreted estradiol. This lack of estradiol production could be due to an abnormality of the ovary such that the cells necessary for estrogen production are missing, due to an abnormal enzyme necessary for the synthesis of estradiol, or due to a lack of production of gonadotropins necessary for stimulation of the ovary.

The most common cause of POF is gonadal dysgenesis. Sixty percent of cases of gonadal dysgenesis are due to structural chromosome abnormalities; 40% of cases are associated with structurally normal chromosomes. Turner's syndrome, described in 1938, is the most common cause of gonadal dysgenesis. It is found in one in 2,500 to 10,000 liveborns (Fig. 13.6). Responsible for one in 15 spontaneous abortions, approximately 99% of cases of Turner's syndrome end in spontaneous abortion. The loss of all or a portion of the

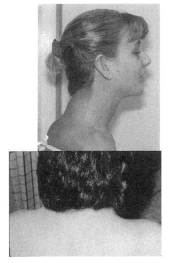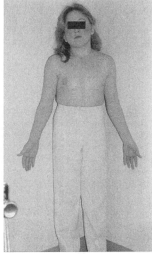

FIG. 13.6. Characteristics of Turner's syndrome, including low-set ears **(top left)**, broad, webbed neck with low-posterior hairline **(bottom left)**, and cubitus valgus with lack of breast development **(right)**. (From Leppert PC, Howard FM. Primary care for women. Philadelphia: Lippincott–Raven, 1997:252, with permission.)

short arm of the X chromosome is responsible for the physical stigmata and ovarian failure of Turner's syndrome. Approximately 60% of cases involve loss of an entire X chromosome (45,XO); 40% involve mosaicism or partial deletions. Unlike trisomy conditions such as Down syndrome, the incidence of Turner's syndrome is not related to maternal age. This is because the chromosome abnormality is due to a postfertilization mitotic nondisjunction event with failure of survival of the corresponding trisomy (47,XXX or 47,XXY) cell line.

Physical abnormalities of Turner's syndrome may first be evident in infancy and include lymphedema of the dorsum of the feet and hand and loose exaggerated skin fold on the posterior neck. These findings in the infant are termed the Bonnevie-Ullrich syndrome and may be recognized during prenatal ultrasounds. Other typical physical findings include short stature (less than 60 inches), high-arched palate, low-set or deformed ears, broad shield-like chest with hypoplastic areolae, low-posterior hairline, short fourth metacarpal, and cubitus valgus. Webbing of the neck is found in 25% to 40% of patients. Potential health concerns of Turner's syndrome include cardiac abnormalities such as aortic coarctation, aortic stenosis, and bicuspid aortic valve; and renal abnormalities such as horseshoe kidney and malpositions. Patients also have an increased risk of diabetes, hypothyroidism, hypertension, recurrent otitis media, and abnormal vascular structures in the small intestines. Unlike many chromosome abnormalities, patients with Turner's syndrome have normal mental development and intelligence. The ovarian failure associated with this syndrome is due to an exaggerated rate of oocyte atresia during fetal life, such that few viable oocytes remain at the time of birth. The gene or genes on the X chromosome controlling oocyte atresia remain to be identified.

Other structural chromosome abnormalities other than 45,XO may result in Turner's syndrome. The presentation of patients with sex chromosome mosaicism may be much more varied. The most common mosaic, 45,XO/46,XX, usually has less severe symptoms depending on the ratio of normal-to-abnormal cells (46). These patients tend to be taller and have more delayed ovarian failure. Onset of puberty at the normal time, ovulatory cycles, and even pregnancies may occur. In contrast, the 45,XO/46,XY mosaic may have many different presentations, varying from females with virilization to males with normal genitalia and vestigial uterus (47). Most cases, which are recognized as female, have ambiguous genitalia. In these cases the gonads may be mixed, such as with a streak gonad on one side and an abnormal testes on the other side, hence the term mixed gonadal dysgenesis. A unilateral testicle may secrete MIF and testosterone, leading to a hemiuterus on one side and wollfian duct structures on the opposite side. As discussed later, these XY gonads are prone to tumor formation. Other chromosomal abnormalities causing Turner's syndrome include an isochromosome of the long arm of one X chromosome (45,XXqi), deletion of the short arm of one X chromosome (46,XXp–), and ring X chromosome (46,XXr).

There are other structural chromosome abnormalities that result in ovarian failure. Deletion of the long arm of one of the X chromosomes results in ovarian failure but no other physical abnormalities. Patients present with sexual infantilism and ultimately may be tall due to the continued linear growth in the absence of estrogen. Finally, approximately 25% of women with triple X syndrome (47,XXX) may exhibit ovarian failure. Ovarian failure may occur before puberty with sexual infantilism or after puberty with primary or secondary amenorrhea (48).

Pure gonadal dysgenesis refers to the syndrome of female phenotype with sexual infantilism, normal stature, female internal genitalia, and bilateral streak gonads. The condition is termed pure gonadal dysgenesis due to the lack of physical stigmata of Turner's syndrome. The karyotype may be 46,XX or 46,XY. Cases with a 46,XX karyotype may be sporadic but also have been identified in families as an autosomal recessive trait (49). This finding has suggested that autosomal genes also play a role in ovarian development. The lack of estrogen production in these individuals results in continued linear growth without appropriate closure of the epiphyseal plates. Thus, these patients ultimately are tall and may manifest an eunuchoid habitus, characterized by an arm span 5 cm greater than height or a sole-to-symphysis length 5 cm greater than the symphysis-to-head length. The ovaries usually are streaks composed of nonfunctioning fibrous tissue. Rarely, active stromal cells may exist in the ovaries and result in mild androgen expression of clitoromegaly. A few cases of complete lack of ovaries, as defined by the inability to find ovarian tissue at laparotomy, have been reported (50,51). Associated abnormalities with XX pure gonadal dysgenesis are not common. Perrault syndrome is a rare combination of sensorineural hearing loss and XX gonadal dysgenesis (52).

Swyer (53) first described the syndrome of pure gonadal dysgenesis with a 46,XY karyotype in 1955. The XY gonads develop as inactive streaks. Normal development of the testes is related to correct expression of the sex-determining region of the Y chromosome (SRY) gene. The protein product of this gene is a DNA transcription factor, thought to initiate the downstream cascade resulting in differentiation of the testes. In a review of 39 cases of Swyer's syndrome, nine were found to have mutations of the SRY gene (54). A greater understanding of all the pathways responsible for testes determination will be necessary to delineate other causes of this syndrome. The dysgenetic gonads do not secrete MIF, so internal female genitalia develop normally. The phenotypic presentation of patients with Swyer's syndrome may be quite heterogeneous. Mild androgen expression may be seen with clitoromegaly present even at birth. Some patients also will have spontaneous, but usually hypoplastic, breast development at the time of expected puberty (55). Some of this variation in presentation may be explained by the high incidence of gonadal tumors, gonadoblastomas (Fig. 13.7). Gonadoblastomas are tumors composed of large germ cells, Sertoli and/or granulosa cells, and stromal cells (theca and/or Leydig cells) that develop within streak gonads of XY karyotype. These tumors may be found in 25% to 50% of cases and are bilateral in approximately one of three patients. Gonadoblastomas may be hormonally active and lead to androgen and estrogen exposure, thus accounting for some of the variations in phenotype. The initiation of breast development around the time of puberty may be due to a responsiveness of the tumor to gonadotropins or to residual active stromal cells within the gonad that are gonadotropin responsive. Gonadoblastomas may occur very early and have been reported in infants as young as 9 months of age. These are benign tumors that do not metastasize. In

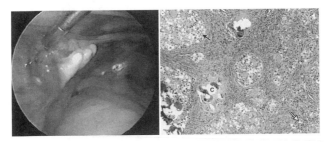

FIG. 13.7. A 16-year-old phenotypic girl with XY pure gonadal dysgenesis. Laparoscopic view of the left gonad with the hypoplastic uterus seen in the background to the **right (left)**. Histology of the gonad shows components of gonadoblastoma *(black arrow)*, microscopic calcification *(C)*, and dysgerminoma *(white arrow)*.

approximately 50% of cases, dysgerminomas will form within the gonadoblastomas. Dysgerminomas are malignant tumors that have metastatic potential.

Gonadal agenesis also occurs with an XY karyotype and may be more frequent than with an XX pattern. Referred to as the vanishing testes syndrome, the phenotype is determined by the age at which the gonads are lost. With very early loss, MIF and testosterone are not secreted and the presentation is the same as pure XY gonadal dysgenesis (56). In other cases, the early testes may produce MIF before the time of regression, resulting in a lack of female internal genitalia (57).

Enzyme Disorders

An enzyme disorder within the ovaries and adrenals may result in an inability to synthesize sex steroids leading to amenorrhea without breast development and a lack of pubic or axillary hair development (Fig. 13.8). A single protein in both the adrenals and ovaries contains the enzyme activities of 17α-hydroxylase and 17,20-lyase. 17α-Hydroxylase converts pregnenolone to 17α-hydroxypregnenolone and progesterone to 17α-hydroxyprogesterone. 17,20-Lyase converts 17α-hydroxypregnenolone

to dehydroepiandrosternedione and 17α-hydroxyprogesterone to androstenedione. A defect leading to inactivity of this protein results in a lack of production of all sex steroids and an overproduction of the mineralocorticoid deoxycorticosterone (DOC). Increased DOC levels result in fluid retention with hypertension and hypokalemia, and compensatory decreases in renin and aldosterone (58). This enzyme deficiency is inherited as an autosomal recessive disorder; thus, it can occur in either sex. Both genetic males and females are born with normal female external genitalia and subsequently fail to develop any secondary sexual characteristics. Genetic males will have intraabdominal testes; they will lack müllerian structures due to the appropriate production of MIF and lack significant wolffian ducts due to the lack of testosterone production. Thus, genetic males will have a blind-ending vagina, whereas genetic females have a hypoplastic uterus. Multiple different defects in the 17α-hydroxylase gene have been reported, with some leading to different presentations. Gene defects may lead to complete protein inactivation with no hydroxylase or lyase activity resulting in the classic presentation discussed earlier (59). Other possibilities include a defect leading to inactivation of the lyase activity only, which results

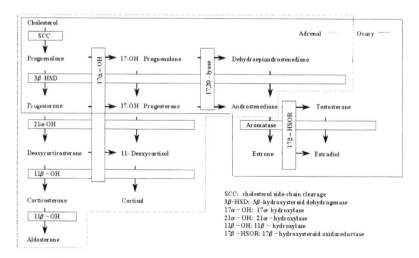

FIG. 13.8. Diagram of adrenal and ovarian steroid biosynthesis.

in a lack of sex steroid production and a lack of hypertension due to normal cortisol production. In addition, a gene defect leading to partial enzyme activity and incomplete virilization in a genetic male has been reported (60).

Two autosomal recessive enzyme deficiencies causing male pseudohermaphroditism may present as female phenotypes with failure to initiate breast development. 5α-Reductase deficiency is responsible for impaired conversion of testosterone to dihydrotestosterone. Genetic males often appear as females at birth, with clitoromegaly, a blind-ending vagina, and varying degrees of labioscrotal fusion. Normal intraabdominal testes lead to a lack of müllerian structures and the presence of wolffian duct structures. At puberty, increased androgen production from the testes causes further growth of the phallus, but breast development and significant body hair growth are absent (Fig. 13.9). The enzyme 17β-hydroxysteroid oxidoreductase is responsible for the conversion of androstenedione to testosterone, and estrone to estradiol. Genetic males are born with varying degrees of ambiguous genitalia, but they may have mild clitoromegaly with a blind-ending vagina. As with 5α-reductase, significant growth of the phallus occurs at puberty but, unlike the former syndrome, it is accompanied by significant sexual hair growth and, in some cases, gynecomastia.

The most recent abnormality in sex steroid synthesis was described in 1991 with the identification of the first gene defect in the enzyme aromatase. Aromatase is a ubiquitous enzyme responsible for the conversion of androgens to estrogens, including testosterone to estradiol and androstenedione to estrone. Abnormalities of the aromatase protein, inherited as an autosomal recessive trait, have been reported in both genetic males and females. Genetic females are born with ambiguous genitalia due to the inability of the placenta to convert maternal and fetal androgens to estrogens. At the time of puberty, girls become virilized due to ovarian androgen production with polycystic ovaries, and they fail to develop breasts. Genetic males are normal at birth and undergo normal sexual development at puberty. Interestingly, both sexes show significant abnormalities in growth and glucose homeostasis. Lack of estrogen leads to an absent pubertal growth spurt, continued long bone growth without epiphyseal closure, and osteoporosis. Hyperinsulinemia and abnormal lipoprotein profiles are seen (61). Roles of estrogen have been further delineated with the identification of an estrogen receptor deficiency in a male in 1994. Characteristics of this man included unusual tallness with delayed bone age, unfused epiphyses, and severe osteoporosis. Despite normal

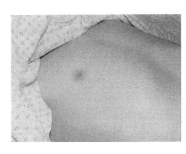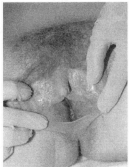

FIG. 13.9. An 18-year-old phenotypic female with 5α-reductase deficiency presented with primary amenorrhea without breast development and clitoromegaly. View of the chest **(left)** shows complete lack of breast development with a male-type nipple. The perineum **(right)** shows extreme clitoral enlargement that occurred at the time of expected puberty. Note the lack of any lower abdominal hirsutism.

androgen levels, gonadotropins were elevated. As with estrogen deficiency, hyperinsulinemia and lipid abnormalities were present. This case illustrated the important roles of estrogen in bone and glucose homeostasis in both sexes (62).

Central Disorders

The cases discussed involve lack of estrogen production from the gonad despite appropriate stimulation from the hypothalamus and pituitary. Congenital lack of gonadotropin production also may occur and has been termed isolated hypogonadotropic hypogonadism or Kallmann's syndrome. Kallmann's syndrome is characterized by the lack of GnRH production associated with anosmia or hyposmia. It occurs at a frequency of one in 10,000 in males and one in 60,000 in females. Reported associated abnormalities include midline facial defects such as cleft lip and palate, mirror movements, nystagmus, sensorineural hearing loss, pes cavus deformity, choanal atresia, unilateral renal agenesis, and short metacarpals (63–65). Abnormalities are more common in males than females. Kallmann's syndrome is caused by a lack of migration of the GnRH neurons from the point of origination in the olfactory placode to the arcuate nucleus of the hypothalamus. In addition, the olfactory neurons fail to migrate to the appropriate location in the brain, resulting in abnormalities of smelling. MRI of the brain in affected patients may be characterized by aplasia or hypoplasia of the olfactory sulcus (66). Inheritance patterns of X-linked, autosomal dominant, and autosomal recessive have all been reported, with X-linked being the most common. X-linked Kallmann's syndrome has been associated with other X-linked diseases of congenital ichthyosis and placental sulfatase deficiency. This form of Kallmann's syndrome is due to a gene defect of a protein KALIG-1. KALIG-1 has significant homology with neural cell adhesion proteins and appears to coordinate the migration of GnRH and olfactory neurons from the olfactory placode to the hypothalamus (67).

Other inheritance patterns for this syndrome suggest that there may be other causes for the lack of GnRH production. Females with Kallmann's syndrome present with lack of breast development. Pubic and axillary hair usually is scant and is influenced only by adrenal androgens. Lack of estrogen leads to tallness with possible eunuchoid characteristics.

Other abnormalities of the hypothalamus and pituitary may lead to lack of puberty, including tumors such as craniopharyngioma, infiltrating diseases such as histiocytosis X, and damage due to trauma or radiation therapy.

Diagnosis and Treatment

Evaluation of women with lack of breast development always begins with an assay of FSH (Fig. 13.10). A high FSH level is compatible with gonadal dysgenesis or an enzyme disorder resulting in estrogen deficiency. With an elevated FSH level, the next test should be a karyotype. An abnormal karyotype establishes the diagnosis. Patients with Turner's syndrome need further evaluation, including echocardiogram and imaging of the aorta, renal imaging, and evaluation for diabetes and thyroid disease. In women with a normal XX karyotype, the differential diagnosis is limited to pure gonadal dysgenesis versus 17α-hydroxylase deficiency. The finding of hypertension and an elevated progesterone level in the latter can separate these two conditions. In women with an XY karyotype, the possible diagnoses include pure gonadal dysgenesis, 17α-hydroxylase deficiency, 5α-reductase deficiency, and 17β-hydroxysteroid oxidoreductase. The diagnosis of XY pure gonadal dysgenesis is established with the finding of a normal vagina, cervix, and uterus. Blind-ending vagina without clitoromegaly in combination with hypertension and elevated progesterone is compatible with 17α-hydroxylase deficiency. The last two enzyme disorders, 5α-reductase deficiency and 17β-hydroxysteroid oxidoreductase deficiency, present with some degree of clitoromegaly that increases at the time of puberty. 5α-reductase deficiency is characterized by lack of breast

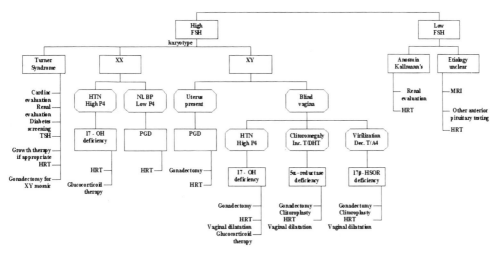

FIG. 13.10. Flow diagram of the diagnosis and treatment of amenorrhea without breast development.

development, lack of significant hirsutism, and an elevated testosterone-to-dihydrotestosterone ratio, which can be exaggerated by hCG administration. 17β-Hydroxysteroid oxidoreductase deficiency differs in that it is associated with more severe virilization, including hirsutism and, in some cases, gynecomastia, at puberty. Laboratory testing demonstrates elevated androstenedione-to-testosterone and estrone-to-estradiol ratios, exaggerated by hCG administration.

Low FSH levels are diagnostic of GnRH insufficiency. Kallmann's syndrome is confirmed by the presence of anosmia and supported by family history. Testing for anosmia should utilize subtle scents such as perfume or fruits. Sensation of harsh substances such as alcohol or ammonia is controlled by different receptors that are not affected by this syndrome. The prevalence of renal abnormalities is high enough in Kallmann's syndrome to warrant renal imaging. If the diagnosis of Kallmann's syndrome is not clear, a brain MRI and testing of other anterior pituitary hormones should be performed.

The treatment for these conditions depends on the karyotype. Phenotypic females with an XY genotype need to have the gonads removed at the time of diagnosis due to the risk of tumor formation. With Turner's syndrome, treatment issues include secondary sexual development and growth. Although growth hormone is not deficient, treatment with growth hormone has been shown to offer benefit to these patients, and consultation with a growth specialist should be arranged for young patients. Estrogen replacement therapy should be initiated at age 11 to 12 years. Therapy should start at low doses, such as 0.3 mg conjugated equine estrogen, to augment growth without leading to early epiphyseal plate closure and to initiate breast development. Estrogen therapy should be increased gradually at 6-month intervals until optimal breast development or a dose of 1.25 to 2.5 mg of conjugated equine estrogen is reached. Cyclic progesterone or a progestin should be initiated if uterine bleeding starts or no later than 1.5 years after starting estrogen. Long-term therapy should include an appropriate dose of estrogen for young women and cyclic progesterone to prevent endometrial hyperplasia. The same treatment for breast development should be used in patients without Turner's syndrome. This strategy comes closest to mimicking the gradual estrogen exposure during puberty. Although never studied, from a theoretical point of view, the use of oral contraceptives is inferior due to downregulation of the estrogen receptor by the chronic progestin exposure. The syndrome of 17α-hydroxylase deficiency requires physiologic cortisol replacement in addition to sex steroid therapy to correct overproduction of DOC.

Fertility is rare in women with these disorders. Spontaneous pregnancies rarely occur in Turner's syndrome, usually with XO/XX mosaicism. Women with Turner's syndrome who conceive have a greater risk of miscarriage and liveborn children with genetic abnormalities of Turner's and Down's syndromes. With the improvements in assisted reproductive technologies, childbearing has now become possible for patients with end-organ failure. Successful pregnancies with donor egg *in vitro* fertilization have been reported in patients with gonadal dysgenesis and 17α-hydroxylase deficiency (68,69). Induction of pregnancy in women with Turner's syndrome creates a high-risk situation and should be carefully considered. Cases of aortic root dissection leading to death have been reported. Fertility may be accomplished in women with Kallmann's syndrome by using exogenous GnRH or gonadotropins. Exogenous GnRH delivered by subcutaneous pump in 60- to 90-minute pulses will reestablish gonadotropin secretion and result in ovulation. This process may take several weeks, because GnRH upregulation of its own receptors on the pituitary is necessary before a response will be noted. In contrast to gonadotropin administration, GnRH treatment is more time consuming, of similar expense, but does result in a lower risk of multiple gestations.

Amenorrhea with Androgen Excess

Functional Disorders

The presence of hirsutism in young women is synonymous with androgen excess. Most commonly, adolescents with disorders leading to androgen excess will have normal to hypoplastic breast development and secondary amenorrhea or oligomenorrhea. Less commonly, patients with these disorders will present with primary amenorrhea.

Polycystic ovarian syndrome (PCOS) is by far the most common cause of menstrual disorders, affecting approximately 5% to 10% of women of reproductive age (Fig. 13.11). Primary amenorrhea occurs in 5% to 10% of subjects with PCOS (70). More commonly, patients experience menarche at the correct time and then have menstrual irregularity that varies from secondary amenorrhea to dysfunctional uterine bleeding. PCOS is classically characterized by hirsutism, ovulatory dysfunction with infertility, obesity, acanthosis nigricans, insulin resistance, and the characteristic ultrasound appearance of multiple peripheral follicles. Hyperthecosis is a variant of PCOS that involves more severe androgen excess and ovarian thecal cell hyperplasia but is still a functional disorder driven by gonadotropins from the brain. Unlike PCOS, mild signs of virilization such as clitoromegaly may be seen with hyperthecosis. Biochemical abnormalities associated with PCOS include excessive androgens, increased LH-to-FSH ratio, and hyperinsulinemia. Androgen excess in women with PCOS is derived from the ovary, the adrenals, and peripheral production in adipose tissue. Typically, women with PCOS will have elevated circulating levels of testosterone, androstenedione, dehydroepiandrostenedione sulfate (DS), and 17-hydroxyprogesterone and decreased levels of sex hormone-binding globulin (SHBG). DS levels that characterize adrenal activity are commonly elevated in PCOS. As shown in Fig. 13.12, the pathology of PCOS is multifactorial. An underlying increase in 17,20-lyase enzyme activity affecting the ovary and adrenal gland leads to increased androstenedione and DS production. Obesity contributes by increasing aromatization of androstenedione to estrone, and further production of androgens via 5α-reductase activity. In addition, central or upper body adiposity results in insulin resistance and compensatory hyperinsulinemia. Insulin activity via the liver results in decreased SHBG and thus increased free testosterone levels. Insulin acting through insulin-like growth factor I receptors stimulates androgen

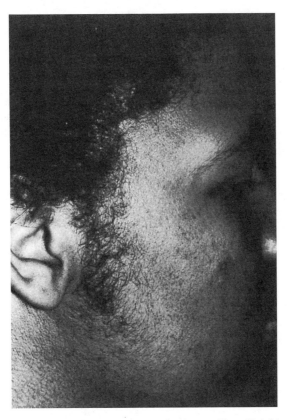

FIG. 13.11. A 17-year-old girl with polycystic ovarian syndrome. Note facial hair and acne due to excess androgens.

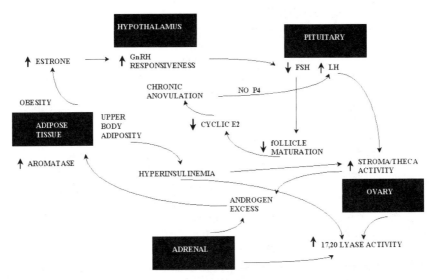

FIG. 13.12. Proposed mechanisms for polycystic ovarian syndrome. (Modified from Yen SCC. Chronic anovulation caused by peripheral endocrine disorders. In: Yen SCC, Jaffe RB, eds. *Reproductive endocrinology.* Philadelphia: WB Saunders, 1986:461, with permission.)

production by theca cells. Recent data suggest that insulin also modulates 17,20-lyase activity in the ovary and probably the adrenal gland (71). High, noncyclic estrone levels result in FSH suppression, and the lack of progesterone production contributes to elevated LH levels. High LH levels stimulate theca cell hyperplasia and androgen production. PCOS definitely has a genetic tendency, but because of the variable presentation and the lack of a definitive marker for the disease, an exact mendelian pattern has not been established.

Two adrenal enzyme disorders, 21α-hydroxylase deficiency and 11β-hydroxylase deficiency, may lead to conditions of androgen excess and menstrual disorders. Both of these disorders are inherited as autosomal recessive traits. The enzyme 21α-hydroxylase is responsible for the conversion of 17-hydroxypregnenolone to DOC, and 17-hydroxyprogesterone to deoxycortisol. Impaired enzyme activity leads to decreased cortisol levels, with compensatory increase in ACTH and overproduction of adrenal androgens. Two genes for this enzyme have been identified on chromosome 6; one is an inactive pseudogene and the other is the active gene. Defects in the two alleles of the active gene determine the phenotype. Gene abnormalities of both alleles lead to complete protein inactivity and cause severe disease presenting as ambiguous genitalia and salt wasting. Gene defects of both alleles cause minor protein impairment, or of one normal allele and one abnormal allele (heterozygote) lead to less severe disease characterized by adult-onset androgen excess. Nonclassic or adult-onset 21α-hydroxylase deficiency is found in approximately one in 100 subjects and is more common in certain ethnic groups, such as Ashkenazi Jews, Eskimos, Yugoslavs, and Hispanics. The presentation of women with adult-onset 21α-hydroxylase deficiency is indistinguishable from PCOS, typified by peripubertal onset of hirsutism, acne, and menstrual irregularity.

11β-Hydroxylase deficiency is approximately 20 times less common than 21α-hydroxylase deficiency. This enzyme is responsible for the conversion of deoxycortisol to cortisol, and DOC to corticosterone. Impairment of enzyme activity leads to increases in adrenal androgens and an increase in the mineralocorticoid DOC. Thus, unlike 21α-hydroxylase deficiency, hypertension is part of the symptomatology. Similar to 21α-hydroxylase, there are two genes for this enzyme on chromosome 8; one is an inactive pseudogene and the other is the active gene. As discussed earlier, different gene mutations of both alleles can result in severe disease with ambiguous genitalia in the newborn or mild disease with adult onset of hirsutism and mild hypertension.

Nonfunctional Disorders

These conditions are all functional disorders due to enzyme disorders within the ovary and/or adrenals. These functional disorders result in hirsutism and occasionally mild clitoromegaly, but rarely do they cause frank virilization. In contrast, the presentation of recent-onset virilization is most consistent with an androgen-producing tumor (Fig. 13.13). In a review of 41 cases of ovarian androgen-producing tumors, 98% had signs of virilization such as temporal balding, deepening of the voice, masculinization of body habitus, and significant clitoromegaly. In this group, 84% of cases had initial testosterone levels greater than 2 ng/mL, and 88% of cases had levels greater than 1.5 ng/mL. When compared to 159 cases of hirsutism due to functional causes, none had testosterone levels greater than 2 ng/mL, and only one patient (0.6%) had a level greater than 1.5 ng/mL (72). In general, the size of virilizing tumors correlates not with circulating levels of testosterone but with the type of tumor. Sertoli-Leydig cell tumors (arrhenoblastoma or androblastoma) are the most common virilizing tumor. Most common in young women, these solid tumors usually are unilateral and most often greater than 5 cm in diameter. These tumors may be malignant 20% of the time and occasionally secrete AFP (alpha fetal protein) (73). Less common tumors that directly secrete androgens include lipoid cell and hilar cell tumors. Hilar cell tumors are most common in perimenopausal and postmenopausal women and can be quite small (74). On rare occasions, granulosa-theca cell tumors will present with symptoms of androgen excess (75). Other ovarian tumors do not directly secret androgens but induce a stromal cell hyperplasia in the affected ovary. Symptoms usually are less severe. Examples include Brenner cell, thecoma, cystadenoma, and cystadenocarcinoma.

Nonfunctional adrenal disorders causing hirsutism and virilization include Cushing's syndrome and adrenocortical tumors. Cushing's syndrome, or overproduction of adrenal glucocorticoids and androgens, may be due to stimulation of the adrenals by ACTH produced by a pituitary tumor (Cushing's disease), by ACTH from an ectopic source, or by an adrenal tumor. Hirsutism, associated with oily skin and acne, is part of the symptomatology in 64% to 81% of cases, with frank virilization being rare. Menstrual disturbances of oligomenorrhea or amenorrhea are seen in 55% to 80% of cases. Other typical symptoms include centripetal obesity, glucose intolerance, hypertension, and proximal muscle weakness (76). Adrenocortical tumors are exceedingly rare, with an estimated incidence of three per million in children less than 20 years of age. Tumors have a 2:1 to 3:1 predominance in females over males and may be either benign adenomas or carcinomas. In a review of 11 cases in children and adolescents, 64% presented with virilization whereas 24% primarily had symptoms of hypercortisolism. Sixty-four percent of the tumors were malignant; the others were adenomas (77).

Diagnosis and Treatment

The diagnosis of PCOS is based on clinical presentation and exclusion of other diseases with similar symptoms. There is no single symptom or test that is diagnostic for this syndrome. Typical laboratory results include an elevated LH-to-FSH ratio of 2:1 to 3:1 and is considered a hallmark of PCOS. This increased ratio is not, however, specific for PCOS and may be seen with other conditions such as CAH. Elevated androgens are found in the majority of patients: androstenedione levels commonly range from 270 to 450 ng/dL, and testosterone levels may range from 50 to 150 ng/dL. Mildly elevated prolactin levels of 20 to 40 ng/mL are found in 15% to 20% of patients. Dehydroepiandrosterone sulfate levels may be elevated in patients with PCOS but usually remain less than 500 μg/dL. Levels above 500 μg/dL suggest the need to evaluate for CAH or an adrenal tumor. The polycystic ovary has a characteristic ultrasound appearance with multiple small peripheral follicles, yet this appearance is not specific for one cause of androgen excess and may be seen with PCOS, hyperprolactinemia, and CAH. Hyperinsulinemia is common in women with PCOS, and the incidence correlates with the severity of upper body obesity. A good indicator of insulin resistance is a

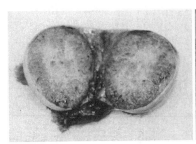 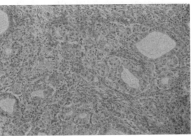

FIG. 13.13. Sertoli-Leydig cell tumor from a 14-year-old girl presenting with secondary amenorrhea and virilization. Gross specimen **(left)** and histology **(right)** after laparoscopic oophorectomy.

fasting glucose-to-insulin ratio less than 4.5 (78).

CAH is evaluated by measuring 17α-hydroxyprogesterone levels in the morning and during the follicular phase in cycling women. A level less than 200 ng/dL is very sensitive for excluding 21α-hydroxylase deficiency. Abnormal screening values should be further evaluated with an ACTH stimulation test, with results interpreted using the nomogram developed by White et al. (79). In contrast, DOC levels should be evaluated in subjects with hypertension to evaluate for 11β-hydroxylase deficiency.

A rapid onset of symptoms and signs of virilization suggest an ovarian androgen-producing tumor. Amenorrhea is more likely with tumors compared to functional disorders. Laboratory findings suggestive of an ovarian tumor include a testosterone level of greater than 200 ng/dL and a low or inverse ratio of androstenedione to testosterone. Normally, androstenedione levels should be three to five times greater than testosterone. Pelvic ultrasound is the next appropriate evaluation for ovarian tumors. The majority of androgen-secreting tumors in premenopausal women are visible on ultrasound. Less commonly, small tumors less than 1 to 2 cm may not be readily visible, and they may be detectable by selective ovarian venous catheterization. In a review of five cases of ovarian tumors not visible with imaging, there was a significantly higher level of testosterone from the ovarian vein of the affected side compared to the normal side. The ratios of testosterone from the affected versus normal sides varied from 1.9 to 12.3. The gradient of venous testosterone levels between the affected ovary and the periphery varied from 1.84 to 14.71 ng/mL. Testosterone secretion always greatly exceeded that of androstenedione. Peripheral ratios of androstenedione to testosterone varied from 0.6 to 2.0 (mean 1.0). In six comparative cases of PCOS, there was no asymmetry to ovarian testosterone secretion, and the peripheral ratios of androstenedione to testosterone varied from 1.87 to 4.76 (mean 3.66) (80).

The best screening test for Cushing's syndrome is a 24-hour urine collection for free cortisol. Abnormal screening tests are followed-up with a standard low-dose dexamethasone suppression test to establish the diagnosis. A high-dose dexamethasone suppression may differentiate between ACTH-dependent and ACTH-independent conditions. Complete evaluation of Cushing's syndrome may be complex and is well described in other text (81). Adrenal tumors associated with virilization often are associated with high DS levels above 500 µg/dL. The vast majority of these tumors are evident by computed tomographic imaging of the adrenals.

Treatment for these various diseases involves addressing multiple problems. In PCOS, treatment is aimed at suppression of androgens for the improvement of hirsutism and acne, endometrial protection from unopposed estrogen, and decreasing cardiovascular risk of insulin resistance and abnormal lipid profiles. The mainstay of therapy remains low-dose oral contraceptives, which suppress ovarian androgens, increase SHBG, and result in orderly uterine withdraw bleeding. More complete ovarian suppression is obtained with GnRH analogue therapy, with the side effects of estrogen deficiency obviated by sex steroid addback therapy. Long-term therapy with this regimen currently is not practical due to the cost of the drug. Additional therapy for hirsutism includes the possible use of receptor antagonists such as spironolactone and flutamide. Inhibition of 5α-reductase by finasteride also improves hirsutism, but its use is contraindicated in women of childbearing potential due to the risk of genital abnormalities. Other therapies for endometrial protection include cyclic natural progesterone or a synthetic progestin such as medroxyprogesterone acetate or norethindrone. Insulin resistance and lipid abnormalities are addressed primarily with weight loss and dietary management. Insulin-sensitizing drugs improve insulin resistance and decrease hyperinsulinemia, but currently are approved only for the treatment of adult-onset diabetes mellitus. Lipid disorders not corrected by diet should be managed with hyperlipidemic drugs.

Treatment of adult-onset 21α-hydroxylase deficiency depends on the severity of the disease. In some cases, suppression of ACTH with low-dose dexamethasone or prednisone is necessary for adequate control of androgen expression. Decreasing the total circulating androgen pool with an oral contraceptive instead of directly targeting the adrenal source may control other milder cases. Preconceptional counseling and prenatal therapy are important considerations with CAH. In susceptible pregnancies, prenatal treatment with dexamethasone should be initiated before the eighth week and continued until the sex of the child and/or the diagnosis of CAH can be established by appropriate testing (82).

Amenorrhea with Hyperprolactinemia

The presentation of hyperprolactinemia depends on the level of the circulating hormone. Mild elevations in prolactin result in luteal phase dysfunction with mild menstrual irregularity. As the level increases, menstrual abnormalities progress to oligomenorrhea and finally to secondary amenorrhea. Rarely, prepubertal hyperprolactinemia leads to pubertal delay and primary amenorrhea. Galactorrhea, not associated with pregnancy, is the hallmark of hyperprolactinemia. Yet, there is significant individual variation of the presence of galactorrhea with hyperprolactinemia. This seems to depend on the degree of estrogen deficiency and the sensitivity of the breast. Thus, analysis of prolactin levels should be included in any evaluation of menstrual dysfunction, irrespective of the presence of galactorrhea.

Causes of hyperprolactinemia include prolactin-secreting tumors and alterations in the normal regulation of prolactin as listed in Table 13.3. Prolactin-secreting adenomas are the most common tumors of the anterior pituitary. In autopsy studies, prolactin-secreting tumors are found in approximately 11% of patients (83). These tumors most commonly develop in the lateral aspect of the gland. Most of these tumors are not true adenomas. Cytochemical studies show that these tumors contain normal dopamine receptors and are capable of appropriate prolactin regulation *in vitro*. Thus, many prolactin-secreting adenomas represent localized growth of lactotrophs due to the lack of appropriate dopamine regulation from abnormalities in the vascular supply. Prolactin levels correlate with the chance of a prolactin-secreting tumor, but there is no threshold that excludes the possibility of a tumor. Tumors have been identified with prolactin levels as low as 27 ng/mL. Prolactin-secreting adenomas tend to be small, usually found as microadenomas (smaller than 10 mm) as opposed to macroadenomas (larger than 10 mm). Microadenomas usually change little with time. In a review of 43 cases of microadenomas followed without long-term treatment, two cases showed tumor enlargement after 2 and 5 years despite no significant change in the degree of prolactin elevation. In contrast, three patients had complete resolution of all symptoms and normalization of prolactin elevation (84). Less commonly, pituitary adenomas may cosecrete both prolactin and growth hormone. Approximately 20% to 40% of cases of acromegaly will have hyperprolactinemia. Rarely, nonpituitary tumors such as mature cystic teratomas of the ovary may cause hyperprolactinemia (85).

Other abnormalities of the hypothalamus/pituitary result in hyperprolactinemia by interfering with the normal inhibition by dopamine. These may include tumors such as craniopharyngioma (86) and other pituitary adenomas. Nontumor conditions include postinflammatory conditions of encephalitis and meningitis; infiltrative conditions of hemochromatosis, sarcoidosis, and histiocytosis; necrosis condition of Sheehan's syndrome; and empty sella syndrome. Empty sella syndrome represents a herniation of the arachnoid through the sella diaphragm with cerebrospinal fluid pressure leading to compression and atrophy of the pituitary. Found in 5% to 6% of random autopsies, empty sella syndrome is most common in middle-aged females (87%) and may be found in 4% to 16%

of cases of hyperprolactinemia. Two thirds of cases have no associated endocrine abnormalities, one in five have growth hormone deficiency, one in ten have abnormalities of TSH or gonadotropin secretion, and less than 5% have panhypopituitarism (87).

Primary hypothyroidism is associated with hyperprolactinemia in 3% to 5% of cases and is due to a thyroid-releasing-hormone-induced alteration of dopamine regulation. Less commonly, primary hypothyroidism may cause significant pituitary hyperplasia leading to the impression of a pituitary tumor with imaging studies (88). Renal failure frequently is associated with hyperprolactinemia due to a decrease in renal excretion of the hormone.

Multiple drugs cause hyperprolactinemia. Synthetic estrogens of oral contraceptives directly stimulate prolactin production and lactotroph hyperplasia. Mild elevations in prolactin are found in approximately 40% of users of 35-μg pills, yet galactorrhea is less common due to the elevated synthetic estrogen levels. Other drugs as outlined in Table 13.3 interfere with different aspects of dopamine production, secretion, or action.

Hyperprolactinemia associated with PCOS is common and not often emphasized in discussions of etiology. Up to one in five patients with PCOS will have mildly elevated prolactin levels probably due to stimulation from chronically elevated estrone levels. Unlike patients with primary hyperprolactinemia, women with PCOS will have ovarian androgen excess and not have evidence of estrogen deficiency.

Diagnosis and Treatment

Measurement of prolactin levels should be an initial part of the evaluation of any case with menstrual abnormalities. Evaluation of hyperprolactinemia then should proceed according to the degree of elevation, supporting history, physical findings, and costs of the testing. If possible, measurements of prolactin should not be performed while patients are taking drugs known to affect the level. All cases of nondrug-induced hyperprolactinemia should have a TSH level measured. Physical examination findings separate primary hyperprolactinemia from hyperprolactinemia associated with PCOS. Primary hyperprolactinemia results in gonadotropin suppression and signs of estrogen deficiency, such as lack of cervical mucus and vaginal dryness. In contrast, patients with hyperprolactinemia associated with PCOS do not have ovarian suppression and present with abundant cervical mucus and signs of ovarian androgen excess. The initial prolactin level is helpful in planning the evaluation. Although there is no absolute level that excludes a pituitary adenoma, the degree of prolactin elevation correlates with the probability of a tumor. Thus, with initial prolactin levels greater than 100 ng/mL, normal TSH, and no obvious cause of hyperprolactinemia, cranial imaging should be the next step. With prolactin levels less than 50 ng/mL, all other causes of hyperprolactinemia should be evaluated before cranial imaging. For example, in a patient with oligomenorrhea and repetitive prolactin levels in the 30 to 40 ng/mL range, elevations of androstenedione and testosterone, physical findings of hirsutism, oily skin, and abundant cervical mucus, the diagnosis is PCOS, and cranial imaging is not necessary. In cases of hyperprolactinemia in which the etiology is not obvious, cranial imaging is best performed with MRI.

The diagnosis of macroadenoma requires further evaluation (Fig. 13.14). Visual field testing by ophthalmology is necessary, in addition to testing of other pituitary function. The thyroid axis is analyzed by assays for TSH, thyroxine, and T_3 uptake; the growth hormone axis is analyzed by assay for insulin-like growth factor I; and the adrenal axis is analyzed by a.m. and p.m. cortisol levels. Abnormal levels may be evaluated further with dynamic testing, such as with stimulation by the corresponding hypothalamic hormones. Further testing of adrenal reserve is possible with a 1-hour ACTH stimulation test or with an insulin tolerance test, which is more sensitive because it tests the complete axis from

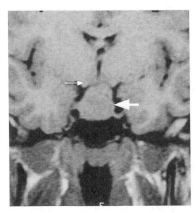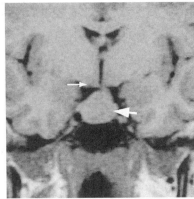

FIG. 13.14. Adolescent presenting with amenorrhea/galactorrhea due to a prolactin-secreting macroadenoma. Despite compression of the optic chiasm *(small arrow)*, visual field testing was normal. Follow-up magnetic resonance imaging 3 months after initiation of dopamine-agonist therapy shows tumor shrinkage away from the chiasm.

hypothalamus to adrenal. However, the test requires careful monitoring and may be quite unpleasant due to the side effects of hypoglycemia. The 1-hour ACTH stimulation test assays the production of cortisol by the adrenal gland. Although the adrenal gland is capable of normal function, chronic lack of stimulation by ACTH will result in subnormal cortisol production with the 1-hour test. Similar screening of pituitary function should be performed in women with hyperprolactinemia thought secondary to empty sella syndrome, inflammatory or infiltrative diseases of the pituitary, or nonpituitary CNS tumors. Screening is not necessary in asymptomatic women with microadenomas. The possibility of pituitary apoplexy should be discussed with patients with macroadenomas. Patients should consider wearing a medical alert bracelet until the tumor has responded to therapy and reduced to a microadenoma.

Treatment of hyperprolactinemia is aimed at correction of the underlying etiology and reestablishment of a normal estrogen status. Dopamine-agonist therapy is the most common treatment of hyperprolactinemia due to a prolactin-secreting adenoma. In this country, the drugs pergolide, bromocriptine, and cabergoline are available for treatment. Cabergoline offers advantages of twice a week dosing, greater effectiveness, and less nausea compared to bromocriptine (89). With treatment, prolactin levels should normalize within 2 to 4 weeks, and this time frame should be used to titrate the necessary dosage. In general, galactorrhea resolves and menses resume within 8 weeks of normalization of prolactin levels. Follow-up imaging of adenomas is necessary even with correction of the hyperprolactinemia. Initial repeat MRI should be done 6 months after the diagnosis of a macroadenoma to evaluate for a decrease in size with therapy. A repeat scan should be done 1 year after the diagnosis of a microadenoma and then repeated in 2 to 3 years to evaluate for change. Referral for surgical consult is necessary if significant visual field defects are present from compression of the optic chiasm by a macroadenoma, if a macroadenoma does not decrease in size with therapy, or if a microadenoma grows significantly while on therapy. Although surgical evacuation is successful for tumor removal, recurrence of hyperprolactinemia is seen in 80% of macroadenomas and up to 40% of microadenomas (90). This probably is not due to residual adenoma but to defects in the microcirculation of the remaining lactotrophs. Adenomas cosecreting growth hormone with signs of acromegaly may not respond to dopamine-agonist therapy.

Other therapy with somatostatin analogues or surgery usually is necessary.

An alternative treatment for idiopathic hyperprolactinemia or due to a microadenoma is hormone replacement therapy. As discussed earlier, the odds of a microadenoma increasing in size is small even without therapy. Hormone therapy prevents the complications of estrogen deficiency, but often it will not resolve galactorrhea. Hormone therapy with low-dose oral contraceptives often is preferable in a young woman without bothersome galactorrhea who requires birth control.

Hyperprolactinemia secondary to primary hypothyroidism will resolve with thyroid replacement and does not require dopamine-agonist therapy.

CONCLUSIONS

Amenorrhea is a symptom of altered function of the hypothalamic-pituitary axis, the ovarian response to gonadotropins, the integrity of the genital outflow tract, or the mechanisms of sexual differentiation. Diagnosis of the etiology of amenorrhea should be based on an understanding of the physiology of puberty, the physiology of the female reproductive cycle, and the hormonal interactions between the hypothalamus, pituitary gland, and ovaries. This chapter suggests a strategy for the evaluation of amenorrhea based on physical characteristics that serve as a bioassay for abnormalities of sex steroids. The history and physical examination should be used to target the applicable disease states. Focused laboratory studies should be used to ascertain and confirm the final diagnosis. Broad, nonspecific laboratory testing is expensive and should not be undertaken. Rather, complex laboratory studies should be carefully selected based on history, physical examination, and initial laboratory studies. Treatment of amenorrhea should be directed to correct the underlying pathophysiology. Hormone replacement is essential for adolescent women with ovarian failure and may be warranted for those with hypothalamic-pituitary dysfunction.

REFERENCES

1. Marshall WA, Tanner JM. Variations in the pattern of pubertal changes in girls. *Arch Dis Child* 1969;44:291.
2. Grumbach MM, Styne DM. Puberty: ontogeny, neuroendocrinology, physiology and disorders. In: Wilson JD, Foster DW, eds. *Williams textbook of endocrinology.* Philadelphia: WB Saunders, 1992:1146.
3. Smith EP, Boyd J, Frank GR, et al. Estrogen resistance caused by a mutation in the estrogen-receptor gene in a man. *N Engl J Med* 1994;331:1056–1061.
4. Apter D, Vihko R. Serum pregnenolone, progesterone, 17-hydroxyprogesterone, testosterone and 5α-dihydrotestosterone during female puberty. *J Clin Endocrinol Metab* 1977;45:1039–1048.
5. Frisch RE, McArthur JW. Menstrual cycles: fatness as a determinant of minimum weight for height necessary for their maintenance at onset. *Science* 1974;185: 949–951.
6. Ahima RS, Dushay J, Flier SN, et al. Leptin accelerates the onset of puberty in normal female mice. *J Clin Invest* 1997;99:391–395.
7. Blum WF, Englaro P, Hanitsch S, et al. Plasma leptin levels in healthy children and adolescents: dependence on body mass index, body fat mass, gender, pubertal stage and testosterone. *J Clin Endocrinol Metab* 1997; 82:2904–2910.
8. Palmert MR, Radovick S, Boepple PA. Leptin levels in children with central precocious puberty. *J Clin Endocrinol Metab* 1998;83:2260–2265.
9. Garcia-Mayor RV, Andrade A, Rios M, et al. Serum leptin levels in normal children: relationship to age, gender, body mass index, pituitary-gonadal hormones and pubertal stage. *J Clin Endocrinol Metab* 1997;82: 2849–2855.
10. Bates GW, Garza DE, Garza MM. Clinical manifestations of hormonal changes in the menstrual cycle. *Obstet Gynecol Clin North Am* 1990;17:289.
11. Winderl LM, Silverman RK. Prenatal diagnosis of congenital imperforate hymen. *Obstet Gynecol* 1995;85: 857–860.
12. Yu TJ, Lin MC. Acute urinary retention in two patients with imperforate hymen. *Scand J Urol Nephrol* 1993; 27:543–544.
13. Rock JA, Zacur HA, Dlugi AM, et al. Pregnancy success following surgical correction of imperforate hymen and complete transverse vaginal septum. *Obstet Gynecol* 1982;59:448–451.
14. Usta IM, Awwad JT, Usta JA, et al. Imperforate hymen: report of an unusual familial occurrence. *Obstet Gynecol* 1993;82:655–656.
15. Suidan FG, Azoury RS. The transverse vaginal septum: a clinicopathological evaluation. *Obstet Gynecol* 1979; 54:278–283.
16. Regenstein AC, Berkeley AS. Discordance of mullerian agenesis in monozygotic twins. *J Reprod Med* 1991; 36:396–397.
17. Rock JA, Baramki TA, Parmley TH, et al. A unilateral functioning uterine anlage with mullerian duct agenesis. *Int J Gynaecol Obstet* 1980;18:99–101.
18. Bader PI, Keye WR, Cowan JT, et al. Mullerian agenesis hypoplasia of distal extremities, unusual dermatoglyphics, and pigmentation. *Obstet Gynecol* 1982;60: 263–266.
19. Massafra C, Bartolozzi M, Bartolozzi P, et al. Rokitan-

sky-Kuster-Hauser syndrome with ectrodactyly. *Acta Obstet Gynecol Scand* 1988;67:557–560.

20. Muechler EK. Mullerian duct agenesis associated with renal and skeletal abnormalities. *Am J Obstet Gynecol* 1975;121:567–568.

21. Griffin JE. Androgen resistance—the clinical and molecular spectrum. *N Engl J Med* 1992;326:611–618.

22. De Bellis A, Quigley CA, Marschke KB, et al. Characterization of mutant androgen receptors causing partial androgen insensitivity syndrome. *J Clin Endocrinol Metab* 1994;78:513–522.

23. Dempsey AT, de Swiet M, Dewhurst J. Premature ovarian failure associated with the candida endocrinopathy syndrome. *Br J Obstet Gynaecol* 1981;88:563–565.

24. Hoek A, Schoemaker J, Drexhage HA. Premature ovarian failure and ovarian autoimmunity. *Endocr Rev* 1997; 18:107–134.

25. Chen S, Sawicka J, Betterle C, et al. Autoantibodies to steroidogenic enzymes in autoimmune polyglandular syndrome, Addison's disease, and premature ovarian failure. *J Clin Endocrinol Metab* 1996;81:1871–1876.

26. Jones GS, de Moraes-Ruehsen M. A new syndrome of amenorrhea in association with hypergonadotropism and apparently normal ovarian follicular apparatus. *Am J Obstet Gynecol* 1969;104:597–600.

27. Conway GS, Kaltsas G, Patel A, et al. Characterization of idiopathic premature ovarian failure. *Fertil Steril* 1996;65:337–341.

28. Kim TJ, Anasti JN, Flack MR, et al. Routine endocrine screening for patients with karyotypically normal spontaneous premature ovarian failure. *Obstet Gynecol* 1997;89:777–779.

29. Kuki S, Morgan RL, Tucci JR. Myasthenia gravis and premature ovarian failure. *Arch Intern Med* 1981;141: 1230–1232.

30. Ayala A, Canales ES, Karchmer S, et al. Premature ovarian failure and hypothyroidism associated with sicca syndrome. *Obstet Gynecol* 1979;53:98S–101S.

31. Fenichel P, Sosset C, Barbarino-Monnier P, et al. Prevalence, specificity and significance of ovarian antibodies during spontaneous premature ovarian failure. *Hum Reprod* 1997;12:2623–2628.

32. Wheatcroft NJ, Salt C, Milford-Ward A, et al. Identification of ovarian antibodies by immunofluorescence, enzyme-linked immunosorbent assay or immunoblotting in premature ovarian failure. *Hum Reprod* 1997; 12:2616–2622.

33. Fraser IS, Russell P, Greco S, et al. Resistant ovary syndrome and premature ovarian failure in young women with galactosaemia. *Clin Reprod Fertil* 1986;4: 133–138.

34. Kaufman FR, Reichardt JKV, Ng WG, et al. Correlation of cognitive, neurologic, and ovarian outcome with the Q188R mutation of the galactose-1-phosphate uridyltransferase gene. *J Pediatr* 1994;125:225–227.

35. Morrison JC, Givens JR, Wiser WL, et al. Mumps oophoritis: a cause of premature menopause. *Fertil Steril* 1975;26:655–659.

36. Chapman RM, Sutcliffe S. The effects of chemotherapy and radiotherapy on fertility and their prevention. *Recent Adv Clin Oncol* 1986;2:239–251.

37. Madsen BL, Giudice L, Donaldson SS. Radiation-induced premature menopause: a misconception. *Int J Radiat Oncol Bio Phys* 1995;32:1461–1464.

38. Wallace WHB, Shalet SM, Crowne EC, et al. Ovarian failure following abdominal irradiation in childhood: natural history and prognosis. *Clin Oncol* 1989;1: 75–79.

39. Kreuser ED, Xiros N, Hetzel WD, et al. Reproductive and endocrine gonadal capacity in patients treated with COPP chemotherapy for Hodgkin's disease. *J Cancer Res Clin Oncol* 1987;113:260–266.

40. Clark ST, Radford JA, Crowther D, et al. Gonadal function following chemotherapy for Hodgkin's disease: a comparative study of MVPP and a seven-drug hybrid regimen. *J Clin Oncol* 1995;13:134–139.

41. Manuel M, Katayama KP, Jones HW. The age of occurrence of gonadal tumors in intersex patients with a Y chromosome. *Am J Obstet Gynecol* 1976;124:293–300.

42. Lindenman E, Shepard MK, Pescovitz OH. Mullerian agenesis: an update. *Obstet Gynecol* 1997;90:307–312.

43. Starup J, Philip J, Sele V. Oestrogen treatment and subsequent pregnancy in two patients with severe hypergonadotrophic ovarian failure. *Acta Endocrinol* 1978;89:149–157.

44. Treissman MJ, Miller D, McComb PF. Laparoscopic lateral ovarian transposition. *Fertil Steril* 1996;65: 1229–1231.

45. Blumenfeld Z, Haim N. Prevention of gonadal damage during cytotoxic therapy. *Ann Med* 1997;29:199–206.

46. Barakat BY, Jones HW. Gynecologic and cytogenetic aspects of gonadal agenesis and dysgenesis. *Obstet Gynecol* 1970:36:368–372.

47. Hung W, Verghese KP, Picciano D, et al. Mixed gonadal dysgenesis with XO/XY mosaicism in multiple tissues. *Obstet Gynecol* 1970;36:373–376.

48. Itu M, Neelam T, Ammini AC, et al. Primary amenorrhea in a triple X female. *Aust N Z J Obstet Gynaecol* 1990;30:386–388.

49. Youlton R, Michelsen H, Be C, et al. Pure XX gonadal dysgenesis in identical twins. *Clin Genet* 1982;21: 262–265.

50. Nazareth HR, Farah LMS, Cunha AJB, et al. Pure gonadal dysgenesis (type XX). *Hum Genet* 1977;37: 117–120.

51. Medlina M, Kofman-Alfaro S, Perez-Palacios G. 46,XX gonadal absence: a variant of the XX pure gonadal dysgenesis? *Acta Endocrinol* 1982;99:585–587.

52. Cruz OLM, Pedalini MEB, Caropreso CA. Sensorineural hearing loss associated to gonadal dysgenesis in sisters: Perrault's syndrome. *Am J Otol* 1992;13: 82–83.

53. Swyer GI. Male pseudohermaphroditism: a hitherto undescribed form. *Br Med J* 1955;2:709.

54. Guidozzi F, Ball J, Spurdle A. 46,XY pure gonadal dysgenesis (Swyer-James Syndrome)—Y or Y not?: a review. *Obstet Gynecol Surv* 1994;49:138–146.

55. Barakat AY, Ances IG, Tang CK, et al. 46,XY gonadal dysgenesis with secondary amenorrhea, virilization, and bilateral gonadoblastomas. *South Med J* 1979;72: 1163–1165.

56. DeMarchi M, Campagnoli C, Ghiringhello B, et al. Gonadal agenesis in a phenotypically normal female with positive H-Y antigen. *Hum Genet* 1981;56:417–419.

57. Wu RH, Boyar RM, Knight R, et al. Endocrine studies in a phenotypic girl with XY gonadal agenesis. *J Clin Endocrinol Metab* 1976;43:506–511.

58. Goldsmith O, Solomon DH, Horton R. Hypogonadism and mineralocorticoid excess. The 17-hydroxylase deficiency syndrome. *N Engl J Med* 1967;277:673–677.

59. Yanase T, Sanders D, Shibata A, et al. Combined 17α-hydroxylase/17,20-lyase deficiency due to a 7-basepair duplication in the N-terminal region of the cytochrome $P450_{17\alpha}$ (CYP17) gene. *J Clin Endocrinol Metab* 1990; 70:1325–1329.

60. Ahlgren R, Yanase T, Simpson ER, et al. Compound heterozygous mutations (Arg 239 → Stop, Pro 342 → Thr) in the CYP17 (P450 17α) gene lead to ambiguous external genitalia in a male patient with partial combined 17α-hydroxylase/17,20-lyase deficiency. *J Clin Endocrinol Metab* 1992;74:667–672.

61. Ito Y, Fisher CR, Conte FA, et al. Molecular basis of aromatase deficiency in an adult female with sexual infantilism and polycystic ovaries. *Proc Natl Acad Sci U S A* 1992;90:11673–11677.

62. MacGillivray MH, Morishima A, Conte F, et al. Pediatric endocrinology update: an overview. *Horm Res* 1998;49:2–8.

63. Molsted K, Kjaer I, Giwercman A, et al. Craniofacial morphology in patients with Kallmann's syndrome with and without cleft lip and palate. *Cleft Palate Craniofac J* 1997;34:417–424.

64. Klein VR, Friedman JM, Brookshire GS, et al. Kallmann syndrome associated with choanal atresia. *Clin Genet* 1987;31:224–227.

65. Hardelin JP, Levilliers J, Blanchard S, et al. Heterogeneity in the mutations responsible for X chromosome-linked Kallmann syndrome. *Hum Mol Genet* 1993;2:373–377.

66. Klingmuller D, Dewes W, Krahe T, et al. Magnetic resonance imaging of the brain in patients with anosmia and hypothalamic hypogonadism (Kallmann's syndrome). *J Clin Endocrinol Metab* 1987;65:581–584.

67. Franco B, Guioli S, Pragliola A, et al. A gene deleted in Kallmann's syndrome shares homology with neural cell adhesion and axonal path-finding molecules. *Nature* 1991;353:529–536.

68. Sauer MV, Lobo RA, Paulson RJ. Successful twin pregnancy after embryo donation to a patient with XY gonadal dysgenesis. *Obstet Gynecol* 1989;161:380–381.

69. Ben-Nun I, Siegal A, Shulman A, et al. Induction of artificial endometrial cycles with oestradiol implants and injectable progesterone: establishment of a viable pregnancy in a woman with 17α-hydroxylase deficiency. *Hum Reprod* 1995;10:2456–2458.

70. Canales ES, Zarate A, Castelazo-Ayala L. Primary amenorrhea associated with polycystic ovaries. *Obstet Gynecol* 1971;37:205–210.

71. Ehrmann DA, Schneider DJ, Sobel BE, et al. Troglitazone improves defects in insulin action, insulin secretion, ovarian steroidogenesis, and fibrinolysis in women with polycystic ovary syndrome. *J Clin Endocrinol Metab* 1997;82:2108–2116.

72. Meldrum DR, Abraham GE. Peripheral and ovarian venous concentrations of various steroid hormones in virilizing ovarian tumors. *Obstet Gynecol* 1979;53:36–43.

73. Larsen WG, Felmar EA, Wallace ME, et al. Sertoli-Leydig cell tumor of the ovary: a rare cause of amenorrhea. *Obstet Gynecol* 1992;79:831–833.

74. Russell JB, Lambert SJ, Taylor KJW, et al. Androgen-producing hilus cell tumor of the ovary. Detection in a postmenopausal woman by duplex doppler scanning. *JAMA* 1987;257:962–963.

75. Martinez L, Salmeron M, Carvia RE, et al. Androgen producing luteinized granulosa cell tumor. *Acta Obstet Gynecol Scand* 1997;76:285–286.

76. Orth DN, Kovacs WJ, DeBold CR. The adrenal cortex. In: Wilson JD, Foster DW, eds. *Williams textbook of endocrinology.* Philadelphia: WB Saunders, 1992:536.

77. Mayer SK, Oligny LL, Deal C, et al. Childhood adrenocortical tumors: case series and reevaluation of prognosis—a 24-year experience. *J Pediatr Surg* 1997;32: 911–915.

78. Legro RS, Finegood D, Dunaif A. Fasting glucose to insulin ratio is a useful measure of insulin sensitivity in women with polycystic ovary syndrome. *J Clin Endocrinol Metab* 1998;83:2694–2698.

79. White PC, New MI, Dupont B. Congenital adrenal hyperplasia. Part 1. *N Engl J Med* 1987;316:1519–1524.

80. Bricaire C, Raynaud A, Benotmane A, et al. Selective venous catheterization in the evaluation of hyperandrogenism. *J Endocrinol Invest* 1991;14:949–956.

81. Thorner MO, Vance ML, Horvath E, et al. The anterior pituitary. In: Wilson JD, Foster DW, eds. *Williams textbook of endocrinology.* Philadelphia: WB Saunders, 1992:283.

82. Wudy SA, Homoki J, Teller WM. Successful prenatal treatment of congenital adrenal hyperplasia due to 21-hydroxylase deficiency. *Eur J Pediatr* 1994;153:556–559.

83. Burrow GN, Wortzman G, Rewcastle NB, et al. Microadenomas of the pituitary and abnormal sellar tomograms in an unselected autopsy series. *N Engl J Med* 1981;304:156–158.

84. March CM, Kletzky OA, Davajan V, et al. Longitudinal evaluation of patients with untreated prolactin-secreting pituitary adenomas. *Am J Obstet Gynecol* 1981;139: 835–844.

85. Palmer PE, Bogojavlensky S, Bhan AK, et al. Prolactinoma in wall of ovarian dermoid cyst with hyperprolactinemia. *Obstet Gynecol* 1990;75:540–543.

86. Nakasu Y, Nakasu S, Handa J, et al. Amenorrhea-galactorrhea syndrome with craniopharyngioma. *Surg Neurol* 1980;13:154–156.

87. Shreefter M, Friedlander RL. Primary empty sella syndrome and amenorrhea. *Obstet Gynecol* 1975;46: 535–538.

88. Keye WR, Yuen BH, Knopf RF, et al. Amenorrhea, hyperprolactinemia, and pituitary enlargement secondary to primary hypothyroidism. *Obstet Gynecol* 1976;48: 697–702.

89. Webster J, Piscitelli G, Polli A, et al. A comparison of cabergoline and bromocriptine in the treatment of hyperprolactinemic amenorrhea. *N Engl J Med* 1994;331: 904–909.

90. Serri O, Rasio E, Beauregard H, et al. Recurrence of hyperprolactinemia after selective transsphenoidal adenomectomy in women with prolactinoma. *N Engl J Med* 1983;309:280.

14

Abnormal Uterine Bleeding

Spencer S. Richlin and John A. Rock

Abnormal vaginal bleeding is a presenting complaint for many gynecologic and nongynecologic conditions, and it is a common problem encountered by physicians providing health care for adolescents. Possible etiologies include (a) organic causes such as pregnancy complications, infections, trauma, cancer lesions and tumors of the genital tract, blood dyscrasias, and endocrine and systemic disorders; (b) abnormal consequences of contraceptive methods such as oral contraceptives and intrauterine devices; and (c) dysfunctional uterine bleeding (DUB), which refers to abnormal uterine bleeding for which no demonstrable organic cause can be found.

In the adolescent, DUB is the most common cause of abnormal bleeding, comprising about 48% to 97% of the causes (1–4). The underlying problem is anovulation or oligoovulation, with the maturational process of the hypothalamic-pituitary-ovarian (HPO) axis often taking 2 to 5 years to complete (5–7). Menarche, which occurs at an average age of 12.8 years in the United States, is an anovulatory bleeding episode, and as many as 82% of the cycles in the first postmenarcheal year (5,6) and up to 28% of the cycles in the fifth postmenarcheal year are anovulatory (6). However, most adolescents who have irregular bleeding in the first and second postmenarcheal years do not require long-term management (2,8). Yet, when irregular bleeding persists after 4 years from the onset of bleeding, serious gynecologic sequelae, such as problematic uterine bleeding, reduced fertility potential, and a high rate (1.3%) of endometrial cancer in women under 40 years of age, were observed (8).

Normal variations in bleeding patterns are important to understand in order to establish when to consider to the bleeding as abnormal. The mean amount of blood loss in a normal cycle is about 35 mL (range 20 to 60 mL). Chronic blood loss of more than 80 mL per cycle results in a high frequency of iron deficiency anemia (9). Outside of research protocols, estimating the amount of blood loss is difficult at best, and frequently the perception of how much blood has been lost is not reliable (10). Even using estimates based on the number of well-soaked regular perineal pads, such as eight, or the number of tampons, such as 12, as upper limits of normal may not correlate with actual blood loss when pads and tampons are changed frequently or blood clots are present (10). The duration of flow averages 3 to 7 days, with more than 7 days considered prolonged. The frequency of bleeding occurs between 24 and 36 days in normal cycles. However, cycle lengths as short as 21 days and as long as 40 days may be normal. In general, an adolescent's established menstrual pattern can serve as a reference to determine how the problematic bleeding differs from her "normal" menstrual flow, but in the absence of previously regular menstrual bleeding, these values may be used as guidelines.

Bleeding abnormalities may be classified according to the amount of flow, duration of flow, and regularity or interval between bleeding episodes. Certain descriptive terms such as "menorrhagia" (hypermenorrhea), "metrorrhagia," and "menometrorrhagia" may be used to classify the types of bleeding and assist in establishing a differential diagnosis. These terms and others are defined in Table 14.1, and some of the possible etiologic conditions are included. With the inherent difficulties in assessing irregular bleeding in the adolescent and the numerous organic causes that must be excluded before DUB can be designated as the etiology, the health care provider is faced with a significant diagnostic challenge. In addition, the physician must be aware of both the treatment options in order to individualize the management as well as the potential psychoemotional impact of the problem on the adolescent and her parents.

MENSTRUAL CYCLE

Before one can understand the abnormalities of the adolescent cycle, a thorough understanding of the normal cycle is needed. Except for the extremes of reproductive life, the menstrual cycle has a medial duration of 28 days due to a 14-day follicular phase and a 14-day luteal phase (11). The cyclic expression of the HPO axis leads to functional and structural changes in several target tissues, particularly the endometrium. In the absence of a conception, the demise of the corpus luteum leads to the withdrawal of ovarian steroids from the endometrium, which in turn leads to an orderly withdrawal menses. Any aberration in this orderly sequence of events can lead to asynchronous development and shedding of the endometrium with subsequent abnormal uterine bleeding.

The actual event responsible for the initiation of puberty and subsequent maturation of the hypothalamus is unknown. Before the onset of puberty, insufficient hypothalamic gonadotropin-releasing hormone (GnRH) stimulation to the pituitary causes low gonadotropin levels and subsequent absent follicular development (7). As the hypothalamus begins to mature, sleep-induced luteinizing hormone (LH) pulses are seen that disappear after puberty (12,13). In early adolescence, follicular recruitment and episodic estrogen secretion lead to development of the endometrium, but this often is followed by an inability of the immature hypothalamus to respond with an LH surge (14). This leads to the frequent occurrence of anovulation and DUB, as described later.

The human menstrual cycle can be divided into three distinct phases. The *follicular phase,* which probably begins in the preceding luteal phase, is characterized by the selection of the dominant follicle and growth of the endometrium under the influence of estrogen. The *ovulatory phase,* which begins with the

TABLE 14.1. *Classification of abnormal uterine bleeding in the adolescent*

Menorrhagia (hypermenorrhea): Excessive uterine bleeding in either the amount or the duration of flow, which occurs at the normal intervals of regular menses. Etiologies may include blood dyscrasias, endometrial polyps, hypothyroidism, chronic endometritis, or submucus myoma.

Polymenorrhea: Regular episodes of uterine bleeding occurring at intervals of <24 days due to either a proliferative phase of <10 days or a secretory phase of <12 days. Endocrine, systemic, or metabolic disorders, or psychogenic causes may be found.

Metrorrhagia: Uterine bleeding occurring at irregular intervals, which may range from spotting to a normal menstrual-like flow. Some causes include anovulation, oligoovulation, blood dyscrasias, complications of pregnancy, breakthrough bleeding with oral contraceptives, benign or malignant pelvic conditions, and thyroid disorders.

Menometrorrhagia: Irregular and frequent bleeding, which may be excessive in amount and/or prolonged induration. Causes are similar to metrorrhagia.

Oligomenorrhea: Irregular bleeding episodes occurring at intervals of >42 days. The most frequent causes are anovulation, recurrent functional ovarian cysts, and pregnancy.

Intermenstrual bleeding: Episodes of uterine bleeding occurring between regular menstrual periods. Ovulatory dysfunctional uterine bleeding, and benign or malignant pelvic conditions are frequent causes.

Postcoital bleeding: Bleeding occurring after sexual intercourse, which frequently indicates a cervical problem such as cervicitis, eversion, erosion, polyp, or cancer.

Hypomenorrhea: Decreased amount of uterine bleeding occurring at regular intervals. Causes include premature ovarian failure, cervical stenosis, intrauterine adhesions (Asherman's syndrome), and endocrine and oral contraceptive effects.

onset of the luteinizing surge, is characterized by a dramatic switch from estrogen to progesterone production and final release of the oocyte. The *luteal phase,* which lasts 13 to 14 days after ovulation, is characterized by preparation of the endometrium for implantation under the influence of the corpus luteum. The HPO axis and the endometrial changes

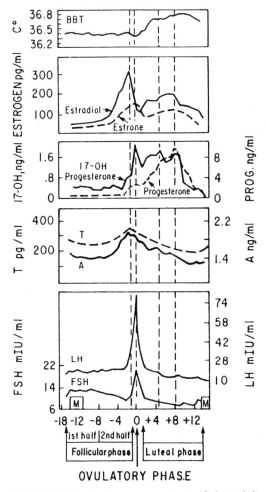

OVULATORY PHASE

FIG. 14.1. Cyclic hormone pattern of the adult human menstrual cycle centered on the day of the luteinizing hormone (LH) peak (day 0). Basal body temperatures (BBT) are shown on the **top,** ovarian steroids are shown in the **center,** and gonadotropin levels are shown on the **bottom.** (From Yen SCC. The menstrual cycle. In: Yen SCC, Jaffe RB, eds. *Reproductive endocrinology,* 2nd ed. Philadelphia: WB Saunders, 1986: 200–236, with permission.)

for each phase will be described in the following section. The hormone pattern of the adult human menstrual cycle is shown in Figs. 14.1–14.2.

Follicular Phase

Hypothalamic-Pituitary-Ovarian Axis

Knobil (15) showed that gonadotropin output by the pituitary is directly controlled by the GnRH pulse generator located in the accurate nucleus of the hypothalamus. Administration of a GnRH agonist leads to rapid pituitary gonadotropin suppression, which is reversed quickly on discontinuation of the drug (16). In the absence of either implantation or exogenous human chorionic gonadotropin (hCG), there is demise of the corpus luteum followed by a fall in serum progesterone. This declining steroid output by the ovary causes an alteration in the GnRH pulse generator, leading to more frequent pulses of GnRH. Decreasing serum steroid levels combined with a change in the pulse generator cause a rise in pituitary follicle-stimulating hormone (FSH) output, which can be detected 1 to 2 days before menses (17). It is this rise in serum FSH that is believed to initiate the subsequent follicular phase.

The first half of the follicular phase is marked by selection of the dominant follicle. At the start of each cycle, there exists a cohort of follicles destined for either atresia or ovulation (18). During the early follicular phase, all follicles show growth up to 10 mm; however, after selection of the dominant follicle, the remaining follicles show a decrease in size (19). The cohort of follicles ranges from 3 to 11 per ovary. The selection of the dominant follicle depends on both its microenvironment and its capacity for estrogen synthesis (20).

Although LH has multiple target sites, FSH appears to act only on the granulosa cells. Before selection of the dominant follicle, increasing levels of FSH causes an increase in the number of FSH receptors and induce granulosa cells to convert androgens to estrogens via an aromatizing enzyme (21). These

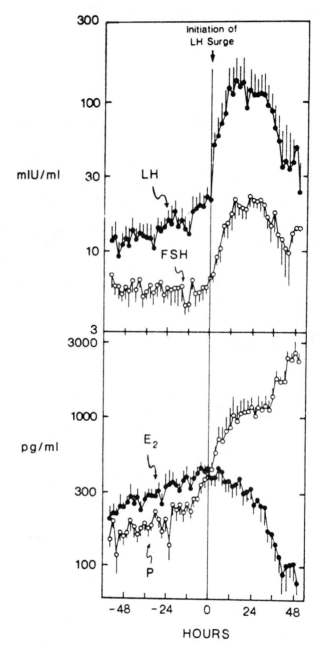

FIG. 14.2. Mean ± luteinizing hormone, follicle-stimulating hormone, estradiol, and progesterone levels measured every 2 hours for 5 days at midcycle in seven studies. Data are centered around the initiation of the gonadotropin surge. Note that the hormone concentrations are plotted on a logarithmic scale. (From Hoff JD, Quilgley ME, Yen SSC. Hormonal dynamics at midcycle: a reevaluation. *J Clin Endocrinol Metab* 1983;57:792–796, with permission.)

two actions lead to an increase in estrogen within the follicle. Estrogen then is able to increase the number of its own receptors. The follicle that is best able to utilize this synergistic relationship between FSH and estrogen is destined to change from an androgenic microenvironment to an estrogenic microenvironment and thus selection as the dominant follicle.

Once the dominant follicle has been selected (day 7), the next half of the follicular phase is marked by growth of the dominant follicle and preparation for ovulation. Declining serum levels of pituitary FSH, secondary to inhibin B production from the dominant follicle, leads to withdrawal of support from the secondary follicles. Thus, the dominant follicle produces the most inhibin B, whereas follicles destined to die produce smaller amounts of inhibin B. At the same time, activin proteins, which augment FSH activity, are produced in higher concentrations in the early follicular period (22). This ensures that only one oocyte will be ovulated each cycle. During the early part of the cycle, FSH has no effect on LH receptors. However, after exposure to increasing levels of estrogen, there is induction of LH receptors in the granulosa cells of the dominant follicle. Although LH stimulation of the theca interna is responsible for androgen production (which subsequently is aromatized to estrogen in the dominant follicle), it is the appearance of LH receptors in the granulosa cells that is responsible for subsequent progesterone production (23,24).

Endometrium

The anatomic changes that occur in the endometrium in response to ovarian steroids have been studied extensively in the human (25). The early follicular phase endometrium (i.e., menstrual endometrium) is marked by tissue breakdown in the form of necrosis, white cell infiltration, and glandular disruption. It is composed primarily of a nonfunctioning basalis component, which is left after the majority of the endometrium has sloughed. If the breakdown is secondary to the programmed withdrawal of progesterone, then the loss is orderly and complete and occurs in all segments of the endometrium.

Once estrogen levels start to rise in response to follicular recruitment, the process of growth and healing begins in the endometrium. The two structures that respond dramatically to estrogen are the glands and spiral arterioles. During the next several days, the endometrium will grow from 0.5 up to 5 mm due to an increase in the number and size of the glands. In stimulated cycles, the number of glands is positively correlated to the serum estrogen level (26). The glandular epithelium, marked by mitosis and pseudostratification, extends to form an epithelial lining facing the endometrial cavity. The spiral vessels also extend through the stroma.

Estrogen has been shown to have a significant effect on endometrial blood vessels (27). When estrogen levels fluctuate, changes can be seen in vessel permeability and fragility. Therefore, in an estrogen-primed endometrium, fluctuations in estrogen levels that are seen in the typical anovulatory cycles during adolescence lead to vessel fragility and incomplete and disorderly endometrial breakdown. This disorderly endometrial breakdown leads to the classic anovulatory uterine bleeding seen in early adolescence.

Ovulatory Phase

Hypothalamic-Pituitary-Ovarian Axis

The increasing amounts of estrogen produced by the dominant follicle exert a positive feedback on the hypothalamic-pituitary axis (28). The onset of the midcycle gonadotropin surge (LH and FSH) is related to the peak estradiol level and lasts roughly 48 hours, as shown in Fig. 14.2. The LH surge is characterized by a rapid ascending limb (accompanied by a rapid decline of serum estradiol) followed by a longer descending limb. The shift in steroidogenesis begins roughly 12 hours before the onset of the LH surge, when progesterone levels start to rise and estradiol levels begin to plateau. During the 48 hours of the LH surge, progesterone abruptly rises as estradiol continues to decline. An abnormal LH surge often is seen in adolescence where the hypothalamic-pituitary axis is unable to respond to the rising estradiol levels (14).

In addition to a shifting of steroidogenesis from estrogen to progesterone in the granulosa cells, the LH surge serves two other important functions. First, it causes resumption of meiosis; and second, it causes an alteration in the follicular environment, which leads to the physical process of ovulation (28). Tissue levels of cAMP rise in the preovulatory follicle and are followed by digestion of the follicular wall (29). Follicular fluid levels of prostaglandins are highest at ovulation (30) and appear to be involved in the actual process of ovulation. Plasminogen activator, which is produced after the LH surge, forms plasmin by granulosa and theca cells. Plasmin and other collagenases degrade the collagen connective tissue in the follicle, which ultimately facilitates follicle rupture (31). Prostaglandins and hydroxyeicosatetraenoic acids, in addition to plasminogen activator, may help facilitate follicular rupture (32,33).

Endometrium

During the 48 hours of the LH surge, the switch to progesterone fixes the height of the endometrium and begins the process of moving glandular secretions to the lumen of the glands. The early secretory endometrium is remarkable for movement of the intracellular vacuoles from the subnuclear region into the lumen. This is most prominent from days 16 to 19. Due to continued growth in fixed structure, the glands and spiral vessels begin to coil. As long as steroid output by the corpus luteum is adequate, the vessels will maintain their structure.

Once follicular recruitment begins and estrogen levels start to rise in early adolescence, the endometrium responds by growth and development of the glands and arterioles. In the absence of an LH surge and subsequent progesterone production, estrogen levels begin to fluctuate, which leads to vessel fragility in the endometrium. This causes incomplete breakdown of the endometrium and prolonged DUB.

Luteal Phase

Hypothalamic-Pituitary-Ovarian Axis

As the most steroidogenically active tissue in the body, the corpus luteum produces about 25 mg of progesterone per day (Table 14.2) (34). This progestogenic dominance serves to slow the GnRH pulse generator, thereby preventing further recruitment of follicles. In addition, inhibin A, mediated by LH, is secreted by the corpus luteum (35) and aids in preventing new follicular development in the luteal phase (36). The corpus luteum progesterone also serves to prepare the endometrium for implantation. Serum prog-

TABLE 14.2. *Production rate of sex steroids in women during the early follicular and midluteal phase*

Sex steroids	Daily production rate[a]	
	Early follicular	Midluteal
Progesterone	1.000	25.000
17-Hydroxyprogesterone	0.500	4.000
Androstenedione	2.600	3.400
Testosterone	0.200	0.170
Estrone	0.050	0.250
Estradiol	0.036	0.250

[a]Expressed as mg/24 h.
*From ref. 34.
From Yen SCC. The menstrual cycle. In: Yen SCC, Jaffe RB, eds. *Reproductive endocrinology*, 2nd ed. Philadelphia: WB Saunders, 1986;200–236, with permission.

esterone levels reach a peak roughly 8 days after the LH peak, and there is a parallel increase of 17-hydroxyprogesterone, estradiol, and estrone levels.

The health of the corpus luteum appears to depend on the preceding follicular phase (i.e., the development of LH receptors on the granulosa cells) (37,38). Selective suppression of FSH during the follicular phase results in a decreased luteal cell mass and a decreased progesterone production by the corpus luteum (39). The health of the corpus luteum also appears to depend on proper vascularization and the delivery of cholesterol for progesterone synthesis (40).

Pituitary LH is vital for the survival of the corpus luteum. This has been demonstrated by several studies. First, in hypophysectomized women, ovulation induction with gonadotropins is followed by low progesterone levels and a short luteal phase (41). Second, administration of a potent GnRH agonist or antagonist in the luteal phase results in a dramatic decline of progesterone (42). Cell culture experiments have shown that luteinized granulosa cells produce large amounts of progesterone, which peaks on day 3 of culture and is greatly increased in the presence of hCG (43). Thus, even though the GnRH pulse generator is slowed, pituitary LH is the vital luteotropic hormone in adult women.

Without hCG or LH stimulation, the lifespan of the human corpus luteum generally is 13 to 14 days. Prostaglandin $F_{2\alpha}$ is but one luteolytic that has been described. It stimulates endothelin 1, which induces luteal regression (44). The process of luteolysis has been further elucidated. Matrix metalloproteinases (MMPs) are zinc-dependent proteolytic enzymes. Tissue inhibitors of metalloproteins (TIMPs) are products of the corpus luteum. They inhibit MMPs. Luteolysis may occur with an increase in MMPs, as TIMPs do not increase during the luteal phase. When a woman becomes pregnant and hCG is exposed to the corpus luteum, "luteal rescue" is associated with a decrease of MMPs (45). With the demise of the corpus luteum, there is a dramatic fall in serum progesterone, estro-gen, and inhibin A (46), with a resultant increase in pulses from the GnRH pulse generator. The increase in GnRH frequency leads to a rise in serum FSH levels and initiation of the next follicular phase with recruitment of a new cohort of follicles.

Endometrium

During the luteal phase, the endometrium continues to prepare for implantation. The vacuoles have moved into the lumen of the glands, the glands have become exhausted, and the stroma has become edematous. Although the precise role of the glandular secretions is unknown, a teleologic view would hold that they provide nourishment for the embryo. The glandular secretions are prominent at a time when the embryo is in the endometrial cavity and preparing for implantation, between 4 and 7 days after ovulation.

Progesterone also has an effect on endometrial stroma cells, leading to edema, decidualization, and prolactin production (47). Around day 22 to 23, the spiral arterioles acquire a cuff of pseudodecidualized stromal cells. This is the earliest predecidual change. Pseudodecidualized stromal cells extend to beneath the epithelium by day 25, and by day 27 the endometrium appears as solid sheets of pseudodecidualized cells (25). Prostaglandin $F_{2\alpha}$ ($PGF_{2\alpha}$), which is believed to be important in the process of both implantation and menstruation, rises in late luteal endometrium (48) and appears to be decreased by the addition of progesterone (49).

Inadequate progesterone production after estrogen priming of the endometrium leads to thin endometrium without stromal edema or decidualization (50). Treatment during the follicular phase with an antiestrogen leads to lower levels of cytoplasmic progesterone receptors in the luteal endometrium (51). This could be a factor leading to lower conception rates in these cycles. Progesterone also has an effect on endometrial vessels and probably acts synergistically with estrogen to maintain an intact endometrium (52). Administration of an antiprogesterone during the early luteal phase results in decreased glandular secretory activity, vascular changes, and accelerated degenerative changes (53). Furthermore, administration of an antiprogesterone during the late luteal phase leads to a prompt withdrawal menses and shortening to the luteal phase (54). Although the precise role of decidualization and endometrial prolactin production is unclear, they may be involved in the initial establishment of an intact fetomaternal unit. Women who have delayed or abnormal decidualization show an increased incidence of both infertility and recurrent pregnancy loss (55,56). Furthermore, embryos implanted in tissue other than the endometrium show an abnormal amount of trophoblastic invasion (57) and abnormal development (57,58).

In the absence of implantation and subsequent hCG, there is demise of the corpus luteum and waning estrogen and progesterone levels. Withdrawal of steroids from the endometrium leads to vessel fragility and spiral arteriole constriction. Tissue necrosis, white cell migration, and menstruation follow. The edematous stoma of the spongiosum is sloughed, leaving behind the basalis and a residual spongiosum. Progesterone withdrawal also leads to an alteration in the GnRH pulse generator and a subsequent rise in FSH levels. This serves to initiate the next follicular phase and aid in the healing process of the endometrium. Menstrual flow stops due to prolonged vasoconstriction, platelet aggregation, and estrogen-induced vessel stability and healing.

CAUSES OF ABNORMAL UTERINE BLEEDING

Anovulatory DUB is the most frequent cause of abnormal bleeding in the adolescent, but its diagnosis requires the exclusion of many disorders (Table 14.3). Less commonly observed is ovulatory DUB, which may present as polymenorrhea, periovulatory (midcycle) bleeding, or premenstrual spotting. Midcycle bleeding may be attributed to the decrease in estrogen before ovulation and occasionally may be due to uterine polyps or fi-

broids. Premenstrual spotting may be seen with luteal phase inadequacy and decreased progesterone effect on the endometrium, although a fairly high association with endometriosis has been observed (59).

The frequency of the other causes of abnormal bleeding is different depending on the presentation. Extremely heavy menses requiring transfusions and beginning with or shortly after menarche is likely to be due to a coagulation disorder. Studies of acute adolescent menorrhagia showed that 3% to 19% of these patients have a coagulation disorder as the etiology for their bleeding (1,60). von Willebrand's disease is the most common inherited blood dyscrasia, affecting 1% of the population (61). Type 1 von Willebrand's disease accounts for 70% of all cases (62) and presents clinically with menorrhagia epistaxis, bruising, and gum bleeding (62). Many of the coagulation disorders are familial; a family history of bleeding problems frequently is elicited. Leukemia may present with either menorrhagia or menometrorrhagia, usually as a result of decreased plasma fibrinogen.

Adolescent pregnancy is an all too common occurrence in the United States. As many as 70% of women have sexual intercourse by age 19 years, and only half used contraception during their first intercourse (63). Consequently, a high index of suspicion of a possible pregnancy complication, such as a threatened or spontaneous abortion and ectopic pregnancy, is required when evaluating abnormal bleeding.

Infections as a cause of abnormal bleeding are more likely in acute episodes, although chronic endometritis may present with menorrhagia. Cervicovaginitis, including trichomoniasis, gonorrhea, herpes, condylomata, and chlamydia, may cause vaginal bleeding. When painful bleeding is observed, pelvic inflammatory disease must be considered as a possible cause. Local irritation and trauma from a foreign body left in the vagina may present with a bloody, malodorous discharge and requires differentiation from an infection. The most common foreign body is a tampon. Atrophic vaginitis from premature

TABLE 14.3. *Causes of abnormal uterine bleeding*

Dysfunctional uterine bleeding	Arteriovenous malformation
Anovulatory	Endometriosis
Ovulatory	Intrauterine device
Blood dyscrasia	Tuberculosis
Idiopathic thrombocytopenia	Disorders of the ovary
von Willebrand's disease	Polycystic ovarian disease
Leukemia	Neoplasia (benign or malignant)
Thrombocytopenia	Premature ovarian failure
Drug-induced	Disorders of the adrenal gland
Thalassemia major	Congenital adrenal hyperplasia
Fanconi's anemia	Cushing's disease
Glanzmann's disease	Addison's disease
Hemophilia	Neoplasia (benign or malignant)
Anticoagulants	Neoplasia of the central nervous system
Complications of pregnancy	Prolactinoma
Spontaneous or induced abortion	Nonsecreting pituitary tumor
Ectopic pregnancy	Craniopharyngioma
Hydatidiform mole	Pelvic inflammatory disease
Disorders of the cervix	Weight disorder
Cervicitis	Malnutrition
Polyps	Excessive exercise
Condylomata	Anorexia nervosa
Erosion	Bulimia
Sarcoma botyroides	Obesity
Mixed mesodermal sarcoma	Thyroid disease
Disorders of the vagina	Hyperthyroidism
Vaginitis	Hypothyroidism
Foreign body	Chronic illness
Coital trauma	Cancer
Sexual abuse	Organ failure (heart, lung, liver, kidney)
Septum	Renal dialysis
Adenosis	Psychogenic factors
Clear cell carcinoma	Medications
Disorders of the uterus	Hormonal
Congenital anomalies	Anticonvulsants
Endometritis	Neuroleptics
Neoplasia	Anabolic steroids
Polyps	Sliding inguinal hernia
Fibroids	
Cancer	

ovarian failure may be seen rarely in the adolescent presenting with spotting and vaginal discharge.

Sexual intercourse and/or abuse may present with vaginal trauma and bleeding. It requires a thorough history and examination for legal documentation when identified or suspected. Neoplasms of the cervix, vagina, uterus, and ovaries are rare causes of bleeding in the adolescent, but because of the often more serious nature of both benign and malignant tumors, a physician should always be concerned about these etiologies when performing an examination.

Endocrine causes most often present with recurrent abnormal bleeding, with thyroid disorders most commonly found. Hypothyroidism often is associated with hypermenorrhea, whereas hyperthyroidism usually results in hypomenorrhea. Signs of hyperandrogenism in the adolescent with abnormal bleeding may occur with polycystic ovarian disease, congenital adrenal hyperplasia, androgen-secreting neoplasms of the ovary or adrenal glands, and Cushing's disease. Anovulatory uterine bleeding frequently results from these endocrinopathies, as is also the case with weight disorders, chronic illnesses, and psychogenic causes. Polycystic ovarian syndrome should be suspected in any adolescent with androgen excess (hirsutism, acne, acanthosis nigricans), virilization, obesity, oligomenorrhea, and anovulatory bleeding. It is one of the most common causes of anovulation in this age group. Ovarian hyperandrogenism and anovulation are due to hyperinsulinemia during puberty (64). These adolescents are at risk for endometrial hyperplasia, cardiovascular disease (65), and noninsulin-dependent diabetes mellitus (Table 14.4) (66).

Endometriosis presents with chronic pelvic pain, dysmenorrhea, and bowel dysfunction. Studies have shown that up to 69% of adoles-

TABLE 14.4. *Evaluation of abnormal bleeding in the adolescent*

I. Essential evaluation
  A. Careful history
    1. Pubertal events/menstrual history
    2. Sexual history
    3. Coagulation disorder
    4. Extremes of weight/exercise
    5. Sexually transmitted diseases
    6. Contraceptive use
    7. Sexual abuse/trauma
    8. CNS tumors (headache, visual changes, weight loss)
    9. Medications
  B. Physical examination
    1. Systemic signs of chronic illness
    2. Systemic signs of coagulopathy
    3. Systemic signs of endocrinopathy
    4. Exact source of bleeding
    5. Vaginal, cervical, or pelvic abnormalities
  C. Laboratory testing
    1. Complete blood count
    2. Coagulation screen: platelet count, prothrombin time, partial thromboplastin time, bleeding time
    3. Pregnancy testing
    4. Pap smear
    5. Endometrial biopsy in selected cases
II. Additional laboratory studies if clinically indicated
  A. Further endocrine workup if anovulatory bleeding persists or clinically indicated
    1. Thyroid studies
    2. Prolactin level
  B. Blood glucose
  C. Screen for sexually transmitted disease
    1. Cervical cultures
    2. Erythrocyte sedimentation rate
  D. Evaluation of hirsutism
    1. DHEAS
    2. Testosterone
    3. 17-OH progesterone
  E. Evaluation of polycystic ovarian disease
    1. LH, FSH, prolactin, TSH
    2. Testosterone and DHEAS
    3. Total cholesterol and high-density lipoprotein
    4. Fasting glucose and insulin
III. Additional evaluation if clinically indicated
  A. Pelvic ultrasound
  B. Computed tomography scan of the pituitary
  C. Hysteroscopy/dilatation and curettage (last resort)
  D. Consultation
    1. Hematologist
    2. Endocrinologist
    3. Psychiatrist
    4. Oncologist

DHEAS, dehydroepiandrosterone sulfate; FSH, follicle-stimulating hormone; LH, luteinizing hormone; TSH, thyroid-stimulating hormone.

cents presenting with pelvic pain will have endometriosis, and 9.4% of these adolescents will have abnormal vaginal bleeding (67).

Congenital anomalies of the reproductive tract, although rare, can cause vaginal bleeding. A transverse septum can bleed after trauma from tampon placement or intercourse. An imperforate transverse vaginal septum with obstruction can lead to hematocolpos. Symptoms include severe cyclic abdominal and pelvic pain, and no menstrual flow with the development of a central pelvic or abdominal mass. If the septum develops a tract, abnormal vaginal bleeding ensues (68). This bleeding will be red during a menstrual cycle then change to brown blood if it appears between periods. In addition to the patient's personal history, the family history is important, as polycystic ovarian syndrome, endometriosis, and blood dyscrasias all have an inherited tendency.

DIAGNOSIS AND EVALUATION

As noted in Table 14.3, the causes of abnormal bleeding in adolescence are numerous. Even though the majority of cases represent anovulatory uterine bleeding, the more serious causes need to be excluded. The investigation of the adolescent with abnormal bleeding consists of three initial phases: history, physical examination, and laboratory tests. Table 14.4 outlines the essential evaluation and additional tests in the evaluation of adolescent bleeding.

As with most presenting complaints, a careful history will enable the clinician to make the diagnosis in the majority of cases. The history should be obtained with and without the patient's parent in the room. The patient's menstrual history needs to be reviewed in detail. Age of first menses and the nature of this first period, along with the frequency, duration, and regularity of their current menstrual cycle, are noted. Coagulopathies, polyps, or submucous myomas may present as heavy menses with no intermenstrual bleeding, whereas endometriosis, infections, congenital anomalies, foreign bodies, and malignancies can present with heavy periods and intermenstrual bleeding.

Reviewing the sequence of pubertal events is important. The absence of secondary sexual characteristics along with uterine bleeding should alert the physician to some of the more unusual and rare causes of abnormal bleeding, because menarche is the final event in puberty and therefore DUB should occur only after the development of secondary sexual characteristics. Systems of systemic progesterone (breast tenderness, mood swings, bloating) should alert the physician to ovulatory cycles and the probable diagnosis of DUB. Even though teenagers are poor at estimating the amount of blood loss, an attempt should be made to determine if the blood loss is excessive.

The remainder of the history should be directed toward the possibility of pregnancy and its complications, coagulation defects, sexually transmitted disease, sexual abuse or trauma, diet and/or exercise extremes, drug and/or medication use, and central nervous system tumors. After a thorough history, the physical examination is performed with these disorders in mind. An initial height and weight will help determine pubertal events, diet abnormalities, and overall health. The general physical examination may reveal systemic signs of a coagulation defect (petechiae or ecchymoses), endocrinopathy (hirsutism, hair changes, obesity, acne, acanthosis nigricans, galactorrhea, virilization, striae), a central nervous system tumor (visual changes) or chronic illness.

The pelvic examination may reveal the exact site of bleeding and may help rule out infection, cervicitis, sexually transmitted diseases, sexual abuse, trauma, and a foreign body. The examination is initiated after the physician has explained to the patient what he or she is planning to do. First, the external genitalia are examined. A young, apprehensive patient might best be placed on her parent's lap with her legs spread over their thighs. An older adolescent can be examined on an examination table with stirrups. In the very young patient, the pelvic examination may need to be performed under anesthesia. Ultrasound can be an integral part of the initial workup before an examination under anesthesia. In the sexually active, emotionally mature adolescent, transvaginal ultrasound can detect immediate pathology; the transabdominal approach is reserved for any nonsexually active female (69).

The vestibule should be examined with gentle labial retraction. The labia minora and majora, mons pubis, clitoral glans, and hood are evaluated along with the urethra, hymen, and posterior forchette. The cervix and vagina are visualized with a speculum or by vaginoscopy. Additionally, the knee-chest position causes the vagina to open.

When a speculum is used, cervical cultures, wet mount, and Pap smear are obtained if warranted. In the pediatric patient who does not tolerate a speculum examination, vaginal irrigation may provide these specimens. A bimanual examination is performed to evaluate the adnexa and uterus of masses and tenderness. If the hymeneal orifice is too small for digital palpation of the cervix, a rectoabdominal examination should be performed.

Following a careful history and physical examination, laboratory tests should be ordered. The essential laboratory evaluation of acute adolescent bleeding should include a complete blood count, which provides an indication of the severity of the bleeding in both acute and chronic loses, and screens for an infectious etiology. Due to the importance of pregnancy complications, a pregnancy test should always be performed. Because many adolescents will have an underlying coagulation defect, blood should be sent for a platelet count, prothrombin time, partial thromboplastin time, von Willebrand antigen, ristocetin cofactor assay, factor VIII antigen, and bleeding time, especially in cases of either acute hemorrhage or where the hemoglobin is less than 10 g/dL. This coagulation screen, if normal, will rule out all but the most unusual forms of coagulation defects and, if abnormal, indicate additional studies and consultation with a hematologist.

In addition to the essential workup as outlined earlier, other laboratory studies such as endocrine testing may be obtained if clinically indicated. Because the majority of anovulatory uterine bleeding in early adolescence will resolve with maturation of the HPO axis, these further tests also are indicated in nonacute cases where the anovulatory uterine bleeding persists long after menarche. Additional testing to evaluate anovulatory uterine bleeding may include thyroid studies, prolactin level, evaluation of hirsutism, and radiologic evaluation of the pituitary. A blood glucose, pelvic ultrasound, or screen for sexually transmitted disease should be obtained when clinically indicated.

Due to the low yield and potential harm, surgical evaluation in the form of hysteroscopy, and dilatation and curettage seldom are necessary in the evaluation of an adolescent and should be used as last resort when medical treatment fails. This is especially true when anovulatory uterine bleeding is the working diagnosis. Surgical evaluation may be useful in cases where a neoplasm or trauma is suspected. It also may be useful in certain pregnancy complications.

In cases where anovulatory uterine bleeding does not appear to be the diagnosis, a consultation with a specialist may be appropriate. The expertise of a hematologist, reproductive endocrinologist, or psychiatrist may be useful in the evaluation of the adolescent with abnormal bleeding refractory to treatment.

TREATMENT

Frequently the evaluation and the treatment of uterine bleeding are being performed concurrently and overlap significantly. Once specific organic causes and blood dyscrasias have been excluded, a designation of DUB may be made. Because the underlying problem is hormonal in DUB, the bleeding can be managed primarily with hormonal preparations and secondarily with adjunctive measures. With organic causes, endocrine causes, and blood dyscrasias, correcting or treating the disorder is foremost whenever possible. Hormonal treatments are reserved for control of heavy refractory uterine bleeding in appropriate cases.

Organic causes may need to be treated surgically, whereas endocrine disorders including hypothyroidism, congenital adrenal hyperplasia, hyperprolactinemia, and polycystic ovarian disease are treated medically. The blood dyscrasia von Willebrand's disease, type 1, can be treated with desmopressin acetate either as a nasal spray or by intravenous injection.

The most common clinical situation that will be seen in adolescents by health care providers is an irregular interval of bleeding that is neither heavier nor longer than a normal menstrual flow. Reassurance, observation, and recording the days and amount of bleeding (menstrual calendar) are sufficient unless a progression of problematic bleeding is observed. Chronic or recurrent episodes of mild-to-moderate bleeding (Table 14.5) are the next most common presentation, followed in decreasing frequency by chronic or recurrent episodes of heavy bleeding, acute heavy bleeding, and acute hemorrhage.

In each presentation of abnormal bleeding, excluding pregnancy is a necessary prerequisite to initiating therapy. In addition, an endometrial sampling should be performed with heavy bleeding, whether acute or chronic, once a pregnancy has been ruled out. Frequently, a physician may decide to forego endometrial sampling when the history strongly suggests DUB or the adolescent cannot be examined adequately. However, use of intravenous sedation may sufficiently reduce apprehension to allow performance of both the examination as well as endometrial sampling in an office setting. In rare instances, examination under general anesthesia may be required when organic causes are strongly suspected.

The value of endometrial sampling lies in both assisting in the immediate management by assessing the quantity of tissue obtained and evaluating pathologic changes causing the bleeding. Very little tissue or a thin endometrial stripe on transvaginal ultrasound suggests a relatively atrophic endometrium or chronic bleeding with only basal endometrium remaining, which would best re-

TABLE 14.5. *Management of abnormal uterine bleeding*

I. Chronic/recurrent episodes of mild-to-moderate bleeding
   Rule out pregnancy
   Examination
   Endometrial sampling, selected cases
   Observation
   Iron replacement
   Prostaglandin synthetase inhibitors
II. Chronic/recurrent episodes of heavy bleeding
   Rule out pregnancy
   Examination
   Endometrial sampling (if not on hormonal medication)
   Hormonal
   Oral estrogen/progestin
   Oral progestin
     Periodic
     Continuous
   Danazol
   Gonadotropin-releasing hormone agonists
   Depo-Progestin
   Prostaglandin synthetase inhibitors
   Antibiotics
   Iron replacement
   Dilatation and curettage (if significant bleeding persists on medical therapy)
   Hysteroscopy
III. Acute heavy bleeding
   Rule out pregnancy
   Examination
   Endometrial sampling
   Hormonal
     Progesterone in oil, intramuscular
     Oral progestin
     Oral estrogen/progestin
     Oral estrogen
   Correction of coagulation abnormalities
   Antinauseants
   Antibiotics
   Dilatation and curettage (if significant bleeding persists after 24–48 h)
IV. Acute hemorrhage
   Rule out pregnancy
   Hospitalization
   Intravenous fluid
   Blood replacement
   Correction of coagulation abnormalities
   Hormonal
     Oral estrogen
     Oral estrogen/progestin
     Intravenous estrogen
   Antibiotics
   Antinauseants
   Observation
   Dilatation and curettage (if significant bleeding persists after 24 h)

spond to estrogen initially. A large amount of tissue is consistent with an unopposed estrogenic milieu and anovulation, which generally responds well to progestin therapy.

The advent of saline infusion sonography (SIS) can aid in differentiating between an organic cause for bleeding and "dysfunctional uterine bleeding." As an office procedure, the physician can detect polyps, myomas, synechiae, hyperplasia, endometrial cancer, and normal uterine cavities (70). In addition, the adnexa can be evaluated. SIS is an excellent office study that can be done without the need for sedation or an operating room. Hysteroscopy with dilatation and curettage should be reserved for abnormal uterine bleeding refractory to hormonal treatment or when a lesion is seen on SIS. Long-term management of bleeding may require iron supplementation to prevent iron deficiency anemia and may include a prostaglandin synthetase inhibitor to reduce blood loss with each episode (71–73). When the amount of bleeding is heavy initially or after a period of observation, hormonal treatment also may be prescribed.

ACUTE BLEEDING

There are several regimens of hormonal therapy that have been used in acute episodes of heavy bleeding. The following discussions on hormonal therapy should be viewed as guidelines to be individualized by the health care provider, not necessarily exclusive of alternative regimens. In adolescents with suspected anovulatory type bleeding, consisting of heavy bleeding and oligomenorrhea, with more than usual amounts of endometrial tissue when sampled, or who have been receiving estrogenic preparations, progestin therapy to produce a secretory change of the endometrium and ultimately a progestin withdrawal bleed should be the initial hormonal intervention. Failure to withdraw bleed warrants a workup.

Progestin therapy may be accomplished using (a) progesterone in oil 100 to 200 mg intramuscular injection followed by 10 to 14 days of oral progestin; (b) medroxyprogesterone ac-

etate (MPA) 10 to 20 mg orally per day for 10 to 14 days; or (c) norethindrone acetate 5 to 10 mg orally per day for 10 to 14 days.

Progesterone in oil offers an immediate progestational effect on a bleeding endometrium, with a decrease in bleeding usually occurring within 12 to 24 hours, but it must be followed by 10 to 14 days of oral progestin. Common errors of progestin therapy are inadequate duration of treatment, which should be a minimum of 10 days, and failure to counsel patients to anticipate bleeding after completing the prescribed course of the progestational agent.

After control of the acute bleeding, periodic progestin therapy of 10 to 14 days each month should be given for up to 6 months before observing the bleeding pattern without medication. This is the treatment of choice for chronic or recurrent bleeding due to anovulation in an adolescent who has withdrawal bleeding when progestins are administered. Anovulatory dysfunctional bleeding in adolescents is due to an immaturity of the hypothalamic-pituitary axis. There is no positive feedback of estradiol, which is needed for ovulation. These patients need a progestin withdrawal bleed monthly until their HPO axis matures to induce an orderly endometrial slough and avoid endometrial hyperplasia.

In adolescents with prolonged moderate bleeding, decreased amount of tissue on endometrial sampling (thin endometrial stripe on ultrasound), or suspected hypoestrogenism, estrogen therapy is used to cause proliferation of an otherwise atrophic or "thinned out" endometrium. Initial regimens of estrogen therapy include (a) conjugated estrogens 0.625 to 1.25 mg orally every 4 to 6 hours, (b) conjugated estrone 0.625 to 1.25 mg orally every 4 to 6 hours, and (c) estradiol 1 to 2 mg orally every 4 to 6 hours.

Once significant bleeding has been stopped, which is usually 24 hours, reduction of the dose to a daily or b.i.d. schedule may be tried. Because of the greater potential for thromboembolic sequelae with high-dose synthetic estrogens such as ethinyl estradiol, these regimens discussed are preferable. With heavy bleeding and acute hemorrhage, attempts may be made to control bleeding rapidly. Conjugated estrogens are given 25 mg intravenously every 4 hours until the bleeding stops or for 24 hours (74). Once bleeding has subsided, patients are placed on 10 mg of oral equine estrogen daily for 21 to 25 days, and oral medroxyprogesterone acetate 10 mg daily with estrogen for the last 7 to 10 days. Once both hormones are withdrawn, the patient will have a heavy withdrawal bleed (61). This intravenous regimen may be used for moderate-to-heavy bleeding adolescents unable to tolerate oral estrogen preparations. Although very rare, deaths have occurred with high-dose intravenous estrogen preparations due to thromboembolic complications.

In a sexually active adolescent, monophasic oral contraceptives may be used to control acute moderate-to-heavy bleeding. Therapy is initiated as one pill twice a day for 5 to 7 days. Therapy is maintained despite cessation of flow within 12 to 24 hours. If flow does not stop, one must rule out other causes (polyps, incomplete abortion, and neoplasia) of continued bleeding. After stopping therapy, patients should anticipate heavy and crampy flow for 2 to 4 days. On the fifth day of flow or on the following Sunday, a low-dose combination oral contraceptive medication (one pill a day) is started. This will be repeated for several 3-week treatments (usually three), followed by 1-week withdrawal flow intervals (75). Once the acute episode of bleeding has been controlled, patients need to be followed closely. With anovulatory bleeding, unopposed estrogen can cause endometrial hyperplasia and continual bouts of recurrent bleeding. As we know, young women in their twenties can develop endometrial adenocarcinoma (76). A periodic withdrawal bleed with oral contraceptives in patients needing contraception or with a progestin regimen is mandatory.

Patients who are clinically hypovolemic with low hemoglobins and active bleeding need to be hospitalized and observed. Complete laboratory evaluation should be initiated, including a workup for blood dyscrasias. Hormonal or even surgical treatments may be needed to stop bleeding. Transfusion is reserved for hypovolemic and unstable patients.

Other important measures in the management of uterine bleeding may be beneficial, such as correction of significant abnormalities in coagulation factors when feasible, the use of antinauseants to improve toleration of high-dose hormonal therapies, and the use of antibiotics when prolonged bleeding, moderate-to-severe dysmenorrhea, or a tender uterus is noted. Chronic endometritis may present with menorrhagia (77), and an ascending secondary infection may occur in heavy prolonged bleeding, resulting in the loss of local homeostatic mechanisms in an inflamed or infected endometrium.

Dilatation and curettage rarely are required in the adolescent and should be performed only after failure of hormonal therapies either acutely or after longer-term treatments, or when a high index of suspicion for an organic cause exists. When curettage is to be performed to identify or exclude a suspected intrauterine lesion, hysteroscopy will offer a higher sensitivity than curettage for the identification of intrauterine pathology (78). Transvaginal sonohysterography can identify polyps and submucous myomas, both of which can cause abnormal bleeding.

Long-term suppression of menses may be advantageous in the adolescent who has moderate-to-severe anemia because of heavy bleeding due to blood dyscrasia, chronic illness, or DUB. Danazol 200 to 800 mg daily has been effective in producing an atrophic endometrium and an amenorrheic state (77). However, the cost and the androgenic side effects frequently limit its use. GnRH agonists have become available to the clinician. They produce a reversible hypoestrogenic state and amenorrhea in most individuals. Hot flushes occur in most individuals but can be alleviated with noerthindrone acetate 2.5 mg (half of a 5-mg tablet) daily. Because of loss of calcium from bone, use of GnRH agonists presently is limited to 6 months. Norethindrone acetate 5 mg daily (half tablet, b.i.d.) also may be used to achieve long-term suppression of uterine bleeding.

The intramuscular depot form of MPA may produce prolonged suppression of the HPO axis; therefore, it should only be used in limited situations in the adolescent, such as mentally retarded or chronically ill individuals with problematic bleeding. This approach generally produces amenorrhea, overcomes any compliance or absorption problems of oral preparations, and provides contraception. Initially, 100 to 150 mg of depot MPA is given intramuscularly on a weekly basis for a month; then monthly for 3 to 4 months; and finally every 2 to 4 months as required to suppress uterine bleeding completely.

There is no single method or approach that will control problematic bleeding in every adolescent. Consequently, to achieve optimal results, thoroughness in evaluating the numerous causes, development of a comprehensive, individualized therapeutic plan, and close surveillance of the responses to treatment are required. Nevertheless, the health care provider should remember the importance of being informative, caring, and supportive to the adolescent and her parents during this often frightening and frustrating process.

REFERENCES

1. Classens EA, Cowell CA. Acute adolescent menorrhagia. *Am J Obstet Gynecol* 1981;139:277–280.
2. Demanest CB. When the teen has irregular periods. *Patient Care* 1984;18:151–163.
3. Pepe F, Iachello PM, Panella M. Dysfunctional uterine bleeding in adolescents. *Clin Exp Obstet Gynecol* 1987; 14:182–184.
4. Giowani GP. Vaginal bleeding in adolescents. *J Reprod Med* 1984;29:417–420.
5. Apter D, Viinkka L, Vihko R. Hormonal pattern of adolescent cycles. *J Clin Endocrinol Metab* 1978;47: 944–954.
6. McDonough PG, Gantt P. Dysfunctional bleeding in the adolescent. In: Barwin BN, Belisle S, eds. *Adolescent gynecology and sexuality.* New York: Masson Publishing, 1982.
7. LeMarchand-Beraud T, Zufferey M, Reymond M, et al. Maturation of the hypothalalmo-pituitary-ovarian axis in adolescent girls. *J Clin Endocrinol Metab* 1982;54: 241–26.
8. Southam AL, Richart RM. The prognosis for adolescents with menstrual abnormalities. *Am J Obstet Gynecol* 1966;94:637–645.
9. Hallberg L, Hogdahl AM, Nelsson L, et al. Menstrual blood loss—a population study. *Acta Obstet Gynecol Scand* 1966;45:320–351.
10. Fraser IS, McCannon G, Markham R. A preliminary study of factors influencing perception of menstrual blood loss volume. *Am J Obstet Gynecol* 1984;149: 788–793.
11. Treloar AE, Boynton RE, Benn BG, et al. Variation of human menstrual cycle through reproductive life. *Int J Fertil* 1967;12:77–126.
12. Boyar R, Finkelstein JW, David R, et al. Twenty-four hour patterns of plasma luteinizing hormone and follicle-stimulating hormone in sexual precocity. *N Engl J Med* 1973;289:282–286.
13. Boyar RM, Finkelstein J, Roffward H, et al. Twenty-four hour luteinizing hormone and follicle-stimulating hormone secretory patterns in gonadal dysgenesis. *J Clin Endocrinol Metab* 1973;37:521–525.
14. Fraser IS, Michie EA, Wide L, et al. Pituitary gonadotropins and ovarian function in adolescent dysfunctional uterine bleeding. *J Clin Endocrinol Metab* 1973; 37:407–414.
15. Knobil E. The neuroendocrine control of the menstrual cycle. *Recent Prog Horm Res* 1980;36:53–88.
16. Bider D, Ben-Rafeal Z, Shalev J, et al. Pituitary and ovarian suppression rate after high dosage of gonadotropin-releasing hormone agonist. *Fertil Steril* 1989;51:578–581.
17. Midgley AR Jr, Jaffee RB. Regulation of human gonadotropins: IV. Correlation of serum concentration of follicle-stimulating and luteinizing hormones during the menstrual cycle. *J Clin Endocrinol Metab* 1968;28: 1699–1703.
18. di Zerega GS, Hodgen GD. Folliculogenesis in the primate ovarian cycle. *Endocr Rev* 1981;2:27–49.
19. Pache TD, Waladimiroff JW, De Jong FH, et al. Growth patterns of nondominant ovarian follicles during the normal menstrual cycle. *Fertil Steril* 1990;54:638–642.
20. Hillier SG, Reichert LE Jr, Van Hall EV. Control of preovulatory follicular estrogen biosynthesis in the human ovary. *J Clin Endocrinol Metab* 1981;52:847–856.
21. Dorrington JH, Armstrong DT. Effects of FSH on gonadal functions. *Recent Prog Horm Res* 1979;35: 301–342.
22. Magoffin DA, Jakimiuk AJ. Inhibin A, inhibin B and activin A in the follicular fluid of regularly cycling women. *Hum Reprod* 1997;12:1714.
23. Welsh TH Jr, Zhuang L-Z, Hsueh AJW. Estroprogestin augmentation of gonadotropin-stimulated progestin biosynthesis in cultured rat granulosa cells. *Endocrinology* 1983;112:1916–1924.
24. McNatty KP, Makris A, DeGrazia C, et al. The production of progesterone, androgens and estrogens by human granulosa cells, thecal tissue and stromal tissue from human ovaries in vitro. *J Clin Endocrinol Metab* 1979; 49:687–699.
25. Noyes RW, Hertig AW, Rock J. Dating the endometrial biopsy. *Fertil Steril* 1950;1:3–25.
26. Bonhoff A, Johannisson E, Bonhnet HG. Morphometric analysis of the endometrium of infertile patients in relation to peripheral hormone levels. *Fertil Steril* 1990;54: 84–89.
27. Schmidt-Matthiesen H. Die vaskularisierung des menschilichen endometriums. *Arch Gynaek* 1962;196: 575–584.
28. Hoff JD, Quilgley ME, Yen SSC. Hormonal dynamics at midcycle: a reevaluation. *J Clin Endocrinol Metab* 1983;57:792–796.

29. Nilsson L, Hillensjo T, Ekholm C. Preovulatory changes in rat follicular cyclic AMP and sensitivity to gonadotropins. *Acta Endocrinol (Copenh)* 1977;86: 384–393.

30. LeMaire WJ, Leidner R, March JM. Pre- and post-ovulatory changes in the concentration of prostaglandins in rat graffian follicles. *Prostaglandins* 1975;9:221–229.

31. Yoshimura Y, Stantulli R, Atlas SJ, et al. The effects of proteolytic enzymes on in vitro ovulation in the rabbit. *Am J Obstet Gynecol* 1987;157;468.

32. Miyazaki T, Katz E, Dharmarajan AM, et al. Do prostaglandins lead to ovulation in the rabbit by stimulating proteolytic enzyme activity? *Fertil Steril* 1991; 55;1182.

33. Espey LL, Tanaka N, Adams RF, et al. Ovarian hydroxyeicosatetraenoic acids compared with prostanoids and steroids during ovulation in rats. *Am J Physiol* 1991; 260;E163.

34. Yen SCC. The menstrual cycle. In: Yen SCC, Jaffe RB, eds. *Reproductive endocrinology*, 2nd ed. Philadelphia: WB Saunders, 1986:200–236.

35. McLachlin RI, Cohen NL, Vale WE, et al. The importance of luteinizing hormone in the control of inhibin and progesterone secretion by the human corpus luteum. *J Clin Endocrinol Metab* 1989;68:1078.

36. Speroff L, Glass RH, Kase NG, eds. *Clinical gynecologic and infertility*, 6th ed. Philadelphia: Lippincott Williams & Wilkins, 1999:201–246.

37. Goodman AL, Hodgen GD. The ovarian triad of the primate menstrual cycle. *Recent Prog Horm Res* 1983;39: 1–73.

38. Di Zerega GS, Hodgen GD. Luteal phase dysfunction infertility: a sequel to aberrant folliculogenesis. *Fertil Steril* 1981;35:489–499.

39. Stoffer RL, Hodgen GD. Induction of luteal phase defect in rhesus monkeys by follicular fluid administration at the onset of the menstrual cycle. *J Clin Endocrinol Metab* 1980;51:669–671.

40. Carr BR, Sadler RK, Rochell DB, et al. Plasma lipoprotein regulation of progesterone biosynthesis by human corpus luteum tissue of organ culture. *J Clin Endocrinol Metab* 1981;52:875–881.

41. VandeWiele R, Bogumil J, Dyrenfurth I, et al. Mechanisms regulating the menstrual cycle in women. *Recent Prog Horm Res* 1970;26:63–103.

42. Yen SSC. Clinical applications of gonadotropin-releasing hormone and gonadotropin-releasing hormone analogs. *Fertil Steril* 1983;39:257–266.

43. Greenberg LH, Stouffer RL, Brenner RM, et al. Are human luteinizing granulosa cells a site of action for progesterone and relaxin? *Fertil Steril* 1990;53:446–453.

44. Girsh E, Wang W, Mamiuk R, et al. Regulation of endothelin-1 expression in the bovine corpus luteum: elevation by prostaglandin F$_{2\alpha}$. *Endocrinology* 1996;137: 5191.

45. Duncan WC, McNeilly AS, Illingworth PJ. The effect of luteal "rescue" on the expression and localization of matrix metalloproteinases and their tissue inhibitors in the human corpus luteum, *J Clin Endocrinol Metab* 1998;83:2470.

46. Welt CK, Martin KM, Taylor AE, et al. Frequency modulation of follicle-stimulating hormone (FSH) during the luteal-follicular transition: evidence for FSH control of inhibin B in normal women. *J Clin Endocrinol Metab* 1997;82:2645.

47. Maslar IA, Riddick DH. Prolactin production by human endometrium during the normal menstrual cycle. *Am J Obstet Gynecol* 1979;135:751–754.

48. Brumsted JR, Chapitis J, Deaton JL, et al. Prostaglandin F$_{2\alpha}$ synthesis and metabolism by luteal phase endometrium in vitro. *Fertil Steril* 1989;52:769–773.

49. Abel MH, Baird DT. The effect of 17β-estradiol and progesterone on prostaglandin production by human endometrium maintained in organ culture. *Endocrinology* 1980;106;1599–1606.

50. Good RG, Moyer DL. Estrogen-progesterone relationships in the development of secretory endometrium. *Fertil Steril* 1969;19:37–49.

51. Molina R, Castilla JA, Vergara F, et al. Luteal cytoplasmic estradiol and progesterone receptors in human endometrium: in vitro fertilization and normal cycles. *Fertil Steril* 1989;51:976–979.

52. Kaiser IH. Newer concepts of menstruation. *Am J Obstet Gynecol* 1948;:1037–1047.

53. Li T-C, Dockery P, Thomas P, et al. The effects of progesterone receptor blockade in the luteal phase of normal fertile women. *Fertil Steril* 1988;50:732–742.

54. Roseff SJ, Kettel LM, Rivier J, et al. Accelerated dissolution of luteal-endometrial integrity by the administration of antagonists of gonadotropin-releasing hormone and progesterone to late-luteal phase women. *Fertil Steril* 1990;54:805–810.

55. Wentz AC. Endometrial biopsy in the evaluation of infertility. *Fertil Steril* 1980;33:121–124.

56. Jones GS. The luteal phase defect. *Fertil Steril* 1976;27: 351–356.

57. Kirby DRS. The influence of the uterine environment on the development of mouse. *J Embryol Exp Morphol* 1962;10:496–506.

58. Kirby DRS. The development of mouse blastocysts transplanted to the scrotal and cryptorchid testis. *J Anat* 1963;97:119–130.

59. Wentz AC. Premenstrual spotting: its association with endometriosis but not luteal phase inadequacy. *Fertil Steril* 1980;33:605–607.

60. Falcone T, Desjardins C, Bourque J, et al. Dysfunctional uterine bleeding in adolescents. *J Reprod Med* 1994;39: 761–764.

61. Chuong CJ, Brenner PF. Management of abnormal uterine bleeding. *Am J Obstet Gynecol* 1996;175[3 Pt 2]: 787–792.

62. Kadir RA, Economides DL, Sabin CA, et al. Frequency of inherited disorders in women with menorrhagia. *Lancet* 1998;351:485–489.

63. Alan Guttmacher Insitute. *Teenage pregnancy: the problem that hasn't gone away*. New York: AGI, 1981.

64. Gordon CM. Menstrual disorders in adolescents. *Pediatr Clin North Am* 1999;46:519–543.

65. Guzick DS, Talbott EO, Sutton-Tyrrell K, et al. Carotid atherosclerosis in women with polycystic ovary syndrome: initial results from a case-control study. *Am J Obstet Gynecol* 1996;174:1224–1232.

66. DeFronzo RA, Ferrannini E. Insulin resistance: a multifaceted syndrome responsible for NIDDM, obesity, hypertension, dyslipidemia, and atherosclerotic cardiovascular disease. *Diabetes Care* 1991;14:173–194.

67. Laufer MR, Goitein L, Bush M, et al. Prevalence of endometriosis in adolescent girls with chronic pelvic pain not responding to conventional therapy. *J Pediatr Adolesc Gynecol* 1997;10:199–202.

68. Isojarvi JI, Laatikainen TJ, Pakarinen AJ, et al. Menstrual disorders in women with epilepsy receiving carbamazepine. *Epilepsia* 1995;36:676–681.

69. Arbel-DeRowe Y, Tepper R, Rosen DJ, et al. The contribution of pelvic ultrasonography to the diagnostic process in pediatric and adolescent gynecology. *J Pediatr Adolesc Gynecol* 1997;10:3–12.

70. Widrich T, Bradley LD, Mitchinson AR, et al. Comparison of saline infusion sonography with office hysteroscopy for the evaluation of the endometrium. *Am J Obstet Gynecol* 1996;174:1327–1334.

71. Fraser IS, Sherman RP, McIlveen J. Efficacy of mefenamic acid in patients with a complaint of menorrhagia. *Obstet Gynecol* 1981;58:543–551.

72. Hall P, MacLachlan W, Thom W, et al. Control of menorrhagia by the cyclo-oxgenase inhibitor naproxen sodium and mefenamic acid. *Br J Obstet Gynecol* 1987;94:554–558.

73. Vargyar JM, Campeau JD, Mishell DR. Treatment of menorrhagia with meclofenamate sodium. *Am J Obstet Gynecol* 1987;157:944–950.

74. DeVore GR, Owens O, Kase W. Use of intravenous Premarin® in the treatment of dysfunctional uterine bleeding—a double-blind randomized study. *Obstet Gynecol* 1982;59:285–291.

75. Speroff L, Glass RH, Kase NG, eds. *Clinical gynecologic and infertility,* 6th ed. Philadelphia: Lippincott Williams & Wilkins, 1999:575–593.

76. Farhi B, Nosanchok J, Silverber S. Endometrial carcinoma in women under 25 years of age. *Obstet Gynecol* 1986;68:741–744.

77. Fraser IS. Treatment of dysfunctional uterine bleeding with danazol. *Aust N Z J Obstet Gynecol* 1985;25:224–226.

78. Valle RF. Office hysteroscopy. *Clin Obstet Gynecol* 1999;42:276–289.

15

Dysmenorrhea

John S. Hesla

Dysmenorrhea, or painful menstruation, is the most common gynecologic complaint of young women (1). This disorder traditionally has been divided into two basic types. Primary dysmenorrhea is defined as pelvic pain that is experienced during menstruation in the absence of gross underlying pelvic pathology. In contrast, the discomfort of secondary dysmenorrhea can be ascribed to the presence of physical alterations in normal pelvic anatomy (Table 15.1). Hence, direct visualization of the peritoneal structures may be necessary for establishment of the etiology of the pain and appropriate categorization of the disorder.

The first dysmenorrheic symptoms typically develop 1 to 3 years after menarche in girls who have established ovulatory menstrual cycles (Fig. 15.1). Spasmodic suprapubic pain usually begins 1 to 4 hours after the onset of menstrual flow and lasts for 24 to 48 hours. Less commonly, the pain may be present 1 to 2 days before menstruation and continue for 2 to 4 days after the onset of flow.

TABLE 15.1. *Causes of secondary dysmenorrhea*

Endometriosis
Pelvic inflammatory disease
Ovarian cyst
Intrauterine device
Congenital malformations of the müllerian system
Cervical stricture
Uterine leiomyomas, uterine polyps[a]
Adenomyosis[a]
Complications of early pregnancy[b]

[a]Rare in adolescents.
[b]Associated with irregular bleeding and pain.

The pelvic cramping may radiate to the back and along the inner aspects of the thighs and is accompanied by one or more systemic symptoms in greater than 50% of patients, including nausea and vomiting (89%), fatigue (85%), lower backache (60%), diarrhea (60%), and headache (45%) (2). Rarely, the severity of pain may cause syncope and collapse. Menstrual pain that arises more than 3 years after menarche is more likely to be caused by an associated pathologic condition, such as infection or endometriosis, rather than the biochemical alteration present in primary dysmenorrhea.

Classification systems that label the degree of disability associated with primary dysmenorrhea vary somewhat among published studies. Nevertheless, the definition of general terms facilitates discussion of the disorder. Dysmenorrhea may be considered mild if pain occurs only on the first day of menstruation, has little or no associated systemic symptoms, and does not inhibit the daily activities of the adolescent (3,4). Moderate dysmenorrhea typically is experienced during the first 2 to 3 days of menses and frequently is accompanied by diarrhea, headache, and fatigue. Some restriction in the daily routine may be necessary during the period of peak discomfort, although absenteeism from school is infrequent. Intense, spasmodic pain may develop before the onset of flow and last 2 to 7 days in patients with severe dysmenorrhea. This pain and associated gastrointestinal symptoms may significantly impinge on the adolescent's ability to carry out her normal activities.

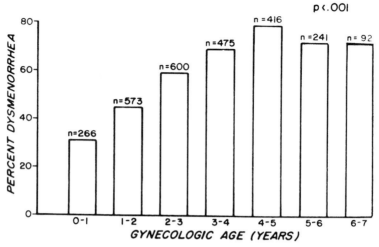

FIG. 15.1. Prevalence of dysmenorrhea in adolescents by gynecologic age. (From Klein JR, Litt IF. Epidemiology of adolescent dysmenorrhea. *Pediatrics* 1981;68:661–664, with permission.)

PREVALENCE

Although there is some variation in the definition and analysis of subjective pain symptoms among epidemiologic studies, a consistently high prevalence of dysmenorrhea has been found to exist irrespective of socioeconomic status and cultural and geographic background. Of 2,699 menarcheal adolescents questioned in the National Health Examination Survey, 59.7% reported some degree of menstrual pain (5). The pain was described as mild by 49%, moderate by 37%, and severe by the remaining 14%. Fourteen percent of the girls reported frequent school absenteeism during the time of menstruation, whereas data extracted from teachers' reports suggested that 25% of all excessive school absences among female pupils were due to dysmenorrhea. These statistics are confirmed by several other studies, where the prevalence of dysmenorrhea among females aged 10 to 20 years ranged from 43% to 90% (3,6–10). Young women who experience a pain episode lasting 3 or more days during menstruation have a 72% probability of having pain lasting at least 2 days during their next menstrual period (11).

The prevalence of dysmenorrhea increases with age and reaches its peak during early adulthood. In a 1979 study of Finnish adolescents aged 13 to 20 years, Widholm (7) reported a 36.2% incidence of occasional or recurring dysmenorrhea during the first gynecologic year compared to a 64.7% incidence during the fifth gynecologic year. The lower incidence in the younger age group has been attributed to an increased proportion of anovulatory cycles during the first years after menarche. Menstrual pain most commonly is experienced between the ages of 20 and 24 years, but it then declines after age 25 as well as after the birth of a child (12).

As one of the leading if not the greatest single cause of lost working hours and school days among young women, dysmenorrhea presents a significant problem from an individual and public health perspective (13). It has been estimated that 140 million hours are lost annually because of the abdominal pain, vomiting, nausea, headache, and other discomfort associated with primary dysmenorrhea (5). In addition, dysmenorrheic women receive lower grades and have more school adjustment problems than do nondysmenorrheic women (14).

ETIOLOGY OF PRIMARY DYSMENORRHEA

The etiology of severe incapacitating pain in the absence of obvious pathology was a matter of great debate until the latter part of the twentieth century. Hippocrates believed that cervical obstruction and stagnation of menstrual blood were responsible for dysmenorrhea. This theory persisted for centuries; it was recognized only recently that dilatation and curettage for presumed cervical stenosis is an ineffective and inappropriate treatment for primary dysmenorrhea (15). Before the discovery of prostaglandins, painful menstruation frequently was thought to be due to a psychosomatic derangement in which the woman was rejecting her femininity. Nonanalytical psychological factors that were proposed to explain this complaint include patient suggestibility, a self-fulfilling prophesy, imitation of the mother, and the benefits of secondary gain. In addition, primitive taboos and lack of education were believed to contribute to an overly negative attitude toward menstruation on the part of the patient and society (16). Dysmenorrhea historically has been associated with severe depression, increased suicide rates, neuroticism, and general maladjustment (17). In accordance with these theories, past treatment regimens included psychotherapy, narcotics, exercise, vitamins, and surgery, including hysterectomy.

Evidence has existed since the 1950s to support the concept that dysmenorrhea arises through the active expulsion of degenerating endometrium during menstruation and that this activity is related to a substance released by the menstrual endometrium into the circulating blood. Pickles (18) was the first investigator to extract a lipid-like smooth muscle stimulant from menstrual fluid in 1957; this substance later was identified as the 20-carbon-chain prostaglandin E (PGE) and prostaglandin F (PGF) (19). Elevated levels of prostaglandin $F_{2\alpha}$ ($PGF_{2\alpha}$) and its metabolites have been found in the menstrual fluid of dysmenorrheic women; the concentration of these substances in the menstrual effluvium and plasma correlate well with the presence of pain (20,21). Direct measurement of prostaglandins in the endometrium and jet washings of the uterus have shown increased concentrations in dysmenorrheic women compared to those who do not experience painful menses

(22,23). In addition, there is a striking similarity between the symptoms of primary dysmenorrhea and the clinical effects created by the administration of exogenous prostaglandin via differing routes for the induction of labor or abortion (13).

The mechanisms by which menstruation, prostaglandin production, and pelvic pain are associated are still being clarified. It appears that a decline in progesterone secretion by the corpus luteum during the perimenstrual time period leads to breakdown of endometrial cell lysosomes and release of phospholipase A_2. This enzyme converts fatty acids into arachidonic acid, a precursor of prostaglandins via the cyclooxygenase enzyme pathway. Arachidonic acid is also a precursor of leukotrienes by the 5-lipoxygenase pathway. Increased production of prostaglandins and leukotrienes results in a rise in resting tone of the uterus and a greater frequency and dysrhythmia of uterine contractions. The intensity of these contractions may be 1.5 to 3 times greater than the peak pressures experienced during labor. The resultant uterine ischemia promotes a heightened sensitivity of pain fibers to the action of bradykinin and other physical stimuli (24,25). Hence, arachidonic acid metabolites modulate blood flow, smooth muscle tone, contractile responses of the uterus, and pain receptor sensitivity.

The posterior pituitary hormone vasopressin has been ascribed an important etiologic role in the myometrial hyperactivity, reduced uterine blood flow, and pain of primary dysmenorrhea. Some preliminary data suggest that there may be an increase in circulating vasopressin levels in this group of women at the time of menstruation (26). If a proportional increase in oxytocin concentration does not accompany this rise, dysrhythmic uterine contractions may occur (27). Nevertheless, serial changes in vasopressin concentration for an individual patient have not been analyzed over the course of the perimenstrual period. One pilot study revealed that parenteral administration of a short-acting vasopressin antagonist was significantly more effective in relieving moderate-to-severe dysmenorrheic symptoms than placebo (26).

Epidemiologic Associations

The severity of dysmenorrhea experienced by the patient is significantly correlated with the duration and amount of menstrual flow (3). The physiologic basis for this association may be explained by recognizing the action of prostaglandins in both the regulation of menstruation and the rise in pain (2). Earlier age at menarche and long menstrual period increased the occurrence, duration, and severity of pain in a survey of women aged 17 to 19 years (11).

Epidemiologic studies also revealed the indicators of unhealthy behavior and poor self-rated health status are almost as strongly associated with a high prevalence of pain as the duration of menstrual flow and gynecologic age of the patient. Teperi and Rimpelä (28) found that girls who smoked daily, consumed alcohol occasionally or frequently, and engaged in little physical activity were found to be at increased risk of severe dysmenorrhea. Nevertheless, a dose-response relationship between smoking and dysmenorrhea could not be demonstrated, and the association between the two became statistically insignificant when alcohol consumption was controlled. However, in one case control investigation, smoking ten or more cigarettes per day increased the odds of having moderate-to-severe dysmenorrhea by about 90% (29). An American study of women aged 17 to 19 years found that smokers had a 50% increase in the odds of having pain lasting more than 2 days per menstrual cycle (11). Hence, most recent studies have suggested an association between tobacco use and dysmenorrhea.

Wood and colleagues (30) attempted to clarify the association between alcohol intake and pelvic pain symptomatology by proposing that alcohol may be used to dull menstrual pain or, alternatively, alcohol may worsen the pain by interfering with the breakdown of prostaglandins. Teperi and Rimpelä (28) did find increased alcohol consumption in patients who described severe dysmenorrhea; nevertheless, the perception of pain by this subgroup of teenagers did not vary as their consumption of alcohol increased. Moreover, the frequency of alcohol use is low in adolescent girls, minimizing the importance of this relationship. Although caffeine intake has been linked with premenstrual symptomatology, the consumption of beverages containing caffeine has not been demonstrated to heighten dysmenorrhea (31).

Studies linking psychological attributes to perimenstrual distress have shown that patients with more pain complaints score higher on measures of depression and anxiety. Metheny and Smith (32) reported in a multivariate analysis that women experiencing higher levels of stress also described more severe menstrual discomfort. The effect of stress on symptom severity overshadowed the influences of optimism and mood. Women who expressed more severe dysmenorrhea generally felt more overwhelmed by life experiences. In addition, subjects with negative expectations about menstruation and a traditional view of the female role reported higher perimenstrual distress than those with opposing views (33). A history of maternal or sibling dysmenorrhea appears to be an important characteristic of adolescents with dysmenorrhea, perhaps due to an inherited increased production of prostaglandins by the menstrual endometrium along with psychological conditioning by the family unit (3,16).

SECONDARY DYSMENORRHEA

Endometriosis and pelvic inflammatory disease are the most frequent causes of secondary dysmenorrhea and chronic pelvic pain in adolescence. Goldstein et al. (34) diagnosed endometriosis in 47 (47%) of 140 postpubertal girls with chronic pelvic pain who underwent diagnostic laparoscopy. Postoperative adhesions and pelvic inflammatory disease were discovered in 18 (13%) and 10 (7%), respectively. Of 47 adolescent females aged 11 to 19 years undergoing laparoscopy for chronic pelvic pain in Milan, 19 (40.4%) had no detectable pelvic abnormalities and 18 (38.3%) were found to have endometriosis (35). The majority of these patients had minimal disease, and many of the lesions were nonpigmented or nonclassic in appearance.

Acquired dysmenorrhea is the most prominent symptom of adolescent patients with laparoscopically confirmed endometriosis. Twenty-two of 28 girls in one surgical series noted such discomfort; even mild and moderate stages of disease may be associated with severe, disabling pelvic pain (36). Whether these cramps are secondary to the early development of endometriosis or whether the greater uterine contractility associated with menstrual pain predisposes these patients to endometriosis is not known. When chronic pelvic pain of at least 3 months' duration is unresponsive to nonsteroidal antiinflammatory drugs (NSAIDs) and oral contraceptive pills, laparoscopy may reveal endometriosis in more than two thirds of such adolescents (37). Genetic factors have been established in its development, as Simpson et al. (38) reported a 6.9% rate of endometriosis in first-degree relatives of women with the disease compared to only 1% of control relatives.

The pain symptoms of endometriosis may be cyclic or acyclic in nature, with the most severe symptoms occurring just before and during the menses. In one study, 64% of girls with endometriosis had cyclic pain and 36% had acyclic pain that initially developed at an average of 2.9 years after menarche (39). The pain tends to increase in severity over time and may begin to occur throughout the month. Rectal pressure and dyspareunia occasionally are reported. Although oral contraceptives and antiprostaglandin agents may ameliorate the discomfort, the pain usually is not totally relieved by these medications and will begin to increase in intensity over subsequent cycles.

Mild-to-moderate tenderness may be the only positive finding on physical examination in the adolescent with endometriosis; this sign is elicited most frequently in the late luteal phase of the menstrual cycle. Uterosacral nodularity and pelvic masses are rare in this age group; in fact, 20% to 30% of patients in the series of Goldstein et al. (39) who were diagnosed with endometriosis had a completely normal pelvic examination at initial assessment.

Most adolescents with endometriosis have minimal or mild stages of disease; however,

girls with obstructing genital tract malformations have a high rate of severe endometriosis, even in the immediate postmenarcheal years (40). The patient with complete obstruction of the lower genital tract presents with primary amenorrhea and cyclic pelvic pain caused by reflux menstruation that begins 2 to 3 years after the onset of breast development. Presumably, endometriotic foci form through peritoneal implantation of the large volumes of refluxed menstrual tissue, as initially hypothesized by Sampson in the 1920s.

Imperforate hymen and complete transverse vaginal septum, two müllerian fusion defects associated with this disorder, are readily diagnosed on pelvic examination. Hematocolpos formation may cause severe pain and a bulging of the introitus. Cervical atresia in conjunction with a functioning endometrium results in hematometra development.

Vertical fusion defects that yield unilateral müllerian obstruction with patency of the contralateral outflow tract are more difficult to detect by physical examination and typically are associated with cyclic menses and increasing dysmenorrhea. The blockage may occur in the lower genital region, such as unilateral vaginal atresia associated with uterus didelphys, or higher as with a noncommunicating rudimentary uterine horn. Palpation of a vaginal or adnexal mass in the patient with a suggestive history is virtually diagnostic of this category of anatomic abnormality.

Other Causes of Secondary Dysmenorrhea

Pelvic adhesions may develop due to previous surgery or an inflammatory process such as salpingitis. Cyclic discomfort at the time of menstruation is unlikely to be caused by mere adhesive disease. Ascending pelvic infections most commonly originate during or shortly after menstruation and may be characterized by increasing pelvic pain despite the resolution of menstrual flow, irregular bleeding, and development of fever.

The occasional young woman with an intrauterine device may note increased dysmenorrhea after placement, particularly if it is not a progestin-containing system. An inflammatory-like response and a heightened production of $PGF_{2\alpha}$ develop in the endometrium immediately adjacent to the device within 1 to 5 months after its insertion (2).

Adenomyosis, endometrial polyps, and uterine leiomyomas are rare in adolescents. Onset of pain with these conditions usually begins after the age of 20 years and has been associated with increased levels of endometrial prostaglandins.

EVALUATION OF THE DYSMENORRHEIC PATIENT

The adolescent patient may spontaneously raise the issue of dysmenorrhea during a routine office visit. Its detection also may be the result of a systematic inquiry that should be a part of the medical history of any postmenarcheal patient (Fig. 15.2).

A complete menstrual history includes the age of menarche, approximate date of the first day of the last menstrual period, regularity of menses, duration and amount of flow, and presence or absence of cramps or other associated symptoms. If dysmenorrhea is present, the patient should be questioned as to when the painful periods began, whether the pain develops before, coincident with, or after the onset of flow, the location and quality of the pain, and whether or not it is associated with other symptoms such as those involving the gastrointestinal, musculoskeletal, and urinary systems. The degree of disruption of daily routine,

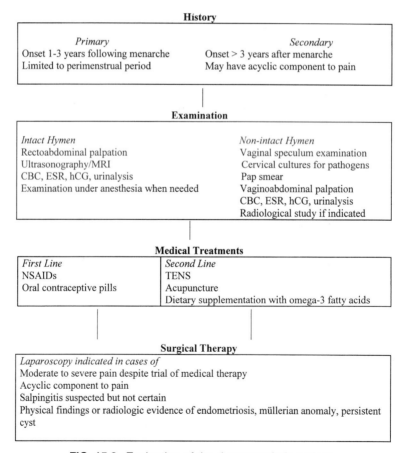

History

Primary	*Secondary*
Onset 1-3 years following menarche	Onset > 3 years after menarche
Limited to perimenstrual period	May have acyclic component to pain

Examination

Intact Hymen	*Non-intact Hymen*
Rectoabdominal palpation	Vaginal speculum examination
Ultrasonography/MRI	Cervical cultures for pathogens
CBC, ESR, hCG, urinalysis	Pap smear
Examination under anesthesia when needed	Vaginoabdominal palpation
	CBC, ESR, hCG, urinalysis
	Radiological study if indicated

Medical Treatments

First Line	*Second Line*
NSAIDs	TENS
Oral contraceptive pills	Acupuncture
	Dietary supplementation with omega-3 fatty acids

Surgical Therapy

Laparoscopy indicated in cases of
Moderate to severe pain despite trial of medical therapy
Acyclic component to pain
Salpingitis suspected but not certain
Physical findings or radiologic evidence of endometriosis, müllerian anomaly, persistent cyst

FIG. 15.2. Evaluation of the dysmenorrheic patient.

including school and social activities, should be elicited. The names, dosages, and treatment schedules of medications used in the past must be obtained. In addition, the adolescent should be asked about any behavior that ameliorates or exacerbates the symptoms. The family and social history, as well as the association of the pain episodes with stressful events, should be detailed. A history of maternal or sibling dysmenorrhea or endometriosis should be noted. An accurate sexual history is essential, including contraceptive method used, if applicable.

Some adolescent girls will be found to have disability related to menstrual cramps that seem out of proportion to the severity of the pain. Occasionally, an underlying psychosocial problem, such as school phobia, sexual abuse, or other serious personal or family problem, may be identified as contributing to the decreased pain tolerance and heightened anxiety centered around the menses.

The diagnosis of dysmenorrhea secondary to pelvic disease depends on recognition of an atypical history or abnormal pelvic examination, such as lateralization of symptoms or signs. Pain onset more than 3 years after menarche, dysfunctional uterine bleeding or change in menstrual pattern, and history of pelvic surgery may suggest secondary etiologies. Pelvic inflammatory disease should be suspected in dysmenorrheic adolescents with a fever as well as those patients whose pelvic pain increases as the menses end. Pelvic infection and abnormal pregnancy are possible causes of acute pain associated with vaginal bleeding in the sexually active young woman.

Examination

The physical examination of the patient with cyclic pain is helpful in excluding causes of secondary dysmenorrhea and will allow the physician to reassure the adolescent of the normality of her genital organs. The abdomen is carefully palpated in search of tenderness, masses, or organomegaly (Fig. 15.2). It often is helpful to ask the patient to point with one finger to the location of the pain. The physician then can attempt to reproduce the pain by the application of gentle pressure.

The approach for the evaluation of the pelvic organs may vary depending on the patient's symptoms and history of sexual activity. If the patient is virginal and her pain is mild and typical of primary dysmenorrhea, a trial of NSAID therapy may be prescribed without examination of the genital tract. Virginal adolescents who have moderate or severe pain that is otherwise characteristic of primary dysmenorrhea should be evaluated more thoroughly. After inspection of the vulva and vaginal introitus, bimanual rectoabdominal examination is performed in the lithotomy position to assess for abnormal pelvic masses or tenderness. The patient may tolerate a vaginal speculum examination and vaginoabdominal bimanual palpation. This will allow a greater appreciation of the uterine size and shape, the presence of cervical or adnexal tenderness, and the identification of adnexal masses or thickening. All adolescents with atypical symptomatology suggestive of secondary dysmenorrhea should have a complete examination, including evaluation of the internal genital tract. Administration of anesthesia may be necessary in some circumstances to ensure patient comfort. Pelvic sonography is helpful to confirm the presence of a mass when the pelvic examination is not completely satisfactory, to identify the presence of free fluid in the cul de sac, and to localize a suspected pregnancy. Magnetic resonance imaging can be used to better characterize a mass or suspected müllerian anomaly.

All dysmenorrheic adolescent women with a history of sexual activity should undergo speculum examination to exclude the presence of congenital abnormalities and to take cervical cultures for *Chlamydia trachomatis* and *Neisseria gonorrhoeae*. A Pap smear is recommended. Bimanual palpation may reveal abnormalities suggestive of associated disease states. Cervical motion tenderness is typical of pelvic inflammatory disease. Adnexal masses, decreased mobility of pelvic structures, and cul-de-sac nodularity may be detected in cases of tuboovarian abscess, hydrosalpinx, ovarian cyst, or endometriosis.

The basic laboratory evaluation of the patient with dysmenorrhea of moderate or severe intensity should include a complete blood count with differential, erythrocyte sedimentation rate, urinalysis, urine culture, pregnancy test, and cervical cultures for gonorrhea and chlamydia.

The finding of leukocytosis or an elevated sedimentation rate suggests the presence of either an infectious or inflammatory process. Less frequently, tissue ischemia that occurs with adnexal torsion or bowel obstruction may cause these hematologic abnormalities. An ectopic pregnancy or abnormal intrauterine pregnancy may present with pain and irregular bleeding.

Diagnostic Laparoscopy

The timely use of laparoscopy for evaluation of undiagnosed pelvic complaints in young women provides a convenient, minimally traumatic, and often definitive method of establishing a diagnosis and at times permits correction of various abnormalities without recourse to major abdominal surgery. Laparoscopy should be considered in the patient with dysmenorrhea unresponsive to the usual therapy with antiprostaglandin agents or ovulation suppression as well as for the confirmation or exclusion of clinically suspected endometriosis, chronic pelvic inflammatory disease, pelvic adhesions, ovarian cysts, and appendiceal disease. Any areas suspicious for endometriosis should be biopsied during laparoscopy. Endometriosis implants may be red, clear, black, gray, blue, yellow, and white in color and may range in appearance from macular to papular to nodular with subperitoneal penetration (36,41). Petechial implants of endometriosis produce twice the amount of PGF than intermediate, brown lesions, which in turn produce more PGF than typical powder-burn implants (42). Hence, dysmenorrhea associated with atypical implants may be related to abnormal prostaglandin and interleukin production, inflammation, and focal bleeding.

The red, superficial lesion is the predominant type of implant in adolescents (43,44). Many early lesions are small and atypical in appearance. Lack of tissue biopsy results in a failure to diagnose or effectively treat endometriosis in a significant proportion of cases (39). Clear vesicles can be differentiated from light reflection by submerging the lesion in question in irrigation fluid (45). Subtle lesions in adolescents may evolve into more classic disease a decade later (46). One recent study suggested that the intensity of menstrual pain is directly related to the number of endometrial implants in patients with endometriosis (47). Deeply invasive lesions are significantly associated with pelvic pain (48) and should be completely excised or ablated.

THERAPY FOR PRIMARY DYSMENORRHEA

NSAIDs have effectively alleviated symptoms of primary dysmenorrhea in 64% to more than 95% of patients studied, although these response rates may be influenced by large variations in methodology and the relatively high placebo response noted in pain therapy (49). These drugs act at two different sites in the arachidonic acid cascade to inhibit prostaglandin synthetase. Type I inhibitors suppress the action of cyclic endoperoxide synthetase at the cyclooxygenase enzyme level, whereas type II inhibitors affect the cyclic endoperoxide cleavage enzymes after the formation of cyclic endoperoxides. Most of the marketed prostaglandin synthetase inhibitors act on cyclooxygenase. Type II inhibitors are less efficacious because they do not significantly suppress the production of cyclic endoperoxides, which are potent uterotonic substances.

Smith and Powell (49) studied one such NSAID, meclofenamate, by correlating uterine activity assessed by intrauterine pressure measurements, plasma drug levels, and subjective scoring of pain intensity. They demonstrated that a reduction in intrauterine pressure and uterine activity during drug treatment results in a reduction in pain associated with primary dysmenorrhea. All parameters that reflected uterine work showed a statistically greater effect of NSAID over placebo. Sixty-three percent of the patients receiving this antiprostaglandin agent experienced a reduction in the number of uterine contraction waves to below 20% of their pretreatment levels. In addition, the intensity of the contractions was diminished and the uterine tonus remained at the basal level for a greater proportion of time compared to nontreated patients. Other studies that examined the effect of flurbiprofen and naproxen sodium described a similar reduction in active pressure, frequency of the pressure cycles, and area under the curve after the oral administration of these NSAIDs (50). Hence, drug therapy acts to prevent pain rather than merely to ameliorate pain.

Nonsteroidal Antiinflammatory Drug Classifications

The NSAIDs may be broadly grouped into several categories according to their chemical structures. These include benzoic acid derivaives (aspirin), butyrophenones (phenylbutazone), indoleacetic acid derivatives (indomethacin), fenamates (mefenamic acid, meclofenamate), oxicams (piroxicam), and arylpropionic acid derivatives (ibuprofen, ketoprofen, naproxen) (Table 15.2).

Aspirin and acetaminophen-containing analgesics, although only marginally effective, constitute very common therapy for the adolescent patient population, primarily because of their ready availability. In a recent Canadian study, 77.8% of junior high school students surveyed had taken acetaminophen for dysmenorrhea in the previous 3 months, whereas only 31.5% had taken ibuprofen (51). More than three fourths of these adolescents chose what type of analgesic to take without consulting an adult. A double-blind crossover study of 32 dysmenorrheic women comparing the analgesic benefit of aspirin, naproxen sodium, and placebo showed no superiority of aspirin to placebo in reducing dysmenorrhea (52). Other published data support these findings, although one study that used a menstrual distress questionnaire noted that pain scores and school absenteeism were significantly lower in patients who took aspirin 600 mg four times a day compared to placebo (53). Acetaminophen was not superior to placebo in the treatment of dysmenorrhea, presumably because of its inability to effectively prevent prostaglandin synthesis (54).

Enolic acid derivatives include phenylbutazone and piroxicam and act by inhibition of the isomerase/reductase step in the production of PGE_2 and $PGF_{2\alpha}$. Due to the high incidence of adverse effects, phenylbutazone is not prescribed for the treatment of dysmenorrhea. Piroxicam, however, has been shown to be efficacious in alleviating symptoms. Single daily doses of piroxicam 20 and 40 mg are as effective as ibuprofen 400 mg four times daily for the relief of primary dysmenorrhea (55). In addition, the incidence of side effects

TABLE 15.2. *Pharmokinetic parameters/dosage recommendations of nonsteroidal antiinflammatory drugs*

	Time to peak levels (h)[a]	Half-life (h)	Usual starting dose	Maximum recommended daily dose (mg)	Frequency
Flurbiprofen	1.5	5.7	50 mg qid	300	bid–qid
Ibuprofen	1–2	1.8–2.5	400 mg q4–6h	3,200	q4–6h
Ketoprofen	0.5–2	2–4	25–50 mg q6–8h	300	tid–qid
Naproxen	2–4	12–15	250 mg q6–8h[c]	1,500	q6–8h
Naproxen sodium	1–2	12–13	275 mg q6–8h[c]	1,375	q6–8h
Meclofenamate	0.5–1	2(3.3)[b]	100 mg tid	400	tid–qid
Mefenamic acid	2–4	2–4	250 mg q6h[c]	1,000	q6h
Piroxicam	3–5	30–86	20 mg qd	40	qd

[a]Food decreases the rate of absorption and may delay the time to peak levels.
[b]Half-life with multiple doses.
[c]Recommended initial loading dose is two times the maintenance dose.

for patients treated with piroxicam 40 mg for 2 days has not been found to be greater than that experienced with ibuprofen.

Indomethacin and other indoles cause gastrointestinal distress in a significant proportion of patients and therefore are not usually prescribed for the treatment of dysmenorrhea.

A recent meta-analysis of the efficacy and safety of ibuprofen, naproxen, mefenamic acid, and aspirin in primary dysmenorrhea concluded that ibuprofen had the most favorable risk-to-benefit ratio (56). The dose must be repeated every 6 hours to maintain effective inhibition of prostaglandin synthetase activity. Ketoprofen and ibuprofen have equivalent duration of action and time to onset of analgesia (57). Ketoprofen exhibits inhibitory effects on prostaglandin and leukotriene synthesis, antibradykinin activity, and lysosomal membrane-stabilizing action.

Naproxen sodium has the dual advantages of being very rapidly absorbed and having a relatively long half-life. This allows a twice per day dosage schedule that often is easier for adolescents to follow than a briefer interval between dosing. Naproxen sodium, the sodium salt, is more rapidly absorbed and reaches peak plasma levels sooner than naproxen. However, naproxen is more likely to cause nausea than ibuprofen in the treatment of primary dysmenorrhea (56).

Mefenamic acid and related drugs have the theoretical advantage in pharmacologic action of both inhibiting prostaglandin synthetase and blocking myometrial receptor sites for already formed prostaglandins (58). The rapid onset of action of these drugs may be useful in patients who experience acute onset of severe discomfort, although mefenamic acid and meclofenamate are not recommended in children less than 14 years of age.

Medication selection should be based on clinical experience, patient convenience, side effects, and cost. If the therapeutic response with one medication is not satisfactory, substitution of a different drug is a reasonable option. Nevertheless, the psychological impact of frequent alterations of therapy must be considered. Hulka et al. (59) reported that the greater the number of drugs prescribed by a physician, the greater the number of drugs discarded by patients and the greater the number of nonprescription drugs taken by patients. A substantial proportion of adolescents with moderate-to-severe dysmenorrhea use over-the-counter medications at lower than the recommended daily doses or do not take any analgesic drugs during pain episodes (60).

When to Begin Nonsteroidal Antiinflammatory Drugs

Because prostaglandin synthesis by the endometrium occurs over an extended period, effective suppression of menstrual prostaglandins can be achieved with rapidly absorbed NSAIDs even when therapy is initiated at the onset of flow. Chan et al. (61) demonstrated that introduction of therapy on cycle Day 1 was as effective in relieving pain as beginning the drug 3 days before the expected onset of the menses. If, during the first cycle of use, some degree of uterine cramping persists after the initial ingestion of drug, the starting dose should be increased by 50% to 100% with the next cycle. Alternatively, a nonsexually active patient with severe cramps accompanied by early vomiting often may benefit from starting the drug 1 or 2 days before the onset of her menses. Nevertheless, a careful medication history must be elicited because the patient may have taken inadequate doses of the drug previously, particularly if it was a nonprescription item.

The NSAID selected for administration should be taken continuously throughout the first 48 hours of menstrual flow to correct the biochemical derangement in excessive production and release of menstrual fluid prostaglandins. A higher failure rate is more likely to be observed if medication is ingested on an as-needed basis rather than regularly during this time period.

Due to the potential placebo effect of any medical regimen introduced for the alleviation of pain, the response of the patient must be followed over the initial cycles of therapy to appreciate fully its efficacy. Fedele et al.

(62) reported that 84% of dysmenorrheic patients noted a favorable response to placebo during the first menstrual cycle of therapy. This was not statistically significant from patients receiving NSAIDs. Nevertheless, the response rate fell to 29% in the second, 16% in the third, and 10% in the fourth placebo treatment cycle. Conversely, the efficacy of antiprostaglandin agents was maintained throughout the course of study. Psychological theories suggest that deterioration of the placebo response may be attributed to deconditioning of the patient. Hence, a single preliminary cycle of NSAID may not distinguish responders from nonresponders. An adjustment of the type and/or dosage of drug over a 3- to 6-month period is reasonable before consideration of ovulatory suppression with oral contraceptives or diagnostic laparoscopy to exclude secondary causes of dysmenorrhea.

Side Effects of Nonsteroidal Antiinflammatory Drugs

Epigastric distress, nausea, vomiting, and diarrhea are occasional side effects of NSAID therapy and probably are caused by suppression of the protective effect of prostaglandins on the gastric mucosa (63). The incidence of such toxicity is highest with aspirin, indomethacin, and phenylbutazone, although these reactions may exist with fenamates and arylpropionic acid derivatives. Other side effects include constipation, anorexia, headache, dizziness, vertigo, and, less commonly, visual disturbances, melena, hearing disturbances, irritability, depression, drowsiness, skin rash, edema, bronchospasm, hepatotoxicity, and nephrotoxicity (64). All NSAIDs can interfere with platelet function and prolong bleeding time and therefore should be avoided in patients with hematologic disorders or in those who are scheduled for surgery. In addition, NSAIDs are contraindicated in patients with a history of aspirin allergy or aspirin-induced bronchospasm.

Acetaminophen in combination with small doses of codeine may be prescribed for girls who cannot take NSAIDs. Adolescents who take codeine-containing medications frequently experience dizziness and nausea.

Leukotriene and Nonsteroidal Antiinflammatory Drug Nonresponders

Preliminary results from ongoing research indicate that the activity of the 5-lipoxygenase pathway is increased in a subgroup of women with primary dysmenorrhea who do not have increased production and release of uterine prostaglandins. *In vitro* culture of endometrial tissues obtained from these patients revealed an increased biosynthesis of leukotrienes (65). These potent hydrocarbons cause vasoconstriction and induce uterine muscle contractions. Because NSAIDs are essentially cyclooxygenase blockers, they may be unable to completely relieve dysmenorrhea in patients with increased activity of the 5-lipoxygenase pathway. Meclofenamate and the other fenamates inhibit the activity of 5-lipoxygenase, but the clinical importance of the inhibition of leukotrienes has not been clearly established.

Oral Contraceptives

Prostaglandin synthetase inhibitors have certain distinct advantages over the alternative option of hormonal manipulation of the dysmenorrheic patient with oral contraceptives, because the former are taken only during 2 to 3 days of the menstrual cycle. Moreover, NSAIDs do not significantly suppress the pituitary-gonadal axis and do not carry the metabolic effects of the birth control pill, which has to be taken for at least 21 of every 28 days. Nevertheless, NSAIDs are not universally effective, and oral contraceptives offer dual benefits in the sexually active, dysmenorrheic adolescent who wishes to prevent conception.

Menstrual fluid prostaglandin levels are reduced to below normal during oral contraceptive therapy. This may occur via two mechanisms. Combination steroid contraceptives suppress endometrial growth and therefore reduce menstrual fluid volume. In addition, the anovulation induced by oral contraceptive therapy creates an endocrine milieu that is not favorable for the production of prostaglandins. The endometrium must be exposed to luteal phase levels of progesterone after it has been adequately estrogenized so as to produce and release $PGF_{2\alpha}$ and PGE_2 in amounts that result in the development of primary dysmenorrhea (13).

Initiation of oral contraceptive therapy in patients with a history of primary dysmenorrhea has been shown to suppress spontaneous uterine activity as reflected by the frequency and amplitude of contractions. In addition, intravenous injections of vasopressin or $PGF_{2\alpha}$ were found to induce less pain after study subjects began taking oral contraceptives, presumably by lessening the uterine sensitivity to these agents that promote tissue ischemia (66). Ninety percent or more of women with primary dysmenorrhea experience symptom relief after initiation of combination oral contraceptive therapy. Maximal benefit is noted after 2 to 3 months of use. There are no significant differences in the prevalence and severity of dysmenorrhea between the users of monophasic oral contraceptives, irrespective of progestin activity, and users of triphasic formulations (67). If the patient has not experienced relief after 3 to 4 months of pill therapy, an NSAID may be added.

The sexually active adolescent with severe dysmenorrhea usually prefers to continue on oral contraceptives for a long-term period. In one study of teenage women attending an inner-city family planning clinic, those who had severe dysmenorrhea and experienced a reduction of dysmenorrhea as a result of oral contraceptives were eight times more likely to be consistent oral contraceptive users than those users with little or no history of pain (68). If contraception is unneeded, the medication may be discontinued after 6 to 12 months of use. The patient may continue to have relief from cramps for several additional, possibly anovulatory, cycles before the baseline menstrual discomfort recurs.

Other Medical Therapies

Calcium antagonists such as nifedipine and verapamil have been shown to reduce prostaglandin-induced uterine hypercontractility and by doing so relieve menstrual pain (69). Oral intake of a single dose of nifedipine 30 to 40 mg markedly reduced or abolished uterine contractions in the majority of otherwise healthy, dysmenorrheic patients as objectively verified by intrauterine pressure recordings. An improvement in pain symptoms occurred simultaneous with a decrease in uterine activity, typically within 15 to 20 minutes of drug intake. Nevertheless, headaches are a troublesome side effect of these preparations; in addition, a slight fall in blood pressure may be measured. Dawood (2) has found nifedipine to be efficacious when used in a limited number of intractable cases of dysmenorrhea without pelvic pathology. However, the prescription of this class of drug is not recommended on a routine basis because of a lack of sufficient clinical trials documenting efficacy and adverse effects.

Ulmsten (70) administered oral nifedipine 30 mg to 12 patients ranging in age from 14 to 22 years and noted an alleviation of pain in nine subjects. Two of the remaining three were found to have a secondary cause for dysmenorrhea on subsequent laparoscopy, and the third patient failed to experience any of the usual peripheral vasodilatory side effects of the medication, perhaps due to incomplete gastrointestinal absorption of the drug. These findings suggest that short-term administration of nifedipine may be a tool to delineate disorders of primary versus secondary dysmenorrhea (70).

The therapeutic benefits of β-adrenergic receptor agonists in alleviating primary dysmenorrhea have been investigated. Terbutaline and related drugs are only partially effective (71), and the results of double-blind studies suggest that they are not significantly better than placebo and carry considerable side effects (13). Their use in dysmenorrhea, therefore, is currently limited and perhaps reserved for only those women in whom more proven methods of therapy have failed or are contraindicated.

Dietary supplementation with omega-3 fatty acids appears to have a beneficial effect on symptoms of primary dysmenorrhea in adolescents (72). Omega-3 fatty acids compete with omega-6 fatty acids for the production of prostaglandins and leukotrienes through incorporation into cell wall phospholipids and through competition at the prostaglandin synthetase level. The daily supplementation of fish oil consisted of eicosapentaenoic acid 1,080 mg, docosapentaenoic acid 720 mg, and vitamin E 1.5 mg, and was administered in two divided doses per day.

Behavioral Therapy

Relaxation training is a common component of all behavioral treatments and has been used successfully in the management of spasmodic pain associated with menstruation (73). In addition, activity scheduling has been shown to reduce symptom severity (74). This operant approach to pain management consists of increasing activity levels through reinforcement principles, reducing pain medications, and increasing social reinforcement for well behavior by family members. Although emotional distress seems to exacerbate perimenstrual symptoms (75), alternative behavioral treatments such as biofeedback have demonstrated limited utility (73).

Regular exercise decreases stress, improves mood, and even lifts depression; nevertheless, the direct effect of exercise on dysmenorrheic symptoms is controversial (28). Although Prior and Vigna (76) reported that habitual physical exercise decreased the severity of some premenstrual symptoms presumably by altering hormonal physiology, Metheny and Smith (32) found that complaints of menstrual discomfort were generally increased in those subjects who exercised regularly. Most studies have suggested a decreased prevalence and/or improved symptoms with exercise (77). Undoubtedly, the impact of physical activity on the symptoms associated with dysmenorrhea is complex and individualized.

Alternative Treatments

In traditional Chinese medicine, acupuncture has long been used during labor and at delivery, as well as for treatment of various gynecologic disorders, including amenorrhea, menorrhagia, dysmenorrhea, and infertility. The peripheral sensory, central, and autonomic nervous systems mediate the activity of acupuncture inputs through dermatomal nerve radiation influences and a complex combination of cutaneovisceral, visceromotor, and viscerocutaneal reflexes, perhaps by activating the endogenous opioid system. Helms (78) recently reported that ten of eleven subjects treated with acupuncture for relief of dysmenorrhea showed an improvement in symptoms compared with four of eleven women treated with placebo acupuncture. In addition to decreasing cramping pain, acupuncture resulted in amelioration of the extragenital symptoms of nausea, headache, and backache, and of the premenstrual symptoms of fluid retention and breast tenderness. The physiologic mechanisms involved in this pain relief are unknown.

Transcutaneous electrical nerve stimulation (TENS) has been found to be an effective and safe method for relieving the pain of primary dysmenorrhea. In a randomized, four-cycle crossover study comparing TENS treatment with sham TENS (placebo) or ibuprofen, Dawood and Ramos (79) found that one third of patients treated with TENS did not require any sort of supplemental pain medication. Among those who required backup ibuprofen, the doses needed were significantly lower than those in placebo TENS cycles or cycles treated with ibuprofen alone. Furthermore, the use of TENS temporally delayed the need for rescue medications. TENS significantly reduced the occurrence of diarrhea, fatigue, menstrual flow, and clot formation compared with placebo TENS. Only a small fraction of patients noticed side effects of muscle vibrations, change in stimulation with movement, tightness, headaches after use, or a slight redness or a burning sensation with TENS treatment (79). Although TENS alone was effective, TENS plus ibuprofen provided the best overall pain relief. The TENS setting used was 100 pulses per second with 100-μs pulse widths.

Most patients treated with TENS in a study by Lundeberg et al. (80) reported that the best site for stimulation was the painful area on the back (T10 through L1). A smaller proportion of patients preferred an abdominal location. About 70% of subjects in this investigation experienced pain reduction when treated with high-frequency (100 Hz) TENS. Low-frequency (2 Hz) TENS was clearly less effective, relieving only about 45%.

Smith and Heltzel (81) recently reported that high-frequency TENS therapy in three patients led to a successful subjective improvement in symptoms at the same time that intrauterine pressure parameters remained steady or showed signs of worsening. Similar results were reported by Milsom and colleagues (82). This suggests that there is a fundamental difference in the mechanism of action between TENS and drug therapy, for with NSAIDs the perception of pain is inextricably linked to the process that causes the pain.

TENS relieves primary dysmenorrhea through three likely mechanisms. With continuous TENS, the preganglionic fibers are bombarded with impulses that saturate the nerve cells of the dorsal horn and therefore block propagation of pain impulses along these fibers. The nerve stimulation also may increase endorphin release by these nerve cells, contributing to the relief of pain. None of the patients in the series by Lundeberg et al. (80) consistently experienced any inhibition of pain reduction with the administration of naloxone, suggesting that the mode of action was not through the release of endogenous opioids. Finally, TENS may decrease myometrial ischemia either by a local increase in blood flow or a decrease in oxygen consumption (82).

TREATMENT OF SECONDARY DYSMENORRHEA

Endometriosis

An NSAID should not be the agent of first choice for managing dysmenorrhea and pelvic pain in the patient with endometriosis.

Treatment of the less advanced stages of endometriosis, those usually encountered in the adolescent patient, includes laparoscopic ablation of lesions with laser, electrocautery, or thermocoagulation, and/or hormonal suppression with oral contraceptives, progestational agents, gonadotropin-releasing hormone (GnRH) analogues, or danazol (83). Severe disease may require resection by laparotomy. Presacral neurectomy may be efficacious for women with recalcitrant chronic midline pain (84), but it may not affect the frequency and duration of dysmenorrhea in women with endometriosis (85).

Goldstein et al. (34) treated adolescent endometriosis patients with surgery alone or surgery with or without subsequent ovulation suppression and followed them after laparoscopy for 1 to 58 months. Of those with endometriosis as the sole pathologic finding at surgery, 71% experienced pain relief with their initial treatment; the remaining 29% reported pain persistence or recurrence. In a study of 49 patients, Davis and colleagues (43) reported that satisfactory resolution of pain and cyclic nausea and diarrhea during menses occurred in 84% of adolescents treated by operative laparoscopy and ovulation suppression with a daily oral contraceptive. GnRH analogues are associated with menopausal symptoms, loss of bone mineral density, and breast regression, sequelae that may be unacceptable to the young patient (86), unless small amounts of estrogen and progestin are coadministered as part of "add-back" therapy (87). Large daily doses of progestins, depot medroxyprogesterone acetate, and danazol have significant adverse side effects and are associated with poor adolescent compliance (39).

Ultrasonography, magnetic resonance imaging, examination under anesthesia, laparoscopy, and hysterosalpingography are useful in defining the anatomy of the young woman with a suspected müllerian anomaly so that appropriate reconstruction can be carried out. Excision of the rudimentary blind horn or creation of a permanent outflow tract in the case of a lower genital obstruction may prevent the development of endometriosis by eliminating menstrual reflux (88). Complete and spontaneous regression of endometriosis has been documented after the creation of an outlet for the menstrual effluvium away from the peritoneal cavity.

Other Categories of Secondary Dysmenorrhea

In patients experiencing dysmenorrhea in association with intrauterine device usage, NSAIDs can effectively suppress the induced prostaglandin production to normal or below-normal levels and thereby minimize the discomfort.

Patients who are diagnosed with pelvic inflammatory disease should have cervical cultures taken for potential pathogens followed by introduction of broad-spectrum antibiotic therapy. Hospitalization frequently is necessary to administer parenteral antibiotics. Therapy for other causes of secondary dysmenorrhea is oriented toward correction of the underlying disease state.

CONCLUSION

Despite the high frequency of occurrence of dysmenorrhea in adolescent females of all backgrounds, only a fraction of patients have an appropriate understanding of the pathophysiology of their condition and the medications available to relieve their symptoms. Over-the-counter aspirin and acetaminophen preparations are the most commonly used medications, even though the antiprostaglandin action of these drugs is minimal. Only 14.7% of girls in one American survey could name an NSAID other than aspirin as potentially effective for dysmenorrhea; 46% of these students were unaware that certain medications existed that could relieve cramps (8). In another study completed before the availability of nonprescription ibuprofen, 49% of dysmenorrheic subjects took medication to relieve symptoms, but only 10% of these used a prescription drug (9).

A mere 15% or so of dysmenorrheic girls in the United States seek consultation with a physician or nurse for their symptoms. This percentage increases to approximately 26% to 29% for young women with more severe conditions resulting in a greater absenteeism from school or work (5,8). When dysmenorrhea is ignored, underlying medical problems and gynecologic diseases such as pelvic infection and endometriosis may be left untreated, leading to potential long-term disability. Hence, this subject should be raised during each health care visit of the adolescent girl.

Education concerning the pathophysiology of primary dysmenorrhea and the availability of antiprostaglandin medications may dispel any misperceptions and lessen the possibility that the patient will fear menstruation or begin to view herself as ill or handicapped. NSAIDs interfere with the pathogenic process, may be limited in administration to the time when an individual suffers the pain, are highly effective and without undue side effects, and have a prompt onset of analgesic action.

The adolescent with primary dysmenorrhea should be seen initially every 3 or 4 months to evaluate the effectiveness of the medication. Such visits also facilitate the rapport between the health care provider and patient that is essential in the treatment of this problem. Those with persistent symptoms after this period despite the introduction of antiprostaglandin agents and/or oral contraceptives should be considered for diagnostic laparoscopy.

REFERENCES

1. Alvin PE, Litt IF. Current status of the etiology and management of dysmenorrhea in adolescence. *Pediatrics* 1982;70:516–525.
2. Dawood MY. Etiology and treatment of dysmenorrhea. *Semin Reprod Endocrinol* 1985;3:283–294.
3. Andersch B, Milsom I. An epidemiologic study of young women with dysmenorrhea. *Am J Obstet Gynecol* 1982; 144:655–660.
4. Coupey SM, Alhstrom P. Common menstrual disorders. *Pediatr Clin North Am* 1989;36:551–571.
5. Klein JR, Litt IF. Epidemiology of adolescent dysmenorrhea. *Pediatrics* 1981;68:661–664.
6. Svanberg L, Ulmsten U. The incidence of primary dysmenorrhea in teenagers. *Arch Gynecol* 1981;230: 173–177.
7. Widholm O. Dysmenorrhea during adolescence. *Acta Obstet Gynecol Scand* 1979;87[Suppl]:61–66.
8. Johnson J. Level of knowledge among adolescent girls

regarding effective treatment for dysmenorrhea. *J Adolesc Health Care* 1988;9:398–402.

9. Wilson C, Emans SJ, Mansfiled J, et al. The relationships of calculated percent body fat, sports participation, age and place of residence on menstrual patterns in healthy adolescent girls at an independent New England high school. *J Adolesc Health Care* 1984;5:248–253.

10. Jamieson DJ, Steege JF. The prevalence of dysmenorrhea, dyspareunia, pelvic pain, and irritable bowel syndrome in primary care practices. *Obstet Gynecol* 1996;1:55–59.

11. Harlow SD, Park M. A longitudinal study of risk factors for the occurrence, duration and severity of menstrual cramps in a cohort of college women. *Br J Obstet Gynaecol* 1996;103:1134–1142.

12. Svennurud S. Dysmenorrhea and absenteeism. *Acta Obstet Gynecol Scand* 1989;38[Suppl 2]:1–88.

13. Ylikorkala O, Dawood MY. New concepts in dysmenorrhea. *Am J Obstet Gynecol* 1989;130:833–847.

14. Frisk M, Widholm O, Hortling H. Dysmenorrhea: psyche and soma in teenagers. *Acta Obstet Gynecol Scand* 1965;44:339–347.

15. Cholst IN, Carlon AT. Oral contraceptives and dysmenorrhea. *J Adolesc Health Care* 1987;8:121–128.

16. Widholm O, Kantero R-L. Correlations of menstrual traits between adolescent girls and their mothers. *Acta Obstet Gynecol Scand* 1971;50[Suppl 14]:30–36.

17. Dawood MY. Nonsteroidal anti-inflammatory drugs and changing attitudes toward dysmenorrhea. *Am J Med* 1988;84:23–29.

18. Pickles VR. A plain-muscle stimulant in the menstruum. *Nature* 1957;180:1198–1199.

19. Pickles VR, Hall WJ, Best FA, et al. Prostaglandins in endometrium and menstrual fluid from normal and dysmenorrhoeic subjects. *J Obstet Gynaecol Br Commonwealth* 1965;72:185–192.

20. Lundström V, Green K. Endogenous levels of prostaglandin F_2 and its main metabolites in plasma and endometrium of normal and dysmenorrheic women. *Am J Obstet Gynecol* 1978;13:640–646.

21. Chan WY, Dawood MY. Prostaglandin levels in menstrual fluid of nondysmenorrheic and of dysmenorrheic subjects with and without oral contraceptive or ibuprofen therapy. *Adv Prostaglandin Thromboxane Leukot Res* 1980;8:1443–1447.

22. Willman EA, Collins WP, Clayton SG. Studies in the involvement of prostaglandins in uterine symptomatology and pathology. *Br J Obstet Gynaecol* 1976;83:337–341.

23. Halbert DR, Demers LM, Fontana J, et al. Prostaglandin levels in endometrial jet wash specimens in patients with dysmenorrhea before and after indomethacin therapy. *Prostaglandins* 1975;10:1047–1056.

24. Csapo AI, Pulkkinen MO, Henzl MR. The effect of naproxen sodium on the intrauterine pressure and menstrual pain of dysmenorrheic subjects. *Prostaglandins* 1977;13:193–199.

25. Åkerlund M. Pathophysiology of dysmenorrhea. *Acta Obstet Gynecol Scand* 1979;87[Suppl]:27–32.

26. Haukttsson A, Åkerlund M, Forsling ML, et al. Plasma concentrations of vasopressin and a prostaglandin $F_{2\alpha}$ metabolite in women with primary dysmenorrhoea before and during treatment with a combined oral contraceptive. *J Endocrinol* 1987;115:355–361.

27. Åkerlund M. Can primary dysmenorrhea be alleviated by a vasopressin antagonist? Results of a pilot study. *Acta Obstet Gynecol Scand* 1987;66:459–461.

28. Teperi J, Rimpelä M. Menstrual pain, health and behaviour in girls. *Soc Sci Med* 1989;29:163–169.

29. Parazzini F, Tozzi L, Mezzopane R, et al. Cigarette smoking, alcohol consumption, and risk of primary dysmenorrhea. *Epidemiology* 1994;5:469–472.

30. Wood C, Larsen L, Williams R. Social and psychological factors in relation to premenstrual tension and menstrual pain. *Aust N Z J Obstet Gynaecol* 1979;19:111–115.

31. MacKay Rossingnol A. Caffeine-containing beverages and premenstrual syndrome in young women. *Am J Public Health* 1985;75:1335–1337.

32. Metheny WP, Smith RP. The relationship among exercise, stress, and primary dysmenorrhea. *J Behav Med* 1989;12:569–586.

33. Aubuchon PG, Calhoun KS. Menstrual cycle symptomatology: the role of social expectancy and experimental demand characteristics. *Psychosom Med* 1985;47:35–45.

34. Goldstein DP, deCholnoky C, Emans SJ, et al. Laparoscopy in the diagnosis and management of pelvic pain in adolescents. *J Reprod Med* 1980;24:251–256.

35. Vercellini P, Fedele L, Arcaini L, et al. Laparoscopy in the diagnosis of chronic pelvic pain in adolescent women. *J Reprod Med* 1989;34:827–830.

36. Chatman DL, Ward AB. Endometriosis in adolescents. *J Reprod Med* 1982;27:156–160.

37. Laufer MR, Goitein L, Bush M, et al. Prevalence of endometriosis in adolescent girls with chronic pelvic pain not responding to conventional therapy. *J Pediatr Adolesc Gynecol* 1997;10:199–202.

38. Simpson JL, Elias S, Malinak LR, et al. Heritable aspects of endometriosis: I. Genetic studies. *Am J Obstet Gynecol* 1980;137:327–331.

39. Goldstein DP, deCholnoky C, Emans SJ. Adolescent endometriosis. *J Adolesc Health Care* 1980;1:37–41.

40. Olive DL, Henderson DY. Endometriosis and mullerian anomalies. *Obstet Gynecol* 1987;69:412–415.

41. Jansen RP, Russell P. Nonpigmented endometriosis: clinical, laparoscopic, and pathologic definition. *Am J Obstet Gynecol* 1986;155:1154–1159.

42. Vernon MW, Beard JS, Graves K, et al. Classification of endometriotic implants by morphologic appearance and capacity to synthesize prostaglandin F. *Fertil Steril* 1986;46:801–806.

43. Davis GD, Thillet E, Lindemann J. Clinical characteristics of adolescent endometriosis. *J Adolesc Health* 1993;14:362–368.

44. Reese KA, Reddy S, Rock JA. Endometriosis in an adolescent population: the Emory experience. *J Pediatr Adolesc Gynecol* 1996;9:125–128.

45. Laufer MR. Identification of clear vesicular lesions of atypical endometriosis: a new technique. *Fertil Steril* 1997;68:739–740.

46. Martin DC, Hubert GD, Vander Zwaag R, et al. Laparoscopic appearance of peritoneal endometriosis. *Fertil Steril* 1989;51:63–67.

47. Perper MM, Nezhat F, Goldstein H, et al. Dysmenorrhea is related to the number of implants in endometriosis patients. *Fertil Steril* 1995;63:500–503.

48. Koninckx PR, Martin DC. Deep endometriosis: a consequence of infiltration or retraction or possibly adenomyosis externa? *Fertil Steril* 1992;58:924–928.

49. Smith RP, Powell JR. Simultaneous objective and subjective evaluation of meclofenamate sodium in the treatment of primary dysmenorrhea. *Am J Obstet Gynecol* 1987;157:611–618.

50. Milson I, Andersch B, Sundell G. The effect of flurbiprofen and naproxen sodium on intrauterine pressure and menstrual pain in patients with primary dysmenorrhea. *Acta Obstet Gynecol Scand* 1988;67:711–716.

51. Chambers CT, Reid GJ, McGrath PJ, et al. Self-administration of over-the-counter medication for pain among adolescents. *Arch Pediatr Adolesc Med* 1997;151: 449–455.

52. Rosenwaks Z, Jones GS, Henzl MR, et al. Naproxen sodium, aspirin, and placebo in primary dysmenorrhea. Reduction of pain and blood levels of Prostaglandin $F_{2\alpha}$ metabolite. *Am J Obstet Gynecol* 19891;140:592–598.

53. Klein JR, Litt IF, Rosenberg A, et al. Effects of aspirin on dysmenorrhea in adolescents. *J Pediatr* 1981;98: 987–990.

54. Janbo T, Lokken P, Nesheim BI. Effect of acetylsalicylic acid, paracetamol, and placebo on pain and blood loss in dysmenorrheic women. *Eur J Clin Pharmacol* 1978;14: 413–416.

55. Pasquale SA, Rathauser R, Dolese HM. A double-blind, placebo-controlled study comparing three single-dose regimens of piroxicam with ibuprofen in patients with primary dysmenorrhea. *Am J Med* 1988;84[Suppl 5A]: 30–34.

56. Zhang WY, Li Wan Po A. Efficacy of minor analgesics in primary dysmenorrhoea: a systematic review. *Br J Obstet Gynaecol* 1998;105:780–789.

57. Mehlisch R. Ketoprofen, ibuprofen, and placebo in the treatment of primary dysmenorrhea: a double-blind crossover comparison. *J Clin Pharmacol* 1988;28:529–533.

58. Budoff PW. Use of mefenamic acid in the treatment of primary dysmenorrhea. *JAMA* 1979;241:2713–2716.

59. Hulka BS, Cassel JC, Kupper LC, et al. Communication, compliance, and concordance between physicians and patients with prescribed medications. *Am J Public Health* 1976;66:847–853.

60. Campbell MA, McGrath PJ. Use of medication by adolescents for the management of menstrual discomfort. *Arch Pediatr Adolesc Med* 1997;151:905–913.

61. Chan WY, Dawood MY, Fuchs F. Prostaglandins in primary dysmenorrhea. *Am J Med* 1981;70:535–541.

62. Fedele L, Marchini M, Acaia B, et al. Dynamics and significance of placebo response in primary dysmenorrhea. *Pain* 1989;36:43–47.

63. Henzl MR, Massey S, Hanson FW, et al. Primary dysmenorrhea, the therapeutic challenge. *J Reprod Med* 1980;25:226–235.

64. Dawood MY. Dysmenorrhea. *Clin Obstet Gynecol* 1990; 33:168–178.

65. Demers LM, Hahn DW, McGuire JL. Newer concepts in dysmenorrhea research: leukotrienes and calcium channel blockers. In: Dawood My, McGuire JL, Demers LM, eds. *Premenstrual syndrome and dysmenorrhea.* Baltimore: Urban and Schwarzenberg, 1985:205–220.

66. Hauksson A, Ekstrom P, Juchnicka E, et al. The influence of a combined oral contraceptive on uterine activity and reactivity to agonists in primary dysmenorrhea. *Acta Obstet Gynecol Scand* 1989;68:31–34.

67. Milsom I, Sundell G, Andersch B. The influence of different combined oral contraceptives on the prevalence and severity of dysmenorrhea. *Contraception* 1990;42: 497–507.

68. Robinson JC, Plichta S, Weisman CS, et al. Dysmenorrhea and use of oral contraceptives in adolescent women attending a family planning clinic. *Am J Obstet Gynecol* 1992;166:578–583.

69. Andersson D-E, Ulmsten U. Effects of nifedipine on myometrial activity and lower abdominal pain in women with primary dysmenorrhea. *Br J Obstet Gynaecol* 1978; 85:142–148.

70. Ulmsten U. Calcium blockade as a rapid pharmacological test to evaluate primary dysmenorrhea. *Gynecol Obstet Invest* 1985;20:78–83.

71. Åkerlund M, Andersson KE, Ingemarsson J. Effects of terbutaline on myometrial activity, uterine blood flow, and lower abdominal pain in women with primary dysmenorrhea. *Br J Obstet Gynaecol* 1976;83:673–678.

72. Harel Z, Biro FM, Kottenhahn RK, et al. Supplementation with omega-3 polyunsaturated fatty acids in the management of dysmenorrhea in adolescents. *Am J Obstet Gynecol* 1996;174:1335–1338.

73. Denny DR, Gerrard M. Behavioral treatments of primary dysmenorrhea: a review. *Behav Res Ther* 1981;19: 303–312.

74. Sigmon ST, Nelson RO. The effectiveness of activity scheduling and relaxation training in the treatment of spasmodic dysmenorrhea. *J Behav Med* 1998;11: 483–495.

75. Logue CM, Moos RH. Perimenstrual symptoms: prevalence and risk factors. *Psychosom Med* 1986;48: 388–414.

76. Prior JC, Vigna Y. Conditioning exercise and premenstrual syndrome. *J Reprod Med* 1987;32:423–428.

77. Golomb LM, Solidum AA, Warren MP. Primary dysmenorrhea and physical activity. *Med Sci Sports Exerc* 1998;30:906–909.

78. Helms JM. Acupuncture for the management of primary dysmenorrhea. *Obstet Gynecol* 1987;69:51–56.

79. Dawood MY, Ramos J. Transcutaneous electrical nerve stimulation (TENS) for the treatment of primary dysmenorrhea: a randomized crossover comparison with placebo TENS and ibuprofen. *Obstet Gynecol* 1990;75: 656–660.

80. Lundeberg T, Bondesson L, Lundström V. Relief of primary dysmenorrhea by transcutaneous electrical nerve stimulation. *Acta Obstet Gynecol Scand* 1985;64: 491–497.

81. Smith RP, Heltzel JA. Interrelations of analgesia and uterine activity in women with primary dysmenorrhea. A preliminary report. *J Reprod Med* 1991;36:260–264.

82. Milsom I, Hedner N, Mannheimer C. A comparative study of the effect of high-intensity transcutaneous nerve stimulation and oral naproxen on intrauterine pressure and menstrual pain in patients with primary dysmenorrhea. *Am J Obstet Gynecol* 1994;170:123–129.

83. Vercellini P, Trespidi L, Colombo A, et al. A gonadotropin-releasing hormone agonist versus a low-dose oral contraceptive for pelvic pain associated with endometriosis. *Fertil Steril* 1993;60:75–79.

84. Chen F-P, Soong Y-K. The efficacy and complications of laparoscopic presacral neurectomy in pelvic pain. *Obstet Gynecol* 1997;90:974–977.

85. Candiani GB, Fedele L, Vercellini P, et al. Presacral neurectomy for the treatment of pelvic pain associated with endometriosis: a controlled study. *Am J Obstet Gynecol* 1992;167:100–103.

86. Reichel RP, Schweppe K-W. Goserelin (Zoladex) Depo for the treatment of endometriosis. *Fertil Steril* 1992; 57:1197–1202.

87. Lubianca JN, Gordon CM, Laufer MR. "Add-back" therapy for endometriosis in adolescents. *J Reprod Med* 1998;43:164–172.

88. Perino A, Chianchiano N, Simonaro C, et al. Endoscopic management of a case of "complete septate uterus with unilateral haematometra." *Hum Reprod* 1995;10: 2171–2173.

16

Premenstrual Syndrome

William R. Keye, Jr.

Although recognized in adult women and often referred to as "the mid-thirties syndrome" (1), premenstrual syndrome (PMS) has been largely unrecognized in adolescents. Premenstrual dysphoria, anger, or withdrawal in adolescents often has been labeled "just adolescence" or "changing hormones." On the other hand, severe premenstrual symptoms have been blamed on other medical or psychiatric diseases or syndromes. Because of this, many adolescents with premenstrual symptoms have been ignored or misdiagnosed and, thus, inappropriately evaluated and treated. Unfortunately, years of untreated premenstrual symptoms may result in unnecessary suffering and psychosocial complications, such as decreased self-esteem and assertiveness, loss of self-confidence, disturbed relationships, unfinished education, or loss of employment (2). Thus, it is important that PMS in the female adolescent be recognized and treated.

PREVALENCE

There has been controversy over whether or not adolescents even experience PMS. A common assumption has been that adolescents suffer with dysmenorrhea and women in their thirties and forties suffer with PMS (3–8). This may have occurred for several reasons. First, researchers such as Golub and Harrington (3) found and reported that normal adolescents do not experience increased anxiety or depression during the premenstrual phase of the menstrual cycle. Second, early essays on PMS by pioneers in reproductive medicine, such as Israel (9), claimed

that premenstrual tension occurs in women between the ages of 20 and 40. Finally, few adolescents complain to their pediatrician, family doctor, or gynecologist about premenstrual symptoms.

However, there is recent evidence that many adolescent women experience premenstrual symptoms. Researchers have reported that many women with PMS retrospectively trace their first symptoms to adolescence (10–13). In addition, surveys of adolescent women have found that many of them experience premenstrual symptoms (2,14–17).

Estimations of the prevalence of PMS in adults and adolescents vary from 4.6% to 89% depending on how symptoms are assessed and how PMS is defined. Whereas mild premenstrual symptoms are common, severe premenstrual symptoms are not.

Fisher et al. (14) administered the Premenstrual Assessment Form (PAF) to 207 adolescent females and found that almost all subjects experienced at least one premenstrual symptom of minimal (96%) or moderate (89%) severity. These figures were similar to those reported by Halbreich and co-workers (18), who administered the PAF to 154 adults and Cleckner-Smith and colleagues (19) who studied 75 adolescents. In their study, Cleckner-Smith et al. found that 100% had at least one minimal symptom and 88% had at least one symptom of moderate severity.

Shye and Jaffe (20) used a structured interview to survey 545 adolescent women and found that 80% commonly experience at least one premenstrual symptom. They also found that those who experience painful periods complain more often of premenstrual symptoms than those who do not experience menstrual cramps.

Whereas most adolescent women experience one or more premenstrual symptoms, fewer report that their symptoms are numerous or severe enough to disrupt their daily activities. Raja and co-workers (21) conducted a longitudinal study of 384 15-year-olds. Each woman completed a shortened form of the Menstrual Distress Questionnaire (MDQ), which rated symptoms in both the premenstrual and postmenstrual phases of the menstrual cycle. Whereas the majority experienced at least one symptom before their period, only 14% met the authors' criteria for PMS. Chau and colleagues (22) used Abraham's Menstrual Symptom Questionnaire in a study of 153 Chinese female high school students and found that 19% met Abraham's diagnostic criteria for PMS (23).

Even fewer adolescent women meet the criteria established for late luteal phase dysphoric disorder established in *Diagnostic Statistical Manual of Mental Disorders, Revised Third Edition (DSM-IIIR)* by the American Psychiatric Association (24). Late luteal phase dysphoric disorder is a subsyndrome of PMS that focuses primarily on cognitive and emotional symptoms that are severe enough to interfere with daily activities or relationships with others. Rivera-Tovar and Frank found that only 4.6% of 217 young women aged 17 to 29 met the criteria for premenstrual dysphoric disorder (PMDD) (24A). However, this was similar to the prevalence in older adult women (2.5%) (25).

Finally, Wilson and Keye (2) reported that 44% of a group of adolescent girls (n = 88) perceived that premenstrual symptoms affected their academic performance, 17% reported class absenteeism as a result of their symptoms, and premenstrual depression was reported by 42% of the adolescent women. They found that as many adolescent women experience premenstrual symptoms as experience dysmenorrhea. Thus, there should be no doubt as to the existence of PMS in adolescents.

DEFINITION AND DIAGNOSTIC CRITERIA

PMS is defined as a combination of physical, emotional, and behavioral symptoms that occur before menstruation but after ovulation (luteal phase) and regress or disappear during menstruation. In addition, the symptoms must not be the result of environmental stress and must be so severe as to interfere with the quality of life or the ability to carry out normal everyday activities. More than 150 symptoms representing every organ system have been reported as part of the syndrome of PMS. These symptoms are overwhelmingly numerous, diverse, complex, and diagnostically nonspecific (26–28). Unfortunately, this conceptual definition is of little help to the health care provider in the usual clinical setting.

Fortunately, there are several sets of specific diagnostic criteria available to aid the clinician. One of the most commonly used are the diagnostic criteria for PMDD now listed in the fourth edition of the *Diagnostic Statistical Manual for Mental Disorders (DSM-IV)* (29). The criteria for PMDD include the requirement that at least five of the following eleven symptoms be present: depressed mood, anxiety, labile mood, irritability, lethargy, change in appetite, sleep disturbance, out of control, lack of interest, and physical symptoms, and must occur in the week before menses during most menstrual cycles. In addition, these symptoms must disappear within a few days of the onset of menses and be absent during the week after menstruation. Furthermore, the criteria require that these symptoms impair social or occupational function or the ability to interact with others. The criteria also require that these symptoms are confirmed by daily prospective self-ratings in at least two consecutive symptomatic menstrual cycles. Although the National Institute of Mental Health (30) has suggested that there should be at least a 30% increase in symptom severity in the 5 days before menses compared with the 5 days after menses, adolescents and women with severe PMS frequently will note at least a doubling of the severity of their symptoms during the premenstrual (luteal) phase of the menstrual cycle. Finally, the symptoms cannot be the result of an underlying physical or psychiatric disease.

CLINICAL FEATURES

PMS in the adolescent is characterized by recurring physical, emotional, and behavioral symptoms or changes during the premenstrual (luteal) part of the menstrual cycle. Common premenstrual physical symptoms include backache, headache, bloating, breast tenderness, headache, acne, joint pain, abdominal discomfort, palpitations, and fatigue. Common emotional and cognitive symptoms among adolescents include anxiety, irritability, depression, paranoia, mood swings, increased sensitivity, impulsive behavior, decreased self-confidence, altered and negative body image, loneliness, dissatisfaction with appearance, and decreased concentration. Finally, the behavioral changes that are common in adolescents with PMS include social withdrawal, emotional or physical abuse, binge eating or consumption of alcoholic beverages, increased sexual activity, and suicidal gestures.

Adolescent premenstrual symptoms are essentially no different than those that occur in adult women, but when superimposed on the stresses of adolescence, they often cause interpersonal and social crises. In addition, because menstrual periods in adolescents are commonly irregular, the association between these symptoms and behavior changes and the premenstrual (luteal) part of the menstrual cycle may not be obvious. As a result, parents and other persons in authority positions, unaware of the underlying cause of the behavior, may either ignore the behavior or react negatively. This can lead to interpersonal conflict and social complications that, in and of themselves, may become problematic. Not frequently, the adolescent with severe behavioral changes will have faced severe criticism from parents, teachers, or law enforcement officers.

ETIOLOGY OF PREMENSTRUAL SYNDROME

Beginning with the description of PMS by Frank (31) in 1931, there has been a succession of authors and researchers who have proposed various etiologies for PMS (32). The etiologies tend to fall into three groups: medical, psychological, and social.

Common medical theories regarding the etiology of PMS include deficiencies or excesses of estrogen and progesterone, imbalances in the ratio of estrogen and progesterone, excess in the production of various other hormones including prolactin, renin-angiotensin, or prostaglandins, deficiencies in hormones such as β-endorphin or thyroxine, or alteration in the growth-hormone–insulin-like-growth-factor axis. Nonhormonal medical theories include infection with various bacteria or yeast, vitamin deficiencies, alteration in the metabolism of essential fatty acids, or abnormalities in neurotransmitter metabolism (33).

Recent studies suggest that PMS occurs in susceptible women from an abnormal response of a vulnerable central nervous system to the normal fluctuations of estrogen and progesterone during the menstrual cycle. The most convincing evidence in support of this hypothesis is the finding reported by Schmidt and co-workers (32) that the administration of estrogen and progesterone to women with a history of PMS whose ovaries were suppressed by leuprolide triggered the development of premenstrual symptoms. In contrast, symptoms did not occur in women without PMS to whom estradiol and progesterone were administered.

The nature of the abnormal response has not yet been elucidated, although abnormal serotonin or γ-aminobutyric acid responses may be involved (25,34,35). These changes may be related to lower concentrations of the 5α reduced metabolite of progesterone, allopregnanolone, in women with PMS compared to women without PMS (36).

Psychological explanations for PMS in adolescents include a rejection of the female role or the possibility that PMS is merely a variation of other common affective disorders. Social explanations for the existence of PMS include the mimicking of the behavior of other significant females in the life of the adolescent, social expectations, or pressure from others (37).

Unfortunately, none of these theories explains PMS in all situations, and none has withstood close and careful scientific scrutiny. As noted earlier, recent research findings suggest that the hormones of the premenstrual (luteal) phase of the menstrual cycle act as triggers to stimulate the development of premenstrual symptoms in women who are predisposed to develop PMS. However, this biologic stimulus, although necessary, appears not to be sufficient for the development of PMS.

A biopsychosocial model of PMS may be useful in understanding PMS in adolescents. This biopsychosocial model is a methodologic tool, germane to all illnesses, all disciplines, and all types of health care professionals. It has been used to recognize and investigate PMS because the syndrome involves the convergence of the disciplines of endocrinology, chronobiology, behavioral phenomenonology, social psychology, neurobiology, and their interactions (38). This model assumes that PMS is a result of reciprocal ongoing interactions of the following factors: biologic, psychological, and social. In addition, it recognizes that psychosocial factors are equally important, if not more so, than biomedical factors in determining the nature and severity of PMS (39).

The biopsychosocial model as seen in Fig. 16.1 proposes that the hormone changes of the premenstrual (luteal) phase of the menstrual cycle, that is, the increase(s) in estradiol and/or progesterone that occurs in the premenstrual (luteal) phase, trigger premenstrual symptoms in women who are biologically or psychologically predisposed to develop PMS (40). Although these hormonal changes appear to be necessary for the development of PMS, they may not be sufficient. It appears that whether or not an individual develops premenstrual symptoms in response to the hormonal change of the menstrual cycle depends on past and present biologic, psychological, or social conditions that may have predisposed the individual to develop PMS. Therefore, one may have a biologic predisposition but experience no premenstrual symptoms because the psychological and social conditions that are necessary for the development of premenstrual symptoms are not present. The benefit of the biopsychosocial model is that it encourages clinicians and health care providers to recognize the contribution to PMS by biologic, psychological, and social factors and provides a logical approach to management, including medical, psychological, and social therapy and support (40).

It is helpful to realize that adolescent development often precipitates a crisis in family-life development (41,42). For example, the onset of menses is a significant biologic event for the female adolescent (43,44). In addition, marked changes occur in cognition and thought organization; there is maturity in interests and attitudes and acceptance of female

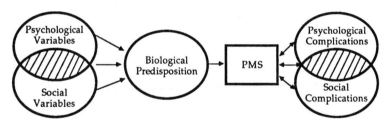

FIG. 16.1. Biopsychosocial model.

role and sexuality (37,42–49). However, research by Peterson (50) indicated that, although the biologic events of puberty are unavoidable, not all adolescents experience problems. Rather, social and environmental factors play a significant role. Examples of these factors include the death of a parent, divorce of parents, change in schools, disruption of peer-group structure, and different achievement expectations. It is in the context of these factors that health care providers must evaluate adolescents with premenstrual symptoms.

EVALUATION OF THE FEMALE ADOLESCENT FOR PREMENSTRUAL SYNDROME

Many professionals find that providing health care to adolescents, although rewarding, can be frustrating, difficult, challenging, and time consuming. The adolescent is in transition between childhood and adulthood, between dependence and independence, never static in her physical, cognitive, and social growth. Thus, the diagnostic evaluation of the adolescent and treatment of PMS poses a dual challenge: the enigmatic complexity of PMS combined with the equally complex nature of adolescent development.

In the assessment of adolescent PMS, the practitioner should realize that the most important need of the adolescent is private and confidential care. At least part of the interview and physical examination should be private. In the end, the findings should be discussed with both the adolescent and parents, if possible. However, if the adolescent requests confidentiality, it is important that the health care provider or practitioner respect this confidence to maintain trust and communication. At times, it may be necessary for the practitioner to ensure that the parents are aware of a problem if it involves a serious health risk. Any serious problems should be discussed with the parents. Such discussion should be with the adolescent's permission with the adolescent present and, ideally, by the adolescent herself (51).

In addition, the initial evaluation may be performed most effectively if the adolescent can be seen once when the adolescent is not suffering from premenstrual symptoms and once when she is so that the clinician can observe any mood or personality changes that may occur.

Finally, the practitioner should be flexible and understanding of adolescent life experience that differs from the adult. For example, whereas the adult woman may be upset that her mother-in-law is visiting her or devastated over a recent divorce, the adolescent may be angry that her brother ate her cereal for breakfast or devastated that she did not win a position on the cheerleading squad.

To assess and diagnose PMS, the following five-step procedure is recommended.

Initial Interview

The patient is asked at the time of the initial interview to describe her physical, emotional, and behavioral symptoms and changes. She also is asked to describe her menstrual period, including the age at which she first menstruated, the interval between her menstrual periods, the duration of her periods, the regularity of her periods, and the presence or absence of pelvic pain during her menstrual periods. She is asked to relate the timing of her symptoms to the onset of her menstrual periods to determine if she perceives a premenstrual occurrence of her symptoms. In addition, her general medical, family, and social history should be obtained. Finally, any previous therapies and their outcomes should be discussed with the patient.

In addition to evaluating the specific symptoms, it is important to determine the impact of behavioral changes and symptoms on the patient's self-esteem, self-image, assertiveness, and relationship with family, friends, coworkers, and fellow students. Adolescence that is complicated by PMS is often a perplexing issue and may lead to a variety of interpersonal problems that need to be considered.

Physical Examination

After the physical symptoms have been described by the patient, it is important to perform a physical examination to rule out underlying diseases that may explain the specific premenstrual symptoms. Such diverse diseases as thyroid abnormalities, autoimmune diseases, or central nervous system disorders may produce symptoms that occur in the premenstrual phase of the menstrual cycle. Pelvic examination of the adolescent is indicated under the following circumstances: (a) menstrual abnormalities, (b) abdominal pain, (c) sexual activity, (d) vaginal discharge, (e) maternal history of diethylstilbestrol (DES) exposure during pregnancy, (f) teenager desires to know that she is "normal," and (g) a history of rape (52).

Utah PMS Calendar II

A premenstrual history of symptoms needs to be confirmed by a prospective gathering of data. The Utah PMS Calendar II is an extremely useful and easy tool for obtaining prospective data. This calendar (Appendix) is a grid that makes it possible for the adolescent or adult woman suffering from premenstrual symptoms to record each day, on a single sheet of paper, the presence and severity of symptoms that she may experience. For simplicity, a three-point rating scale of symptoms can be used, where 1 = mild, 2 = moderate, and 3 = severe.

The adolescent should record her weight several times in the first and second parts of her menstrual cycle. If there is a question of whether or not she is ovulating, she can take her basal body temperature on awakening in the morning and record it on the calendar. In addition, she can record on the calendar the use of medications and the presence of other significant events in her life that may influence the presence of symptoms. After 1 to 2 months of charting information on the calendar, the patient should be interviewed again. The calendar then is evaluated to determine if there is a premenstrual pattern to her symptoms.

It is important to realize that not all of the symptoms that the adolescent reports are necessarily related to PMS. It is not uncommon for an adolescent or an adult woman to experience some symptoms premenstrually and some symptoms throughout the menstrual cycle that may be exacerbated premenstrually. A premenstrual pattern of symptoms is displayed in the sample calendar in the Appendix.

Psychosocial Evaluation

The clinician should consider a psychosocial evaluation of the adolescent who displays or complains of marked behavioral changes or emotional symptoms in the premenstrual phase of the menstrual cycle (53–55). Psychometric tests that are designed to evaluate the absence of depression or anxiety can be used. Alternatively, an interview by a trained social worker or psychologist may be very useful. Many of the common psychiatric disorders may be confused with PMS. Therefore, it is important that psychometric or psychosocial evaluations should be performed once during the follicular (postmenstrual) phase of the menstrual cycle and once during the premenstrual (luteal) phase of the menstrual cycle. If one interviews or evaluates an adolescent with PMS during only one of these phases, one may be left on the one hand with the impression that the adolescent is completely free of any emotional distresses or on the other hand that she suffers from a chronic affective disorder or other significant psychiatric illness. In addition to determining that there is a significant change in the psychological status from the follicular (postmenstrual) to luteal (premenstrual) phase, the psychometric tests and/or interview should be designed to determine the severity of any psychosocial complications that may have occurred as a result of recurring premenstrual symptoms.

Review and Diagnostic Session

At the conclusion of the evaluation, it is useful to sit down with the adolescent and her parents (if appropriate) to review the results of the findings from previous visits and evaluations. It is important that this diagnostic session be held during the follicular (postmenstrual) phase of the menstrual cycle because the patient may be angry, depressed, or confused during the premenstrual (luteal) phase of the menstrual cycle and unable to cooperate or concentrate during the session. It is during this visit that the findings are reviewed, the diagnosis is discussed, and a practical approach to the management of PMS is established.

THERAPY OF PREMENSTRUAL SYNDROME IN THE ADOLESCENT

Validation

The therapy of PMS in the adolescent begins with the process of evaluation. Often the adolescent is unable to understand why she engages in socially unacceptable behavior, such as rapidly changing, destructive mood swings. As a result, she may feel inadequate and have self-doubts, feelings that are reinforced by authority figures in her life. By evaluating her behavior and her feelings in medical terms, the burden of guilt often is removed from her shoulders. Ultimately, if PMS is diagnosed, her self-worth and emotional strength are validated. Ultimately, her improved self-image may decrease the severity or impact of her premenstrual symptoms.

Reassuring the adolescent that her experiences are real and that she is not "going crazy" can have a powerful therapeutic effect. In addition, if a social worker or psychologist demonstrates through standardized psychometric tests that the patient is suffering from PMS and is emotionally stable and healthy the other days of the month, the adolescent with PMS may begin the long process of healing and recovery.

Education

It is important that the female adolescent with PMS and her family be told that certain behaviors and feelings may be due to PMS. However, they also need to know that there are other times when negative or unpleasant emotional feelings are appropriate and represent the healthy, normal range of human feelings. Thus, the adolescent should be told that it is appropriate to express feelings of anger or sadness under certain circumstances and that she should not feel guilty about these feelings. In addition, the adolescent and her parents should be convinced that neither the adolescent nor her family and friends should use PMS as a scapegoat for unacceptable behavior.

Lifestyle Changes

Mild premenstrual symptoms are often amenable to a number of self-help measures, including adequate rest and sleep, stress management, aerobic exercise, and good nutrition. Many of the daily activities of the adolescent tend to aggravate the severity of premenstrual symptoms. For example, long periods of fasting in an attempt to maintain or lose body weight may aggravate the symptoms of PMS. Although there is little scientific evidence to document the value of adequate nutrition in the treatment of PMS, some adolescent and adult women relate that they experience fewer and less severe premenstrual symptoms if they follow a diet that includes frequent, small meals to avoid fasting; the incorporation of complex carbohydrates; a decrease in the amount of simple sugars, salt, caffeine, and alcohol; and the avoidance of fat-free diets that can create metabolic abnormalities that may aggravate the symptoms of PMS.

Aerobic exercise has been shown to reduce the severity of premenstrual symptoms (56). Whether this is because the adolescent is distracted from her emotional feelings or because the exercise increases the level of β-endorphins is uncertain. However, some women report that 20 to 30 minutes of aerobic exercise performed 3 to 7 days per week during the premenstrual (luteal) phase of the menstrual cycle is beneficial. By learning how to manage her symptoms through diet and exercise, she learns how to manage her PMS instead of being victimized by it. This principle is one that the adolescent female may find helpful in other areas of her daily life.

The adolescent who is diagnosed with PMS and is given medication or a variety of self-help measures to decrease the severity and frequency of her symptoms may find it difficult to be compliant if she does not have the support and acceptance of her family, friends, and school authority figures. Family members or friends may undermine or sabotage the success of the adolescent's therapy and may discourage her from complying with the recommendations of the health care professional. It is important to educate those in the immediate family so that they can be supportive of the adolescent and make it easier for her to comply with medical recommendations.

Eliminating Contributing Factors

Often the severity of PMS is influenced by psychological and social dysfunction within the family unit. An adolescent who experiences premenstrual symptoms but has to live in a household dominated by an alcoholic or abusive parent may continue to experience significant premenstrual symptoms in addition to other psychophysiologic reactions. Therefore, it is important to identify and help the adolescent control those negative social and psychological forces in her life. It may be necessary to recommend that the family seek counseling or therapy for issues unrelated to PMS so that the adolescent can recover in a relatively stress-free environment.

Medical Therapy

The medical therapies available to the adolescent with PMS can be divided into three categories: (i) symptomatic therapies, (ii) therapies that cause anovulation and amenorrhea, (iii) miscellaneous therapies.

Symptomatic Therapies

Among the symptomatic therapies, there are a number of over-the-counter medications that are available and promoted for the reduc-

tion of symptoms of PMS. Commonly, they contain a diuretic, analgesic, and antihistamine. Women and adolescents with mild premenstrual symptoms and premenstrual molimina may experience relief of their symptoms when using these symptomatic medications. For the adolescent who has a single specific premenstrual symptom, symptomatic therapy may be beneficial. For example, if premenstrual headaches are experienced, the use of appropriate analgesics or antiprostaglandins may be recommended after a thorough neurologic evaluation has ruled out underlying disease.

Although physical symptoms are common, psychological symptoms such as depression, anxiety, and irritability are the most common symptoms for which women seek care. Therefore, antidepressants and anxiolytics sometimes are useful when the symptoms are severe enough to warrant therapy. Well-designed studies showed that alprazolam 0.25 mg and the selective serotonin reuptake inhibitors are very effective in reducing the severity of premenstrual mood changes in adults (57–60). For example, in a multicentered study of fluoxetine, 52% of women experienced at least a 50% reduction in symptom severity compared to only 27% of women who received a placebo (58).

In a similar study of paroxetine, 64% who received the drug reported that they were enormously or much improved, whereas only 38% of those who received a placebo reported similar improvement (59).

Finally, a recent study demonstrated that 62% of women who received sertraline reported much or very much improvement, whereas only 34% of those who received the placebo noted as much improvement (60). In addition, 38% noted improvement in their productivity (13% in the placebo group), 38% noted improved social activity (17% in the placebo group), and 42% reported improved interpersonal relationships (15% in the placebo group).

The decision to use an antidepressant often should be made in collaboration with a psychiatrist who works with adolescent mood disorders and is familiar with the use of selective serotonin reuptake inhibitors and other psychotropic drugs in adolescents.

Anovulatory Therapy

The second approach to therapy creates anovulation. The most common medication used to create anovulation in the adolescent is an oral contraceptive. Whereas approximately two thirds of adult women with PMS are intolerant of birth control pills, adolescents with premenstrual symptoms may have a positive response. Therefore, the administration of a low-dose oral contraceptive for 21 days of each month will not only regulate the sometimes irregular menstrual periods of the adolescent but also may reduce the severity of her symptoms. Alternatively, medroxyprogesterone acetate 10 mg two to three times a day used continuously may cause anovulation and amenorrhea and reduce premenstrual symptoms. Unfortunately, some women have significant fluid retention and may experience mild headache or depression while taking medroxyprogesterone acetate or birth control pills and therefore discontinue their use. The use of other drugs, such as danazol or gonadotropin-releasing hormone agonists to interfere with ovulation is safe only for a brief time and is not useful for long-term therapy.

Miscellaneous Therapies

The third category of medical therapies, although based on the clinical observations of physicians, have not been studied or proven to be useful in randomized clinical trials. Although they may be unproven in scientific studies, they nonetheless may help reduce the frequency and severity of symptoms in some women.

Among these approaches to therapy are combination multiple vitamins that are rich in vitamin B_6 and magnesium. However, the use of megadoses of vitamins should be discouraged because significant side effects may occur. A recent study demonstrated that the daily use of calcium carbonate 1,200 mg was more effective than placebo in reducing premenstrual symptoms (61). Nutritional supplementation with oil of evening primrose, which is rich in γ-linolenic acid, may be helpful, although results of controlled scientific studies have been contradictory. Finally, progesterone has been endorsed for the treatment of adolescent premenstrual symptoms by Dr. Katharina Dalton in England. In her vast experience, she has noted and reported significant reduction of premenstrual symptoms in the adolescent after the administration of progesterone. There have been a number of double-blind, placebo-controlled, crossover studies that have been inconsistent. Studies using vaginal suppositories have failed to demonstrate a benefit of progesterone over placebo. However, a single study using oral micronized progesterone demonstrated an effect of the progesterone that cannot be accounted for by the placebo (62). Micronized progesterone 100-mg capsules administered in doses of 100 mg in the morning and by 200 mg in the evening significantly decreased premenstrual symptoms.

In addition to these therapies, there are a number of other medical therapies based on alternative theories of PMS (63). These include the use of antibiotics, antifungal agents, immunotherapy, nutritional therapies, or muscle and joint manipulations. The value of these alternative therapies is yet unproven (63).

CONCLUSION

The patient, as well as her family and friends, should realize that ignoring PMS can cause a series of spiraling multidimensional problems that may impact health and quality of life. The patient may lose self-confidence and experience a decrease in her self-esteem. She may develop an altered body image while feelings of inadequacy increase. She may lose her willingness to be assertive, a characteristic much needed to resist adolescent peer pressure. Relationships with significant others may deteriorate, and other close relationships may become strained or nonexistent. The PMS sufferer's functional level can regress and deteriorate if she is unable to cope emotionally, maintain a job, or pursue educational goals, particularly if she becomes withdrawn or socially isolated.

Health care providers need to be understanding and sensitive to the physical, psychological, and social dynamics of the adolescent. As medicine becomes more specialized, the practitioner may lose sight of the "whole" person. Thus, it often may be necessary for the practitioner to collaborate with other professionals who are trained in different disciplines to provide needed multidisciplinary care. The appropriate support team may consist of physician assistants, health educators, nurses, social workers, gynecologists, psychiatrists, and psychologists.

Confidential, empathetic, entrusted care for the adolescent is essential. Health education is critical. The female adolescent with PMS has an opportunity to learn healthy lifestyle habits that may control her PMS or prevent it from worsening. The woman in her mid-thirties who has not exercised or applied preventive care to her lifestyle has an extremely difficult time changing her behavior. However, the adolescent is flexible and teachable, and adverse habits usually are not yet well established.

Providers of adolescent female health care face the challenge of understanding, preventing, detecting, and treating PMS. Hopefully, the controversies surrounding the etiology and pathophysiology of PMS will be unraveled as we focus on the female adolescent. The reward will be manifested in the women of the future—women who will suffer less—women who will live happier, healthier, more productive lives.

REFERENCES

1. Lloyd TS. The mid-thirties syndrome. *Va Med Mnthly* 1963;90:51.
2. Wilson CA, Keye WR Jr. A survey of adolescent dysmenorrhea and premenstrual symptom frequency: a model program for prevention, detection and treatment. *J Adolesc Health Care* 1989;10:317–322.
3. Golub S, Harrington D. Premenstrual and menstrual mood changes in adolescent women. *J Pers Soc Psychol* 1981;41:961–965.
4. Logue C, Moos R. Premenstrual symptoms: prevalence and risk factors. *Psychosom Med* 1986;48:388–414.
5. Moos RH. Typology of menstrual cycle symptoms. *Gynecology* 1969;103:390–402.
6. Rosenwaks Z, Seegar-Jones G. Menstrual pain: its origin and pathogenesis. *J Reprod Med* 1980;25:207–212.
7. Rubinow D, Roy-Byrne P. Premenstrual syndrome: overview from a methodologic perspective. *Am J Psychiatry* 1984;141:163–172.
8. World Health Organization. A cross-cultural study of menstruation: implications for contraceptive development and use. *Stud Fam Plann* 1981;12:3–16.
9. Israel SL. Premenstrual tension. *JAMA* 1938;110: 1721–1723.
10. Dalton K. *Once a month.* New York: Hunter House, 1983.
11. Keye WR Jr. Premenstrual symptoms: evaluation and treatment. *Compr Ther* 1988;14:19–26.
12. Norris RV, Sullivan C. *PMS.* New York: Rawson Associates, 1983.
13. Woods NF, Lentz MJ, Mitchell ES. Arousal and stress response across the menstrual cycle in women with three perimenstrual symptom patterns. *Res Nurs Health* 1994;17:99–110.
14. Fisher M, Trieller RN, Napolitano B. Premenstrual symptoms in adolescents. *J Adolesc Health Care* 1989; 10:369–375.
15. Widholm O. Dysmenorrhea during adolescence. *Acta Obstet Gynecol Scand Suppl* 1979;87:61.
16. Widholm O, Kantero RL. Menstrual patterns in adolescent girls according to the chronological gynecological ages. *Acta Obstet Gynecol Soc Suppl* 1971;14:19–29.
17. Wilson C, Emans S, Mansfield J. The relationship of calculated percent body fat, sports participation, age and place of residence on menstrual patterns in healthy adolescent girls at an independent New England high school. *J Adolesc Health Care* 1988;5:248–253.
18. Halbreich U, Endicott J, Schacht S, et al. The diversity of premenstrual changes as reflected in the premenstrual assessment form. *Acta Psychiatr Scand* 1982;65: 46–65.
19. Cleckner-Smith CS, Doughty AS, Grossman JA. Premenstrual symptoms: prevalence and severity in an adolescent sample. *J Adolesc Health* 1998;22:403–408.
20. Shye D, Jaffe B. Prevalence and correlates of perimenstrual symptoms: a study of Israeli teenage girls. *J Adolesc Health* 1991;12:217–224.
21. Raja SN, Feehan M, Stanton WR, et al. Prevalence and correlates of the premenstrual syndrome in adolescents. *J Am Acad Child Adolesc Psychiatry* 1992;92:783–789.
22. Chau JPC, Chang AM, Chang AMZ. Relationship between premenstrual tension syndrome and anxiety in Chinese adolescents. *J Adolesc Med* 1998;22:247–249.
23. Abraham GE. Nutritional factors in the etiology of the premenstrual tension syndrome. *J Reprod Med* 1983; 28:446–464.
24. American Psychiatric Association. *Diagnostic and statistical manual of mental disorders,* 3rd ed, revised. Washington, DC: American Psychiatric Association, 1987.
24A. Rivera-Tovar AD, Frank E. Late luteal phase dysphoric disorder in young women. *Am J Psychiatry* 1990;147: 1634–1636.
25. Mortola JF. Premenstrual syndrome: a pathophysiologic consideration. *N Engl J Med* 1998;338:256–257.
26. Dalton K. *The premenstrual syndrome.* Springfield: Charles C Thomas, 1964.

27. Moos RH. The development of a menstrual distress questionnaire. *Psychosom Med* 1968;30:853–867.
28. Rubinow D, Hoban C, Grover G. Medical and psychiatric perspectives. In: Keye WR Jr, ed. *The premenstrual syndrome.* Philadelphia: WB Saunders, 1988:27–43.
29. American Psychiatric Association. *Diagnostic and statistical manual of mental disorders,* 4th ed. Washington, DC: American Psychiatric Association, 1994.
30. National Institute of Mental Health. *Workshop on premenstrual syndrome.* Rockville, MD: National Institute of Mental Health, 1983.
31. Frank RT. The hormonal causes of premenstrual tension. *Arch Neurol Psychiatry* 1937;26:1053–1057.
32. Schmidt PJ, Nieman LK, Danaceau MA, et al. Differential behavioral effects of gonadal steroids in women with and in women without premenstrual syndrome. *N Engl J Med* 1998;338:209–216.
33. Reid R. Etiology: medical theories. In: Keye WR Jr, ed. *The premenstrual syndrome.* Philadelphia: WB Saunders, 1988:66–93.
34. Halbreich U, Tworek H. Altered serotonergic activity in women with dysphoric premenstrual syndromes. *Int J Psychiatry Med* 1993;23:1–7.
35. Halbreich U, Petty F, Yonkers K, et al. Low plasma γ-aminobutyric acid levels during the late luteal phase of women with premenstrual dysphoric disorder. *Am J Psychiatry* 1996;153:718–720.
36. Rapkin AJ, Morgan M, Goldman L, et al. Progesterone metabolitic allopregnanolone in women with premenstrual syndrome. *Obstet Gynecol* 1997;90:709–714.
37. Abplanalp J. Psychosocial theories. In: Keye WR Jr, ed. *The premenstrual syndrome.* Philadelphia: WB Saunders, 1988:94–112.
38. Keye WR Jr, Trunnell E. A biopsychosocial model of premenstrual syndrome. *Int J Infertil* 1986;31:259–262.
39. Trunnell E, Turner C, Keye WR Jr. A comparison of the psychological and hormonal factors in women with and without premenstrual syndrome. *J Abnorm Psychol* 1988;97:1.
40. Trunnell EP, White GL, Pedersen DM, et al. Biopsychosocial model for premenstrual syndrome. *Physician Assist* 1989;13:45–52.
41. Blos P. *On adolescence:* a psychoanalytic interpretation. New York: Free Press, 1971.
42. Erickson EH. *Identity and the life cycle.* New York: International Universities Press, 1959.
43. Danza R. Menarche: its effects on mother-daughter and father-daughter interactions. In: Golub S, ed. *Menarche.* Lexington: Lexington Books, 1983.
44. Kestenberg J. *Menarche in adolescents: psychoanalytic approach to problems and therapy.* New York: Harper and Brothers, 1961.
45. Koff E, Rierdan H, Silverstone E. Changes in representation of body image as a function of menarcheal status. *Dev Psychol* 1978;14:635–642.
46. Whisant L, Zegans L. A study of attitudes toward menarche in white middle-class American adolescent girls. *Am J Psychiatry* 1975;132:809–814.
47. Davis BL. Attitudes towards school among early and late maturing adolescent girls. *J Genet Psychol* 1977; 131:261–266.
48. Stone CP, Barker RG. The attitudes and interests of premenarcheal and postmenarcheal girls. *J Genet Psychol* 1939;54:27–71.
49. Lambert G, Rothchild B, Altand R, et al. *Adolescence.* Monterey: Brooks/Cole, 1972.
50. Peterson AC. Those gangly years. *Psychol Today* 1981; September:28–34.
51. Coupey SM. The challenge of providing health care to adolescents. *Womens Health* 1984;9:1–14.
52. Hein K. The first gynecologic examination. *Diagnosis* 1981;3:32–52.
53. Keye WR Jr, Hammond C, Strong T. Medical and psychologic characteristics of women presenting with premenstrual symptoms. *Obstet Gynecol* 1986;68: 634–637.
54. Hammond DC, Keye WR Jr. Premenstrual syndrome. *N Engl J Med* 1985;312:920.
55. Hammond DC. The psychosocial consequences. In: Keye WR Jr, ed. *The premenstrual syndrome.* Philadelphia: WB Saunders, 1988:128–141.
56. Prior JC, Vigna Y, Sciarreta D. Conditioning exercise decreases premenstrual symptoms: a prospective, controlled 6-month trial. *Fertil Steril* 1987;47:402–408.
57. Freeman DW, Rickels K. Sondheimer SJ, et al. A double-blind trial of oral progesterone, alprazolam, and placebo in treatment of severe premenstrual syndrome. *JAMA* 1995;274:51–57.
58. Steiner M, Steinberg S, Stewart D. Fluoxetine in the treatment of premenstrual dysphoria. *N Engl J Med* 1995;332:1529–1534.
59. Eriksson E, Hedberg MA, Andersch B, et al. The serotonin reuptake inhibitor paroxetine is superior to the noradrenaline reuptake inhibitor maprotiline in the treatment of premenstrual syndrome. *Neuropsychopharmacology* 1995;12:169–176.
60. Yonkers KA, Halbreich U, Freeman E. Symptomatic improvement of premenstrual dysphoric disorder with sertraline treatment: a randomized controlled trial. *JAMA* 1997;278:983–988.
61. Thys-Jacobs S, Starkey P, Berstein D, et al. Calcium carbonate and the premenstrual syndrome: effects on premenstrual and menstrual syndrome. *Am J Obstet Gynecol* 1998;179:444–452.
62. Dennerstein L, Spencer-Gardner C, Gotts, G. Progesterone and the premenstrual syndrome: a double blind crossover trial. *Br Med J* 1985;290:1617.
63. Carter J, Verhoef MJ. Efficacy of self-help and alternative treatments of premenstrual syndrome. *Womens Health Issues* 1994;4:130–137.

17

Hirsutism in the Pediatric or Adolescent Patient

Ricardo Azziz

The chapter will outline the normal pubertal development and metabolism of androgens; the normal physiology and pathophysiology of hair growth; and the differential diagnosis, workup, and treatment of hirsutism in the pediatric and adolescent patient.

NORMAL ANDROGEN METABOLISM

Androgens are C-19 steroids (containing 19 carbons) derived from cholesterol and are secreted by the adrenal cortex and ovaries. Androgens also may be derived (not secreted) from the conversion of other steroids by the liver and some peripheral tissues (e.g., adipose tissue, muscle, skin). Principal circulating androgens include testosterone (T) and its metabolite dihydrotestosterone (DHT), androstenedione (A4), and dehydroepiandrosterone (DHA) and its metabolite dehydroepiandrosterone sulfate (DHS) (Fig. 17.1). Androgens act through a specific cytoplasmic/nuclear intracellular receptor.

After puberty, T originates approximately 25% from the ovary, 25% from the adrenal, and 50% from the peripheral conversion of A4 (1). Testosterone and A4 are metabolized to DHT, the most potent of androgens, through the action of the enzyme 5α-reductase in the liver and skin. DHT is primarily formed from the peripheral nonhepatic 5α-reduction of T in men and from A4 in women (2,3).

Androstenedione is produced equally from the ovary and the adrenal cortex. Approximately 90% of DHA and 99% of DHS are produced by the adrenal cortex. DHA, DHS, and A4 exhibit a circadian rhythm similar to

that of cortisol, with peak serum concentrations in early morning and the nadir in late evening (4–6). Although DHS is the most abundant androgen in circulation, at a concentration approximately 80,000 to 10,000 times that of T, these three steroids are very weak androgens compared to T and DHT, and under normal circumstances they have a very limited androgenic effect.

T and DHT circulate tightly bound to a hepatic α-globulin called sex hormone-binding globulin (SHBG; or testosterone binding globulin [TeBG]) and, to lesser extent, to albumin. Androstenedione is only weakly bound, whereas DHA and DHS circulate mostly unbound (7,8). Because only free (unbound) steroid is able to act on the androgen receptor, the action of T and DHT is greatly influenced by the circulating SHBG level. If the SHBG level is low, the free fractions of T and DHT are going to be higher and their effect greater (9). In addition, the SHBG level influences the clearance of T and DHT from circulation (10), because only free androgen can be metabolized by the liver and peripheral tissues. The circulating SHBG level is decreased by androgens and increased by estrogens (11–14). Thus, if the circulating level of androgens increases, the SHBG concentration will drop, resulting in a higher T and DHT clearance. The final result may be that although the total T level remains relatively normal, T production and its free (active or unbound) fraction are increased (9).

Androgen production and clearance are affected by various physiologic states. In obesity, androgen production and clearance are

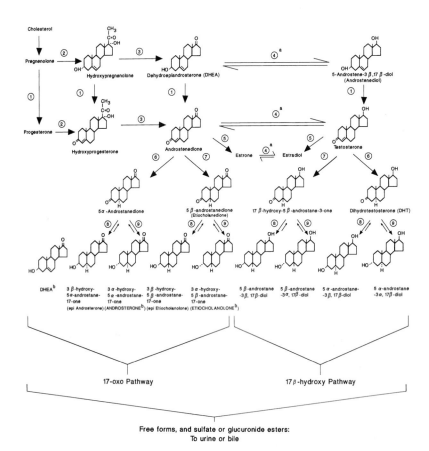

FIG. 17.1. Principal pathways of androgen synthesis and catabolism. Enzymes: (1) 3β-hydroxy-steroid dehydrogenase; (2) 17β-hydroxylase; (3) 17,20-lyase; (4) 17β-hydroxysteroid dehydroge-nase; (5) aromatase; (6) 5α-reductase; (7) 5β-reductase; (8) 3β-oxoreductase; (9) 3α-reductase. [a]In the gonads the 17β-hydroxysteroid dehydrogenase activity predominantly yields 17β-dehydro-genated products (androstenediol and testosterone), whereas the reverse is true in peripheral tis-sues. [b]Aldosterone, etiocholanolone, and dehydroepiandrosterone (DHEA) are the principal urinary metabolites of androgens. (From Azziz R. Reproductive endocrinologic alteration in female asymp-tomatic obesity. *Fertil Steril* 1989;52:703–725, with permission.)

accelerated (15). The increased clearance is, in part, due to an obesity-related decrease in SHBG, which leads to higher levels of rapidly metabolizable free T and DHT. In addition, because steroids are fat soluble, the increased amount of adipose tissue in obese women tends to "trap" androgens, increasing their extravascular pool. In obesity, a greater per-centage of the androgens are metabolized to estrogens, through the action of aromatase, present in the stroma of adipose tissue. Because androgen levels in obese women gen-erally are normal or only slightly decreased,

their production rate must be increased to compensate for their higher clearance. How-ever, the exact mechanism(s) by which andro-gen production increases in obesity remains unclear.

ANDROGENS AND PUBERTY

Circulating Androgens Throughout Puberty

Circulating androgen levels increase throughout puberty, with such changes being evident before the appearance of clinical features of pubertal maturation.

Total and Free Testosterone, and Androstenedione

It is important to understand the changes in serum androgen levels and adrenal function that take place at puberty to clearly diagnose syndromes of androgen excess during this period of time. Total T levels in prepubertal boys and girls are approximately equal, increasing fourfold in girls to reach a mean of 38 ng/dL (range 20 to 85 ng/dL) in Tanner stage V (16–20). In comparison, boys in

Tanner stage V have T levels ranging from 200 to 1,000 ng/dL (Fig. 17.2) (16,17). DHT concentrations increase similarly in normal girls, from a mean of 6 ng/dL in Tanner stage I to 17 ng/dL at the completion of puberty (20). Free T also increases during this period of time, from a mean of 3.8 pg/mL (range 2 to 6 pg/mL) to 8.8 pg/mL (range 5 to 13 pg/mL) (19).

Androstenedione levels increase throughout puberty in a similar fashion in both boys and girls, from a mean of 35 ng/dL (range 10 to 100 ng/dL) to approximately 141 ng/dL (range 58 to 224 ng/dL) in Tanner stage V (16,21,22). The pubertal increases in T and

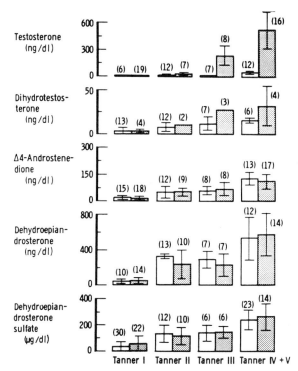

FIG. 17.2. Mean (± SD) serum concentrations of testosterone, dihydrotestosterone, Δ4-androstenedione, dehydroepiandrosterone, and dehydroepiandrosterone sulfate in normal boys and girls according to pubarchal development (Tanner I, II, III, and IV+V). Testosterone was higher in boys in stages II, III, and IV+V ($p < 0.001$). Dihydrotestosterone was higher in boys in stages III and IV+V ($p < 0.01$). In both sexes, differences between stages I and II are significant for all steroids ($p < 0.001$). Differences between stages II and III are significant in boys for testosterone ($p < 0.001$). Differences between stages III and IV+V are significant for all steroids, except dehydroepiandrosterone, in girls. (From Korth-Schultz S, Levine LS, New MI. Serum androgens in normal prepubertal and pubertal children and in children with precocious adrenarche. *J Clin Endocrinol Metab* 1976;42:117–124, with permission.)

A4 throughout puberty appear to be mostly of ovarian origin. In Turner's syndrome patients, the increase in serum T and A are minimal. At the age of 15 years, the concentrations of these androgens were 50% and 60%, respectively, for the corresponding levels in normal girls of the same age (18).

Sex Hormone-binding Globulin

It is speculated that the increase in androgen levels during female puberty would offset any positive effect that the increase in estrogens may have on circulating SHBG levels. Consistent with this hypothesis, SHBG concentrations during female puberty have been reported to change little (19), although other investigators reported a decrease (23,24). Cunningham and colleagues (24) noted a decrease in SHBG levels with chronologic age, regardless of androgen status, in four normal men and their two 46,XY androgen-insensitive siblings, suggesting that the decrease in SHBG in puberty is independent of androgen activity and may be under the regulation of other factors, such as insulin (24).

Dehydroepiandrosterone and Dehydroepiandrosterone Sulfate

A marked increase in serum DHA and DHS concentrations is noted beginning at about the age of 5 years and continuing throughout puberty (Fig. 17.2) (17,18,21,22, 25–28). The levels of these adrenal steroids rise similarly in both boys and girls, from a mean of 133 ng/dL (range 19 to 300 ng/dL) to 741 ng/dL (range 389 to 1,093 ng/dL) for DHA, and from 43 μg/dL (range 24 to 86 μg/dL) to 120 μg/dL (range 78 to 163 μg/dL) for DHS. In patients after 13 years of age with Turner's syndrome, the mean serum DHA concentration was slightly, but significantly, lower (20% to 30%) than that of normal girls of the same age, suggesting that this steroid is produced in part by the ovary (18).

Adrenarche

The increased adrenal secretion of androgens and estrogens begins 2 to 3 years before the onset of puberty and is termed pubarche or adrenarche. Histopathologically, adrenarche correlates with the appearance of a continuous reticularis zone in the adrenal cortex. Focal development of the reticularis begins at about the age of 5 years. By 8 years of age it usually is present as a continuous zone (29). The measurement of urinary or serum androgens and their metabolites (30), the steroid response to adrenal stimulation (31), and in vitro studies of adrenal microsomal activity (32) suggest that the relative efficiency (activity) of 3β-hydroxysteroid dehydrogenase (3β-HSD) activity decreases and that of 17,20-lyase and, to a lesser extent, 17-hydroxylase increases during adrenarche. However, we have reported that a rise in DHS occurs before any observable increase in circulating DHA, or its response to adrenocorticotropic hormone (ACTH) stimulation, suggesting that an increase in sulfotransferase activity may precede changes in adrenocortical 17,20-lyase and 3β-HSD activity (33). Some investigators also observed a doubling in 21-hydroxylase (21-OH) activity in vitro (32), and a fall in 11β-hydroxylase (11-OH) by measurement of urinary steroid metabolites (30). It should be noted that these alterations do not lead to a change in circulating cortisol levels, which remain stable throughout puberty (28).

The mechanisms responsible for initiating and controlling adrenarche are not clear. Adrenarche appears to occur independently of gonadal maturation (34). Some investigators have proposed that the development of the continuous reticularis and the changes in adrenocortical biosynthesis are under the control of both ACTH and an as yet unidentified pituitary regulatory factor, the adrenal androgen-stimulating hormone (AASH) or cortical androgen-stimulating hormone (CASH) (35,36). Experimental evidence for such a substance rests on the observation that bovine and human pituitary extracts stimulate a greater secretion of DHA relative to cortisol, from dog and human adrenals *in vitro* and *in vivo* (36). The sequence of this peptide has been proposed to be identical to a portion of the joining peptide of the pro-opiomelanocortin molecule (37), although this remains to be confirmed. Clinical evidence for the presence of a non-ACTH pituitary factor controlling adrenal maturation and androgen production include the following (38):

- The pattern of plasma androgens in premature adrenarche is different from that seen in children after protracted ACTH stimulation.
- Circulating levels of androgens do not exert a negative feedback on the pituitary secretion of ACTH.
- There is no difference in ACTH release after metyrapone administration between adults and children.
- There are numerous instances of a divergence in the secretion of cortisol and adrenal androgens, including alternative day glucocorticoid administration (39), and surgical trauma or severe burns (40,41).

Alternatively, other investigators suggested that much, if not all, of the changes in adrenal androgen production at puberty can be explained by alterations in the intrinsic adrenocortical hormonal milieu and the progressive development of the reticularis. Rich and colleagues (31) suggested that the increase in DHA levels noted at adrenarche results from a combination of changes in the response of the adrenal cortex to ACTH. More of the precursor 17-hydroxypregnenolone is available, and the percentage of this steroid converted to DHA increases as the result of an apparent improvement in 17,20-lyase activity, while DHA is less efficiently converted to A4 because of an apparent decrease in 3β-HSD activity. These authors noted that the resultant increase in DHA after ACTH stimulation, together with acquisition of sulfotransferase activity by the adrenal, was sufficient to explain the adrenarchal rise in DHS.

That ACTH is one of the principal hormones regulating adrenal androgen secretion in prepubertal and pubertal girls also was noted by Pintor and colleagues (22), who reported that, in these children, short-term dexamethasone administration decreased the circulating levels of cortisol, pregnenolone, DHA, progesterone, 17-hydroxyprogesterone (17-HP), A4, T, and estradiol (22). Alternatively, Kreitzer and colleagues (42) were not able to suppress the circulating DHS level in preadrenarchal children with the administration of high doses of prednisone for 1 week, although the same regimen was able to reduce circulating DHS levels by 70% in postadrenarchal children. These data suggested that there may be two distinct regulatory pathways leading to DHS production, one of which is independent of ACTH.

Dickerman and colleagues (43) observed that the shift in the relative activities of 3β-HSD and 17,20-lyase at adrenarche were associated with changes in the steroidal microenvironment of the adrenal cortex, and that the age-related changes in adrenal size are accompanied by significant changes in intraadrenal steroid concentrations of sufficient magnitude to influence steroidogenesis. These investigators suggested that the developmental changes in adrenal androgen secretion could be explained in terms of shifts in relative enzyme activities induced solely by the necessity to maintain stable cortisol secretion in face of continued adrenal growth, without the need to invoke the action of a pituitary androgen-stimulating hormone. Hornsby and Aldern (44) reported that cultured human fetal definitive zone cells (which will result in the fasciculata-reticularis zone in the adult) produced cortisol and DHS (via DHA) about equally from 17-hydroxypregnenolone after ACTH administration. When compared to bovine adrenocortical cells (which secrete only minimal amounts of DHS), the difference in DHS production between species was believed to be secondary to differences in the intrinsic activity of 3β-HSD and not the presence of an extrinsic adrenal androgen-stimulating factor(s).

Overall, it still remains unclear the extent to which adrenarche and adrenal androgen secretion the result of changes in intraadrenal hormonal milieu, adrenocortical cell mass, and adrenal response to ACTH, or the result of the secretion of a specific androgen-stimulating pituitary hormone.

SIGNS AND SYMPTOMS OF ANDROGEN EXCESS

In young girls or adolescents, the most common signs of androgen excess include hirsutism, acne, or oligoovulation. Rarely, androgen excess may present as virilization or masculinization.

Excess Hair Growth

Following is a review of the normal physiology of hair development and growth, and the appearance of hirsutism.

Normal Hair Physiology

Hair follicles cover the entire body with the exception of the soles of the feet, the palms of the hands, and the lips. Most hair follicles are present at birth; very few new ones are formed thereafter (45). Hair follicles are lost in a generalized fashion beginning in the mid to late forties leading to the thinning of hair noted thereafter. Although there are racial and ethnic differences in follicle numbers, there is no difference between genders within each race/ethnic group. The visible differences between men and women do not relate to the number of hair follicles, but rather to the type of hair arising from these follicles. White individuals have a higher density of hair follicles than blacks, who in turn have more follicles than Asian patients (45–47).

In general there are three types of hair. *Lanugo* is the soft unmedullated hair covering the surface of the fetus, which is shed sometime in late gestation or the early postpartum period. *Vellus hairs* are short (2 to 5 mm), soft, fine, unmedullated, and usually nonpigmented, and cover the apparently "hairless" areas of the body. *Terminal hairs* are long, coarse, and medullated; they make up the eyebrows, eyelashes, and scalp, and pubic and axillary hair. Whereas in women many of the hair follicles produce vellus hairs, in men these same follicles produce terminal hairs leading to the appearance of visible facial, chest, and abdominal hair.

The hair growth cycle can be divided into three phases (45). The hair grows actively during the *anagen phase,* associated with downward progression of the dermal papilla (Fig. 17.3). During the *catagen phase,* the hair follicle involutes, followed by the *telogen phase,* in which the hair is eventually shed. Whereas in many animal species the growth cycles of all hair follicles are in synchrony, in humans this is not the case, which accounts for the impression that hair continuously grows. Occasionally a greater number of hair follicles shift into synchrony, as in pregnancy, menopause, or after delivery, or when starting or stopping oral contraceptive medications, which eventually leads to the temporary shedding of excessive numbers of hairs, without an actual reduction in the number of hair follicles (e.g., telogen effluvium). This is a temporary situation that eventually reverts to normal.

There are a number of hormones that control hair growth. Thyroid and growth hormone produce a generalized growth in hair. Hyperthyroidism yields a fine friable hair that is easily lost; hypothyroidism produces a coarse brittle hair that also is easily lost. Of the reproductive hormones, progesterone has a minimal effect, whereas estrogens basically oppose the effect of androgens, most importantly by increasing circulating SHBG leading to a decrease in free T and DHT. Androgens, in turn, are the most important determinant of the type and distribution of hairs throughout the body.

Circulating androgens, particularly T and A4, are converted in the hair follicle to DHT through the action of 5α-reductase. DHT then acts on the dermal papilla and sebaceous gland (which compose the pilosebaceous unit) to increase the growth rate and thickness of terminal hairs and increase sebum production. Androgens also transform vellus-producing follicles to terminal hair-producing follicles, an irreversible process. The effect of androgens on the hair follicle will be specific to the

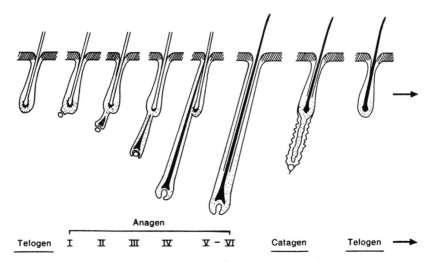

Anagen

Telogen   I   II   III   IV   V – VI   Catagen   Telogen ⟶

FIG. 17.3. Growth cycle of a hair follicle. Depicted is a club hair (in white) in telogen, early anagen (I–IV) follicles, and a new hair (in black) in late anagen (V–VI). Involution (catagen) of the hair follicle follows the anagen (active growth) phase. (From Uno H. Biology of hair growth. *Semin Reprod Endocrinol* 1986;4:131–141, with permission.)

area of skin in which it is located (45). Some skin areas (e.g., eyelashes, eyebrows, lateral and occipital aspects of the scalp) appear to be relatively independent of the effects of androgens and are designated as *nonsexual skin.* Other areas are very sensitive to the effect of even low levels of androgens, due to their high 5α-reductase activity, and include the lower pubic triangle and the axilla, which are designated as *ambosexual areas.* The hair follicles in these areas develop terminal hairs early in puberty, accompanying the minimal increases in adrenal androgens. Other parts of the skin contain lower levels of 5α-reductase and respond only to high concentrations of androgens, including the chest, lower abdomen, lower back, upper thighs, upper arms, chin, face, and upper pelvic triangle, and are designated as *sexual areas.* Terminal hair growth in these areas is characteristically masculine and, if present in women, is considered *hirsutism.*

Hirsutism

Hirsutism is the presence of terminal hairs in women in a male-like pattern. The areas affected are the upper lip, chin, chest, upper and lower abdomen and back, thighs, and upper arms. Excessive growth of coarse hairs of the lower forearms and lower legs alone does not constitute hirsutism. However, a woman suffering from hirsutism also may note an increase in the pigmentation and growth rate of hairs on the lower forearm and leg. Although hirsutism usually is obvious, it may be important to standardize the examination for future reference by using a standardized scoring system (Fig. 17.4). It also is important to remember that not all hyperandrogenic women demonstrate hirsutism (e.g., women of Asian extraction rarely do so) (48,49), whereas some patients with obvious hirsutism have normal circulating androgen levels (see section on Idiopathic Hirsutism on page 262).

Acne

The pilosebaceous unit, in addition to the hair follicle, also contains a sebaceous gland that produces an oily protective secretion, sebum, in response to androgen action. The excessive production of sebum leads to oily skin (seborrhea), clogged hair follicles, folliculitis, and subsequent acne. Although all androgens may lead to acne, the sole presence of acne without hirsutism often is associated with ex-

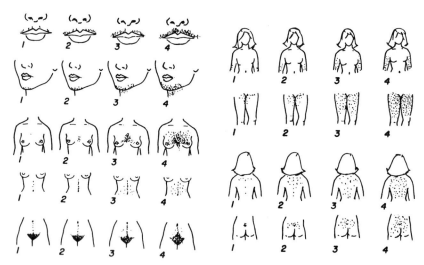

FIG. 17.4. Example of one method to score the extent of hirsutism, modified from that originally reported by Ferriman and Gallwey. The values in each of nine body areas are summed to produce a total hirsutism score. (From Hatch R, Rosenfeld RL, Kim MH, et al. Hirsutism: implications, etiology, and management. *Am J Obstet Gynecol* 1981;140:815–830, with permission.)

cessive levels of the adrenal androgens DHA and/or DHS (50–53). Although these steroids are relatively weak in their stimulation of terminal hair growth, they are relatively effective in increasing sebum production. Elevations in other serum androgen levels have been noted (54–58), particularly in patients with acne and hirsutism, although not all investigators agree (59–62). Other investigators observed that although serum androgen levels may be relatively normal, the metabolism of such androgens by the affected skin is increased (63–65).

Although, intuitively, persistent acne in adults may be considered to be related to elevated androgen levels more frequently than acne in adolescents, we were unable to confirm this supposition. In fact, we reported that approximately 45% of females with acne only had two or more abnormal androgen values, regardless of age (66). Consistent with its androgenic nature, acne frequently improves after treatment with oral contraceptives, glucocorticoid suppression, spironolactone, or cyproterone acetate (67–73).

Oligoovulation or Anovulation

Clinical evidence suggests that excessive androgen levels can directly disrupt the hypo-

thalamic-pituitary-ovarian axis and inhibit follicular development, as noted in female-to-male transsexual patients receiving exogenous androgens (74). Adolescent oligomenorrhea is frequently hyperandrogenic in nature (75,76). Approximately one half of these children will go on to develop persistent hyperandrogenemia, with all its consequences (77).

The risk that adolescent oligoovulation will lead to persistent hyperandrogenic oligoovulation, as, for example, the polycystic ovary syndrome (PCOS), remains unclear. Nonetheless, a few high-risk populations have been identified, such as adolescents with oligomenorrhea and persistently elevated luteinizing hormone (LH) levels (77,78). Furthermore, a 13-year follow-up study by Apter and Vihko (79) reported that hyperandrogenemia observed in early adolescence frequently persisted into adulthood and that higher serum androgen levels increased the risk of subfertility. If hyperandrogenic features are to develop, it appears that such abnormalities will already be evident in girls ages 14 to 18 years. For example, adolescent girls with oligomenorrhea frequently demonstrate elevated circulating androgen levels (75–77). In addition, hyperandrogenic adolescents have been reported to demonstrate enlarged multicystic ovaries (77), hyperinsulinism (80,81), and an exaggerated 24-hour LH pulsatility and LH/follicle-stimulating hormone (FSH) ratio (82), much like adult patients with PCOS. These data suggest that PCOS frequently is associated with persistent adolescent oligo-menorrhea, and that the typical gonadotropic and metabolic features of the disorder are already established during this period of life.

Virilization and/or Masculinization

If the androgen levels are extremely elevated and present before puberty, the patient's body habitus may become masculinized with amenorrhea, absence of breast development, increase in muscle mass, upper body obesity, and virilization. Virilization includes temporal and frontal balding, clitoromegaly, reduction in breast size, and severe hirsutism. In general, virilization or masculinization should raise the suspicion of an androgen-producing tumor or congenital adrenal hyperplasia. Occasionally girls with severe hyperthecosis or who suffer from severe insulin resistance syndrome (see later) may exhibit a moderate degree of virilization.

DIFFERENTIAL DIAGNOSIS OF ANDROGEN EXCESS

Common Androgenic Causes

Most commonly, hirsutism is the result of disorders of androgen action, either peripherally, centrally, or both. The vast majority of hyperandrogenic girls suffer from PCOS; a lesser fraction suffers from idiopathic hirsutism (IH); even less suffer from the hyperandrogenic insulin-resistant acanthosis nigricans (HAIRAN) syndrome or 21-OH deficient nonclassic adrenal hyperplasia (NCAH). Finally, rare patients will suffer from androgen-secreting tumors.

Polycystic Ovary Syndrome

PCOS affects approximately 4% of U.S. women, regardless of race, making it one of the most common endocrinologic abnormalities (83). PCOS is the most common cause of hirsutism, accounting for 60% and 85% of patients, depending on definition. PCOS is a heterogeneous disorder of unknown etiology. Overall, the diagnosis is one of exclusion, having eliminated other causes of hyperandrogenemia. We prefer to use the recommendations of a preliminary consensus conference sponsored by the National Institute of Child Health and Human Development (NICHD) in April 1990 (84). The conference concluded "that the major criteria for [PCOS] should include (in order of importance) (i) hyperandrogenism and/or hyperandrogenemia, (ii) oligo-ovulation, [and] (iii) exclusion of other known disorders, such as Cushing's syndrome, hyperprolactinemia, or congenital [non-classic] adrenal hyperplasia." The presence of "polycystic ovaries on ultrasound" also was noted as a possible inclusion criterion, although this was believed to be "particularly controversial" and not necessary for the diagnosis of these patients.

Patients with PCOS have varied clinical features. They generally demonstrate elevated circulating levels of free T and a reduction in SHBG, accompanied by variable increases in total T (9,85,86). Approximately 50% will demonstrate an abnormally high DHS level, although rarely above 6,000 ng/mL (87). Prolactin usually is normal, although up to 15% of such patients may demonstrate mild elevations (generally less than 80 ng/mL, depending on the assay) without any other apparent cause (88,89). The LH/FSH ratio usually is 3:1 or greater (90–92), which is observed in approximately 60% of these patients.

Pathologically, the ovarian cortex contains multiple intermediate and atretic follicles measuring 2 to 5 mm in diameter, which give the ovary its "polycystic" appearance at sonography or laparoscopy. However, not all PCOS patients demonstrate ovaries that are "polycystic," nor are "polycystic" ovaries diagnostic for PCOS (93–96). Approximately 40% of PCOS patients are obese, 60% are amenorrheic, and 15% have regular menses (97). One should note that not all patients with

PCOS demonstrate hirsutism (48,97–99). These patients do not generally present with virilization or masculinization. PCOS may result in primary amenorrhea (100,101) and present as early as age 12 years (102).

Insulin resistance and the development of compensatory hyperinsulinemia are frequent findings in PCOS, affecting approximately 30% to 80% of these patients (49,103). The insulin resistance of PCOS appears to be associated with abnormal cellular glucose transport in insulin-responsive tissues, most likely due to postreceptor signaling aberrations. In turn, the insulin resistance results in compensatory hyperinsulinemia, with the excess insulin causing an exaggerated effect in other, less traditionally responsive, tissues. For example, insulin excess stimulates androgen secretion by the ovarian theca; excess growth of the basal cells of the skin, resulting in acanthosis nigricans; increased vascular and endothelial reactivity; and abnormal hepatic and peripheral lipid metabolism. That the insulin resistance of PCOS patients underlies many of the features of this disorder is highlighted by the finding that the administration of insulin-sensitizing agents, principally metformin and troglitazone, have been found to improve these features in many patients (104–108).

As noted, the resistance to the action of insulin in PCOS refers to the impaired action of this hormone on glucose transport and antilipolysis, primarily in adipocytes, in the presence of normal insulin binding (108–112). It should be noted that the insulin resistance of PCOS differs from that observed in Type 2 diabetes mellitus (DM) and simple obesity, because these latter disorders demonstrate reductions in both insulin receptor binding and glucose transport (113). However, in Type 2 DM and obesity, if glucose transport is corrected by insulin receptor number, insulin sensitivity then is found to be normal (113). The metabolic dysfunction of PCOS has been associated with an increased risk of developing Type 2 DM, gestational diabetes, hypertension, dyslipidemia, and possibly cardiovascular disease (114,115).

There is a strong genetic effect in PCOS, which results in an increased risk of the disorder among female relatives of an affected individual. For example, approximately 50% of sisters of patients with PCOS will have the disorder (116), a fact that requires counseling families. As always, early detection and treatment of PCOS in female relatives will minimize the severity and improve the prognosis of the disorder.

Few prospective longitudinal studies determining the early developmental aspects of PCOS are available, in part because it has been difficult to identify sufficient individuals at risk. One such high-risk group has been girls with either premature adrenarche (117), or central precocity and an exaggerated adrenal response to ACTH (118), where up to 40% of patients develop a PCOS-like phenotype postpubertally. Another group of at risk patients are adolescents with oligomenorrhea and persistently elevated LH levels (77,78). If hyperandrogenic features are to develop, it appears that androgenemic, gonadotropic, metabolic, and ovarian abnormalities similar to those of adult patients with PCOS will already be evident in girls ages 14 to 18 years (73–77,80–82).

Idiopathic Hirsutism

The diagnosis of IH is reached only when a patient is obviously hirsute, but has regular ovulation. These patients also generally have normal circulating androgen levels. Approximately 15% of hirsute women will have this diagnosis (119). It should be noted that approximately 40% of hirsute patients with apparent eumenorrhea actually are oligoanovulatory when evaluated by basal body temperatures and luteal phase progesterone levels (119). In addition, many of these patients simply demonstrate degrees of hyperandrogenemia that are not detectable by routine clinical androgen assays and, in fact, may more accurately reflect a nonsensitive laboratory assay.

It has been suggested that some women with IH have excessive 5α-reductase activity of the hair follicle, which leads to hirsutism in the face of "normal" circulating androgen levels (120). The measurement of serum 3α-androstanediol-glucuronide (3α-Adiol-G), a metabolite of DHT, has been proposed to help to confirm the "hyperfunction" of this enzyme (120,121). Nevertheless, the diagnosis of IH is usually a diagnosis of exclusion, when normal androgen levels (at least free and total T and DHS) and normal ovulatory function are encountered in a patient with obvious hirsutism, and other disorders such as NCAH are excluded. Patients with IH should not be designated as having "familial hirsutism," because this implies that IH is not treatable, ignores the fact that PCOS is also highly inherited, and serious diseases (e.g., Type 2 DM and cardiovascular disease) also have an inherited component. Finally, treatment of IH requires an antiandrogen, usually in combination with an oral contraceptive.

Adrenal Hyperplasias

Adrenal hyperplasias are disorders arising from defects in the action of enzymes necessary for the biosynthesis of glucocorticoids and sometimes mineralocorticoids. The adrenal in many of these individuals is under persistent and excessive ACTH stimulation in compensation for the deficient production of cortisol, which results in hyperplasia of the zona reticularis/fasciculata of the adrenal cortex and the excessive accumulation of enzymatic precursors. Defects of 3β-HSD and 11-OH have been reported to cause hyperandrogenic adrenal hyperplasia, although over 95% of all patients seen exhibit varying defects of 21-OH action. The adrenal hyperplasias can be subdivided, according to age of presentation, into those disorders that are considered "classic," with symptoms evident at or near birth; and "nonclassic," with symptoms appearing peripubertally or postpubertally. Following is a brief review of these disorders.

Classic Adrenal Hyperplasia

Also called the adrenogenital syndrome or congenital adrenal hyperplasia, classic adrenal hyperplasia (CAH) represents one of the most common autosomal recessive disorders, affecting one of every 5,000 to 10,000 newborns (122). The disorder generally results from the inherited deficiency of P450c21, which determines intraadrenal 21-OH activity (Fig. 17.5), an enzyme necessary for the adrenocortical biosynthesis of cortisol.

The signs and symptoms of these disorders will depend on the severity and location of the enzymatic block. If the defect is extremely severe (as in the total absence of enzymatic activity), cortisol and aldosterone may not be produced in sufficient quantities. This leads to the development of polyuria, dehydration, hypokalemia, and seizures ("adrenal crisis"), resulting in death if left untreated (122). The accumulation of very high levels of progesterone, 17-HP, and particularly A4 and T generally leads to severe degrees of masculinization of the female genitalia *in utero*. These patients are designated as "salt wasters." Alternatively, in "simple virilizing" CAH patients, cortisol is produced in amounts sufficient to sustain life and androgens accumulate to lesser degrees, producing less disfiguring genital abnormalities in girls.

Girls with CAH will develop amenorrhea, acne, hirsutism, and virilization if untreated. Simple virilizing CAH may remain undiagnosed, although fortunately rarely, and results in progressive clitoromegaly, hirsutism, amenorrhea, and even masculinization. The diagnosis can be established by the measurement of basal 17-HP and A4 levels, with basal 17-HP levels usually exceeding 200 ng/mL (123). An electrolyte panel and renin activity level should be obtained in all patients suspected of suffering from CAH. Once the diagnosis is established, corticosteroid (with prednisone or hydrocortisone) and, if necessary, mineralocorticoid (with fluorocortisone) replacement will suffice. Nevertheless, the hirsutism may not improve completely, requiring the addition of antiandrogens. Some simple virilizing CAH patients also may require low doses of mineralocorticoids in the event their basal renin measurements are elevated (124).

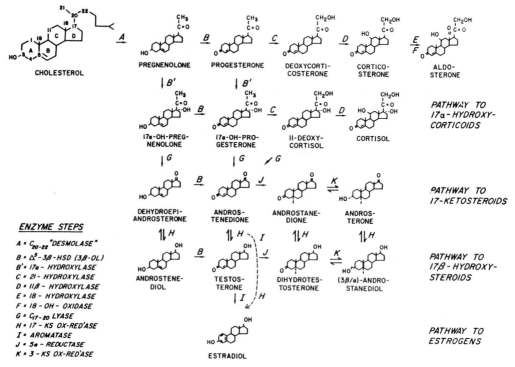

FIG. 17.5. Mayor pathways off steroid biosynthesis from cholesterol. The flow of hormonogenesis usually is to the right and downward. Note that C$_{20-22}$ "desmolase" (enzyme step A) also is known as the cholesterol cleavage enzyme. (From Hatch R, Rosenfeld RL, Kim MH, et al. Hirsutism: implications, etiology, and management. *Am J Obstet Gynecol* 1981;140:815–830, with permission.)

Fertility is possible and will depend on the extent of genital virilization (125), which will determine the overall coital success after reconstructive surgery (126) and the degree of progesterone excess. Persistently elevated levels of progesterone and 17-HP of adrenal origin may result in chronic atrophy of the endometrium and thickened cervical mucus, regardless of circulating estrogen levels. Persistent progesterone and 17-HP excess can be very difficult to treat, often not responding even to the highest doses of glucocorticoid suppression and necessitating adrenalectomy for adequate treatment.

Nonclassic Adrenal Hyperplasia

Between 1% and 10% of hyperandrogenic women suffer from 21-OH deficient NCAH (127). In contrast to CAH, where the enzyme deficiency is so severe that the symptoms of cortisol deficiency and/or androgen excess are present in the newborn or in childhood, patients with NCAH are clinically indistinguishable from other hyperandrogenic patients and usually present peripubertally or postpubertally (127–130).

Serum levels of the exclusive adrenal androgen DHS are not any higher than levels of other hyperandrogenic women (128–130). Although levels of A4 are higher than in other hyperandrogenic patients, the overlap is sufficient to make the measurement of this steroid useless for screening purposes. Fortunately, measurement of a morning 17-HP level in the follicular phase of the menstrual cycle can be used to screen for this disorder (130). If the baseline 17-HP is higher than 2 ng/mL (or 200 ng/dL), then the patient should undergo an ACTH stimulation test to rule out the disorder (see later). Nonetheless, it is important to note that the false-positive rate is as high as

50% if the 17-HP measurement is obtained in the luteal (postovulatory) phase.

Patients with NCAH can be treated with corticosteroid replacement (dexamethasone 0.5 mg daily or every other day, prednisone 5 to 10 mg daily, or hydrocortisone 20 to 30 mg daily). Nevertheless, if long-standing, their hirsutism and ovulatory disorder may not respond solely to corticosteroids, requiring the addition of antiandrogens or oral contraceptives (131) (see later).

Hyperandrogenic Insulin-resistant Acanthosis Nigricans Syndrome

Between 1% and 5% of hyperandrogenic women suffer from this disorder. It is characterized by extremely high circulating levels of insulin, generally greater than 80 μU/mL in the fasting state and greater than 300 μU/mL after an oral glucose tolerance test (132–134). In young patients, fasting glucose levels usually will be normal. Measuring the 2-hour postprandial glucose and insulin response, the responses to an oral glucose tolerance test may be required for detection in some patients. The high levels of insulin usually are due to an inherited defect of the insulin receptor action or more commonly postreceptor signaling (135–141). Rarely some of these women demonstrate circulating antiinsulin receptor antibodies (142,143). This syndrome should not be confused with the insulin resistance noted among many patients with PCOS, where the increase in insulin levels generally is mild.

In spite of the relative resistance of insulin for glycemic control, the resultant hyperinsulinemia affects other organs. For example, in the epidermis of the skin, acanthosis nigricans will develop, with hyperplasia of the basal layers of the epidermis. This results in a velvety, hyperpigmented change of the crural areas of the skin, particularly the nape of the neck. Likewise, significant dyslipidemia and hypertension may be present, secondary to as yet undetermined mechanisms. At the ovarian level, insulin acts synergistically with LH to stimulate increased androgen production by the theca-stroma cells, resulting in hyperandrogenemia and clinical hyperandrogenism. These girls can be severely hyperandrogenic and can even be masculinized.

These patients usually respond to standard therapy with antiandrogens and oral contraceptives, although some patients may require the administration of ketoconazole (KTZ) or long-acting GnRH analogues (144–146). KTZ is an antifungal agent that has been found to block androgen synthesis by inhibiting, among others, P450c17α (which determines 17,20-lyase activity). Long-acting GnRH analogues inhibit LH-dependent androgen production by reducing circulating gonadotropins to castrate levels. At least 3 to 6 months of gonadotropin suppression are required to achieve full androgen suppression in HAIRAN syndrome (Fig. 17.6) (146). If standard therapy fails, a bilateral ovarian wedge resection or even oophorectomy may be considered.

It should be noted that hyperthecosis usually is found in the ovaries of patients with severe insulin resistance (147–149). Hyperthecosis is not an endocrinologic diagnostic entity onto itself, rather it is a histopathologic finding, where islands of hyperplastic luteinized theca cells are noted throughout the stroma. In general and in contrast to the ovaries of women with PCOS, hyperthecotic ovaries contain relatively few small atretic follicles (147–152). These patients usually are severely androgenized and may even be virilized, and they have very high levels of circulating T, often greater than 200 ng/dL (147–154). Patients with hyperthecosis may be particularly difficult to treat, as many do not respond to conventional therapy. These patients may require extensive ovarian wedge resection or oophorectomy, although the use of long-acting GnRH agonists appears to be promising (155,156).

Androgen-secreting Tumors

Androgenic tumors are relatively rare. They should be suspected when the onset of androgenic symptoms is rapid and sudden, and when virilization and masculinization ensue.

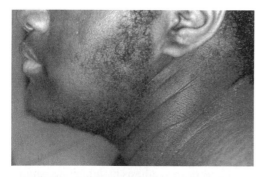

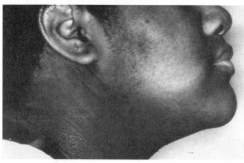

FIG. 17.6. Thirteen-year-old patient with hyperandrogenic insulin-resistant acanthosis nigricans (HAIRAN) syndrome, before **(A)** and after 6 months of treatment with leuprolide **(B)**. Note acanthosis nigricans and marked improvement in hirsutism after treatment with the long-acting gonadotropin-releasing hormone agonist.

Steroid-secreting neoplasms may be associated with other systemic symptoms, including weight loss, anorexia, abdominal bloating, and back pain. These tumors are usually of ovarian or adrenal origin. Suppression and stimulation tests (including corticosteroid, oral contraceptive, human chorionic gonadotropin, and ACTH administration) can be misleading and are not encouraged for the screening or diagnosis of these neoplasms (157).

Androgen-producing tumors of the adrenal are relatively rare. The appearance of cushingoid features and/or virilization along with hirsutism should arouse suspicion (158). The diagnosis usually is established by a computed tomographic (CT) scan of the adrenal, with images obtained at 0.5-cm intervals. Adrenal carcinomas usually are associated with cushingoid features and generally are greater than 6 cm and irregular on CT scan.

Unfortunately, their prognosis is very poor. Androgen-secreting adrenocortical adenomas are even more rare. They are distinguishable from carcinomas by their smaller size and regular borders on radiographic study and by the lack of glucocorticoid excess features. Although these adrenal tumors may be suspected when the serum DHS level exceeds 6,600 ng/mL and/or the T level exceeds 200 ng/dL (159), the most useful tool for detection is the history and physical examination (158).

In general, the diagnosis of excessive cortisol production (Cushing's syndrome) can best be established by a 24-hour urine free cortisol. A more simple screening method is the measurement of a morning fasting cortisol after administering dexamethasone 1 mg the evening before, although the false-positive rate for this test can be as high as 15% among obese women or depressed patients, with a false-negative rate of approximately 2%.

Ovarian tumors are somewhat more common, occurring in one in 300 to 1,000 unselected hyperandrogenic patients in our experience (160). They are usually palpable on pelvic examination and/or are associated with a unilateral ovarian enlargement on pelvic ultrasonography. They frequently are not malignant and include Sertoli-Leydig cell tumors and lipoid cell tumors. Although it has been suggested that ovarian tumors should be suspected when the circulating T levels are greater than 200 ng/dL (161), it is important to understand that 20% to 50% of androgen-producing ovarian tumors may have T levels below this value (161), and that the majority of women with T levels over 200 ng/dL have HAIRAN syndrome, hyperthecosis, or PCOS, and not an ovarian tumor (160,162).

Uncommon Causes of Androgen Excess

Uncommon causes of androgen excess include some forms of male pseudohermaphroditism, use or abuse of androgenic drugs, and Cushing's disease. For example, accidental or deliberate ingestion or overingestion of danazol, methyltestosterone, or stanozolol, particularly in young women engaged in body building, can result in the development of acne, hirsutism, and oligomenorrhea.

The peripubertal onset of hirsutism, breast development, and clitoromegaly accompanied by primary amenorrhea can suggest the presence of incomplete androgen insensitivity syndrome (i.e., testicular feminization) or a Y-bearing dysgenetic gonad (163). If undiagnosed, progressive masculinization may result. On examination, these individuals will demonstrate a blind vaginal pouch and varying degrees of clitoromegaly. These patients also may demonstrate bilateral or unilateral vulvar swelling secondary to descent of one or both gonads. In some patients with XY gonadal dysgenesis, a uterine remnant may be present, invariably accompanied by some degree of genital asymmetry.

Pituitary Cushing's (Cushing's disease) can lead to excessive glucocorticoid, adrenal androgen hypersecretion, and hyperandrogenemia. However, the incidence of this disorder presenting as hirsutism is rare. Of approximately 1,000 hyperandrogenic patients seen by this investigator, only one was diagnosed with Cushing's disease. Most of these patients will present with typical cushingoid features, including "yoke-like" centripetal obesity, thinning and striae of the skin, muscle wasting, glucose intolerance, and osteoporosis. However, some patients with ectopic ACTH tumor or adrenal carcinoma may demonstrate few of these signs, presenting as malnourished and/or cachectic. In these patients, diagnosis of glucocorticoid excess can be established as noted earlier.

Nonandrogenic Causes

In rare cases, hirsutism will arise as a result of nonandrogenic causes. Acromegalic women may demonstrate a generalized increase in hair growth and sebum production and may present with hirsutism (164). Accompanying the hirsutism will be enlargement of the hands and feet and coarsening of the facial features. This cause of hirsutism is extremely rare, and the diagnosis is based on determination of excessive growth hormone secretion.

Teleologically, hairs protect the skin. Chronic irritation of the skin secondary to depilating agents, environmental toxins, and other factors can lead to a local increase in hair growth, as well as the increased transformation of vellus to terminal hairs (45).

Certain anabolic medications cause a generalized growth of many tissues, particularly hair, and include phenytoin (Dilantin), norethandrolone (Nilevar), and oxandrolone (Anavar). However, these drugs generally lead to overgrowth of vellus hairs (vellus hypertrichosis) and not hirsutism.

EVALUATION OF ANDROGEN EXCESS

Evaluation of hirsute patients consists of assessing the history, physical examination, and if needed, laboratory and radiologic studies (Fig. 17.7).

History

The pace of pubertal development and its relation to the onset of hirsutism, acne, and/or obesity should be established. History of drug or medication use, and exposure or use of skin irritants should be elicited. Menstrual history, onset and progression of hirsutism and/or acne, change in extremity or head, change in face contour, and balding and hair loss should be noted. A family history of similar signs and symptoms is a powerful clue to the inherited basis of the disorder, although it should be remembered that a strong inherited tendency is observed equally for PCOS, IH, and HAIRAN syndrome. Because NCAH is an autosomal recessive disorder, the frequency of inherited relatives may be less in women with this disorder. The etiology of hirsutism often can be established from the history alone.

Physical Examination

The type and pattern of excessive hair growth and/or acne should be noted and scored. The presence of galactorrhea, viriliza-

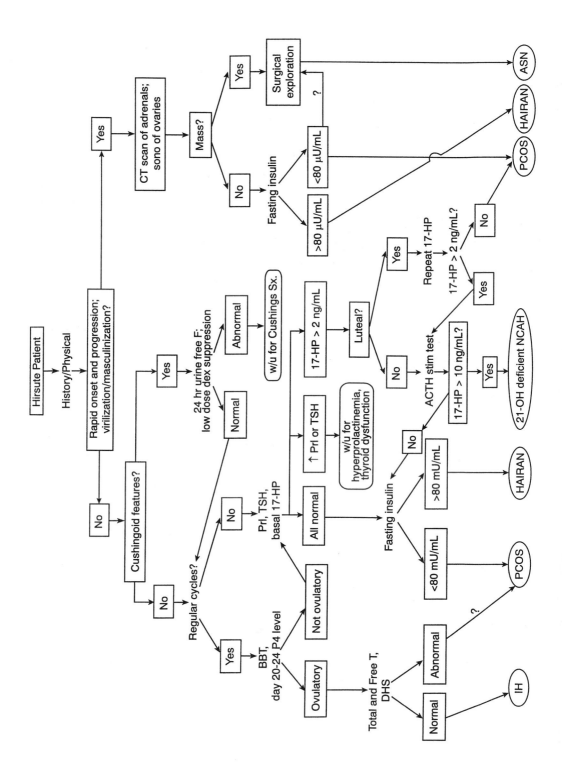

tion, masculinization, clitoromegaly, pelvic and abdominal masses, obesity, cushingoid features, "bluntness" of facial features, thyroid enlargement, or signs of systemic illness should be sought. If the patient is premenarchal or suffers from primary amenorrhea, the upper/lower body and span/height ratios should be determined. If there has been a delay in epiphyseal closure due to insufficient sex steroid availability in the face of physiologic growth hormone exposure, the upper/lower body ratio will be decreased (less than one) and the span/height ratio increased (greater than one). Tanner staging of pubertal and breast development should be noted.

It is most important to determine whether hirsutism is truly present and whether it is related to other endocrinologic features. The excessive growth of vellus hairs, producing a "fuzzy" appearance, is called *vellus hypertrichosis* and should not be considered hirsutism. Although a number of medical problems or medications can lead to hypertrichosis, it is more commonly ethnic, in individuals of Mediterranean or Scandinavian extraction.

Laboratory Assessment

The value of the laboratory in assessing the hyperandrogenic patient is unclear. It is clear that laboratory measurements are valuable in excluding related disorders. For example, in

---

FIG. 17.7. Algorithm outlining the evaluation of the hirsute patient. It should be remembered that, as all algorithms, the figure depicts only generalizations, and clinical judgment and acuity are the keys to diagnosing of the hirsute patient. ASN, androgen-secreting neoplasms; BBT, basal body temperature chart; CT scan, computerized axial tomography; Cushings Sx, Cushing's syndrome; DEX, dexamethasone; F, cortisol; HAIRAN, hyperandrogenic insulin-resistant acanthosis nigricans syndrome; 17-HP, 17α-hydroxyprogesterone; IH, idiopathic hirsutism; 21-OH deficient NCAH, 21-hydroxylase deficient nonclassic adrenal hyperplasia; PCOS, polycystic ovary syndrome; Prl, prolactin; sono, sonogram; TSH, thyroid-stimulating hormone; w/u, work-up.

patients who are oligoanovulatory, measurements of thyroid function (thyroid-stimulating hormone assessed by a third-generation assay, and a free thyroxine level) and prolactin are indicated. As noted previously, hirsute patients claiming to have "regular menstrual cycles" should be studied more carefully for evidence of normal ovulatory function by basal body temperature charting, although the measurement of a progesterone level on days 20 to 24 of the cycle will be easier to obtain in the younger patient. Although an LH/FSH ratio of three or higher appears to be evident in approximately 40% to 60% of PCOS patients, it is neither diagnostic nor specific enough to be of value, unless measured repeatedly. A 24-hour urine for free cortisol (and creatinine to verify the adequacy of collection) is useful in patients suspected of having Cushing's syndrome and should be less than 100 μg per 24 hours. In the rare patient suspected of suffering from male pseudohermaphroditism or XY gonadal dysgenesis, a karyotype should be obtained.

A 17-HP level will help exclude 21-OH deficient NCAH. Approximately 90% of patients with NCAH will have a 17-HP level above 2 ng/mL, if obtained in the follicular phase of the menstrual cycle. It should be noted that if the measurement is obtained in the luteal phase, approximately 50% of normal patients will have a 17-HP level above 2 ng/mL. If the patient demonstrates a follicular 17-HP level above 2 ng/mL, she should undergo an acute adrenal stimulation test to rule out NCAH. One vial of Cortrosyn (1-24 ACTH) 250 μg is administered intravenously, and the blood is sampled before and 60 minutes afterward. If the poststimulation 17-HP level is greater than 10 ng/mL, the diagnosis of 21-OH deficient NCAH is established (Fig. 17.8) (127).

In patients with acanthosis nigricans or severe hyperandrogenism, measurements of fasting insulin and glucose levels are indicated; levels are normally less than 30 μU/mL and 110 mg/dL, respectively. However, exact screening criteria for insulin resistance/hyperinsulinemia in hyperandrogenic patients is

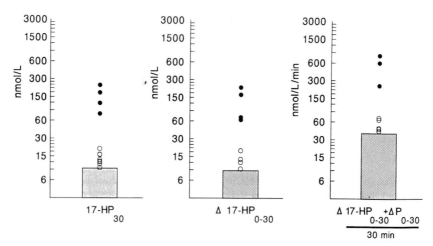

FIG. 17.8. Estimating 21-hydroxylase activity in a population of 164 consecutive hyperandrogenic patients, using the 17α-hydroxyprogesterone (17-HP) and progesterone (P) response to a 30-minute acute ACTH-(1-24) stimulation test. Note that hormonal values are plotted on a logarithmic scale. Measures include the 17-HP level 30 minutes after ACTH administration (17-HP_{30}); the net increment in 17-HP from baseline to 30 minutes (Δ17-HP_{0-30}); and the sum of the increments in 17-HP and P divided by the stimulation time ([Δ17-HP_{0-30} + ΔP_{0-30}]/30 min), to yield the rate of rise of these two steroids. The *boxed area* represents the control response (up to the 95th percentile of normal). ●, NCAH; ○, hyperandrogenic patients with a mild exaggeration in their 17-HP response to ACTH-(1-24). (From Azziz R, Zacur HA. 21-Hydroxylase deficiency in female hyperandrogenism: screening and diagnosis. *J Clin Endocrinol Metab* 1989;69:577–584, with permission.)

still lacking. In general, few normoovulatory patients demonstrate significant insulin resistance (and hyperinsulinemia), and screening may be restricted to those patients with oligo-anovulation. Furthermore, it appears that approximately 40% to 50% of hyperinsulinemic patients may require insulin and glucose measurement after a glucose challenge for detection. Finally, it should be remembered that measurements of insulin and glucose levels do not directly assess the degree of insulin resistance, rather the compensatory hypersecretion of insulin by the pancreatic islet cells. Hence, if β-cell dysfunction is evident, as in patients with glucose intolerance or NIDDM, the value of insulin and glucose levels as a screening tool for insulin resistance is void.

In contrast to those tests excluding related disorders, the value of androgen measures in patients who demonstrate obvious androgenic signs and symptoms is less clear. For example, although some have proposed total T and DHS levels as a screening tool for the detection of androgenic tumors, we found these tests to have a very limited predictive value (160). However, measurements of free T and DHS may be useful for establishing the presence of hyperandrogenemia in a patient with oligoovulation and minimal peripheral features of androgen excess. Although A4 is easily measured, it is of limited value in most patients, but it may be useful in monitoring therapy in patients with NCAH.

TREATMENT OF HIRSUTISM

The treatment of hirsutism should be undertaken *as soon as the diagnosis is established.* Although in young children or adolescents the degree of hair growth may not be as severe as that encountered in adult women, it must be remembered that these disorders usually are progressive and the appearance of terminal hairs not readily reversible. Any terminal hairs remaining after 6 months of adequate suppression with medical therapy must be removed by electrolysis, which can be painful and costly. Hirsutism is not only cosmetically disfiguring, but it can become a significant handicap to a young woman's social life and emotional stability. Furthermore, diagnosing patients with PCOS or the HAIRAN syndrome can have profound medical implications, because these disorders are associated with an increased risk of Type 2 DM, dyslipidemia, hypertension, and cardiovascular disease (114,115). Hyperandrogenic oligomenorrhea also can lead to the development of endometrial hyperplasia and subsequent carcinoma at a young age (165–167). Overall, 30% to 50% of adolescents with oligomenorrhea demonstrate hyperandrogenemia, which may be persistent in 50% of these girls (75–77).

The prime objective of hormonal treatment of hirsutism is stopping the development of new terminal hairs. Hormonal therapy also slows the growth and reduces the diameter and pigmentation of terminal hairs already present. However, it is slow to reverse the transformation of vellus to terminal hairs, and this will be incomplete at best. It is important to emphasize that therapy for hirsutism may take up to 6 months before a clinical response is noted. Hormonal therapy should be combined with mechanical methods of hair control.

Mechanical/Cosmetic Means of Hair Growth Control

Mechanical means of hair removal by themselves do little to affect the long-term course of hirsutism. However, while awaiting the full effect of hormonal therapy, it may be best to encourage the patient to *shave* (either with a blade or a machine) because this causes the least trauma to the skin. Although shaving can lead to a blunt hair end, which may feel "stubble-like," it does not lead to a worsening of hirsutism. It is surprising what satisfactory cosmetic results shaving and the proper application of make-up can produce. Recording the interval between shavings before each office visit also provides a relatively simple way to monitor the efficacy of treatment. *Plucking* or *waxing* should be discouraged because they may stimulate the growth of surrounding follicles and may lead to folliculitis with subsequent development of ingrown hairs. *Depilating agents,* particularly on the face, can lead to skin irritation and worsening of hirsutism. *Electrolysis* is the only method available for the irreversible destruction of hair follicles. It may not be applicable to large areas of the body including sensitive areas, such as the periareolar region. As indicated earlier, electrolysis should be combined with hormonal therapy, after a clinical response has been observed, for maximum cosmetic benefit. Most recently, the use of lasers have been proposed for the treatment of unwanted hairs, although their efficacy remains to be demonstrated.

Hormonal Therapy

Hormonal therapy consists of drugs that primarily suppress androgen secretion from the ovary, the adrenal, or both; and drugs that primarily inhibit the action of androgens at the periphery, i.e., the skin.

Suppression of Androgen Secretion

Oral Contraceptives

The mainstay of androgen excess treatment are oral concentrative pills (OCPs) that, by suppressing the secretion of gonadotropins (LH and FSH), lead to a decrease in ovarian androgen production (168). Full suppression usually is seen within the month. OCPs also decrease adrenal androgen production by a mechanism not yet clear, but may be related to a decrease in circulating ACTH. The progestin in OCPs can also compete for 5α-reductase and the androgen receptor. The estrogen fraction in the OCPs increases circulating SHBG, with a subsequent decrease in free T levels. Because the progestin in OCPs may in turn decrease SHBG, it is most important to select a pill whose progestin is the least androgenic (e.g., ethynodiol diacetate, desogesterel, norethindrone acetate). Birth control pills should be administered in the usual cyclic fashion, and the circulating androgen levels should be checked periodically to assess the adequacy of hormonal suppression.

Retrospective studies of women developing postpill amenorrhea have observed that between 37% and 63% of these patients had a history of oligomenorrhea (169,170), which appears to be higher than the incidence in the general population and has led to the recommendation that OCP administration be contraindicated in oligomenorrheic adolescents. However, the incidence of postpill amenorrhea appears to be relatively low, occurring in less than 0.5% of women taking OCPs (169). Furthermore, the incidence of hyperandrogenemia in adolescent amenorrhea is high (75,76,171) and OCP administration leads to a suppression of their androgen levels (171), although after cessation of therapy androgen levels return to pretreatment levels. It is probable that oligomenorrheic patients who develop postpill amenorrhea simply demonstrate a recurrence of their original pathology, and OCP use actually suppresses the coexisting hyperandrogenemia, with a consequent delay in the appearance of clinical signs such as acne and hirsutism.

Long-acting Gonadotropin-releasing Hormone Analogues

A long-acting GnRH agonist (e.g., leuprolide acetate [Lupron] depot 3.75 mg per month) may be required to suppress the hypothalamic-pituitary-ovarian axis in severely androgenized patients (145,155,156). This drug is particularly useful in patients with low circulating levels of LH and high levels of T, presumed to arise from nonneoplastic ovaries. As noted earlier, most of these patients have severe insulin resistance and hyperinsulinism. It may take 2 or 3 months for the full suppressive effect of the agonist to occur. Long-acting GnRH agonist treatment should be accompanied by estrogen/progestin replacement or an oral contraceptive to reduce the hypoestrogenic side effects (hot flushes, genital dryness, osteoporosis) and

increase circulating SHBG levels. This therapy can be combined with an antiandrogen (see later) for maximum control of hair growth (146,156).

Glucocorticoids

Dexamethasone 0.25 to 0.5 mg every evening to every other evening or prednisone 5 to 10 mg daily can be used as an adjuvant for the treatment of hirsutism (172–176), particularly in patients suffering from NCAH or CAH or in those with significant acne. However, glucocorticoids alone appear to have a limited effect on ovulatory dysfunction (177) or hair growth (172,178). They may be associated with the development of weight gain and osteoporosis.

Ketoconazole

KTZ, an imidazole antimycotic agent, is a known inhibitor of P450 steroidogenic enzymes, specifically $P450_{ssc}$, $P45017\alpha$, and $P450_{arom}$. Vidal-Puig and colleagues (179) prospectively treated 26 women with hirsutism, acne, and oligomenorrhea using low-dose KTZ (400 mg per day) for 9 months. All patients experienced a significant decrease in hirsutism and reduction in circulating total T, DHS, A4, and LH, but little change in circulating SHBG, estradiol, and cortisol. Side effects, including dyspepsia, dysfunctional uterine bleeding, alopecia, and elevated transaminase levels, caused the withdrawal of 30% of the patients from one of these studies. These problems generally normalize after discontinuation of KTZ (144).

Insulin-sensitizing Agents

Because up to 70% of hirsute patients have PCOS or hairan syndrome with overt insulin resistance, hyperinsulinism and dyslipidemia, the administration of insulin-sensitizing agents, principally metformin and troglitazone, have been proposed as treatment. These agents have various potential advantages over traditional therapies, including (i) correcting both the metabolic and the endocrinologic aberrations of the disorder; (ii) permitting the resumption of normal endogenous ovulatory function, with little or no risk of ovarian hyperstimulation and multiple gestation; and (iii) possibly decreasing the long-term risk of NIDDM and cardiovascular disease. Nonetheless, it is important to note that only small studies and/or preliminary data on the use of these agents in PCOS have been published (104–108). Conclusive data regarding outcome, patient selection, and risks and complications, although in the process of being collected, are not yet available.

Peripheral Androgen Suppression

Spironolactone

Spironolactone (SPA) is an aldosterone antagonist and a mild diuretic. It is an effective therapy for hirsutism (180–186), competing for the androgen receptor 5α-reductase and the binding of T to SHBG (187). Furthermore, SPA blocks the action of various enzymes involved in androgen biosynthesis (187–189). Initially a dose as high as 200 mg per day can be used. If the dose is slowly increased from 25 to 200 mg per day, by 25-mg increments every 3 days or so, patients will develop a minimum of side effects. The side effects most commonly associated with SPA use include dyspepsia, nausea, polyuria, fatigue, headaches, and irregular menses. The incidence of metrorrhagia may be decreased by administering the SPA days 4 through 21 of the menstrual cycle (190). Hypertensive patients on a potassium-saving diuretic may rarely develop hyperkalemia.

SPA is extremely effective for treating hirsutism, particularly IH. Treatment should be continued for at least 1 year with a subsequent reduction in dose. Because SPA acts through mechanisms different from that of OCPs, it is possible to improve the overall therapeutic effectiveness by combining these medications (191,192). Furthermore, the use of OCPs or estrogen/progestin therapy in combination with SPA minimize the problems with dysfunctional uterine bleeding or worsening

oligomenorrhea often observed in women using SPA alone, while providing adequate contraception (191–193).

Flutamide

Flutamide is an androgen receptor blocker approved by the Food and Drug Administration (FDA) as adjuvant treatment for prostate cancer. It appears to be an effective treatment for hirsutism when given in doses of 250 to 500 mg daily (194–196). Side effects include liver enzyme abnormalities, appearance of greenish urine, and excessive dryness of skin or scalp hair. It has some teratogenic potential, as does SPA. It appears to be as effective as SPA in randomized trials (194,195).

Cyproterone Acetate

Cyproterone acetate (CPA) is a strong progestin and antiandrogen, and it is an effective treatment for hirsutism (197). It produces a decrease in circulating T and A levels through a reduction in LH. Furthermore, CPA antagonizes the effect of androgens at the androgen receptor level. Side effects may include adrenal insufficiency and loss of libido. This drug currently is not available in the United States.

Finasteride

Finasteride is a 5α-reductase inhibitor approved by the FDA for treatment of benign prostatic hyperplasia. When given at 5 mg per day, it may be useful for treatment of hirsutism in women (198), despite a paradoxic increase in circulating T levels. Teratogenicity (i.e., feminization of a male infant) is a major concern.

Surgical Treatment of Androgen Excess

In the past, ovarian wedge resection has been used with satisfactory results (199,200). More recently, laparoscopic wedge resection (201) or fulguration of multiple areas of the ovarian cortex has been proposed (202–204), although long-term controlled follow-up information is lacking. In general, these destructive procedures should be used as line of last defense, because they frequently lead to ovarian adhesions. It is a rare patient who requires a bilateral ovarian wedge resection, particularly an adolescent. The use of a long-acting GnRH agonist may be a better method of treating these patients, because the agonist produces a medical "oophorectomy" without the surgical risk or possibility of adnexal adhesions. Rarely are individuals so affected that a bilateral oophorectomy need be considered, although this may be applicable in some severely affected young girls who have little hope of improvement otherwise (e.g., those with HAIRAN syndrome). However, these patients are very much the exception.

Therapeutic Goals and Long-term Expectations

It is important to emphasize that therapy for hirsutism may take 6 or 8 months for a difference to be observed. Furthermore, the purpose of hormonal therapy is to correct the underlying problem, to stop new hairs from growing, and *potentially* to slow the growth of terminal hairs already present. Hormonal therapy alone sometimes will produce a thinning and a loss of pigmentation of terminal hairs; however, it usually will not reverse vellus to terminal hair transformation. In general, acne improves more readily than hirsutism, observable within 2 to 8 weeks.

During therapy, circulating androgen and SHBG levels may be monitored to assess the adequacy of hormonal therapy. Oral contraceptives and estrogen should result in an increase in SHBG levels. Oral contraceptives, GnRH analogues, progestins, and estrogens should normalize the circulating level of T; corticosteroids will suppress DHS levels.

It is important to stress that improvement will be slow and that terminal hairs already present will not disappear. The total removal of these already androgenized hair follicles will require electrolysis, once hormonal therapy has exerted its effect, usually after approximately 6 months of therapy. Finally, patients who suffer from hirsutism require long-term follow-up counseling and emotional support because this problem can be particularly distressing. Because androgen excess is an endocrine disorder with metabolic ramifications, patients with this disorder should be counseled that they are at increased risk for other problems, notably heart disease and diabetes.

REFERENCES

1. James VHT, Goodall A. Androgen production in women. In: Jeffcoate SL, ed. *Androgens and anti-androgen therapy.* New York: John Wiley & Sons, 1982;23–40.
2. Mahoudeau JA, Bardin CW, Lipsett MB. The metabolic clearance rate and origin of plasma dihydrotestosterone in man and its conversion to the 5-alpha-androstenediols. *J Clin Invest* 1971;50:1338–1344.
3. Ito T, Horton R. The source of plasma dihydrotestosterone in man. *J Clin Invest* 1971;50:1621–1627.
4. Rosenfeld RS, Rosenberg BJ, Fukushima DK, et al. 24-Hour secretory pattern of dehydroisoandrosterone and dehydro-isoandrosterone sulfate. *J Clin Endocrinol Metab* 1975;40:850–855.
5. Huq MS, Pfaff M, Jespersen D, et al. Concurrence of aldosterone, androgen and cortisol secretion in adrenal venous effluents. *J Clin Endocrinol Metab* 1976;42:230–238.
6. Suzuki T. Circadian rhythm of adrenocortical secretory activity. In: Suzuki T, ed. *Physiology of adrenocortical secretion.* New York: Karger, 1983;72–191.
7. Kato T, Horton R. Studies of testosterone binding globulin. *J Clin Endocrinol Metab* 1968;28:1160–1168.
8. Dunn JF, Nisula BC, Rodbard D. Transport of steroid hormones: binding of 21 endogenous steroids to both testosterone-binding globulin and corticosteroid-binding globulin in human plasma. *J Clin Endocrinol Metab* 1981;53:58–68.
9. Rosenfield RL. Plasma testosterone binding globulin and indexes of the concentration of unbound plasma androgens in normal and hirsute subjects. *J Clin Endocrinol Metab* 1971;32:717–728.
10. Vermeulen A, Verdonck L, Van der Straeten M, et al. Capacity of the testosterone-binding globulin in human plasma and influence of specific binding of testosterone on its metabolic clearance rate. *J Clin Endocrinol Metab* 1969;29:1470–1480.
11. Plymate R, Leonard JM, Paulsen CA, et al. Sex hormone-binding globulin changes with androgen replacement. *J Clin Endocrinol Metab* 1983;57:645–648.
12. Tochimoto S, Olivo J, Southren AL, et al. Studies of plasma β-globulin: sex difference and effect of ethinyl estradiol and testosterone. *Proc Soc Exp Biol Med* 1970;134:700–702.
13. Musa BU, Doe RP, Seal US. Serum protein alterations produced in women by synthetic estrogens. *J Clin Endocrinol Metab* 1967;27:1463–1469.
14. Chetkowski RJ, Meldrum DR, Steingold KA, et al. Biologic effects of transdermal estradiol. *N Engl J Med* 1986;314:1615–1620.
15. Azziz R. Reproductive endocrinologic alteration in female asymptomatic obesity. *Fertil Steril* 1989;52:703–725.

16. Ducharme JR, Collu R. Pubertal development: normal, precocious and delayed. In: Ducharme JR, Collu R, eds. *Clinics in endocrinology and metabolism,* vol. 11. Philadelphia: WB Saunders, 1982:57–87.

17. Korth-Schultz S, Levine LS, New MI. Serum androgens in normal prepubertal and pubertal children and in children with precocious adrenarche. *J Clin Endocrinol Metab* 1976;42:117–124.

18. Apter D, Lenko HL, Perheentupa J, et al. Subnormal pubertal increases of serum androgens in Turner's Syndrome. *Horm Res* 1982;16:164–173.

19. Moll GW Jr, Rosenfield RL. Plasma free testosterone in the diagnosis of adolescent polycystic ovary syndrome. *J Pediatr* 1983;102:461–464.

20. Apter D, Vihko R. Serum pregnenolone, progesterone, 17-hydroxyprogesterone, testosterone and 5α-dihydrotestosterone during female puberty. *J Clin Endocrinol Metab* 1977;45:1039–1048.

21. Collu R, Ducharme R. Role of adrenal steroids in the initiation of pubertal mechanisms. In: James VHT, Giusti MS, Giusti G, et al, eds. *The endocrine function of the human adrenal cortex. Proceedings of the Serono Symposia,* vol. 18. New York: Academic Press, 1978: 547–559.

22. Pintor C, Facchinetti F, Puggioni R, et al. Effect of short dexamethasone suppression on plasma steroids in prepubertal and pubertal girls. *J Endocrinol Invest* 1980;3: 25–28.

23. Belgorosky A, Rivarola MA. Progressive increase in nonsex hormone-binding globulin-bound testosterone and estradiol from infancy to late prepuberty in girls. *J Clin Endocrinol Metab* 1988;67:234–237.

24. Cunningham SK, Loughlin T, Culliton M, et al. Plasma sex hormone-binding globulin levels decrease during the second decade of life irrespective of pubertal status. *J Clin Endocrinol Metab* 1984;58:915–918.

25. De Peretti E, Forest MG. Unconjugated dehydroepiandrosterone plasma levels in normal subjects from birth to adolescence in human: the use of a sensitive radioimmunoassay. *J Clin Endocrinol Metab* 1976;43:982–991.

26. Sizonenko PC, Paunier L. Hormonal changes in puberty III: correlation of plasma dehydroepiandrosterone, testosterone, FSH, and LH with stages of puberty and bone age in normal boys and girls and in patients with Addison's disease or hypogonadism or with premature or late adrenarche. *J Clin Endocrinol Metab* 1975;41:894–904.

27. Korth-Schutz S, Levine LS, New MI. Dehydroepiandrosterone sulfate (DS) levels, a rapid test for abnormal adrenal androgen secretion. *J Clin Endocrinol Metab* 1976;42:1005–1013.

28. Pintor C, Genazzani AR, Carboni G, et al. Adrenal androgens and pubertal development in physiological and pathological conditions. In: Genazzani AR, et al, eds. *Adrenal androgens.* New York: Raven Press, 1980: 173–181.

29. Dhom G. The prepuberal and puberal growth of the adrenal (adrenarche). *Beitr Path Bd* 1973;150:357–377.

30. Kelnar CJH, Brook CGD. A mixed longitudinal study of adrenal steroid excretion in childhood and the mechanism of adrenarche. *Clin Endocrinol (Oxf)* 1983;19: 117–129.

31. Rich BH, Rosenfield RL, Lucky AW, et al. Adrenarche: changing adrenal response to adrenocorticotropin. *J Clin Endocrinol Metab* 1981;52:1129–1136.

32. Schiebinger RJ, Albertson BD, Cassorla FG, et al. The developmental changes in plasma adrenal androgens during infancy and adrenarche are associated with changing activities of adrenal microsomal 17-hydroxylase and 17,20-desmolase. *J Clin Invest* 1981;67: 1177–1182.

33. Farah LA, Knochenhauer ES, Boots LR, et al. Normal adrenarche: a longitudinal study. 46th Annual Meeting of the Society for Gynecologic Investigation, Atlanta, GA, March 10–13, 1999, abstract P-495.

34. Counts DR, Pescovitz OH, Barnes KM, et al. Dissociation of adrenarche and gonadarche in precocious puberty and in isolated hypogonadotropic hypogonadism. *J Clin Endocrinol Metab* 1987;64:1174–1178.

35. Grumbach MM, Richards GE, Conte FA, et al. Clinical disorders of adrenal function and puberty: an assessment of the role of the adrenal cortex in normal and abnormal puberty in man and evidence for an ACTH-like pituitary adrenal androgen stimulating hormone. In: James VHT, Giusti MS, Giusti G, et al, eds. *The endocrine function of the human adrenal cortex. Proceedings of the Serono Symposia,* vol. 18. New York: Academic Press, 1978:583–612.

36. Parker LN, Odell WD. Control of adrenal androgen secretion. *Endocr Rev* 1980;1:392–410.

37. Parker L, Lifrak E, Shively JE, et al. Human adrenal gland cortical androgen-stimulating hormone (CASH) is identical with a portion of the joining peptide of pituitary pro-opiomelanocortin (POMC). 71st Endocrine Society Annual Meeting, 1989, Seattle, WA, abstract 299.

38. Forest MG, de Peretti E, Bertrand J. Developmental patterns of the plasma levels of testosterone, Δ^4–androstenedione, 17α-hydroxyprogesterone, dehydroepiandrosterone and its sulfate in normal infants and prepubertal children. In: James VHT, Giusti MS, Giusti G, et al, eds. *The endocrine function of the human adrenal cortex. Proceedings of the Serono Symposia,* vol. 18. New York: Academic Press, 1978:561–582.

39. Avgerinos PC, Butler Jr, GB, Tsokos GC, et al. Dissociation between cortisol and adrenal androgen secretion in patients receiving alternate day prednisone therapy. *J Clin Endocrinol Metab* 1987;65:24–29.

40. Parker CR Jr, Baxter CR. Divergence in adrenal steroid secretory pattern after thermal injury in adult patients. *J Trauma* 1985;25:508–510.

41. Lephart ED, Baxter CR, Parker CR Jr. Effect of burn trauma on adrenal and testicular steroid hormone production. *J Clin Endocrinol Metab* 1987;64:842–848.

42. Kreitzer PM, Blethen SL, Festa RS, et al. Dehydroepiandrosterone sulfate levels are not suppressible by glucocorticoids before adrenarche. *J Clin Endocrinol Metab* 1989;69:1309–1311.

43. Dickerman Z, Grant DR, Faiman C, et al. Intraadrenal steroid concentrations in man: zonal differences and developmental changes. *J Clin Endocrinol Metab* 1984; 59:1031–1036.

44. Hornsby PJ, Aldern KA. Steroidogenic enzyme activities in cultured human definitive zone adrenocortical cells: comparison with bovine adrenocortical cells and resultant differences in adrenal androgen synthesis. *J Clin Endocrinol Metab* 1984;58:121–127.

45. Uno H. Biology of hair growth. *Semin Reprod Endocrinol* 1986;4:131–141.

46. Bernstein RM, Rassaman WR. The aesthetics of follicular transplantation. *Dermatol Surg* 1997;23:785–799.

47. Bernstein RM, Rassaman WR. Follicular transplantation: patient evaluation and surgical planning. *Dermatol Surg* 1997;23:771–784.

48. McKenna TJ, Loughlin T, Daly L, et al. Variable clinical and hormonal manifestations of hyperandrogenemia. *Metabolism* 1984;33:714–717.

49. Carmina E, Koyama T, Chang L, et al. Does ethnicity influence the prevalence of adrenal hyperandrogenism and insulin resistance in polycystic ovary syndrome? *Am J Obstet Gynecol* 1992;167:1807–1812.

50. Ginsberg GS, Birnbaum MD, Rose LI. Androgen abnormalities in acne vulgaris. *Acta Derm Venereol* 1981;61: 431–434.

51. Marynick SP, Chakmakjian ZH, McCaffree DL, et al. Androgen excess in cystic acne. *N Engl J Med* 1983; 308:981–1025.

52. Vexiau P, Husson C, Chivot M, et al. Androgen excess in women with acne alone compared with women with acne and/or hirsutism. *J Invest Dermatol* 1990;94:279–283.

53. Pekkarinen A, Sonck CE. Adrenocortical reserves in acne vulgaris. *Acta Derm Venereol* 1962;42:200–210.

54. Darley CR, Moore JW, Besser GM, et al. Androgen status in women with late onset or persistent acne vulgaris. *Clin Exp Dermatol* 1984;9:28–35.

55. Steinberger E, Rodriguez-Rigau LJ, Smith KD, et al. The menstrual cycle and plasma testosterone levels in women with acne. *J Am Acad Dermatol* 1981;4:54–58.

56. Lucky AW, McGuire J, Rosenfield RL, et al. Plasma androgens in women with acne vulgaris. *J Invest Dermatol* 1983;81:70–74.

57. Lawrence DM, Katz M, Robinson TWE, et al. Reduced sex hormone binding globulin and derived free testosterone levels in women with severe acne. *Clin Endocrinol (Oxf)* 1981;15:87–91.

58. Held BL, Nader S, Rodriguez-Rigau LJ, et al. Acne and hyperandrogenism. *J Am Acad Dermatol* 1984;10:112–226.

59. van der Meeren HLM, Thijssen JHH. Circulating androgens in male acne. *Br J Dermatol* 1984;110:609–611.

60. Sultan C, Oliel V, Audran F, et al. Free and total plasma testosterone in men and women with acne. *Acta Derm Venereol* 1986;66:301–304.

61. Sheehan-Dare RA, Hughes BR, Cunliffe WJ. Clinical markers of androgenicity in acne vulgaris. *Br J Dermatol* 1988;119:723–730.

62. Levell MJ, Cawood ML, Burke B, et al. Acne is not associated with abnormal plasma androgens. *Br J Dermatol* 1989;120:649–654.

63. Sansone G, Reisner RM. Differential rates of conversion of testosterone to dihydrotestosterone in acne and in normal human skin—a possible pathogenic factor in acne. *J Invest Dermatol* 1971;56:366–372.

64. Lookingbill DP, Horton R, Demers LM, et al. Tissue production of androgens in women with acne. *J Am Acad Dermatol* 1985;12:481–487.

65. Hay JB, Hodgins MB. Metabolism of androgens by human skin in acne. *Br J Dermatol* 1974;91:123–133.

66. Slayden SM, Sams WM Jr, Azziz R. Hyperandrogenemia (HA) is a frequent cause of acne, regardless of age of presentation. Proceedings of the 52nd Annual Meeting of the American Society of Reproductive Medicine, Nov. 2–6, 1996;546.

67. Palatsi R, Reinila M, Kivinen S. Pituitary function and DHEA-S in male acne and DHEA-S, prolactin and cortisol before and after oral contraceptive treatment in female acne. *Acta Derm Venereol* 1986;66:225–230.

68. Hammerstein J, Moltz L, Schwartz U. Antiandrogens in the treatment of acne and hirsutism. *J Steroid Biochem* 1983;19:591–597.

69. Darley CR, Moore JW, Besser GM, et al. Low dose prednisolone or oestrogen in the treatment of women with late onset or persistent acne vulgaris. *Br J Dermatol* 1983;108:345–353.

70. Goodfellow A, Alaghband-Zadeh J, Carter G, et al. Oral spironolactone improves acne vulgaris and reduces sebum excretion. *Br J Dermatol* 1984;II:209–214.

71. Muhlemann MF, Carter GD, Cream JJ, et al. Oral spironolactone: an effective treatment for acne vulgaris in women. *Br J Dermatol* 1986;115:227–232.

72. Nader S, Rodriguez-Rigau LJ, Smith KD, et al. Acne and hyperandrogenism: impact of lowering androgen levels with glucocorticoid treatment. *J Am Acad Dermatol* 1984;11:256–259.

73. Ettinger B, Goldfield B, Burrill E, et al. Plasma testosterone stimulation-suppression dynamics in hirsute women. *Am J Med* 1973;54:195–200.

74. Futterweit W, Deligdisch L. Histopathological effects of exogenously administered testosterone in 19 female to male transsexuals. *J Clin Endocrinol Metab* 1986;62: 16–21.

75. Siegberg R, Nilsson CG, Stenman UH, et al. Endocrinologic features of oligomenorrheic adolescent girls. *Fertil Steril* 1986;46:852–857.

76. Emans SJ, Grace E, Goldstein DP. Oligomenorrhea in adolescent girls. *J Pediatr* 1980;97:815–819.

77. Venturoli S, Porcu E, Fabbri R, et al. Postmenarchal evolution of endocrine pattern and ovarian aspects in adolescents with menstrual irregularities. *Fertil Steril* 1987;48:78–85.

78. Venturoli S, Porcu E, Fabbri R, et al. Longitudinal evaluation of different gonadotropin pulsatile patterns in anovulatory cycles of young girls. *J Clin Endocrinol Metab* 1992;74:836–841.

79. Apter D, Vihko R. Endocrine determinants of fertility: serum androgen concentrations during follow-up of adolescents into the third decade of life. *J Clin Endocrinol Metab* 1990;71:970–974.

80. Ibanez L, Potau N, Zampolli M, et al. Hyperinsulinemia in postpubertal girls with a history of premature pubarche and functional ovarian hyperandrogenism. *J Clin Endocrinol Metab* 1996;81:1237–1243.

81. Apter D, Butzow T, Laughlin GA, et al. Metabolic features of polycystic ovary syndrome are found in adolescent girls with hyperandrogenism. *J Clin Endocrinol Metab* 1995;80:2966–2973.

82. Apter D, Butzow T, Laughlin GA, et al. Accelerated 24-hour luteinizing hormone pulsatile activity in adolescent girls with ovarian hyperandrogenism: relevance to the developmental phase of polycystic ovarian syndrome. *J Clin Endocrinol Metab* 1994;79:970–974.

83. Knochenhauer ES, Key TJ, Kahsar-Miller M, et al. Prevalence of the polycystic ovarian syndrome in unselected Black and White women of the Southeastern United States: a prospective study. *J Clin Endocrinol Metab* 1998;83:3078–3082.

84. Zawadzki JK, Dunaif A. Diagnostic criteria for polycystic ovary syndrome: towards a rational approach. In: Dunaif A, Givens JR, Haseltine F, et al, eds. *Polycystic ovary syndrome.* Boston: Blackwell Scientific Publications, 1992:377–384.

85. Mathur RS, Moody LO, Landgrebe S, et al. Plasma androgens and sex hormone-binding globulin in the evaluation of hirsute females. *Fertil Steril* 1981;35: 29–35.

86. Vermeulen A, Stoica T, Verdonck L. The apparent free testosterone concentration, an index of androgenicity. *J Clin Endocrinol* 1971;33:759–767.

87. Hoffman DI, Klove K, Lobo RA. The prevalence and significance of elevated dehydroepiandrosterone sulfate levels in anovulatory women. *Fertil Steril* 1984; 42:76–81.

88. Luciano AA, Chapler FK, Sherman BM. Hyperprolactinemia in polycystic ovary syndrome. *Fertil Steril* 1984;41:719–725.

89. Carmina E, Rosato F, Maggiore M, et al. Prolactin secretion in polycystic ovary syndrome (PCO): correlation with the steroid pattern. *Acta Endocrinol (Copenh)* 1984;105:99–104.

90. Taymor ML, Barnard R. Luteinizing hormone excretion in the polycystic ovary syndrome. *Fertil Steril* 1962;13:501–512.

91. Yen SSC, Vela P, Rankin J. Inappropriate secretion of follicle-stimulating hormone and luteinizing hormone in polycystic ovarian disease. *J Clin Endocrinol Metab* 1970;30:435–442.

92. Kazer RR, Kessel B, Yen SSC. Circulating luteinizing hormone pulse frequency in women with polycystic ovary syndrome. *J Clin Endocrinol Metab* 1987;65: 233–236.

93. Swanson M, Sauerbrei EE, Cooperberg PL. Medical implications of ultrasonically detected polycystic ovaries. *J Clin Ultrasound* 1981;9:219–222.

94. Polson DW, Wadsworth J, Adams J, et al. Polycystic ovaries—a common finding in normal women. *Lancet* 1988;1:870–872.

95. el Tabbakh GH, Lotfy I, Azab I, et al. Correlation of the ultrasonic appearance of the ovaries in polycystic ovarian disease and the clinical, hormonal, and laparoscopic findings. *Am J Obstet Gynecol* 1986;154: 892–895.

96. Orsini LF, Venturoli S, Lorusso R, et al. Ultrasonic findings in polycystic ovarian disease. *Fertil Steril* 1985;43:709–714.

97. Goldzieher JW, Green JA. The polycystic ovary. I. Clinical and histologic features. *J Clin Endocrinol Metab* 1962;22:325–338.

98. Hosseinian AH, Kim MH, Rosenfield RL. Obesity and oligomenorrhea are associated with hyperandrogenism independent of hirsutism. *J Clin Endocrinol Metab* 1976;42:765–769.

99. Lobo RA, Goebelsmann U, Horton R. Evidence for the importance of peripheral tissue events in the development of hirsutism in polycystic ovary syndrome. *J Clin Endocrinol Metab* 1983;57:393–397.

100. Stanhope R, Adams J, Brook CGD. Evolution of polycystic ovaries in a girl with delayed menarche. *J Reprod Med* 1988;33:482–484.

101. Canales ES, Zarate A, Castelazo-Ayala L. Primary amenorrhea associated with polycystic ovaries. *Obstet Gynecol* 1971;37:205–210.

102. Rao JK, Chihal HJ, Johnson CM. Primary polycystic ovary syndrome in a premenarchal girl. *J Reprod Med* 1985;30:361–365.

103. Dunaif A. Insulin resistance and the polycystic ovary syndrome: mechanism and implications for pathogenesis. *Endocr Rev* 1997;18:774–800.

104. Velazquez EM, Mendoza S, Hamer T, et al. Metformin therapy in polycystic ovary syndrome reduced hyperinsulinemia, insulin resistance, hyperandrogenemia, and systolic blood pressure, while facilitating normal menses and pregnancy. *Metabolism* 1994;43:647–654.

105. Velasquez E, Acosta A, Mendoza SG. Menstrual cyclicity after metformin therapy in polycystic ovary syndrome. *Obstet Gynecol* 1997;90:392–395.

106. Dunaif A, Scott D, Finegood D, et al. The insulin-sensitizing agent troglitazone improves metabolic and reproductive abnormalities in the polycystic ovary syndrome. *J Clin Endocrinol Metab* 1996;81:3299–3306.

107. Ehrmann DA, Schneider DJ, Sobel BE, et al. Troglitazone improves defects in insulin action, insulin secretion, ovarian steroidogenesis, and fibrinolysis in women with polycystic ovary syndrome. *J Clin Endocrinol Metab* 1997;82:2108–2116.

108. Nestler JE, Jakubowicz DJ, Evans WS, et al. Effects of metformin on spontaneous and clomiphene-induced ovulation in the polycystic ovary syndrome. *N Engl J Med* 1998;338:1876–1880.

109. Ciaraldi TM, El-Roeiy A, Madar Z, et al. Cellular mechanisms of insulin resistance in polycystic ovarian syndrome. *J Clin Endocrinol Metab* 1992;75:577–583.

110. Dunaif A, Xia J, Book C-B, et al. Excessive insulin receptor phosphorylation in cultured fibroblasts and in skeletal muscle: a potential mechanism for insulin resistance in the polycystic ovary syndrome. *J Clin Invest* 1995;96:801–810.

111. Marsden PJ, Murdoch A, Taylor R. Severe impairment of insulin action in adipocytes from amenorrheic subjects with polycystic ovary syndrome. *Metab Clin Exp* 1994;43:1536–1542.

112. Ciaraldi TP, Morales AJ, Hickman MG, et al. Cellular insulin resistance in adipocytes from obese polycystic ovary syndrome subjects involves adenosine modulation of insulin sensitivity. *J Clin Endocrinol Metab* 1997;82:1421–1425.

113. Olefsky JM, Ciaraldi TP, Kolterman OG, et al. Mechanism of insulin resistance in obesity and non-insulin-dependent diabetes mellitus: role of receptor and post-receptor defects. In: Skyler JS, ed. *Insulin update*. Amsterdam, The Netherlands: Excerpta Medica, 1982:41–73.

114. Dahlgren E, Johansson S, Lindstedt G, et al. Women with polycystic ovary syndrome wedge resected in 1956 to 1965: a long-term follow-up focusing on natural history and circulating hormones. *Fertil Steril* 1992;57:505–513.

115. Legro RS, Kunselman AR, Dodson WC, et al. Prevalence and predictors of risk for type 2 diabetes mellitus and impaired glucose tolerance in polycystic ovary syndrome: a prospective, controlled study in 254 affected women. *J Clin Endocrinol Metab* 1999;84:165–169.

116. Kahsar-Miller M, Azziz R. The development of the polycystic ovary syndrome: family history as a risk factor. *Trends Endocrinol Metab* 1998;9:55–61.

117. Ibanez L, Potau N, Fabbri R, et al. Postpubertal outcome in girls diagnosed of premature pubarche during childhood: increase frequency of functional ovarian hyperandrogenism. *J Clin Endocrinol Metab* 1993;76: 1599–1603.

118. Lazar L, Kauli R, Bruchis C, et al. Early polycystic ovary-like syndrome in girls with central precocious puberty and exaggerated adrenal response. *Eur J Endocrinol* 1995;133:403–406.

119. Azziz R, Waggoner WT, Ochoa T, et al. Idiopathic hirsutism: an uncommon cause of hirsutism in Alabama. *Fertil Steril* 1998;70:274–278.

120. Gompel A, Wright F, Kuttenn F, et al. Contribution of plasma androstenedione to 5α-androstanediol glucuronide in women with idiopathic hirsutism. *J Clin Endocrinol Metab* 1986;62:441–444.

121. Greep N, Hoopes M, Horton R. Androstanediol glucuronide plasma clearance and production rates in normal and hirsute women. *J Clin Endocrinol Metab* 1986;62:22–27.

122. New MI, Levine LS. *Congenital adrenal hyperplasia.* New York: Springer-Verlag, 1984.

123. Giusti G, Manelli M, Forti G, et al. Plasma steroid values in congenital adrenocortical hyperplasia. In: James VHT, Giusti MS, Giusti G, et al, eds. *The endocrine function of the human adrenal cortex,* vol. 18. New York: Academic Press, 1978:271–287.

124. Griffiths KD, Anderson JM, Rudd BT, et al. Plasma renin activity in the management of congenital adrenal hyperplasia. *Arch Dis Child* 1984;59:360–365.

125. Mulaikal RM, Migeon CJ, Rock JA. Fertility rates in female patients with congenital adrenal hyperplasia due to 21-hydroxylase deficiency. *N Engl J Med* 1987; 316:178–182.

126. Azziz R, Mulaikal RM, Migeon CJ, et al. Congenital adrenal hyperplasia: long-term results following vaginal reconstruction. *Fertil Steril* 1986;46:1011–1014.

127. Azziz R, Dewailly D, Owerbach D. Non-classic adrenal hyperplasia: current concepts. *J Clin Endocrinol Metab* 1994;78:810–815.

128. Kuttenn F, Couillin P, Girard F, et al. Late-onset adrenal hyperplasia in hirsutism. *N Engl J Med* 1985;313: 224–231.

129. Dewailly D, Vantyghem-Haudiquet MC, Sainsard C, et al. Clinical and biological phenotypes in late-onset 21-hydroxylase deficiency. *J Clin Endocrinol Metab* 1986;63:418–423.

130. Azziz R, Zacur HA. 21-Hydroxylase deficiency in female hyperandrogenism: screening and diagnosis. *J Clin Endocrinol Metab* 1989;69:577–584.

131. Spritzer P, Billaud L, Thalabard JC, et al. Cyproterone acetate versus hydrocortisone treatment in late-onset adrenal hyperplasia. *J Clin Endocrinol Metab* 1990; 70:642–646.

132. Barbieri RL, Ryan KJ. Hyperandrogenism, insulin resistance, and acanthosis nigricans syndrome: a common endocrinopathy with distinct pathophysiologic features. *Am J Obstet Gynecol* 1983;147:90–101.

133. Barth JH, Ng LL, Wojnarowska F, et al. Acanthosis nigricans, insulin resistance and cutaneous virilism. *Br J Dermatol* 1988;118:613–619.

134. Richards GE, Cavallo A, Meyer WJ III, et al. Obesity, acanthosis nigricans, insulin resistance, and hyperandrogenemia: pediatric perspective and natural history. *J Pediatr* 1985;7:893–897.

135. Kahn CR, Flier JS, Bar RS, et al. The syndromes of insulin resistance and acanthosis nigricans. *N Engl J Med* 1976;14:739–745.

136. Bar RS, Muggeo M, Roth J, et al. Insulin resistance, acanthosis nigricans, and normal insulin receptors in a young woman: evidence for a postreceptor defect. *J Clin Endocrinol Metab* 1978;47:620–625.

137. Bar RS, Muggeo M, Kahn CR, et al. Characterization of insulin receptors in patients with the syndromes of insulin resistance and acanthosis nigricans. *Diabetologia* 1980;18:209–216.

138. Peters EJ, Stuart CA, Prince MJ. Acanthosis nigricans and obesity: acquired and intrinsic defects in insulin action. *Metabolism* 1986;9:807–813.

139. Moller DE, Flier JS. Detection of an alteration in the insulin-receptor gene in a patient with insulin resistance, acanthosis nigricans, and the polycystic ovary syndrome (type A insulin resistance). *N Engl J Med* 1988;319:1526–1529.

140. Kadowaki T, Bevins CL, Cama A, et al. Two mutant alleles of the insulin receptor gene in a patient with extreme insulin resistance. *Science* 1988;240: 787–790.

141. Moller DE, Cohen O, Yamaguchi Y, et al. Prevalence of mutations in the insulin receptor gene in subjects with features of the type A syndrome of insulin resistance. *Diabetes* 1994;43:247–255.

142. Taylor SI, Dons RF, Hernandez E, et al. Insulin resistance associated with androgen excess in women with autoantibodies to the insulin receptor. *Ann Intern Med* 1982;97:851–855.

143. Kellett HA, Collier A, Raylor R, et al. Hyperandrogenism, insulin resistance, acanthosis nigricans, and systemic lupus erythematosis associated with insulin receptor antibodies. *Metabolism* 1988;7:656–659.

144. Pepper GM, Poretsky L, Gabrilove JL, et al. Ketoconazole reverses hyperandrogenism in a patient with insulin resistance and acanthosis nigricans. *J Clin Endocrinol Metab* 1987;65:1047–1051.

145. Azziz R. The hyperandrogenic-insulin resistant-acanthosis nigricans (HAIRAN) syndrome: therapeutic response. *Fertil Steril* 1994;61:570–572.

146. Corenblum B, Baylis BW. Medical therapy for the syndrome of familial virilization, insulin resistance, and acanthosis nigricans. *Fertil Steril* 1990;53:421–425.

147. Dunaif A, Hoffman AR, Scully RE, et al. Clinical, biochemical, and ovarian morphologic features in women with acanthosis nigricans and masculinization. *Obstet Gynecol* 1985;66:545–552.

148. Nagamani M, Van Dinh T, Kelver ME. Hyperinsulinemia in hyperthecosis of the ovaries. *Am J Obstet Gynecol* 1986;154:384–389.

149. Mantzoros CS, Lawrence WD, Levy J. Insulin resistance in a patient with ovarian stromal hyperthecosis and the hyperandrogenism, insulin resistance and acanthosis nigricans syndrome. Report of a case with a possible endogenous ovarian factor. *J Reprod Med* 1995; 40:491–494.

150. Judd HL, Scully RE, Herbst AL, et al. Familial hyperthecosis: comparison of endocrinologic and histologic findings with polycystic ovarian disease. *Am J Obstet Gynecol* 1973;117:976–982.

151. Scully RE. Correspondence: reply to Dr. Fienberg. *Am J Obstet Gynecol* 1974;119:864–865.

152. Wentz AC, Gutai JP, Jones GS, et al. Ovarian hyperthecosis in the adolescent patient. *J Pediatr* 1976;88: 488–493.

153. Aiman J, Edman CD, Worley RJ, et al. Androgen and estrogen formation in women with ovarian hyperthecosis. *Obstet Gynecol* 1978;51:1–9.

154. Nagamani M, Lingold JC, Gomez LG, et al. Clinical and hormonal studies in hyperthecosis of the ovaries. *Fertil Steril* 1981;36:326–332.

155. Pascale MM, Pugeat M, Roberts M, et al. Androgen suppressive effect of GnRH agonist in ovarian hyperthecosis and virilizing tumours. *Clin Endocrinol* 1994; 41:571–576.

156. Steingold KA, Judd HL, Nieberg RK, et al. Treatment of severe androgen excess due to ovarian hyperthecosis with a long-acting gonadotropin-releasing hormone agonist. *Am J Obstet Gynecol* 1986;154:1241–1248.

157. Padilla SL. Androgen-producing tumors in children and adolescents. *Adolesc Pediatr Gynecol* 1989;2:135–142.

158. Derksen J, Nagesser SK, Meinders AE, et al. Identification of virilizing adrenal tumors in hirsute women. *N Engl J Med* 1994;331:968–973.

159. Yuen BH, Moon YS, Mincey EK, et al. Adrenal and sex steroid hormone production by a virilizing adrenal adenoma and its diagnosis with computerized tomography. *Am J Obstet Gynecol* 1983;145:164–169.

160. Waggoner W, Boots LR, Azziz R. Total testosterone and DHEAS levels as predictors of androgen-secreting neoplasms: a populational study. *Gynecol Endocrinol* 1999;13:1–7.

161. Meldrum DR, Abraham G. Peripheral and ovarian venous concentrations of various steroid hormones in virilizing ovarian tumors. *Obstet Gynecol* 1979;53:36–43.

162. Friedman CI, Schmidt GE, Kim MH, et al. Serum testosterone concentrations in the evaluation of androgen-producing tumors. *Am J Obstet Gynecol* 1985;153:44–49.

163. Philip J, Trolle D. Familial male hermaphroditism with delayed and partial masculinization. *Am J Obstet Gynecol* 1965;93:1076–1083.

164. Materlik H, Slowko T, Jedrzejczak A. Skin changes in acromegaly. *Pol Med J* 1968;23:1522–1527.

165. Jackson RL, Dockerty MB. The Stein-Leventhal syndrome: analysis of 43 cases with special reference to association with endometrial carcinoma. *Am J Obstet Gynecol* 1957;73:161–173.

166. Wood GP, Boronow RC. Endometrial adenocarcinoma and the polycystic ovary syndrome. *Am J Obstet Gynecol* 1976;124:140–142.

167. Farhi DC, Nosanchuk J, Silverberg SG. Endometrial adenocarcinoma in women under 25 years of age. *Obstet Gynecol* 1986;68:741–745.

168. Azziz R, Gay F. The treatment of hyperandrogenism with oral contraceptives. *Semin Reprod Endocrinol* 1989;7:246–254.

169. Steele SJ, Mason B, Brett A. Amenorrhoea after discontinuing Oestrogen-progestogen oral contraceptives. *Br Med J* 1973;4:343–345.

170. Buttram VC, Vanderheyden, JD, Besch PK, et al. Post pill amenorrhea. *Int J Fertil* 1974;19:37–44.

171. Siegberg R, Nilsson CG, Stenman U-H, et al. Sex hormone profiles in oligomenorrheic adolescent girls and the effect of oral contraceptives. *Fertil Steril* 1984;41:888–893.

172. Emans SJ, Grace E, Woods ER, et al. Treatment with dexamethasone of androgen excess in adolescent patients. *J Pediatr* 1988;112:821–826.

173. Ettinger B, Goldfield B, Burrill K, et al. Plasma testosterone stimulation-suppression dynamics in hirsute women. *Am J Med* 1973;54:195–200.

174. Steinberger E, Rodriguez-Rigau LJ, Smith KD. The prognostic value of acute adrenal suppression and stimulation tests in hyperandrogenic women. *Fertil Steril* 1982;37:187–192.

175. Abraham GE, Maroulis GB, Boyers SP, et al. Dexamethasone suppression test in the management of hyperandrogenized patients. *Obstet Gynecol* 1981;57:158–165.

176. Casey JH, Burger HG, Kent JR, et al. Treatment of hirsutism by adrenal and ovarian suppression. *J Clin Endocrinol Metab* 1966;26:1370–1374.

177. Azziz R, Black VY, Hines GA, et al. Glucocorticoid suppression of adrenal androgens in the polycystic ovary syndrome: limited impact on the associated oligo-ovulation. *J Clin Endocrinol Metab* 1999;84:946–950.

178. Rittmaster RS, Givner ML. Effect of daily and alternate day low dose prednisone on serum cortisol and adrenal androgens in hirsute women. *J Clin Endocrinol Metab* 1988;67:400–403.

179. Vidal-Puig AJ, Munos-Torres M, Joder-Gimeno E, et al. Ketoconazole therapy: hormonal and clinical effects in non-tumoral hyperandrogenism. *Eur J Endocrinol* 1994;130:333–338.

180. Ober KP, Hennessy JF. Spironolactone therapy for hirsutism in hyperandrogenic woman. *Ann Intern Med* 1978;89:643–644.

181. Boisselle A, Tremblay RR. New therapeutic approach to the hirsute patient. *Fertil Steril* 1979;32:276–279.

182. Shapiro G, Evron S. A novel use of spironolactone: treatment of hirsutism. *J Clin Endocrinol Metab* 1980;51:429–432.

183. Cumming DC, Yang JC, Rebar RW, et al. Treatment of hirsutism with spironolactone. *JAMA* 1982;247:1295–1298.

184. Lobo RA, Shoupe D, Serafini P, et al. The effects of two doses of spironolactone on serum androgens and anagen hair in hirsute women. *Fertil Steril* 1985;43:200–205.

185. Ylostalo P, Heikkinen J, Kauppila A, et al. Low-dose spironolactone in the treatment of female hirsutism. *Int J Fertil* 1987;32:41–45.

186. Barth JH, Cherry CA, Wojnarowska F, et al. Spironolactone is an effective and well tolerated systemic antiandrogen therapy for hirsute women. *J Clin Endocrinol Metab* 1989;68:966–970.

187. Taylor A, Pita JC, Santen R. Spironolactone and endocrine dysfunction. *Ann Intern Med* 1976;85:630–636.

188. Young RL, Goldzieher JW, Elkind-Hirsch K. The endocrine effects of spironolactone used as an antiandrogen. *Fertil Steril* 1987;48:223–228.

189. Serafini P, Lobo RA. The effects of spironolactone on adrenal steroidogenesis in hirsute women. *Fertil Steril* 1985;44:595–599.

190. Helfer EL, Miller JL, Rose LI. Side-effects of spironolactone therapy in the hirsute woman. *J Clin Endocrinol Metab* 1988;66:208–211.

191. Pittaway DE, Mazson WS, Wentz AC. Spironolactone in combination drug therapy for unresponsive hirsutism. *Fertil Steril* 1985;43:878–882.

192. Chapman MG, Dowsett M, Dewhurst CJ, et al. Spironolactone in combination with an oral contraceptive: an alternative treatment for hirsutism. *Br J Obstet Gynaecol* 1984;92:983–985.

193. Board JA, Rosenberg SM, Smeltzer JS. Spironolactone and estrogen-progestin therapy for hirsutism. *South Med J* 1987;80:483–486.

194. Cusan L, Dupont A, Gomez JL, et al. Comparison of flutamide and spirolactone in the treatment of hirsutism: a randomized controlled trial. *Fertil Steril* 1994;61:281–287.

195. Erenus M, Gurbuz O, Durmusoglu F, et al. Compari-

son of the efficacy of spironolactone verses flutamide in the treatment of hirsutism. *Fertil Steril* 1994;61: 613–616.

196. Marugo M, Bernasconi D, Meozzi M, et al. The use of flutamide in the management of hirsutism. *J Endocrinol Invest* 1994;17:195–199.

197. Belisle S, Love EJ. Clinical efficacy and safety of cyproterone acetate in severe hirsutism: results of a multi-centered Canadian study. *Fertil Steril* 1986;46: 1015–1020.

198. Rittmaster RS. Finasteride. *N Engl J Med* 1994;330: 120–125.

199. Adashi EY, Rock RA, Guzick D, et al. Fertility following bilateral ovarian wedge resection: a critical analysis of 90 consecutive cases of the polycystic ovary syndrome. *Fertil Steril* 1981;36:320–325.

200. Lunde O. Polycystic ovarian syndrome: a retrospective study of the therapeutic effect of ovarian wedge resection after unsuccessful treatment with clomiphene citrate. *Ann Chir Gynaecol* 1982;71:330–333.

201. Campo S, Garcea N, Caruso A, et al. Effect of celioscopic ovarian resection in patients with polycystic ovaries. *Gynecol Obstet Invest* 1983;15:213–222.

202. Greenblatt E, Casper RF. Endocrine changes after laparoscopic ovarian cautery in polycystic ovarian syndrome. *Am J Obstet Gynecol* 1987;156:279–285.

203. Sumioki H, Utsunomyiya T, Matsuoka K, et al. The effect of laparoscopic multiple punch resection of the ovary on hypothalamo-pituitary axis in polycystic ovary syndrome. *Fertil Steril* 1988;50:567–572.

204. Sakata M, Tasaka K, Kurachi H, et al. Changes of bioactive luteinizing hormone after laparoscopic ovarian cautery in patients with polycystic ovarian syndrome. *Fertil Steril* 1990;53:610–613.

18

Pelvic Pain in Children and Adolescents

Betsy Schroeder and Joseph S. Sanfilippo

Pelvic pain in the child and adolescent typically is challenging for the physician, the patient, and her family. As in adults, the pain may be categorized as acute, having been present for less than 3 months and usually attributable to a readily identified etiology, or chronic, having been present for at least 6 months. Chronic pelvic pain often is difficult to diagnose and treat.

A multiorgan system approach, including the reproductive, gastrointestinal, urologic, musculoskeletal, neurologic, and psychological, is required, because any one or combination of these systems may be responsible for, or contribute to, the pain. The clinician must recognize that, although common among adolescents, gynecologic pathology is rare but does occur in prepubertal girls. Conditions related to sexual activity occur in peripubertal girls as well, so they must be part of the differential diagnosis.

ACUTE PELVIC PAIN

Etiologies of acute pelvic pain in the pediatric and adolescent age groups are extensive and varied. Some of the more common causes are listed in Table 18.1. In the prepubertal age group, gastrointestinal conditions, including appendicitis, gastroenteritis, and constipation, are frequent, but rare conditions including omental torsion (1) and deep venous thrombosis (2) have been reported. Among teenage girls, gastrointestinal conditions are still frequent causes of acute abdominal pain, with appendicitis being the most common (3); however, the reproductive tract is much more likely to be involved.

TABLE 18.1. *Differential diagnosis of acute pelvic pain*

Gastrointestinal	Gynecologic
Appendicitis	Pelvic inflammatory disease
Gastroenteritis	Ruptured follicular/corpus luteum cyst
Obstruction	Adnexal torsion
Constipation	Ectopic pregnancy
Volvulus	Outflow tract obstruction
Perforation	Dysmenorrhea
Musculoskeletal	Urologic
Muscle-tendon injury	Nephrolithiasis
Contusions	Cystitis
Growth plate injury	Pyelonephritis
Ligamentous injury	Urethritis
Avulsion fracture	Other
Other fracture	Diabetic ketoacidosis
Inguinal hernia	Sickle cell crisis
Intervertebral disc herniation	Malingering Munchausen syndrome

Diagnosis begins with a thorough history. Location, quality, onset, timing, and radiation of the pain, as well as exacerbating and alleviating factors and associated symptoms, should be determined. Intermittent, colicky pain is indicative of a distended viscous such as in nephrolithiasis. Acute onset of pain may be due to rupture of an organ (such as the appendix), ectopic pregnancy, or ovarian cyst. Pain of gradual onset, often with fever, is likely the result of an inflammatory process, as in pelvic inflammatory disease (PID).

The relationship between the pain and menstruation should be determined. Pregnancy-related conditions are associated with amenorrhea or abnormal vaginal bleeding. PID often develops shortly after menstruation. Problems resulting from ovarian cysts are most common at either the middle or end of the menstrual cycle. A premenarcheal adolescent who began breast development 2 to 3 years earlier may have an outflow tract obstruction, whereas those who have pain with each menstrual cycle may have a partial outflow tract obstruction. These conditions may even present as an acute abdomen (4,5).

A pelvic examination is necessary in the assessment of the adolescent with pelvic pain, and a sexual history is essential. All too often, teenagers with PID are taken to the operating room with a presumptive diagnosis of appendicitis because these important aspects of the assessment were overlooked. If done properly, even a perimenarcheal virgin can tolerate a bimanual examination and a speculum exam with a Huffman speculum. A rectal examination also provides valuable information. In prepubertal girls, the internal pelvic examination should not be performed but should be replaced by the rectoabdominal examination.

Laboratory tests should include a sensitive pregnancy test in addition to those indicated by findings on the history and physical examinations. Ultrasound often is helpful in the evaluation of pelvic pain in the adolescent and prepubertal girl. In cases of uncertain diagnosis, laparoscopy may be warranted for diagnostic purposes, with a 93% to 100% likelihood of making a definitive diagnosis (6–10).

Select Etiologies

Adnexal Torsion

Torsion may occur in any age group, including prepubertal girls (11–14). Making the diagnosis often is challenging, and it must be included in the differential diagnosis for girls and adolescents with acute pelvic pain.

Adnexal torsion may involve the ovary, fallopian tube (15,16), or both. Often it is associated with ovarian pathology resulting in ovarian enlargement, but it also has been found in women with normal ovaries. Involvement of normal ovaries is more common in children (17). Factors that may favor torsion in the normal ovary or fallopian tube include abdominal trauma, previous gynecologic surgery, elongation of the mesosalpingeal vessels, tubal spasm, and a redundant tube (18).

The most common symptom is acute onset of lower abdominal pain (19). With intermittent torsion, the pain will be repetitive. The right side is affected more frequently than the left (20,21). Nausea and vomiting are frequent symptoms. Occasionally, fever and leukocytosis are present. Because symptoms are nonspecific, the diagnosis may be confused with PID (22) or appendicitis (23).

The gold standard radiologic evaluation for possible adnexal torsion is ultrasound with or without Doppler. The most common ultrasonographic findings include cystic, solid, or complex ovarian masses (24). Graif and Itzchak (25) described multiple 8- to 12-mm follicles in the cortical portions of a unilaterally enlarged ovary in seven of eleven patients with ovarian torsion. These findings were confirmed by others (26). Sensitivity improves with the use of Doppler, which may show absent or reverse flow to the ovary. Fleischer et al. (27) were able to distinguish viable from nonviable ovaries with the use of color Doppler. In the viable group, central venous flow was present in three of three cases; in the nonviable group, central venous flow was absent in ten of ten cases. Typical findings with computed tomographic scans and magnetic resonance images have been described (28,29), and these may provide a noninvasive diagnosis in cases where the diagnosis is otherwise uncertain.

Due to the high potential for adnexal loss in cases of torsion, when the diagnosis cannot otherwise be ruled out, definitive diagnosis via laparoscopy should not be delayed. Ben-Arie and co-workers (30) found that only the time interval from admission to diagnosis and treatment affected operative results and preservation of fertility, with those cases receiving more rapid treatment having less harm to the reproductive organ involved. The treatment of choice is laparoscopic detorsion (with cystectomy when applicable) to maximize reproductive potential. Although until fairly recently detorsion was not advocated for fear of thrombotic emboli from the ovarian vein (31), several authors have reported safety and efficacy of detorsion in both adults and children (32,33). Ovarian function with follicular development has been reported following detorsion (34). If the ovary does not respond to detorsion and remains dusky and necrotic, oophorectomy is required.

Because sequential ovarian torsion has been described (35,36), several authors recommend oophoropexy of the contralateral ovary at the initial episode of torsion (37,38). This may be accomplished laparoscopically. Prevention of recurrent torsion in this manner is of particular value in those in whom oophorectomy is required due to necrosis or other ovarian pathology.

Pelvic Inflammatory Disease

PID is an important etiologic factor in acute pelvic pain in the adolescent population. It comprises a spectrum of inflammatory disorders of the female upper genital tract and may include any combination of endometritis (uterus), salpingitis (fallopian tubes), tubo-ovarian abscess (TOA), and pelvic peritonitis (39). It is the second most serious consequence of sexually transmitted diseases (STDs) occurring among adolescents, behind only acquired immunodeficiency syndrome (40). It results from an ascending infection, and it often is polymicrobial in nature. Common organisms include *Neisseria gonorrhea*; *Chlamydia trachomatis*; peptococcus, bacteroides, and peptostreptococcus species; *Escherichia coli*; *Streptococcus*; *Haemophilus influenzae*; and others. Long-term consequences include chronic pelvic pain, infertility, and ectopic pregnancy.

The incidence of PID is higher among sexually active adolescents than any other age group. One third of the one million women affected annually are 18 years or younger (41). In those 15 to 19 years old, the likelihood of having PID is one in eight, compared to one in 80 in women 25 to 29 years of age (42). Early age at first coitus, multiple partners, and intrauterine device use are commonly accepted risk factors. Other risk factors include parity, more than one sexual partner in the previous 30 days, sex during the previous menses, and lack of contraception (43). Hillis and co-workers (44) reported that women who had three or more chlamydial infections were 6.6 times more likely to be hospitalized for PID than those who had a history of only one chlamydial infection.

Cervical instrumentation is also a risk factor in the development of PID. In adolescents, cervical procedures for dysplasia are common and may increase the risk of PID. Hillard et al. (45) reported a 9% incidence of PID within 1 month of cryotherapy in adolescents. Harel and Riggs (46) calculated that the risk of colposcopic biopsy-induced PID is much lower, with a rate of one in 1,000. In spite of the lower rate found in this study, the authors still recommend STD screening in all adolescents undergoing colposcopy to prevent the often devastating sequelae of PID.

Oral contraceptive pill (OCP) use may have a protective benefit against chlamydial PID (47,48). This may be due to a modified immune response as well as thickening of the cervical mucus, inhibiting ascension of the cervical infection. Another possible protective factor against PID is pregnancy. Although there are case reports of surgically verified coexistence of PID in pregnancy (49,50), only one study has looked at the possibility of coexistence of the two conditions in adolescents (51). In this report, 24 (42.1%) of 57

TABLE 18.2. *Criteria for diagnosis of pelvic inflammatory disease*

Minimum criteria
  Lower abdominal tenderness
  Adnexal tenderness
  Cervical motion tenderness
Additional criteria
  Oral temperature >101°F (38.3°C)
  Abnormal cervical or vaginal discharge
  Elevated erythrocyte sedimentation rate
  Elevated C-reactive protein
  Laboratory documentation of cervical infection with
    Neisseria gonorrhoeae or *Chlamydia trachomatis*
Definitive criteria
  Histopathologic evidence of endometritis on
    endometrial biopsy
  Transvaginal sonography showing thickened fluid-
    filled tubes with or without free pelvic fluid or
    tuboovarian abscess
  Laparoscopic abnormalities consistent with pelvic
    inflammatory disease

Adapted from Centers for Disease Control and Prevention: 1998 guidelines for treatment of sexually transmitted diseases. *MMWR* 1997;47:80.

patients admitted to the hospital with pregnancy and a diagnosis of PID met diagnostic criteria for PID; none of these patients had a surgically confirmed diagnosis. Clearly, more research needs to be done in this area.

Symptoms of PID often are nonspecific and may range from minimal to severe. Lower abdominal pain is the most common complaint. The pain may range from sharp and stabbing to dull and crampy. It may be localized to the lower abdomen in the midline or more on one side than the other, or it may be diffuse abdominal pain. There may or may not be peritoneal signs. Diagnostic criteria are listed in Table 18.2. All three minimum plus at least one additional criteria, or one of the definitive criteria, must be present. If the pain is greatest in the right lower quadrant, it may be difficult to distinguish it from appendicitis. If the diagnosis is uncertain, diagnostic laparoscopy should be performed.

Ultrasonography may be helpful in establishing the diagnosis. It may suggest the presence of a different problem that presents with similar symptoms, such as adnexal torsion or a ruptured ovarian cyst, or it may confirm the diagnosis of PID. In a study by Taipale et al. (52), transvaginal ultrasound was performed

in patients with PID. Twenty-seven percent had fluid in the cul de sac, and 36% had fluid-filled fallopian tubes. This group had three subgroups: those with cystic thick-walled tubes, those with cystic thick-walled tubes with layered echogenic contents consistent with pyosalpinx, and those with poorly echogenic, thin-walled tubes consistent with hydrosalpinx. Although the sensitivity in detecting PID may be low, it also may differentiate simple PID from TOAs.

Clinically differentiating PID from a TOA may be difficult, especially because one may not be able to perform an adequate pelvic examination due to tenderness from the disease. Slap and co-workers (53) evaluated adolescents hospitalized with PID, all of whom had an ultrasound. Those who had ultrasound findings consistent with TOAs were more likely than those who did not to have a palpable adnexal mass (13% vs. 3%), white blood cell count greater than 10,500/mL, erythrocyte sedimentation rate greater than 15 mm/h, heart rate greater than 90/min, and last menstrual period more than 18 days before admission. Adolescent patients with TOAs were less likely to have signs of acute illness than those without TOAs, but no single finding or cluster of signs and symptoms was specific to the diagnosis of a TOA, making ultrasound a particularly valuable tool in this patient population. By ultrasound, a TOA will typically appear as a complex cystic adnexal or cul-de-sac mass with thick, irregular walls, septations, and internal debris and echoes. Sensitivity is 93% and specificity is 98.6% (54). Ultrasonography is extremely useful in the evaluation of patients with suspected PID.

Treatment should be initiated as soon as the diagnosis is suspected. Most cases of mild PID are treated in the outpatient setting. In the past, it was recommended that all adolescents with PID be hospitalized for intravenous antibiotics; however, the most recent Centers for Disease Control and Prevention guidelines no longer advocate this, stating that there are no efficacy data comparing oral with parenteral therapy (39). Instead, decision about hospitalization is left to the discretion of the health

TABLE 18.3. *Criteria for hospitalization for pelvic inflammatory disease*

Surgical emergencies cannot be excluded
Patient is pregnant
Failed oral antibiotic therapy
    No response
    Unable to comply
Severe illness with nausea, vomiting, or high fever
Tuboovarian abscess
Immunodeficiency

Adapted from Centers for Disease Control and Prevention: 1998 guidelines for treatment of sexually transmitted diseases. *MMWR* 1997;47:81–82.

TABLE 18.4. *Treatment regimens for pelvic inflammatory disease*

Parenteral regimens
1a. Cefotetan 2 g IV q12h
    or
    Cefoxitin 2 g IV q6h
    plus
    Doxycycline 100 mg IV or PO q12h
2b. Clindamycin 900 mg IV q8h
    plus
    Gentamicin loading dose IV or IM (2 mg/kg body weight) followed by a maintenance dose 1.5 mg/kg 98h. (single daily dosing may be substituted)
Oral regimens
1a. Ofloxacin 400 mg PO bid × 14 d
    plus
    Metronidazole 500 mg PO bid × 14 d
2b. Ceftriaxone 250 mg IM once
    or
    Cefoxitin 2 g IM plus probenecid 1 g PO in a single dose
    or
    Other parenteral third-generation cephalosporin
    plus
    Doxycycline 100 mg PO bid × 14 d

Adapted from Centers for Disease Control and Prevention: 1998 guidelines for treatment of sexually transmitted diseases. *MMWR* 1997;47:82–84.

care provider. Current recommendations for hospitalization are listed in Table 18.3, and some of the antibiotic regimens for treatment are listed in Table 18.4. Although ofloxacin is listed as first-line outpatient treatment, it is contraindicated in those less than 18 years of age and in those who are pregnant, due to the potential risk of osteochondrosis. Tetracycline also should be avoided in pregnant women and children under 8 years of age. Alternative regimens should be used in these patients. Intravenous antibiotics should be given for a minimum of 24 to 48 hours until clinically the patient responds and then may be switched to oral antibiotics to complete a total antibiotic course of 14 days. Patients with TOAs should receive a minimum of 7 days of parenteral antibiotics before making the transition to oral antibiotics.

In patients who do not respond to parenteral antibiotics within 48 hours, surgical intervention may be warranted. In the vast majority of patients who do not respond, there is either a TOA or the diagnosis of PID was incorrect. If the diagnosis is in question, diagnostic laparoscopy is indicated, and, in cases of a known TOA, drainage may be performed laparoscopically or under ultrasound guidance. In adolescents, conservative management is the treatment of choice. It is successful in up to 80% of cases (55), making salpingo-oophorectomy and hysterectomy rare in this age group.

Because PID is a sexually transmitted disease, partners of affected patients should be treated for both gonorrhea and chlamydia. Follow-up testing for reinfection should be performed, and the opportunity to teach the patient about STD prevention should not be missed.

Ovarian Cysts

Although common findings in adult and adolescent patients, ovarian cysts are unusual in the prepubertal child after the first year of life. In this age group, cysts are a rare cause of pelvic pain unless they undergo torsion. Hemorrhage also is uncommon in the absence of torsion.

In adolescents, acute onset of lower abdominal pain is much more likely due to complications of an ovarian cyst, including rupture, hemorrhage, and torsion. Physiologic follicular cysts rupture midcycle when ovulation occurs; occasionally this causes lower abdominal pain, and this is known as mittelschmirtz. The pain occurs in the midline or on the side of the ovulating ovary, and it is usually short lived with spontaneous symptom resolution within 1 to 2 days. Nonsteroidal antiinflammatory drugs (NSAIDs) may be used for pain control. For those who have recurrent pain with each menstrual cycle, inhibition of ovulation with OCPs or medroxyprogesterone acetate (Depo-Provera) may prove effective.

Hemorrhagic cysts may be derived from follicular or corpus luteum cysts. Hemorrhagic follicular cysts present in the first 3 weeks of the menstrual cycle; hemorrhagic corpus luteum cysts are more common in the fourth menstrual week. Symptoms include acute-onset lower abdominal pain in the midline, on the side of the cyst, or throughout the abdomen. Nausea and vomiting occur in up to 80% of cases (56). Bleeding may be significant, as noted in a report by Kayaba et al. (57) in which 900 cc of hemoperitoneum was found on laparotomy in a 12-year-old girl with a ruptured hemorrhagic ovarian cyst. There may be accompanying vaginal bleeding, peritoneal signs, and evidence of hypovolemia in cases with significant bleeding.

As with other gynecologic conditions, ultrasonography is extremely helpful in diagnosing ovarian cysts and may differentiate different cyst types. Hemorrhagic ovarian cysts appear primarily as complex cystic masses or cystic masses with a diffuse homogeneous echo pattern (58). There also may be free fluid in the cul de sac. Guerriero et al. (59) reported a sensitivity of 83% and specificity of 89% in differentiating endometriomas from other ovarian masses.

If the patient is hemodynamically stable, management of ruptured ovarian cysts is medical and similar to the management of mittelschmirtz. With time, symptoms will resolve spontaneously. NSAIDs may be used for pain control, and suppression of ovulation with OCPS or medroxyprogesterone acetate may be used to prevent recurrence. In cases of uncertain diagnosis, laparoscopy should be performed to rule out more serious conditions such as ovarian torsion or appendicitis. If there is significant bleeding with hemodynamic instability, a laparotomy may be indicated.

Ectopic Pregnancy

In all adolescent females with acute onset of lower abdominal pain, the diagnosis of ectopic pregnancy must be included in the differential. This is the leading cause of maternal death during the first trimester and the second overall cause of maternal death in the United States (60).

Established risk factors for ectopic pregnancy include tubal (61) or other pelvic/ abdominal (62) surgery, PID (63) and other sexually transmitted diseases, increased maternal age, smoking (64), intrauterine device use (65), and previous ectopic pregnancy. Other risk factors, such as a history of induced abortion, are controversial (66,67).

Presenting symptoms consist of the classic triad of lower abdominal pain (98%), amenorrhea (90%), and vaginal bleeding (64%); other symptoms include pregnancy-related symptoms such as nausea and vomiting or breast tenderness (41%) and syncope (5%) (62). The abdominal pain may be sharp and acute in onset, or it may be an achy, crampy pain. It usually is localized to the side of the ectopic, but it may be in the midline or on the opposite side. Bleeding is most often scant and described as spotting, but it may be profuse in cases of ruptured ectopic pregnancies. Bleeding may be intraperitoneal, and, in severe cases, the patient will be hypovolemic or in shock.

On physical examination, vital signs may be normal or, as stated earlier, there may be tachycardia and hypotension. The patient will be afebrile. The abdomen may be soft with mild lower abdominal tenderness, or there may be an acute abdomen with rigidity, rebound, and guarding. The pelvic examination may be normal with or without vaginal bleeding, or there may be a palpable adnexal mass and adnexal tenderness.

Laboratory evaluation should include a quantitative β-human chorionic gonadotropin (hCG), complete blood count, and type and screen. If the pregnancy test is positive and the patient is stable, an ultrasound should be performed. In those cases in which an intrauterine pregnancy could not be identified, Shalev et al. (68) reported that transvaginal ultrasonography is 87% sensitive and 94% specific for the diagnosis of an ectopic pregnancy. In those cases in which neither an intrauterine pregnancy nor an ectopic pregnancy can be detected, if the patient is stable, serial β-hCG levels can be followed until a definitive diagnosis is made.

Medical management of ectopic pregnancy with methotrexate is an effective alternative to surgical management in select patients. Stika et al. (69) reported a 64% success rate with single-dose methotrexate; 14% required a second or third dose, for a total success rate of 78%. The 22% who required surgical intervention developed acute abdominal pain, and most underwent salpingectomy via laparoscopy or laparotomy.

Methotrexate has been found to be a reasonable treatment option for adolescents with ectopic pregnancies. McCord and co-workers (70) prospectively followed adolescents with ectopic pregnancies who were appropriate candidates for medical management and compared them to a control group of adult women meeting the same criteria. They found that there was no significant difference in compliance between the teens and the adults, and 85% required no surgical intervention.

Those patients who are not appropriate candidates for methotrexate should undergo surgical treatment. Laparoscopy has been found to be an effective, minimally invasive procedure with a high success rate for the management of ectopic pregnancies (71,72). Linear salpingostomy is the treatment of choice in those who desire future fertility, but occasionally salpingectomy is required.

CHRONIC PELVIC PAIN

Chronic pelvic pain is defined as constant or intermittent discomfort involving one or both lower quadrants lasting for 6 months or more (73). Initial evaluation requires a detailed history and physical examination. Inquiries should be made with respect to any system that may be involved, including gastrointestinal, genitourinary, gynecologic, psychiatric and psychological, and musculoskeletal etiologies, because any or all of these may be contributing factors (Table 18.5). Inquiries should be made with respect to the presence of dysmenorrhea. Any abnormal uterine bleeding is important in the assessment of pelvic pain. Entities such as endomyometritis may be associated with pelvic pain as well as other causes of abnormal uterine bleeding. Concern for pregnancy should always be considered.

The pubertal developmental milestones should be determined, and any evidence of an outflow tract obstruction should be considered with pelvic pain. Childhood diseases, although rarely a cause of pelvic pain, should be considered because entities such as mumps oophoritis can be a source of chronic pelvic pain.

A general physical examination as well as pelvic examination should be performed to determine whether the pelvic area is tender and to elicit any pelvic masses. Evaluation of the cul de sac on bimanual examination is an integral part of the assessment, as is perform-

TABLE 18.5. *Differential diagnosis of chronic pelvic pain*

Gastrointestinal	Gynecologic
Inflammatory bowel disease	Chronic pelvic inflammatory disease
Chronic appendicitis	Endometriosis
Obstruction	Adhesions
Constipation	Leiomyomata
Irritable bowel syndrome	Outflow tract obstruction
Musculoskeletal	Dysmenorrhea
Intervertebral disc herniation	Other
Myofascial pain	Abuse
Strains/sprains	Psychosocial stress
Fibromyositis	Psychiatric disorders
Inguinal hernia	Porphyria
Scoliosis	Substance abuse
	Heavy metal poisoning

ing a careful rectovaginal assessment, to rule out any significant pelvic abnormality.

Laboratory testing should be a reflection of the history and physical examination findings. Depending on the circumstance and response to medical therapy, diagnostic laparoscopy may become an integral part of the assessment of pelvic pain in this age group. Goldstein and co-workers (74), using laparoscopy to examine 109 adolescent girls between the ages of 10.5 and 19 years with unexplained chronic pelvic pain, noted that the youngest documented patient to have endometriosis was 10.8 years of age. This patient had reached menarche 5 months earlier.

Select Etiologies

Psychological

Psychological aspects of chronic pelvic pain should be considered. Work by Gross and co-workers (75) evaluated 25 patients, including adolescents. Each patient was noted to have a normal pelvic examination. Psychological assessment determined that the most frequent diagnosis was "significant pathology with borderline syndrome and hysterical character disorder." A significant incidence of early childhood family dysfunction and incest was noted. Psychological testing corroborated the high incidence of psychopathology. Differences between organic and psychogenic functional pelvic pain have been found (72). Organic pain frequently is sharp and "crampy" and wakes the patient at night, whereas psychogenic pain usually is absent during sleep. The onset of pelvic pain can be linked to a stressful event or life crisis (72). Treatment of chronic pelvic pain often involves reassuring the patient that there is no obvious pelvic abnormality. The adolescent must be apprised of the role of stress in her pain experience, and she must be allowed the proper forum to express anger or frustration.

Determination as to whether or not childhood sexual abuse has occurred and is a contributing factor to chronic pelvic pain is in order. Appropriate inquiry should be made with respect to the adolescent's past history, and any suspicion for prior sexual abuse should be thoroughly evaluated by a psychologist and/or psychiatrist.

Musculoskeletal

Musculoskeletal or abdominal wall etiologies for pelvic pain have received little attention in our literature. However, musculoskeletal dysfunction can be a primary cause of chronic pelvic pain. Aftimos (76) reported two girls ages 11 and 13 years with musculoskeletal pelvic and abdominal pain who were misdiagnosed with a conversion disorder and constipation. Other authors evaluated 106 patients with chronic pelvic pain and found trigger points in 26 (24%) (77). Furthermore, Slocum (78) identified trigger points in 74% of patients with chronic pelvic pain.

Trigger points are areas of hyperirritability that are locally tender on compression and cause referred pain and tenderness. The myofascial pain syndrome occurs with taut bands of skeletal muscle causing pain (79). Most of the theories about the development of trigger points involve noxious stimuli that affect fascia and muscle. Sustained muscle contraction, as in cases of poor posture or response to an injury, may be a triggering factor. Cold or damp weather, especially after a viral illness, or a new physical activity in a previously sedentary individual also may be an etiologic factor (76).

Acute and chronic pelvic pain may be the result of trigger point problems identified in the abdominal wall, vagina, or sacrum. The referred pain often is visceral, resembling dysmenorrhea, or it may present as dyspareunia or with urologic or gastrointestinal symptoms. Although the trigger points are distinct areas on physical examination, the referred pain often is poorly localized and may not follow dermatomal patterns.

Treatment with bupivacaine (0.25%) or procaine (1%) into the trigger points often produces lasting relief (79). Stretching also has been advocated to provide relief. The affected area is sprayed with a local anesthetic before application of fluoromethane or ethyl chloride. The muscle then is massaged and passively stretched, but not to the point at which it is painful. This treatment may be complemented with the use of transcutaneous electrical nerve stimulation (76).

Endometriosis

Endometriosis is the presence of endometrial glands and stroma outside of the normal intrauterine endometrial cavity. Several theories have been proposed to explain its pathogenesis, including coelomic metaplasia, retrograde menstruation, and hematogenous or lymphatic spread, but none of them explains all cases. Immunologic susceptibility may be involved, and there is strong evidence of a genetic influence. Simpson et al. (80) reported a 6.9-fold increase in the rate of endometriosis in women who had a close relative with endometriosis compared to those without a family history.

The incidence of endometriosis in adolescents is higher than previously believed. With the availability of laparoscopy and the growing awareness of the possibility of endometriosis in this population, more accurate assessments are becoming available. Reported rates range from 19% to 65% among teens with chronic pelvic pain (81–86). More recent studies addressed the incidence of endometriosis in adolescents with chronic pelvic pain that is unresponsive to traditional medical management (OCPs and NSAIDs), and findings range from 69.6% to 73% (87,88). Interestingly, there are case reports of premenarcheal patients (88) as well as those that have primary amenorrhea (89) with endometriosis, so menarche is not a prerequisite for the development of the disease.

Symptoms in adolescents often differ from those in adults. The most common presentation leading to diagnosis is pelvic pain with or without dysmenorrhea. Symptoms are worse around the time of menses and may not respond to NSAIDs and OCPs, which distinguishes endometriosis from primary dysmenorrhea. Other symptoms are listed in Table 18.6. Findings on physical examination often

TABLE 18.6. *Presenting symptoms in adolescents with endometriosis*

Cyclic and acyclic pain
Acyclic pain
Dysmenorrhea
Dyspareunia
Menstrual irregularity
Abdominal pain/nausea
Urinary symptoms

are unremarkable, but mild-to-moderate tenderness may be noted. The adnexa usually are normal, without masses. Endometriomas are rare in this age group.

When standard treatment of primary dysmenorrhea is ineffective, symptomatic patients should be evaluated laparoscopically. Diagnosis should not be delayed so as to preserve fertility and to arrest progression of the disease as well as to ameliorate symptoms. Stovall et al. (90) found that more advanced disease at time of diagnosis is associated with greater pain at follow-up, with a mean interval from initial treatment to follow-up of 15.7 years in an historical prospective study. Unfortunately, laparoscopy often is not performed in teenagers for several years after the onset of symptoms.

Treatment may be medical, surgical, or a combination of the two. In teenagers, surgical treatment usually is conservative, consisting of laparoscopic ablation of endometrial implants. This generally is followed with medical management, consisting of hormonal suppression. A number of regimens are available, including OCPs, danazol, depot medroxyprogesterone acetate, and gonadotropin-releasing hormone agonists.

CONCLUSION

Pelvic pain in children and adolescents may be caused by a multitude of conditions involving several different organ systems. It requires a comprehensive and thorough multidisciplinary approach, and it may be particularly difficult to make the appropriate diagnosis and treat effectively. Surgical intervention, primarily in the form of laparoscopy, should be the last resort when the medical assessment and management alternatives have been thoroughly considered and used as appropriate.

REFERENCES

1. Oguzkurt P, Kotiloglu E, Tanyel FC, et al. Primary omental torsion in a 6-year-old girl. *J Pediatr Surg* 1995;30:1700–1701.
2. Schwartz DS, Keller MS. Deep venous thrombosis as a cause of pelvic pain in children. *J Ultrasound Med* 1997;16:281–283.
3. Mollitt DL, Dokler ML. The teenage girl. *Semin Pediatr Surg* 1997;6:100–104.
4. Kinjo K, Kasai T, Ogawa K. Hematometra and ruptured hematosalpinx with ipsilateral renal agenesis presenting as diffuse peritonitis: a case report. *Intensive Care Med* 1997;23:354.
5. Amara DP, Nezhat F, Giudice L, et al. Laparoscopic management of a noncommunicating uterine horn in a patient with an acute abdomen. *Surg Laparosc Endosc* 1997;7:56–59.
6. Salky BA, Edye MB. The role of laparoscopy in the diagnosis and treatment of abdominal pain syndromes. *Surg Endosc* 1998;12:911–914.
7. Navez B, d'Udekem Y, Cambier E, et al. Laparoscopy for management of nontraumatic acute abdomen. *World J Surg* 1995;19:382–386.
8. Cueto J, Diaz O, Garteiz D, et al. The efficacy of laparoscopic surgery in the diagnosis and treatment of peritonitis. *Surg Endosc* 1997;11:366–370.
9. Kontoravdis A, Chryssikopoulos A, Hassiakos D, et al. The diagnostic value of laparoscopy in 2365 patients with acute and chronic pelvic pain. *Int J Gynecol Obstet* 1996;52:243–248.
10. Taylor EW, Kennedy CA, Dunham RH, et al. Diagnostic laparoscopy in women with acute abdominal pain. *Surg Laparosc Endosc* 1995;2:125–128.
11. Ben-Arie A, Lurie S, Graf G, et al. Adnexal torsion in adolescents: prompt diagnosis and treatment may save the adnexa. *Eur J Obstet Gynecol Reprod Biol* 1995;63:169–173.
12. Fleischer AC, Stein SM, Cullinan JA, et al. Color Doppler sonography of adnexal torsion. *J Ultrasound Med* 1995;14:523–528.
13. Bader T, Ranner G, Haberlik A. Torsion of normal adnexa in a premenarcheal girl: MRI findings. *Eur Radiol* 1996;6:704–706.
14. Cohen Z, Shinhar D, Kopernik G, et al. The laparoscopic approach to uterine adnexal torsion in childhood. *J Pediatr Surg* 1996;31:1557–1559.
15. Ferrera PC, Kass LE, Verdile VP. Torsion of the fallopian tube. *Am J Emerg Med* 1995;13:312–314.
16. Isenberg JS, Silich R. Isolated torsion of the normal fallopian tube in premenarchial girls. *Surg Gynecol Obstet* 1990;170:353–354.
17. Helvie MA, Silver TM. Ovarian torsion: sonographic evaluation. *J Clin Ultrasound* 1989;17:327.
18. Mordehai J, Mares AJ, Barki I, et al. Torsion of uterine adnexae in neonates and children: a report of 20 cases. *J Pediatr Surg* 1991;26:1195–1199.
19. Baker TE, Copas PR. Adnexal torsion: a clinical dilemma. *J Reprod Med* 1995;40:447–449.
20. Steyaert H, Meynol F, Valla JS. Torsion of the adnexa in children: the value of laparoscopy. *Pediatr Surg Int* 1998;13:384–387.
21. Hibbard LT. Adnexal torsion. *Am J Obstet Gynecol* 1985;152:456–461.
22. Maynard SR, Peipert JF, Brody JM. Tubal torsion appearing as acute pelvic inflammatory disease. *J Am Assoc Gynecol Laparosc* 1996;3:431–433.
23. Shust NM, Hendricksen DK. Ovarian torsion: an unusual case of abdominal pain in a young girl. *Am J Emerg Med* 1995;13:307–309.
24. Davis LG, Gerscovich EO, Anderson MW, et al. Ultrasound and Doppler in the diagnosis of ovarian torsion. *Eur J Radiol* 1995;20:133–136.
25. Graif M, Itzchak Y. Sonographic evaluation of ovarian torsion in children and adolescents. *Am J Radiol* 1988;150:647–649.
26. Meyer JS, Harmon CM, Harty MP, et al. Ovarian torsion: clinical and imaging presentation in children. *J Pediatr Surg* 1995;30:1433–1436.
27. Fleischer AC, Stein SM, Cullinan JA, et al. Color Doppler sonography of adnexal torsion. *J Ultrasound Med* 1995;14:523–528.
28. Bader T, Ranner G, Haberlik A. Torsion of normal adnexa in a premenarcheal girl: MRI findings. *Eur Radiol* 1996;6:704–706.
29. Kimura I, Togashi K, Kawakami S, et al. Ovarian torsion: CT and MRI imaging appearances. *Radiology* 1994;190:337–341.
30. Ben-Arie A, Lurie S, Graf G, et al. Adnexal torsion in adolescents: prompt diagnosis and treatment may save the adnexa. *Eur J Obstet Gynecol* 1995;63:169–173.
31. Wagaman R, Williams R. Conservative therapy for adnexal torsion. *J Reprod Med* 1990;35:833–834.
32. Cohen Z, Shinhar D, Kopernik G, et al. The laparoscopic approach to uterine adnexal torsion in childhood. *J Pediatr Surg* 1996;31:1557–1559.
33. Chapron C, Capella-Allouc S, Dubuisson JB. Treatment of adnexal torsion using operative laparoscopy. *Hum Reprod* 1996;11:998–1003.
34. Shalev E, Bustan M, Yarom I, et al. Recovery of ovarian function after laparoscopic detorsion. *Hum Reprod* 1995;10:2965–2966.
35. Davis AJ, Feins NR. Subsequent asynchronous torsion of normal adnexa in children. *J Pediatr Surg* 1990;25:687–689.
36. Worthington-Kirsh RL, Raptopoulos V, Cohen IT. Sequential bilateral torsion of ovaries in a child. *J Ultrasound Med* 1986;5:663–664.
37. Nagel TC, Sebastian J, Malo JW. Oophoropexy to prevent sequential or recurrent torsion. *J Am Assoc Gynecol Laparosc* 1997;4:495–498.
38. Germain M, Rarick T, Robins E. Management of intermittent torsion by laparoscopic oophoropexy. *Obstet Gynecol* 1996;88:715–717.
39. Centers for Disease Control and Prevention. 1998 Guidelines for treatment of sexually transmitted diseases. *MMWR* 1997;47:79–85.
40. Wald ER. Pelvic inflammatory disease in adolescents. *Curr Probl Pediatr* 1996;26:86–97.
41. Kottmann LM. Pelvic inflammatory disease: clinical overview. *J Obstet Gynecol Neonatal Nurs* 1995;24:759–767.
42. Eschenback DA. Epidemiology and diagnosis of acute

pelvic inflammatory disease. *Obstet Gynecol* 1980;55 [Suppl]:142S–152S.

43. Jossens MOR, Eskenazi B, Schachter J, et al. Risk factors for pelvic inflammatory disease: a case control study. *Sex Transm Dis* 1996;23:239–247.

44. Hillis SD, Owens LM, Marchbanks PA, et al. Recurrent chlamydial infections increase the risk for ectopic pregnancy and pelvic inflammatory disease. *Am J Obstet Gynecol* 1997;176:103–107.

45. Hillard PA, Biro FM, Wildey L. Complications of cervical cryotherapy in adolescents. *J Reprod Med* 1991; 36:711–716.

46. Harel Z, Riggs S. On the need to screen for Chlamydia and Gonorrhea infections prior to colposcopy in adolescents. *J Adolesc Health* 1997;21:87–90.

47. Spinillo A, Gorini G, Piazzi G, et al. The impact of oral contraception on chlamydial infection among patients with pelvic inflammatory disease. *Contraception* 1996; 54:163–168.

48. Wonler-Hansenn P, Eschembach DA, Paavonen J, et al. Decreased risk of symptomatic chlamydial pelvic inflammatory disease associated with oral contraceptive use. *JAMA* 1990;263:54–59.

49. Kouyoumdjian A, Kirkpatrick J. Coexistence of an intrauterine pregnancy with both an ectopic pregnancy and salpingitis in the right fallopian tube. *J Reprod Med* 1990;35:824.

50. Yip L, Sweeney P, Bock F. Acute suppurative salpingitis with concomitant intrauterine pregnancy. *Am J Emerg Med* 1993;11:476.

51. Acquavella AP, Rubin A, D'Angelo LJ. The coincident diagnosis of pelvic inflammatory disease in pregnancy: are they compatible? *J Pediatr Adolesc Gynecol* 1996;9: 129–132.

52. Taipale P, Tarjanne H, Ylostalo P. Transvaginal sonography in suspected pelvic inflammatory disease. *Ultrasound Obstet Gynecol* 1995;6:430–434.

53. Slap GB, Forke CM, Cnaan A, et al. Recognition of tubo-ovarian abscess in adolescents with pelvic inflammatory disease. *J Adolesc Health* 1996;18: 397–403.

54. Murthy JHK, Hiremagalur SR. Differentiation of tubo-ovarian abscess from pelvic inflammatory disease, and recent trends in the management of tubo-ovarian abscess. *J Tenn Med Assoc* 1995;88:136–138.

55. Blythe MJ. Pelvic inflammatory disease in the adolescent population. *Semin Pediatr Surg* 1998;7:43–51.

56. Grise RF, Morton CB. Acute abdominal symptoms from the bleeding ovary: analysis of eighty-four proved cases. *Surgery* 1950;29:117–123.

57. Kayaba H, Tamura H, Shirayama K, et al. Hemorrhagic ovarian cyst in childhood: a case report. *J Pediatr Surg* 1996;31:978–979.

58. Reynolds T, Hill MC, Glassman LM. Sonography of hemorrhagic ovarian cysts. *J Clin Ultrasound* 1986;14: 449–453.

59. Guerriero S, Mais V, Ajossa S, et al. The role of endovaginal ultrasound in differentiating endometriomas from other ovarian cysts. *Clin Exp Obstet Gynecol* 1995;22: 20–22.

60. Ectopic pregnancy—United States, 1988–1989. *MMWR* 1992;41:591–594.

61. Peterson HB, Xia Z, Hughes JM, et al. The risk of ectopic pregnancy after tubal sterilization. *N Engl J Med* 1997;336:762–767.

62. Tsai HD, Chen HY, Yeh LS. A 12 year survey of 681 ectopic pregnancies. *Chin Med J* 1995;55: 457–462.

63. Simms I, Rogers PA, Nicoll A. The influence of demographic change and cumulative risk of pelvic inflammatory disease on the incidence of ectopic pregnancy. *Epidemiol Infect* 1997;119:49–52.

64. Saraiya M, Berg CJ, Kendrick JS, et al. Cigarette smoking as a risk factor for ectopic pregnancy. *Am J Obstet Gynecol* 1998;178:493–498.

65. Parazzini F, Farraroni M, Tozzi L, et al. Past contraceptive method use and risk of ectopic pregnancy. *Contraception* 1995;52:93–98.

66. Atrash HK, Strauss LT, Kendrick JS, et al. The relation between induced abortion and ectopic pregnancy. *Obstet Gynecol* 1997;89:512–518.

67. Parazzini F, Ferranroni M, Tozzi L, et al. Induced abortions and the risk of ectopic pregnancy. *Hum Reprod* 1995;10:1841–1844.

68. Shalev E, Yarom I, Bustan M, et al. Transvaginal sonography as the ultimate diagnostic tool for the management of ectopic pregnancy: experience with 840 cases. *Fertil Steril* 1998;69:62–65.

69. Stika CS, Anderson L, Fredericksen MC. Single-dose methotrexate for the treatment of ectopic pregnancy: Northwestern Memorial Hospital three-year experience. *Am J Obstet Gynecol* 1996;174:1840–1848.

70. McCord ML, Muram D, Lipscomb GH, et al. Methotrexate therapy for ectopic pregnancy in adolescents. *J Pediatr Adolesc Gynecol* 1996;9:71–73.

71. Tan HK, Tay SK. Laparoscopic treatment of ectopic pregnancies—a study of 100 cases. *Ann Acad Med Singapore* 1996;25:665–667.

72. Clasen K, Camus M, Tournay H, et al. Ectopic pregnancy: let's cut! Strict laparoscopic approach to 194 consecutive cases and review of the literature on alternatives. *Human Reprod* 1997;12:596–601.

73. Glinter K. Chronic pelvic pain. *J Am Osteopath Assoc* 1974;74:335–341.

74. Goldstein D, DeCholnoky C, Leventhal J, et al. New insights into the old problem of chronic pelvic pain. *J Pediatr Surg* 1979;14:675–680.

75. Gross R, Doer RH, Caldirola D, et al. Borderline symptom and incest in chronic pelvic pain patients. *Int J Psychiatr Med* 1987;10:79–96.

76. Aftimos S. Myofascial pain in children. *N Z Med J* 1989;102:440.

77. Peters A, vanDorst E, Jellis B, et al. A randomized clinical trial to compare two different approaches to women with chronic pelvic pain. *Obstet Gynecol* 1991; 77:740.

78. Slocum JC. Neurological factors in chronic pelvic pain: trigger points and the abdominal pelvic pain syndrome. *Am J Obstet Gynecol* 1984;149:536.

79. Ling FW, Slocum JC. Use of trigger point injections in chronic pelvic pain. *Obstet Gynecol Clin North Am* 1993;20:809.

80. Simpson JL, Elias J, Malinak LR, et al. Heritable aspects of endometriosis. *Am J Obstet Gynecol* 1980; 137:327.

81. Bandera CA, Brown LR, Laufer MR. Adolescents and endometriosis. *Clin Consult Obstet Gynecol* 1995;7: 200.

82. Chatman D, Ward A. Endometriosis in adolescents. *J Reprod Med* 1982;27:156.

83. Goldstein DP, deCholnoky C, Emans SJ. Adolescent endometriosis. *J Adolesc Health Care* 1980;1:37.

84. Goldstein DP, deCholoky C, Emans SJ, et al. Laparoscopy in the diagnosis and management of pelvic pain in adolescents. *J Reprod Med* 1980;24:251.

85. Vercellini P, Fedele L, Arcaini L, et al. Laparoscopy in the diagnosis of pelvic pain in adolescent women. *J Reprod Med* 1989;34:827.

86. Wolfman W, Kreutner K. Laparoscopy in children and adolescents. *J Adolesc Health Care* 1984;5:261.

87. Laufer MR, Goitein L, Bush M, et al. Prevalence of endometriosis in adolescent girls with chronic pelvic pain not responding to conventional therapy. *J Pediatr Adolesc Gynecol* 1997;10:199.

88. Reese KA, Reddy S, Rock JA. Endometriosis in an adolescent population: the Emery experience. *J Pediatr Adolesc Gynecol* 1996;9:125.

89. Whitehouse H. Endometriosis invading the bladder removed from a patient who had never menstruated. *Proc R Soc Med* 1925–1926;19:15.

90. Stovall DW, Bowser LM, Archer DF, et al. Endometriosis associated pelvic pain: evidence for an association between the stage of disease and a history of chronic pelvic pain. *Fertil Steril* 1997;68:13.

19

Sexually Transmitted Infections

Jean Anderson

An estimated 15.3 million new cases of sexually transmitted infections (STIs) occur each year in the United States, with economic costs of approximately $10 billion per year, excluding human immunodeficiency virus (HIV). At least one fourth of STIs are in adolescents, and approximately two thirds of Americans who acquire STIs are younger than 25 years of age (1–3).

Women are more vulnerable to STIs. Anatomically, hormonally, and socially, STIs are more difficult to diagnose in women, because they are more commonly asymptomatic and often require speculum examination. Furthermore, vaginal flora and cervical mucous may complicate specimen collection and the sensitivity and specificity of diagnostic techniques. Women also suffer more frequent and severe adverse consequences, including infertility, genital tract cancer, and ectopic pregnancy. Finally, STIs occurring in pregnant women may result in adverse pregnancy outcomes or congenital infection (4,5).

For adolescent females at the beginning of their reproductive life, there are additional characteristics that make them particularly vulnerable to STIs and their serious consequences.

PHYSIOLOGIC SUSCEPTIBILITY

Although the clinical manifestations of STIs are similar in adolescents and adults, adolescents have some physiologic characteristics that make them more susceptible to certain infections if they are sexually active.

Against the background of earlier sexual maturation, as evidenced by decreasing age of menarche over the past century (6), up to 15%

of women are having anovulatory cycles 6 years after menarche (7). The estrogen dominance in these cycles stimulates copious cervical mucous production, but the mucous is thinner and more permeable than in older women (8). Therefore, pathogens may be more likely to attach to epithelial surfaces or to ascend and cause upper tract infection in these women.

Cervical ectopy is a characteristic of early puberty, with extension of columnar epithelium from the endocervical canal onto the vaginal surface of the cervix. Columnar epithelium is particularly vulnerable to infection with gonorrhea and chlamydia (8,9) and possibly HIV (10). In young adolescent girls, therefore, there is a greater surface area favorable for colonization with these pathogens. With age, metaplastic transformation takes place, and the transformation zone is formed, with less vulnerable, multilayered squamous epithelium replacing the fragile single layer of columnar epithelium.

Adolescents just starting sexual activity may be more likely to experience coital trauma of vaginal or cervical mucosa (including trauma to the more fragile columnar epithelium and cervical ectopy). This increases susceptibility to pathogens such as HIV.

The presence and/or role of specific immune mechanisms may be a factor but is not well understood.

SEXUAL BEHAVIOR

Against a background of increasing rates of sexual activity in adolescents in the 1970s and 1980s, recent data suggest a reversal of this

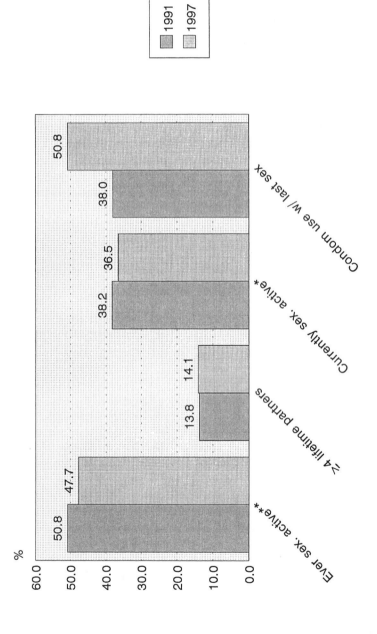

FIG. 19.1. Sexual behavior among high school girls in the United States from 1991 to 1997. (From CDC. Trends in sexual risk behaviors among high school students—United States, 1991–1997. *MMWR* 1998;47:749–752, with permission.)

*preceeding 3 months
**sexual activity defined as sexual intercourse
MMWR 1998;47:749-752

trend. Among female high school students, the proportion who had ever had sexual intercourse decreased from a high of 52.1% in 1995 to 47.7% in 1997. Of high school girls, 14.1% had four or more sex partners during their lifetime, and 36.5% were currently sexually active; slightly more than half had used condoms during their last sexual intercourse as compared to only 38% in 1991 (Fig. 19.1). The rates of sexual activity, multiple sexual partners, and current sexual activity (within the previous 3 months) were significantly higher among black adolescents than white or Hispanic youths; however, rates of condom use also were higher. More than 60% of all twelfth graders have been sexually active, 46% within the previous 3 months (11).

These behavioral changes are consistent with recent reports documenting national decreases in rates of gonorrhea as well as pregnancy (12,13). These decreases in sexual risk behaviors also correlate with an increase in the percentage of high school students who received HIV/acquired immunodeficiency syndrome (AIDS) education in school, from 83.3% in 1991 to 91.5% in 1997 (11).

Although the frequency of intercourse in adolescent females is significantly lower than in adult women, their sexual partners tend to be males 2 to 3 years older than themselves (14). These men generally have greater sexual experience and represent increased risk of STI transmission to their younger female partners.

There are two primary patterns of sexual activity in adolescents. The first pattern is serial monogamy—one relationship at a time, often with deep emotional attachments. However, there are data suggesting that perceptions of the strength of the relationship in heterosexual couples vary dramatically between males and females, with women more likely to perceive the relationship as strong (15). This, coupled with the fact that relationships are initiated at an age when individuals are psychologically unable to make a stable commitment, explains why these relationships are generally short lived. The majority of adolescent females fit into this pattern of sexual behavior (14). The second pattern is that of

sexual adventurers—multiple concurrent sexual partners and/or single sexual relationships in rapid sequence. Approximately 13% of sexually active adolescent women fit into this classification (16).

Contraceptive use affects risk of infection. Oral contraceptives and the male condom are the forms of contraception most commonly used by adolescents (17). Oral contraceptives have been associated with an increased risk of cervical infection with chlamydia (18). Furthermore, there is evidence that adolescents who use hormonal contraception are less likely to use condoms than other sexually active teens (17,19). Although condom use is increasing among adolescents, the majority do not use condoms consistently. There is also evidence that adolescents at greatest risk for STIs appear to use condoms least. Adolescent males who are substance abusers or who have paid for sex are among the least likely to have used condoms at last intercourse (20). Having greater numbers of sexual partners has been associated with less consistent condom use with either primary or secondary partners (21). A high pregnancy rate, even among those using contraception, further emphasizes the frequency of inconsistent or incorrect usage. It also has been found that the frequency with which contraception is used varies inversely with the level of emotional commitment to the relationship (15). Sexual encounters that are more casual (and with possibly higher risks for transmission of infection) are less likely to be associated with use of a contraceptive method that might be protective against the acquisition of infection. On the other hand, young women often believe that their steady partners would view a request to use a condom as indicating a lack of trust or trustworthiness.

These behaviors are partially explained by the unique place in which adolescents find themselves in term of both physical and psychosocial development. Adolescence is a time of rapid physical growth and maturation, often outpacing cognitive and social development. Because of the nature of these changes, along with the rapidity and differing time rates, adolescence is a time of marked psychological stress. During adolescence, there is increasing mobility and independence from parents, and greater identification with peers. Adolescents tend to associate with peers whose values and behavior are similar to what is learned and observed within their own family (22,23). However, peer pressure can be especially significant when the home environment lacks clearly expressed values or exhibits values that are inflexible and authoritarian, or when behavior at home is inconsistent. Adolescents also often have a sense of being invulnerable, believing that bad things will not happen to them or will be easily fixed, and thus they may be unable to fully comprehend the consequences of their actions. The psychic turmoil of adolescence contributes to frequent discrepancy between beliefs or attitudes and behavior. In a study of 3,500 inner city junior and senior high school students, Zabin et al. (15) found that 83% of those who had been sexually active cited the best age for first intercourse older than the age at which they themselves initiated intercourse. Furthermore, 43% stated the best age of first intercourse older than their current age. Behaviors also are affected by cultural setting. Geography, ethnicity, and social class all affect behavior. In certain populations, early sexual activity and childbearing are more accepted and even expected (24). In cultures where machismo has a strong influence, condom usage is less accepted (25).

Finally, the changes in sexual behavior documented over the past several decades must be seen against a background of increasing urbanization, changing sexual mores, and intense media bombardment with often explicit sexual content. From 1963 to 1975, the percentage of U.S. adults accepting premarital intercourse increased from approximately 20% to 70% (26). By the time the average American teenager has finished high school, it is estimated that he or she will have spent 15,000 hours watching television and only 12,000 in formal classroom instruction. It is not surprising that teens have ranked television as a major source of information about sex (27,28).

Incarcerated youths, runaways (many of whom wind up in prostitution), and youths who are victims of sexual assault or were abused constitute groups at particularly high risk for unsafe sexual behaviors and STIs (8).

USE OF AND ACCESS TO HEALTH CARE

The final factor that impacts on the adolescent's risk for an STI involves issues surrounding use of and access to care. The cost of health care and contraceptives, concerns about confidentiality, spoken or unspoken judgmental attitudes from health care providers, and feelings of embarrassment and shame often conspire to prevent adequate health care delivery to adolescents. More than 37% of tenth grade students did not know where to get treated for STIs, and more than 40% stated that they would be embarrassed to ask a doctor about symptoms related to the genitourinary tract (29).

Surveys have shown that adolescents are concerned about STIs and would like more information from their health care providers (30); however, a survey of college freshmen found that almost 80% had never received any counseling about STIs (31). It may be important for the health care provider to initiate these discussions, because adolescents may be too shy to do so themselves. Education about sexuality, contraception, and STIs necessitates use of easily understood and clearly defined terms, including current slang. Questioning should be direct, sensitive, and nonjudgmental. Confidentiality is a critical issue for adolescents. Parental consent is not required for evaluation and treatment of STIs in any state (32); nevertheless, the goal of the health care provider should be to aid adolescents in communicating with their parents and enlisting parental support for the adolescent. The severity of the infection, the need of the teenager for adult assistance to receive adequate medical care, and the developmental maturity of the adolescent all impact on decisions about confidentiality. Once an infection is diagnosed, compliance with prescribed treatment can be poor in adolescents and seems to vary with the nature of the illness and the clinical setting (33). Special considerations regarding metabolism or effectiveness of drugs used to treat STIs in adolescents have not been defined. Single-dose or short-course regimens may be especially helpful. Furthermore, new diagnostic techniques such as DNA amplification tests for gonorrhea and chlamydia, which can be performed on urine, will simplify screening and diagnosis. School-based clinics that provide reproductive health services are one of the few sources for accessible and affordable care for adolescents.

VIRAL INFECTIONS

Human Immunodeficiency Virus

Epidemiology

Through December 1998, Centers for Disease Control and Prevention (CDC) statistics revealed that 4% of AIDS cases and 18% of HIV infections (excluding AIDS) were in 13- to 24-year-olds (34). The number of AIDS cases among 15- to 19-year-olds diagnosed in the years 1993 to 1995 was 177% greater than the number diagnosed from 1988 to 1992 (35). Furthermore, recent calculations suggest that, during the period from 1987 to 1991, approximately 25% of HIV infections were acquired before the age of 22 (36). Prevalence of HIV infection in a number of studies frequently exceeded 1% among adolescents seen at sexually transmitted disease (STD) clinics, in shelters for homeless and runaways, and in those confined to correctional facilities (8). Females account for a larger proportion of adolescent AIDS cases than in older populations. In 1998, 50.5% of AIDS cases in adolescents 13 to 19 years old were in teenage girls compared to 39.6% of cases in those 20 to 24 years old and 22% of cases in those 25 years or older. In 1998, the male-to-female ratio in HIV infections among those 13 to 19 years old was 0.6 (34). Between 1988 and 1993, HIV prevalence in women aged 20 years rose by 36% (37). These trends of increasing HIV/AIDS in young women are fueled by increasing heterosexual transmission. Through 1998, heterosexual transmission accounted for 53% of AIDS cases in female teenagers 13 to 19 years old (Fig.

19.2) (34). The factors noted at the beginning of this chapter resulting in increased risk for other STIs apply to HIV infection as well. Furthermore, the presence of ulcerative and nonulcerative STIs increase the risk of transmission or acquisition of HIV two- to five-fold (38). Although HIV infection attributable to injection drug use has decreased among adolescents, drug use, both injection and noninjection, continues to play a major role in the epidemiology of this disease. In 1995, 7% of high school students had used cocaine at some time during their lives, according to a national survey (39). Cocaine may be used intravenously or intranasally and frequently is combined with other illicit drugs or alcohol; however, even in the absence of injection drug use, there is increased risk for HIV infection in those using cocaine and other drugs of abuse, probably secondary to exchange of sex for money or drugs and disinhibited sexual behavior when "high" (40,41). In several large urban areas with high HIV prevalence, greater than 30% of the injection drug using population may be HIV positive (42). For adolescents involved in drug use, that population may constitute the pool from which the majority of their sexual partners come, forming another link in their chain of risks.

As HIV is increasingly transmitted heterosexually, fewer individuals will know that they are at risk. In an 1988 report, Quinn et al. (43) found that almost three fourths of HIV-positive women under the age of 25 attending the Baltimore City STD clinics denied recognized risk factors. Nationally, investigation of adolescent and adult women with AIDS and no identified risk for exposure revealed that approximately two thirds are reclassified to the heterosexual exposure category. Ethnic and racial minorities constitute more than two thirds of adolescent AIDS cases (34).

Clinical Presentation

Because the average time from acquisition of HIV infection to diagnosis of AIDS is approximately 10 years or more, most adolescents will not develop AIDS and the majority

Exposure Category	13-19 years		20-24 years	
	N	%	N	%
Injection drug use	190	14	1,827	28
Hemophilia	12	1	13	<1
Heterosexual contact	708	53	3,614	54
Transfusion recipient	88	7	114	2
Other/undetermined*	350	26	1,072	16
Total	1,348	100	6,640	100

* Includes patients whose medical record review is pending; patients who died, were lost to follow-up, or declined interview; and patients with other or undetermined modes of exposure

FIG. 19.2. Acquired immunodeficiency syndrome (AIDS) cases in female adolescents and young adults, by exposure category, through 1998 in the United States. (From the Centers for Disease Control and Prevention. HIV/AIDS surveillance in adolescents slide series, with permission.)

will be asymptomatic. Within 2 to 6 weeks of infection, approximately one half of individuals infected with HIV have an acute mononucleosis-like syndrome with nonspecific signs and symptoms (44,45), which often is unrecognized. Primary HIV infection is associated with high levels of viremia and increased risk of transmission to others. The signs and symptoms associated with initial infection resolve spontaneously, and the individual becomes asymptomatic. Although they may remain clinically asymptomatic for many years, CD4-positive T-lymphocytes begin a slow decline, mirroring progressive immunologic dysfunction. Ultimately, in the majority and perhaps all of those who are HIV infected, CD4-positive cells drop below critical levels, viral burden increases, and the individual becomes symptomatic. Symptoms and signs at this stage of illness often include lymphadenopathy, chronic and/or recurrent mucocutaneous candidiasis (including vaginal), and recurrent atypical herpetic infection (46). Finally, patients become so immunocompromised that they develop opportunistic infections and/or an AIDS-associated malignancy. The most common AIDS defining illness and cause of death in patients is pneumocystis pneumonia (Fig. 19.3) (47). Recent advances in therapy (see Treatment) have interrupted this natural history with significant declines in mortality and morbidity secondary to AIDS (48).

Diagnosis

The diagnosis of HIV-1 infection is made by detecting antibodies to the virus, by detecting p24 antigen (an HIV core antigen), or by detecting virus with nucleic acid-based tests or culture (49). The most commonly used test is serology for antibody detection with an enzyme immunoassay (EIA) screening assay and a confirming Western blot on EIA-positive specimens. The Western blot assay identifies antibodies specific for different HIV viral antigens and yields a profile of viral bands characteristic of HIV when incubated with antibody positive serum. Results are reported as positive or reactive, negative, or indetermi-

nant. Overall sensitivity is 99.3%, with specificity of 99.7% (50). The most common cause of a false-negative test is testing during the "window period," after viral transmission but before seroconversion. This is a period that is generally in the range of 3 to 12 weeks and rarely exceeds 6 months (51). Newer, more sensitive antibody tests reduce the typical window period 3 to 4 weeks (52). Indeterminant tests usually result from a positive enzyme-linked immunosorbent assay and a single band on Western blot. Causes of indeterminant results include seroconversion in process; the presence of autoantibodies as seen in collagen vascular disease, autoimmune diseases, and malignancy; and cross-reacting antibodies from pregnancy, blood transfusion, or organ transplantation (53a,53b,54).

A home testing kit for HIV detection is now available in which blood is obtained by a lancet, and a filter strip with blotted blood is mailed for testing in a protective envelope and using an anonymous code. Sensitivity and specificity approach 100%. Negative test results are given through a prerecorded message. Callers who have positive results receive counseling and health care referral from a counselor. There are now three Food and Drug Administration (FDA)-licensed rapid tests that can give results in less than 10 minutes. Sensitivity approaches 100% and specificity is 99.6%; therefore, positive results should be confirmed with routine serology (54). These tests may be especially useful in situations where immediate results are needed or where follow-up visits may be difficult or compliance with follow-up is poor. There also are two FDA-approved tests for HIV detection using urine and saliva, respectively, for antibody detection. Orasure, which uses saliva, has a sensitivity of 99.9% and specificity of 99% (55); advantages of this test over standard serologic testing include ease of specimen collection, reduced cost, and better patient acceptability, all of which may be issues for adolescents.

HIV viral culture is not used for routine diagnosis of HIV because of its cost and complexity. DNA or RNA polymerase chain reac-

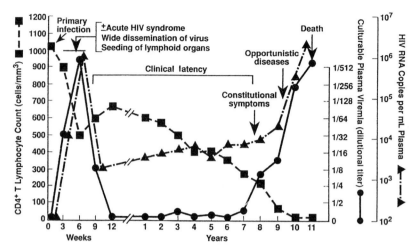

FIG. 19.3. Natural history of untreated human immunodeficiency virus (HIV) infection. (From Fauci AS, Pantaleo G, Stanley S, et al. Immunopathogenic mechanisms of HIV infection. *Ann Intern Med* 1996;124:654–663, with permission.)

tion (PCR) are other viral detection methods to diagnose HIV infection. They generally are not used for routine diagnosis but may be helpful in certain situations, such as primary HIV infection or with challenged or indeterminant serologic testing. Quantitative HIV RNA is the standard test for staging and therapeutic monitoring of HIV infection.

HIV testing should always be preceded by counseling. This should include risk assessment, prevention counseling, issues related to confidentiality, and discussion of what a positive and negative test means. Testing should be voluntary. Informed consent is required in most states and generally is recommended. States vary in their statutes allowing minors to consent to HIV testing (56). HIV testing increased by 44% in 13- to 17-year-olds in Connecticut after removal of a parental consent requirement (57). Posttest counseling should be provided, whether the test result is positive or negative. A negative result will allow an opportunity to intervene when high-risk behaviors have been identified and possibly prevent HIV transmission. When HIV testing is positive, it is essential that appropri-

ate referrals for comprehensive care be made available.

Treatment

Follow-up of the HIV-infected individual requires a comprehensive and multidisciplinary approach. Counseling about safer sexual practices, including the consistent use of male or female condoms and adequate contraception, should be ongoing. Screening for other STIs should be performed regularly in HIV-infected adolescents who are sexually active. Vaginal candidiasis, genital herpes, human papilloma virus (HPV) infection, and squamous intraepithelial lesions are seen more commonly in HIV-infected individuals and may increase in frequency or severity with declining immune function (58–62). CD4 cell counts and HIV RNA levels are followed at 3- to 4-month intervals as indicators of immune function and viral replication. After becoming the third leading cause of death among women 25 to 44 years old in 1994 to 1995 (63), HIV infection has now dropped to fourth overall, although it still remains the second leading cause of death for young black and Hispanic women (64). Along with the decline in mortality, there has been a significant drop in incidence of opportunistic infections and hospitalizations secondary to AIDS (65). These dramatic advances are secondary to better understanding of the natural history of HIV, the ability to measure viral replication and monitor therapeutic response with HIV RNA levels, and, most significantly, the availability of multiple new antiretroviral agents. These agents, commonly given in three drug combinations to maximally suppress viral replication and reduce the emergence of resistant mutants, have dramatically affected longevity and quality of life for HIV-infected individuals. However, these agents offer special challenges in terms of drug toxicity and side effects, interactions with other medications, complexity of regimens, cost, and adherence to therapy (66). The most common cause of failure for these regimens is lack of adherence to therapy. Adolescents with HIV require extensive counseling about the issues of taking antiretroviral therapy and receiving support from their families and health care providers to enable them to take these therapies consistently and correctly. Feelings of invulnerability, rebelliousness, and stigmatization may place adolescents at greater risk for nonadherence and treatment failure. With progression of HIV infection and decline in CD4 cell count below 200/mm^3, HIV-infected individuals should be treated prophylactically with sulfamethoxazole/trimethoprim (Bactrim), dapsone, or aerosolized pentamidine to prevent pneumocystis pneumonia, the most common AIDS indicator condition. Prophylaxis of other common opportunistic infections is indicated with further immunocompromise (47).

Human Papilloma Virus

Epidemiology

HPV infection of the genital tract is the most common STI in the United States, with an estimated incidence of 5.5 million new cases every year and approximately 20 million people currently infected (1). Prevalence of HPV-DNA positivity in adolescent populations ranges from 13% to 38% (67). Using cervicovaginal lavage for cell collection and Southern blot DNA hybridization, Rosenfeld et al. (68) compared 71 teenagers aged 13 to 18 years who had multiple lifetime sexual partners and 74 teenagers in the same age group who had only one lifetime sexual partner. HPV prevalence was 54% and 34%, respectively. However, no such differences in HPV prevalence were found between older adolescents with and without multiple partners, suggesting that some degree of immunity may develop in older women who have been exposed to HPV, or that sexual partners or behaviors are less risky than those of younger women (68).

A recent U.S. study among female college students found that approximately 14% were infected each year and 43% of the women in the study were infected with HPV over the 3-year study period (69). Prevalence of HPV infection for women under the age of 25 years is as high as 46% (70,71).

Clinical Presentation

There are more than 80 distinct types of HPV. At least one third of these have been found to infect the lower genital tract. These infections may be symptomatic and clinically apparent or, more commonly, asymptomatic and invisible to gross inspection. HPV infection is multicentric in the lower genital tract in more than 80% of cases (72). Different sites may be infected with more than one virus type (73). HPV is the etiologic agent for genital warts, which may appear in four different morphologic types: (i) condyloma acuminata, which are cauliflower-shaped growths (Fig. 19.4); (ii) smooth 1- to 4-mm papular lesions that are dome shaped and usually skin colored; (iii) keratotic warts with a thick horny layer, commonly resembling warts found on other parts of the body; and (iv) flat or slightly raised flat-topped papules (74). Genital warts

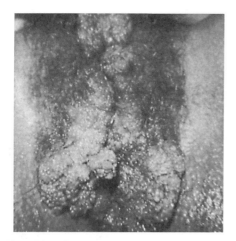

FIG. 19.4. Condyloma acuminata of human papilloma virus infection.

appears to be an important risk factor for progression. It is likely that progression of HPV-induced lesions to malignancy requires a cofactor(s). Suggested cofactor(s) thought to possibly influence the natural history of HPV infection include herpes simplex virus (HSV) or other STIs, cigarette smoking, and immunosuppression (80,81) The risk of becoming infected with HPV or developing genital warts after sexual contact is not known. Genital warts may develop 1 to 2 months after initial exposure, although subsequent recurrences are largely unpredictable. Infectivity may be greater for persons who have clinically apparent genital warts than for those with subclinical HPV infection.

are usually asymptomatic, but they can cause great concern and embarrassment by their presence. Depending on size, number, location, and presence of superinfection, they may be painful, friable, or pruritic. Rarely, HPV infection may be transmitted during delivery to a newborn infant, resulting in laryngeal or vulvar papillomatosis.

Natural History

Evidence from prospective follow-up of women infected with HPV and from correlation of histopathologic evaluation with nucleic acid hybridization data from neoplastic lesions clearly and consistently points to an association between HPV and lower genital tract neoplasia, both intraepithelial and invasive (75,76). HPV types are divided into high, intermediate, and low risk based on their association with anogenital cancer. HPV type 16 accounts for more than 50% of cervical cancers and high-grade lesions. HPV types 16, 18, 31, and 45 account for 80% of cervical cancers (77,78). HPV also has been linked to vulvar, vaginal, and anal neoplasia.

Most HPV infections appear to be transient. Persistence of the infection over time, which is more common with higher risk types and immunosuppression, and in older women (79),

Diagnosis

Diagnosis of HPV infection may be made on clinical examination if the lesion is clinically apparent. Bright lighting and magnification may aid visual examination. Application of a 3% to 10% acetic acid solution, resulting in a whitening of HPV-infected tissues, has a low positive predictive value and is not routinely recommended. Biopsy of lesions should be considered when lesions are atypical; the diagnosis is in doubt; there is progression of disease during treatment; there are prompt and/or frequent recurrences; warts appear pigmented, ulcerated, or fixed; or there are very large individual warts (larger than 1 cm). Subclinical infection has been recognized with cytology, colposcopy, histopathology, and more directly and sensitively with DNA hybridization and amplification. PCR is currently the most sensitive technique for HPV detection. The role of sensitive molecular techniques for HPV detection and typing in diagnosis and management of HPV infection has not yet been defined. Because the diagnosis and treatment of genital warts is not influenced by HPV type, routine HPV-DNA detection and typing of genital warts is not currently recommended (74).

HPV infection and HPV-associated neoplasia of the anogenital tract occur much more frequently in immunodeficient patients, particularly those with defects in cell-mediated immunity, than in the general population. Furthermore, HPV infection and neoplasia in these patients may have an accelerated clinical course, are more extensive in area, and recur more frequently, paralleling the severity of immunocompromise (82,83).

Treatment

There is no currently available therapy to effectively eradicate the presence of HPV in the lower genital tract. When grossly visible disease is present, genital warts may resolve spontaneously, remain unchanged, or increase in size and number. There are several available treatments for genital warts, divided into patient-applied or provider-administered therapies. No single treatment modality is ideal for all patients, and none appears to be clearly superior in terms of efficacy. Size, location, and number of genital warts will affect treatment decisions, as will coexisting medical conditions. Because most treatments disrupt skin integrity to some degree, the patient may be at increased risk for acquiring or transmitting other STIs during the healing process.

Patient-applied therapies include podofilox 0.5% solution or gel, an antimitotic agent, or imiquimod (Aldara), an immune response enhancer. Imiquimod is an inducer of interferon α and other cytokines, including tumor necrosis factor α and interleukin 6. These agents are used by serial application to external genital warts; use on mucosal services should be avoided. Localized signs and symptoms of skin irritation are the most common side effects. Approximately 40% to 80% of patients obtain total clearance of the warts with either of these therapies (74).

Provider-administered treatments include topical applications of bichloroacetic acid (BCA) or trichloroacetic acid (TCA) (80% to 90% concentration), or applications of podophyllin as a 10% to 25% suspension in tincture of benzoin. Repetitive applications of these agents usually are required. Unlike podophyllin, TCA or BCA may be applied intravaginally or to the cervix, as well as during pregnancy. Both can cause local skin irritation. Podophyllin should be washed off within a few hours after application, and TCA/BCA can be neutralized with soap or sodium bicarbonate if necessary. Clearance rates range from 19% to 80% for podophyllin and 50% to 100% for BCA/TCA (74). Cryotherapy, electrocautery, or simple office excision are other simple provider-administered therapies. Intralesional injection of interferon may be effective in the eradication of warts in some cases, but it is costly and has a high frequency of systemic adverse side effects, including flu-like symptoms, leukopenia, thrombocytopenia, and elevated liver enzymes.

Topical or office-based therapies are less likely to be successful when there is a large volume or bulk of genital warts. Vaporization with the CO_2 laser may be the most effective tool in these patients. The external genitalia, perianal region, vagina, and cervix can be treated concurrently. Urethroscopy and anoscopy, which can be easily performed at the time of laser therapy, is helpful to rule out disease in these areas, especially in patients with extensive lower genital tract involvement. Laser therapy is expensive and usually requires general or regional anesthesia; however, it is the treatment of choice in patients with extensive condylomata or HPV disease that has been refractory to other therapy.

As noted earlier, no method of treatment is clearly superior to any other, and there are no clear guidelines concerning which treatments to use first and when to change therapies. When using local topical therapies, it is reasonable to consider changing treatment when three treatment sessions have passed without significant improvement, complete clearance has not occurred after six treatment sessions, or the manufacturer's recommendations for duration of patient-applied therapy have been reached (74). There is no evidence that combining therapies increases effectiveness but may increase complication rates. Regardless of the methods used, recurrence rates are high. Therapies in development include 5-fluorouracil (5-FU)/epinephrine/bovine collagen gel implants and cidofovir. The implants combine the antimetabolite 5-FU with a vasoconstrictor and a biodegradable stabilizing gel that is injected directly below the wart. Because 5-FU is a mutagen and teratogen, it is important that women use effective contraception while being treated; it should be avoided in pregnant women. Cidofovir is a newly developed nucleoside phosphate analogue with broad-spectrum antiviral activity against DNA viruses. It is currently under investigation.

Choice of treatment modality in adolescents should include consideration of their cognitive and emotional development, willingness and ability to use patient-applied therapies, tolerance of minor side effects, and the need to use effective contraception with certain modalities.

It should be reemphasized that none of these methods, despite their frequent efficacy in eliminating gross disease, has been shown to eradicate the presence of HPV. Recurrence is frequent, and the patient should still be considered at potentially increased risk for lower genital tract neoplasia. Pap smear screening should be performed at least annually and colposcopic evaluation of the entire lower genital tract used when cytologic abnormalities are identified. Sexual partners may have clinical or subclinical HPV disease as well; however, treatment of partners has not been shown to prevent recurrences in females with HPV. Patients should be counseled about the implications of HPV, the possible long-term sequelae, and the possibility of transmitting infection to their sexual partners. Condom use should be encouraged and should reduce the risk of transmission; however, transmission of HPV may still occur in condom users by skin-to-skin contact of areas not covered by the condom. Ultimately, the best hope in preventing transmission will be development of a prophylactic vaccine, which is now under active development.

Herpes Simplex Virus

Epidemiology

Using type-specific antibody testing in a national population-based survey, the seroprevalence of HSV-2 in children 12 years of age or older in the United States was 21.9% from 1988 to 1994, which is a 30% increase from the late 1970s (84). The recent seroprevalence survey of adolescents recruited from an urban hospital-based adolescent clinic and a Job Corps site found that 64% of the adolescent girls studied were seropositive for HSV-1 and 14% were seropositive for HSV-2. Girls were more likely than boys to be seropositive for HSV-2 and, in this study, acquired HSV-2 infection at a young age; the seroprevalence rate in girls under age 16 years was 16%. In this study, risk factors for seropositivity included the number of sexual partners and being of African-American race (85). In other studies, early age at first intercourse and history of an STI have been associated with HSV-2 infection (86–88).

HSV transmission generally occurs through close contact with an individual shedding virus at a peripheral site or mucosal surface or in secretions. The virus then is inoculated onto susceptible mucosal surfaces or through small skin abrasions. At the time of the initial infection, the virus ascends peripheral nerves and establishes latency in sensory or autonomic nerve root ganglia. HSV-2 is the most common cause of genital herpes, although 1% to 30% of primary episodes are with HSV-1 (89). Incidence rates for HSV infections were assessed in a 15-year study of 839 adolescent women in Sweden and demonstrated that 50% had acquired HSV-1 and 22% had acquired HSV-2 by the end of the study (90). In addition to higher seroprevalence, women also have a higher rate of acquisition of HSV-2. In one study of serodiscordant couples, the attack rate among seronegative women was approximately 30% per year (91). Most episodes of transmission occur with subclinical shedding.

Clinical Presentation

Clinical manifestations of genital herpes vary with viral type and host factors, such as previous episodes or serologic evidence of past exposure to HSV-1 or HSV-2. In prospective studies, 70% of initial infections with HSV-2 develop genitourinary complaints around the time of acquisition; however, many of these symptoms may be mild or atypical and therefore go unrecognized (89).

More than 50% of women with primary genital HSV-2 infection (no serologic evidence of past HSV-1 or HSV-2) have constitutional symptoms with fever, headache, malaise, and myalgias. These symptoms appear early in the course of disease, peak within 3 to 4 days after the onset of lesions, and gradually recede over the subsequent 3 to 4 days. The classic hallmark signs of primary herpes are widespread painful lesions on the external genitalia. Beginning as papules or vesicles, these lesions become pustular and then ulcerate, eventually healing with crusting and reepithelialization without residual scarring (Fig. 19.5). Duration

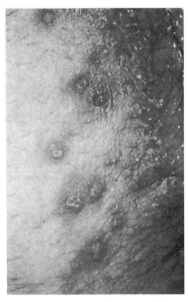

FIG. 19.5. Vulvar papules and ulcers associated with herpes simplex infection.

of viral shedding is approximately 12 days. Other common local symptoms include itching, dysuria, vaginal or urethral discharge, and tender inguinal adenopathy. Concomitant HSV cervicitis appears in 70% to 90% of those experiencing primary infection (92). Complications of primary genital herpes infection occur more commonly in women and include central nervous system involvement, pharyngitis, and extragenital lesions.

Patients with first episode but nonprimary infection with HSV (serologic evidence of past HSV-1 or HSV-2) are less likely to have systemic symptoms and tend to have a milder and shorter duration of local signs and symptoms than persons with true primary infection.

Recurrent genital herpes is characterized by signs and symptoms localized to the genital region, usually unilaterally. Approximately 50% of persons develop prodomal symptoms before the appearance of lesions; these symptoms range from mild tingling to lancinating pains in the buttocks or hips. Symptoms are milder compared to primary infection. Mean duration of lesions is 9 to 10 days, with viral shedding lasting about 4 days from the onset of lesions. Some 15% to 30% of women have concomitant HSV viral shedding from the cervix (89). Recurrence rate depends on viral type, severity of initial episode, and host immune response. Ninety percent of patients have recurrence in the first year after primary episode with HSV-2 versus 60% who have primary HSV-1 infection (93). Patients with a more prolonged initial episode develop higher titers of HSV-2 neutralizing antibody in convalescent sera and are more likely to have recurrence than those who do not develop neutralizing antibody (94,95), possibly reflecting the degree of antigenic exposure during the primary episode and/or a large number of latently infected cells in nerve root ganglia. Recurrence rates vary between individuals and within a given individual over time.

Asymptomatic viral shedding can occur from the cervix, vulva, anus, and urethra. Subclinical shedding is most likely to occur close in temporal proximity to recurrences, and frequent recurrences are associated with frequent subclinical shedding. Subclinical HSV reactivation is seen most commonly in the 6 months after acquisition of infection.

Immunocompromised individuals, including those with HIV infection, often have more atypical, more frequent, and more prolonged genital herpetic outbreaks. As immune function diminishes, viral shedding is increased. In addition, recurrent episodes may have characteristics more similar to primary infection, with systemic symptoms and widespread lesions (96–98).

A major concern in pregnant women with HSV infection is the possibility of transmission to the fetus or neonate. Neonatal herpes, although rare (one of 3,000 to one of 20,000 live births) is a disease of high morbidity and mortality (99). Primary genital herpes in pregnancy carries a risk of perinatal transmission of approximately 50%, whereas transmission with recurrent disease is less than 1% (89). More than 70% of infants with neonatal herpes infections were born to mothers without signs or symptoms at delivery (99,100). Transplacental transmission may occur with primary infection, but most neonatal herpes infection is acquired by contact with the infected maternal genital tract during the intrapartum period. Therefore, women who have clinical evidence of infection or prodromal symptoms at the time of labor should be delivered by cesarean section. Patients with a history of HSV infection but without signs and symptoms of HSV at the time of labor may be allowed to deliver vaginally, although a culture should be obtained from the cervix and vulva to further identify those infants who may be exposed to asymptomatic HSV shedding.

Diagnosis

Viral culture is considered the gold standard for documenting a diagnosis of genital herpes, and it can distinguish between HSV-1 and HSV-2. HSV-DNA detection with PCR promises exquisite sensitivity and the ability to quantitate viral shedding, and it should be available commercially in the near future. Rapid detection methods, including immunofluorescent, immunoperoxidase, and EIA techniques for detecting viral antigen, and DNA hybridization, have sensitivities approaching that of culture when genital lesions are present but reduced sensitivity for asymptomatic viral shedding (101). Type-specific serologic methods, not yet commercially available, can determine if a person is an asymptomatic HSV carrier, but they are not helpful in making a definitive diagnosis in the presence of genital lesions. Cytologic detection has good specificity but poor sensitivity.

Treatment

In first-episode genital herpes, acyclovir 200 mg PO five times a day or 400 mg PO three times a day markedly reduces the duration of symptoms and viral shedding and speeds healing. More recently, valacyclovir, which is almost completely converted to acyclovir by hepatic and intestinal enzymes and significantly increases the bioavailability of acyclovir, has shown comparable effectiveness at a dose of 1,000 mg b.i.d. Famciclovir, a prodrug of penciclovir, is also effective (250 mg PO t.i.d.) and well tolerated. These are generally given for 7 to 10 days. They have no effect on subsequent natural history of the infection. Recommended regimens for episodic recurrent infection include acyclovir 400 mg t.i.d.; acyclovir 200 mg five times a day; acyclovir 800 mg b.i.d.; famciclovir 125 mg b.i.d.; or valacyclovir 500 mg b.i.d., all given for 5 days (102,103). Patient-initiated therapy early in the course of a recurrent episode has some benefit in shortening the duration of lesion and viral shedding (104).

Daily suppressive therapy reduces frequency of genital herpes recurrences by 75% or more among patients who have six or more recurrences per year. Regimens used for suppression include acyclovir 400 mg b.i.d., famciclovir 250 mg b.i.d., valacyclovir 500 mg q.d., and valacyclovir 1,000 mg q.d. (should be used as the valacyclovir preferred dose regimen in patients with more than ten episodes per year). Safety and effectiveness of acyclovir when used for daily suppressive therapy has now been documented for more than 6 years and for more than 1 year with the newer drugs (102,103).

Hepatitis C

Epidemiology

Hepatitis C is the most common chronic bloodborne infection in the United States. It is estimated that some 3.9 million individuals in the United States have been infected with the hepatitis C virus (HCV), resulting in approximately 8,000 to 10,000 deaths each year (105). Although HCV is transmitted primarily through direct percutaneous exposures to blood, case control studies have reported an association between sexual exposure to a partner who has history of hepatitis or history of multiple sexual partners and acquisition of hepatitis C (106,107). Fifteen to twenty percent of patients with acute hepatitis C reported to the CDC have no risk factors other than sexual exposure (105). There is evidence that sexual transmission of HCV from male to female is more likely than from female to male (108).

Clinical Presentation

Acute HCV infection is asymptomatic in approximately two thirds of individuals; the remainder have a mild clinical illness with jaundice and/or nonspecific symptoms. Fifteen to twenty-five percent of individuals subsequently resolve their infection without sequelae, but chronic HCV infection develops in the remainder; approximately two thirds of those with chronic HCV infection have ongoing active liver disease. The course of chronic liver disease is insidious, with development of cirrhosis in 10% to 20% over a period of 20 to 30 years and hepatocellular carcinoma in 1% to 5% (105).

Diagnosis

The only test currently approved by the U.S. FDA for diagnosis of HCV infection measures HCV antibody by EIA with supplemental testing by the more specific recombinant immunoblot assay. These tests detect HCV antibody in more than 97% of infected patients but cannot distinguish among acute, chronic, or resolved infection (105).

Both qualitative and quantitative PCR techniques for detection of HCV RNA are available. They are not recommended as primary tests to confirm or exclude the diagnosis.

Treatment

In patients who are HCV positive, evaluation for presence of chronic liver disease includes multiple measurements of alanine aminotransferase levels at regular intervals. Antiviral therapy is recommended for patients with chronic HCV infection who have persistently elevated alanine aminotransferase levels, detectable HCV RNA, and a liver biopsy revealing portal or bridging fibrosis or moderate or greater degrees of inflammation and necrosis (105). Therapy for hepatitis C involves interferon with or without ribavirin, a nucleoside analogue. These therapies currently are not approved by the FDA for patients under the age of 18 years.

Hepatitis B

Epidemiology

Hepatitis B virus (HBV) affects an estimated 200,000 persons each year in the United States; of these cases, 120,000 are thought secondary to sexual transmission; most are young adults (109). High-risk heterosexual practices, including more than one sexual partner in the previous 6 months or a history of other STIs, are estimated to account for 40% of acute hepatitis B infections (110). In those acquiring infection through heterosexual contact, risk increases with numbers of previous sexual partners. The overall age-adjusted prevalence of HBV infection as determined by data from the National Health and Nutrition Examination Surveys (NHANES II 1976–1980 and NHANES III 1988–1994) was 5.5% in NHANES II compared with 4.9% in NHANES III, with the highest prevalence in black participants (111). This demonstrates that there has been no significant decrease in HBV infection despite the availability of hepatitis B vaccine. It is currently estimated that 417,000 individuals are living with HBV in the United States (110).

Clinical Presentation

After an incubation period of 40 to 110 days, HBV presents insidiously with anorexia, malaise, nausea, vomiting, abdominal pain, and jaundice. Skin rash, arthralgias, and arthritis are less common findings. Many individuals infected with HBV probably have silent infections. In most cases, infection resolves uneventfully. Less than 1% die of an acute infection, and 1% to 6% will become chronic carriers of infection. An estimated 25% of carriers develop chronic active hepatitis, often progressing to cirrhosis. Primary hepatocellular carcinoma is up to 300 times more common in HBV carriers than in the general population (103,112).

Diagnosis

Specific serologic markers are used to make a diagnosis of HBV infection. Hepatitis B surface antigen (HBsAg) can be identified in serum 1 to 2 months after exposure to HBV and persists for a variable period of time. Antibody to the core antigen develops in all HBV infections and persists indefinitely. The immunoglobulin M (IgM) antibody fraction is indicative of recent infection. The presence of hepatitis Be antigen correlates with viral replication and high infectivity. Chronic carrier status is documented by sustained positivity for HBsAg. The appearance of antibody to HBsAg (anti-HBs) indicates resolution of the infection and is protective against reinfection.

Treatment

There is no specific treatment for acute HBV infection, other than supportive care and monitoring. For postexposure prophylaxis after sexual exposure to an individual who is HBsAg positive, a single dose of hepatitis B immune globulin is 75% effective if it is given within 2 weeks of sexual exposure (112).

Ongoing sexual contacts of patients with acute or chronic HBV and those with a history of multiple sexual partners or who have recently acquired another STD should be considered for vaccination. The recommended series of three intramuscular injections of hepatitis B vaccine induces an adequate antibody response in more than 95% of adolescents. Universal prenatal screening now is recommended for pregnant women as a means of preventing perinatal transmission. Universal vaccination of infants and adolescents now also is recommended as an additional strategy for gaining control over this disease (113). Use of condoms may reduce sexual transmission.

Hepatitis A

Hepatitis A is primarily transmitted by fecal contamination and oral ingestion, but transmission may be facilitated by sexual contact, particularly sexual practices including oral-anal contact. The average incubation period is 28 days, and greatest infectivity occurs 2 weeks immediately preceding the onset of jaundice. No chronic carrier state exists with infection by the hepatitis A virus (HAV). Diagnosis of acute infection is made by finding IgM anti-HAV in serum. Immune globulin contains antibodies against HAV and is protective against infection when given preexposure or during the incubation period of the virus. It is recommended for all sexual contacts of persons with hepatitis A. Hepatitis A vaccines are now available and are given on a two-dose schedule, with 6 to 12 months between doses. Protective levels of antibodies to HAV are produced 2 to 4 weeks after active immunization, and efficacy in prevention of HAV is 94% to 100% (114).

Cytomegalovirus

Cytomegalovirus infection is a prevalent infection spread most commonly by sexual transmission, maternal-fetal transmission, and transfusion-associated transmission. Most infections are asymptomatic, although a mononucleosis-like illness may occur. Congenital cytomegalovirus infection, however, may be associated with significant morbidity, including neurologic abnormalities, jaundice, and chorioretinitis (115). Antigen detection or assays of viral DNA are the most useful tests for diagnosis. Vaccination holds promise for future preventive efforts.

Molluscum Contagiosum

Molluscum contagiosum is an infection caused by a member of the pox virus family involving the skin and mucous membranes. Infection can be spread by both sexual and non-sexual roots of transmission through direct contact with the skin of infected person or fomites (116,117). After an incubation period averaging 2 to 3 months, a number of smooth firm papules form with characteristic central umbilications (Fig. 19.6). Most lesions occur on the thighs, lower abdominal wall, or genital region, and most are asymptomatic. Normal hosts have 10 to 20 lesions, but immunocompromised individuals may develop hundreds of lesions, usually at extragenital sites (118). Diagnosis may be made by identifying the characteristic intracytoplasmic molluscum bodies in cytologic or histologic specimens.

The infection is benign and self-limited. Individual lesions usually resolve within 2 months. Treatment usually consists of destruction of lesions with dermal curettage, cryotherapy, or expression of the core of the papule with direct pressure. Alternatively, application of a chemical irritant, such as podophyllin, trichloroacetic acid, or silver nitrate, has been used but may require more than one treatment. Recurrences are common.

BACTERIAL AND CHLAMYDIAL INFECTIONS

Chlamydia

Epidemiology

Chlamydia trachomatis is the most commonly reported STI in the United States, with an estimated three million new cases annually (119). However, chlamydia seems to be declining overall because of better screening and treatment of women. Adolescent females

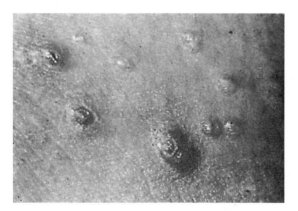

FIG. 19.6. Characteristic papular lesions of molluscum contagiosum with central umbilications.

have the highest age-specific rates of chlamydia. Chlamydia prevalence among sexually active teenage girls often exceeds 10%. A 1997 study of female military recruits found a prevalence of chlamydia of 12.2% among 17-year-olds (120). A 1998 school-based screening program among high school students in New Orleans found that nearly 13% of girls were infected with chlamydia (121).

Almost 21% of 415 attending adolescent clinics were infected with chlamydia, with a higher prevalence found in those who douched at least monthly (122). Chlamydia is a coexistent pathogen in up to 30% to 50% of women with gonorrhea (123). Oral contraceptive use has been associated with increased risk of cervical *C. trachomatis* infection, probably because their use tends to increase cervical ectopy (124).

Clinical Presentation

Approximately 75% of chlamydial infections are asymptomatic (125). When symptoms occur, they are likely to include abnormal vaginal discharge, dysuria, frequency, and abnormal vaginal bleeding. On examination, mucopurulent discharge (more than ten polymorphonuclear leukocytes, × 1,000 field), cervical edema, erythema, and friability often are found. Mucopurulent discharge will appear yellow or green on an endocervical swab. Unfortunately, these simple findings do not have sufficient sensitivity or specificity to adequately make a diagnosis of chlamydial infection.

When women are cultured from both cervix and urethra, 50% of those with positive cultures are positive from both sites and 25% from either site alone (126). Chlamydial urethritis has been implicated as a cause of urethral syndrome (dysuria, frequency, pyuria without bacteriuria). Chlamydia also may produce infection in Bartholin's gland. Histologic evidence of endometritis is present in about 50% of patients with chlamydial cervicitis (127).

Chlamydial infection in pregnancy has been associated with preterm delivery and/or low birth weight and postpartum endometritis. Disease can be transmitted vertically and results in neonatal conjunctivitis and/or pneumonia.

The most common and most serious complication of lower genital tract chlamydial infection is upper genital tract infection or pelvic inflammatory disease (PID), discussed more fully later. Up to 40% of women with untreated cervical chlamydial infection will develop PID (110). Because of the high prevalence of chlamydia in sexually active adolescents, this population should be routinely screened using one of the specific diagnostic techniques discussed in the following section.

Diagnosis

Isolation of *C. trachomatis* is complicated by the fact that it is an obligate intracellular parasite and has a unique lifecycle. It alternates between two morphologically separate forms: the elementary body, which is relatively resistant to extracellular environment and responsible for cell-to-cell and host-to-host infection but metabolically inactive; and the reticulate body, which requires a intracellular environment and is metabolically active but not infectious.

Culture has long been considered the gold standard for the diagnosis for *C. trachomatis.* It requires collection of cells (specimens composed totally of white blood cells or discharge are inadequate). For cervical specimens, a cytobrush may increase sensitivity of culture because more cells are collected. However, the cost, turnaround time, and fastidious collection and transport requirements are real disadvantages in using culture. Development of nonculture tests has been a major priority over the past 15 years.

There are three primary types of nonculture tests for detection of chlamydia. Antigen detection tests include direct immunofluorescent techniques and EIAs. When obtained from the cervix, these tests have a sensitivity between 60% and 85% relative to culture

(125). Test results usually are available in 1 to 2 days.

The next generation of chlamydia tests use nucleic acid hybridization (e.g., Gen Probe), which has performance characteristics with endocervical and urethral specimens comparable to that of the most sensitive antigen detection tests. Both antigen detection and nucleic acid hybridization tests have less stringent transport and maintenance of specimen requirements and are lower in cost.

The newest and most exciting advances in chlamydial testing are methods for the detection of amplified *C. trachomatis* DNA or RNA, which may be especially useful in asymptomatic individuals with lower numbers of organisms. The two most widely used methods are ligase chain reaction (LCR) and PCR. Both of these tests can be used not only for cervical and urethral specimens but also with urine. Simultaneous detection of both chlamydia and gonorrhea is possible using amplification techniques. Specificity has consistently been greater than 99%. Most recent studies demonstrate sensitivity of LCR and PCR ranging from 80% to 96% on first-void urine, using an expanded gold standard. Sensitivity with endocervical swab specimens is generally 90% to 100% with LCR and somewhat lower with PCR in some studies, thought possibly secondary to the presence of inhibitors in cervical mucus (122,125,128–132). Compared with cell culture, LCR is thought to detect 15% to 40% more infections in females (124).

Treatment

Recommended treatment of uncomplicated lower genital infection with *C. trachomatis* includes azithromycin 1 g orally in a single dose or a 7-day course of doxycycline 100 mg orally twice a day. CDC-recommended alternative therapies include erythromycin or ofloxacin for 7 days. Azithromycin offers the advantages of single-dose, directly observed therapy, which significantly enhances compliance. It is the treatment of choice in adoles-cents. Single-dose regimens with penicillins or cephalosporins used to treat gonorrhea do not effectively eradicate concomitant chlamydial infection. Sexual partners should be treated, and women who are sexual partners of men with nongonococcal urethritis should be treated empirically. Because of the high efficacy of these therapies, follow-up chlamydial testing is not necessary after treatment with doxycycline or azithromycin unless symptoms persist or reinfection is suspected (103).

Gonorrhea

Epidemiology

Despite the decline in gonorrhea during the past few decades, rates of infection remain high among adolescents and young adults. The highest age-specific rates are in 15- to 19-year-old girls (718 per 100,000 population in 1997) (133). Demographic risk factors include low socioeconomic status, early onset of sexual activity, illicit drug use, prostitution, and nonwhite race. Approximately 25% of sexually active 16- to 18-year-old African-American females living in low socioeconomic urban census tracts in Seattle acquired gonorrhea each year in 1986 and 1987 (134). It is estimated that 50% to 90% of women who are sexual consorts of men with gonococcal (GC) urethritis will be infected (135, 136).

Clinical Presentation

The majority of uncomplicated gonococcal infections in women probably are asymptomatic, although some studies suggest that gonococcal infections are more apt to be symptomatic than chlamydial infections. Urethritis and cervicitis are the most common clinical syndromes. Urethral colonization is present in 70% to 90% of infected women (137,138), but usually is accompanied by endocervical infection. Signs and symptoms are the same as those noted with symptomatic chlamydial infection. Some 35% to 50% of women with gonococcal cervicitis also have

GC isolated from the rectum, although this usually is asymptomatic (139). Most rectal infections in women occur without an acknowledged history of anal intercourse and are believed to be secondary to rectal contamination with infected cervical and vaginal secretions. Pharyngeal infection with GC occurs in 10% to 20% of women but is the sole site of infection in less than 5% (140,141). More than 90% of pharyngeal infections are asymptomatic, and the spontaneous cure rate approaches 100% within 12 weeks of infection (140–142). However, one study noted a possible increased risk of disseminated gonorrhea in persons with pharyngeal GC (140).

Gonorrheal infection occurring during pregnancy may result in septic abortion, preterm delivery, premature rupture of membranes, or prolonged rupture of membranes and chorioamnionitis. Transmission to the newborn can occur, with the development of ophthalmia neonatorum and, infrequently, gonococcal septicemia.

PID is the most common complication of gonorrhea in women and occurs in a estimated 10% to 20% of those with lower genital tract gonorrhea (139).

Disseminated gonococcal infection is the most common systemic complication of acute gonorrhea and occurs in up to 3% of patients. It usually is manifested clinically as an arthritis/dermatitis syndrome and is more common in women (143). Some 20% to 30% of women infected with gonorrhea are coinfected with chlamydia (139).

Diagnosis

Isolation of gonorrhea is the "gold standard" for diagnosis of gonococcal infection. Antibiotic-containing selected media are preferred for culturing the endocervix, rectum, and pharynx to suppress other bacteria that usually outnumber gonorrhea in these locations. Single cultures will detect 80% to 90% of endocervical infections. Sensitivity may be increased by duplicate cervical cultures or combined cervical and urethral cultures (144). The need to culture areas other than the cervix depends on symptoms and sites exposed. Culture techniques also are used for regional monitoring of antimicrobial susceptibility to guide therapy.

Gram-stained smears from the endocervix are highly specific for gonorrhea when typical gram-negative diplococci are seen within polymorphonuclear leukocytes, and such findings facilitate immediate treatment. Their sensitivity is reported to be only 50% to 70% with uncomplicated gonorrhea. The predictive value is disappointing in asymptomatic women with normal physical examination (139).

As with chlamydia, there has been a significant increase in development and use of non-culture-based diagnosis using both DNA hybridization and amplified nucleic acid detection tests. The nonamplified DNA probe tests are widely used and have sensitivities of 89% to 97% with a specificity of 99%, performing comparably to culture (139). LCR has been found to have sensitivities in the 94% to 98% range both with endocervical swabs and first-void urine specimens (130, 145,146). Other amplified nucleic acid tests, including PCR and transcription-mediated amplification, are becoming available or are in development. A significant advantage of both the amplified and nonamplified nucleic acid tests are that a single specimen can be tested for both gonorrhea and chlamydia.

Treatment

Development of antibiotic resistance has been the primary force driving the changing recommendations for adequate gonococcal therapy. Resistance may be of two types: (i) chromosomally mediated resistance requiring incremental increases in dosages of various antibiotics for curative treatment, and (ii) plasmid-mediated resistance encoding for high-level resistance to certain antibiotic classes. Gonococcal resistance to tetracyclines, erythromycin, spectinomycin, and, most recently,

TABLE 19.1. *1998 Centers for Disease Control and Prevention treatment guidelines for uncomplicated gonorrhea*

Recommended regimens
  Cefixime 400 mg po
  Ceftriaxone 125 mg IM
  Ciprofloxacin 500 mg po
  Ofloxacin 400 mg po
    plus[a]
  Azithromycin 1 g po
  or
  Doxycycline 100 mg po bid × 7 d

[a]To treat possible coexisting chlamydia infection.

fluoroquinolones has been described. In 1997, data from the Gonoccoccal Isolate Surveillance Project found that overall 33.4% of isolates were resistant to penicillin, tetracycline, or both (133). Current CDC-recommended first-line treatment guidelines for uncomplicated gonorrhea are listed in Table 19.1.

Pelvic Inflammatory Disease

Epidemiology and Pathogenesis

PID occurs in 1% of women ages 15 to 25 years in the United States, and teenagers may account for up to 20% of cases of PID reported annually in this country (147–149). The sexually active 15-year-old has a ten times greater risk for developing pelvic infection than does a 24-year-old woman (150). Two major factors contributing to the development of PID include recurrent or persistent chlamydial infection of the cervix and delays in and detection and treatment of cervical infection. A recent study found that women with two chlamydial infections were four times as likely to be hospitalized for PID, and women with three or more chlamydial infections had a six- to seven-fold increased probability of hospitalization for PID (151). Young age, nonwhite race/ethnicity, and low socioeconomic status appear to be risk factors for recurrent cervical infection with both gonorrhea and chlamydia (152). Adolescents are at greater risk for delays in seeking care for reasons already noted, including concerns about confidentiality and insurance/access issues.

In a study comparing adolescents with young adult women diagnosed with PID, adolescents sought health care an average of 2 days later in the course of their illness (153). Other behavioral correlates of PID include smoking, douching, frequent intercourse, and sex during menses. Use of oral contraceptives appears to have a protective effect on development of PID (152).

In the absence of recent pregnancy or instrumentation of the genital tract, PID generally is a polymicrobial sexually transmitted disease. Under certain predisposing circumstances, the ecology of the vaginal environment has changed, such that the mechanical and immunologic barrier of the cervix is breached and infected organisms gain access to the upper genital tract.

Gonorrhea is isolated from the cervix in 40% to 80% of patients with PID in the United States. It is isolated from tubal specimens in approximately 16% of total cases and 42% of cases where gonorrhea is cultured from the cervix. Similarly, U.S. studies show recovery rates of chlamydia from the cervix ranging from 5% to 26% of women with PID; tubal specimens recover chlamydia in 9% of cases overall and in 39% of cases in which chlamydia has been cultured from the cervix (154). Apart from gonorrhea and chlamydia, a variety of other endogenous and miscellaneous organisms have been isolated from upper genital tract specimens of women with acute PID. These include Mycoplasma hominis and a variety of facultative and anaerobic bacteria, including bacteroides species, prevotella bivia, *Escherichia coli, Gardnerella vaginalis,* peptostreptococcus species, staphylococci, streptococcus groups B to D, and *Actinomyces israelii.* Respiratory pathogens including *Haemophilus influenzae, Streptococcus pneumoniae,* and group A streptococci occasionally are isolated from tubal specimens in women with salpingitis (154). Recent evidence supports a role for bacterial vaginosis (BV)-associated organisms in the pathogenesis of PID. These organisms frequently are recovered from upper genital tract cul-de-sac specimens of women with PID (155). BV has been associated with both a clinical diagnosis of PID and with histologic endometritis (156,157), even when controlling for the presence of gonorrhea or chlamydia. There is an increased seroprevalence of HIV in patients with acute PID, and the diagnosis of PID should prompt HIV counseling and offering of testing (158,159). Patients who have PID and are coinfected with HIV may have an altered clinical course, including more frequent diagnosis of tuboovarian abscesses, more frequent need for surgical intervention, and longer hospital stays (160–162).

Clinical Presentation and Diagnosis

Clinical diagnosis of PID is hampered by the lack of specificity of traditional signs and symptoms. Only 65% of women diagnosed clinically have PID confirmed when laparoscopy is performed; 23% of women have normal pelvic findings (163). Furthermore, pelvic infection may produce no symptoms at all or only very mild ones. In one series, 6% of patients with PID diagnosed laparoscopically had not complained of abdominal pain; only 41% of PID patients had temperature greater than 38°C (163). Seroepidemiologic studies confirmed the significant relationship between tubal infertility and the presence of serum antibodies to *C. trachomatis* and *Neisseria gonorrhea,* even in patients without a history of PID (164–166).

Clinicians should consider the diagnosis of PID in any adolescent girl with abdominal pain. Diagnosis of PID also should be suspected with mild or nonspecific symptoms, such as abnormal bleeding, dyspareunia, and abnormal vaginal discharge. Symptoms with documented chlamydial infection appear to be milder, with more indolent onset, whereas infection initiated by GC is associated with more severe symptoms and a more fulminant course. When nausea and vomiting are prominent symptoms, gastrointestinal disease should be considered in the differential diagnosis. In a minority of cases, right upper quadrant pain because of a concomitant perihepatitis (Fitz-Hugh–Curtis syndrome) may be the dominating symptom and has been reported as an obscure cause of abdominal pain in adolescents without other symptoms of pelvic infection (167).

On physical examination, fever, pelvic and abdominal tenderness, and abnormal cervical secretions are the hallmark findings associated with PID. This combination of signs, however, was found by Jacobson and Westrom (163) in only 20% of laparoscopically confirmed cases of PID and in 14% of women with a clinical diagnosis of PID but normal tubes at laparoscopy. A palpable adnexal fullness or mass is a common finding and correlates with severity of inflammation as determined by the laparoscope but also is reported not infrequently in women with normal findings on laparoscopy (154). Because of the ascending pathogenesis of PID, women with this diagnosis also should have objective evidence of lower genital tract infection, and the presence of normal cervicovaginal secretions should call the diagnosis of PID into question. Approximately two thirds of patients with acute PID have peripheral white blood cell counts greater than 10,000/mL. An elevated erythrocyte sedimentation rate has been found in more than three fourths of patients with PID (163). C-reactive protein usually is elevated, and the level appears to reflect the severity of laparoscopically proven PID. This appears to be a more sensitive and specific predictor than erythrocyte sedimentation rate (168). Other serum markers, including specific genital isoamylases, have been studied in patients with PID but remain investigational. As with findings on history and physical examination, laboratory tests are relatively nonspecific and often discriminate poorly between upper genital tract infection and lower genital tract infection alone. Pregnancy testing should be performed in all cases of PID to exclude the possibility of ectopic pregnancy. Testing for endocervical gonorrhea and chlamydia should be performed.

Ultrasound cannot reliably confirm or exclude PID as a diagnosis. It is an important tool, however, in identifying the presence of tuboovarian abscess (occurring in 7% to 16% of females with acute PID) (169) or dilated fallopian tubes suggestive of pyosalpinx in cases of severe PID. In one study, vaginal probe ultrasound showing dilated tubes, thickening of the wall of the tube, or fluid within the tube was 85% sensitive and 100% specific compared to endometritis diagnosed on biopsy (170).

Other more invasive diagnostic techniques include culdocentesis with aspiration of purulent material or peritoneal fluid with an increased white blood cell level. Endometrial biopsy demonstrating endometritis based on detection of plasma cells and intraepithelial polymorphonuclear leukocytes had a sensitivity of 92% and a specificity of 87% compared to laparoscopy in one study (171). Endometrial biopsy may be better tolerated in an adolescent with paracervical block.

Laparoscopy is considered the "gold standard" for the diagnosis of PID. It should be used liberally when a diagnosis is in question or when the patient fails to respond appropriately to treatment. A laparoscopic grading system for severity of infection (Table 19.2) is helpful in determining prognosis and predicting rapidity of response to treatment (172). Laparoscopy also can help to prevent inaccurate diagnosis of pelvic pain and allow early treatment of other conditions, such as appendicitis or endometriosis. Once diagnosis of PID is made, future episodes of pelvic or

TABLE 19.2. *Severity of pelvic inflammatory disease by laparoscopic examination*

Degree	Findings
Mild	Erythema, edema, no spontaneous purulent exudate, tubes freely movable
Moderate	Gross purulent material evident; more marked erythema and edema; tubes may not be freely movable and/or patent
Severe	Pyosalpinx or inflammatory complex, abscess (size should be measured)

From Hager WD, Eschenbach PA, Spence MR, et al. Criteria for diagnosis and grading of salpingitis. *Obstet Gynecol* 1983;61:113.

TABLE 19.3. *1998 Centers for Disease Control and Prevention treatment guidelines for pelvic inflammatory disease*

Parenteral regimens
1. Cefotetan 2 gm IV q12h
    or
    Cefoxitin 2 g IV q6h
    plus
    Doxycycline 100 mg IV or PO q12h
2. Clindamycin 900 mg IV q8h
    plus
    Gentamicin loading dose 2 mg/kg with maintenance dose
        1.5 mg/kg q8h (may substitute single daily dosing)
Oral regimens
1. Ofloxacin 400 mg PO bid × 14 d
    plus
    Metronidazole 500 mg PO bid × 14 d
2. Ceftriazone 250 mg IM
    or
    Cefoxitin 2 gm IM plus probenecid 1 g po
    or
    Other parenteral third-generation cephalosporin
    plus
    Doxycycline 100 mg PO bid × 14 d

Adapted from Centers for Disease Control and Prevention: 1998 guidelines for treatment of sexually transmitted diseases. *MMWR* 1997;47:82–84.

lower abdominal pain are likely to be labeled, perhaps inappropriately, as recurrent PID. If PID has been diagnosed clinically and the patient has recurrent episodes, laparoscopy may be considered for definitive diagnosis.

Current CDC-recommended criteria for diagnosis of PID (Table 19.3) attempt to maximize sensitivity by recommending empiric treatment in the presence of all three minimum criteria (103). Additional criteria are used to increase specificity to avoid incorrect diagnoses and prevent unnecessary morbidity from treatment. Patients who are more seriously ill, or when the diagnosis is in question, warrant more definitive criteria to ensure accurate diagnosis and timely treatment.

Treatment

The ultimate objectives of treatment are to preserve fertility and prevent the complications and long-term sequelae resulting from PID.

There is evidence that early appropriate treatment will reduce damage to the fallopian tubes, the incidence of post-PID infertility, and possibly other sequelae (173).

Hospitalization for inpatient treatment should be considered in all adolescents because of their greater number of reproductive years at risk and because of issues of compliance. There are currently no efficacy data regarding either clinical or long-term outcomes with inpatient versus outpatient PID therapy. Appropriate antibiotic therapy must take into account the polymicrobial nature of PID and should cover the most frequently expected microorganisms, including gonorrhea, chlamydia, and common aerobic and anaerobic isolates.

Currently CDC-recommended primary regimens for parenteral and oral treatment of acute PID are listed in Table 19.3. Pooled cure rates of clinical trials using these regimens show roughly equivalent short-term clinical and microbiologic cure rates in approximately 90% to 100% (174). There have been relatively few studies of oral outpatient regimens, but cure rates appear comparable. In addition to considerations related to patient age, outpatient therapy generally is contraindicated in the following situations: (a) surgical emergency cannot be excluded; (b) pregnancy; (c) failure to respond clinically to outpatient therapy; (d) unable to follow or tolerate an outpatient regimen; (e) severe illness with nausea, vomiting, or high fever; (f) presence of a tuboovarian abscess; and (g) immunodeficiency (103). Intravenous antibiotic therapy should be continued for at least 24 to 48 hours after significant clinical improvement, and oral therapy should be used to complete a 14-day total course. Repeat bimanual examination and examination of endocervical secretions may help confirm a satisfactory response to therapy before discharge from the hospital. The patient should be clinically reevaluated 1 to 2 weeks later, at which time repeat cultures from the lower genital tract may be obtained.

An essential adjunct to effective treatment of PID is evaluation and treatment of the woman's sexual partners. In one study, up to 71% of male partners of women with PID who were located had GC or nongonococcal urethritis (175). Furthermore, 20% to 92% of patients with GC or chlamydial urethritis are asymptomatic (176–179). It is important to treat these male partners with a regimen effective against both organisms, regardless of culture results.

Surgical treatment in PID is indicated when rupture of a pelvic abscess occurs or when medical therapy fails. When surgery is necessary, it should be as conservative as possible. Rarely is hysterectomy and removal of bilateral adnexa indicated. Removal of unilateral adnexa or abscess drainage at laparotomy or laparoscopy usually is sufficient and allows the possibility of future pregnancy. Percutaneous abscess drainage is successful in approximately 90% of cases (180,181) and may prevent the need for surgery unless abscess rupture is suspected.

Complications and Sequelae

The most common long-term complications of PID include recurrent infection, chronic pelvic/abdominal pain, ectopic pregnancy, and infertility. Approximately one fourth of all women with their first episode of PID eventually develop one or more other infections, and women below the age of 20 years are reinfected twice as frequently as are older women (182).

Almost one fifth of patients eventually have chronic abdominal/pelvic pain of more than 6 months' duration; this has been correlated with pelvic adhesive disease and with infertility (182,183).

The incidence of ectopic pregnancy has risen dramatically in the past 30 years, paralleling the increase in PID (154). Ectopic pregnancy occurs in one of 24 women after an episode of PID as compared to one of 147 control women (183). Antichlamydial antibodies are more prevalent and of higher titer in women with ectopic pregnancy than age-matched controls with intrauterine pregnancies (184,185). The second leading cause of maternal mortality in the United States is ectopic gestation, and women 15 to 19 years of age have the highest mortality rates in this group (186).

PID has long been recognized as a major cause of infertility. Although infertility rates are significantly lower in women having their first episode of PID before the age of 25 years, chances of infertility increase at all ages with severity of disease and number of episodes. For adolescents having one episode of severe PID, 27.3% subsequently will be unable to conceive; after three or more episodes, more than one half will be infertile (187).

The need for subsequent gynecologic operations is increased in women who had PID compared to controls (188). Finally, although mortality from PID is rare in developed countries, mortality is approximately 3% to 8% if a pelvic abscess ruptures and generalized peritonitis occurs (189,190).

Bacterial Vaginosis

Epidemiology

BV, previously known as nonspecific vaginitis, gardnerella vaginitis, or haemophilus vaginitis, is the most prevalent vaginal infection, accounting for approximately one third of all cases in women of childbearing age.

In BV, the normal equilibrium of the vaginal microenvironment is disturbed. There is an overgrowth of both aerobic and anaerobic organisms, most notably *G. vaginalis, M. hominis,* and bacteroides and mobiluncus species. The concentration of gardnerella and anaerobes in vaginal secretions is 100 to 1,000 times greater in this syndrome than in control women without evidence of vaginal infection (191). The role of sexual transmission is unclear, and BV should be considered sexually associated rather than exclusively sexually transmitted. Sexually inexperienced postpubertal women have significantly lower prevalence of BV compared with those who have been sexually active (192). Male part-

ners of women with BV have been found to have an increased rate of *G. vaginalis* and anaerobic isolation from the urethra (193,194).

Clinical Presentation

Up to 50% of women with BV may be asymptomatic (195). Abnormal vaginal discharge and malodor are the most common complaints; irritative symptoms usually are absent or minimal.

Diagnosis

Diagnosis of BV generally is made on the basis of a composite of three of the following four clinical criteria (192): (i) homogeneous vaginal discharge; (ii) vaginal pH greater than 4.5; (iii) clue cells on wet mount representing greater than 20% of vaginal epithelial cells; and (iv) fishy odor on alkalinization of vaginal secretions. In addition, gram stain of vaginal secretions showing a predominance of mixed bacterial types with absent or small numbers of lactobacillus morphotypes is highly correlated with this syndrome (196). Several methods based on detection of the metabolic products of the various microorganisms found in BV have been described but they primarily are research tools at the present time.

Treatment

Treatment alternatives for BV include metronidazole 500 mg b.i.d. for 7 days, clindamycin cream 2% one applicator-full per vagina q.h.s. for 7 days, or metronidazole gel 0.75% one applicator-full per vagina b.i.d. for 5 days. CDC-recommended alternatives are metronidazole 2 g in a single dose orally or clindamycin 300 mg orally b.i.d. for 7 days (103). Routine treatment of sexual partners has not been shown to decrease rates of recurrence and is not routinely recommended.

Pregnant women at high risk for preterm delivery and who have BV have a reduction in preterm deliveries when treated with oral metronidazole (197,198). Meta-analysis of studies addressing the use of metronidazole during pregnancy revealed no evidence of teratogenicity (199). The role of routine screening for, and treatment of, asymptomatic BV is still undefined.

Lymphogranuloma Venereum

Lymphogranuloma venereum is an infection caused by certain serovars of *C. trachomatis.* Although it is considered a "minor" STD in North America, it is endemic in much of the developing world (200). The primary lesion is a small papular ulcer, which is relatively asymptomatic and often unnoticed. The secondary stage is characterized by either inflammation and swelling of inguinal lymph nodes (inguinal syndrome) or, more commonly in women, acute proctocolitis with fever, rectal pain, and tenesmus (anogenital rectal syndrome). Even without treatment, most infections resolve after this stage. In a small minority of patients, however, a chronic inflammatory response leads to development of genital ulcers, genital elephantiasis, and rectal strictures (201,202).

Correct diagnosis is suggested by the clinical picture but may be confirmed by chlamydial isolation from infected tissue or appropriate serologic tests. Currently, recommended treatment is doxycycline 100 mg b.i.d. for 21 days or erythromycin base 500 mg orally q.i.d. for 21 days as an alternative (103).

Chancroid

Chancroid is a sexually transmitted genital ulcerative infection associated with infection by *Haemophilus ducreyi.* Much more prevalent in men than women, the incidence of this infection increased significantly in the United States after 1980 (203,204).

The incubation period usually is between 4 and 7 days, with the initial clinical manifestation being a tender papule, which over the course of 1 to 2 days becomes pustular and then ulcerative. The ulcer classically has ragged undermined edges, is well demarcated,

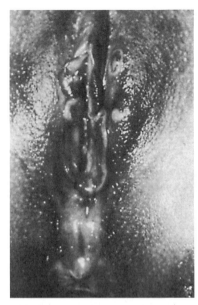

FIG. 19.7. Ulcerated lesion of the vulva caused by chancroid.

and is without induration (Fig. 19.7). The base of the ulcer is friable and covered with necrotic purulent debris. Depending on the site of the ulcer, symptoms in women may include pain with urination or defecation, vaginal discharge, dyspareunia, and rectal bleeding. Symptoms in women are often more subclinical than in men. Painful, generally unilateral, and sometimes suppurative, inguinal lymphadenopathy is a characteristic feature but is less common in women (205).

A "probable" diagnosis can be made using the following criteria: (a) one or more painful genital ulcers; (b) HSV and syphilis are excluded; and (c) the clinical presentation is typical.

Laboratory confirmation of this diagnosis depends on isolation of *H. ducreyi* from a genital ulcer or inguinal node, and PCR will soon be commercially available. Gram stain of exudate from the ulcer base shows typical gram-negative bacilli in a "school of fish" pattern and may aid in diagnosis. Recommended treatment includes azithromycin 1 g PO, ceftriaxone 250 mg IM, ciprofloxacin 500 mg PO b.i.d. for 3 days, or erythromycin base 500 mg orally q.i.d. for 7 days (103). Sexual partners should be treated simultaneously and abstinence encouraged until lesions have healed.

Granuloma Inguinale

Granuloma inguinale, also known as donovanosis, is a chronic and progressively destructive infection of the genital region caused by the bacterium *Calymmatobacterium granulomatis.* Most common in tropical and subtropical environments, granuloma inguinale has been described in adolescents in the United States (206). The role of sexual transmission is controversial (207). There is some evidence that the causative organism may be a normal inhabitant of the intestinal tract and may be autoinoculated into the vagina. Clinical disease then occurs after sexual or nonsexual trauma of sites harboring *C. granulomatis* (208).

The incubation period is not well defined, but it appears to be in the range from 8 to 80 days. The initial lesion is a small subcutaneous nodule(s), which erodes to the skin and forms a painless, beefy red, hypertrophic well-defined ulcerative lesion, which bleeds on contact. Lesions slowly enlarge and often coalesce. In women, most lesions are found on the labia but also have been described in the vagina or on the cervix. Fibrosis and lymphedema of surrounding tissue occur with progressive disease. The clinical picture has not infrequently been confused with carcinoma (206).

Diagnosis is easily confirmed by stained crushed preparation from the lesion with demonstration of Donovan bodies, deep-staining clusters of organisms with a "safety pin" appearance in the cytoplasm of large mononuclear cells. First-line treatment consists of trimethoprim-sulfamethoxazole DS b.i.d. orally or doxycycline 100 mg orally b.i.d. until lesions have completely healed, for a minimum of 3 weeks. Ciprofloxacin and erythromycin base are alternative therapies (103).

SPIROCHETE INFECTION

Syphilis

Epidemiology

From a peak incidence in 1990, syphilis rates declined 84% to 3.2 per 100,000 in 1997. Rates of primary and secondary syphilis are highest in women 20 to 24 years old, at 8.2 per 100,000 population; in 1997 rates in girls 15 to 19 years old were 5.8 per 100,000. There is significant racial and ethnic disparity in syphilis rate, with rates in African-Americans reaching 31.8 per 100,000 in girls 15 to 19 years old and 47.9 per 100,000 in women 20 to 24 years old. More than 1,000 cases of congenital syphilis were reported in 1997, and the incidence of congenital syphilis closely follows rates and trends in primary and secondary disease in women. Geographically, the most recent statistics show syphilis cases are concentrated in the southeastern United States (110,133).

Clinical Presentation

Approximately 30% of women who have sexual contact with a partner who has early syphilis will themselves become infected. The lesion of primary syphilis, the chancre, occurs at the portal of entry of the treponeme an average of 3 weeks after exposure (Fig. 19.8). It typically is single, indurated, and painless, and usually is associated with regional adenopathy. It heals within a few weeks with or without treatment.

With widespread hematogenous and lymphatic dissemination of *Treponema pallidum,* a variable systemic illness develops weeks to months after the disappearance of the chancre. A flu-like illness, with low-grade fever, malaise, headache, sore throat, myalgias, and adenopathy, is common. The presence of a papular rash involving the palms and soles should heighten suspicion for secondary syphilis. Condylomata lata are moist confluent papular lesions of secondary syphilis in intertriginous areas and contain large numbers of spirochetes (Fig. 19.9).

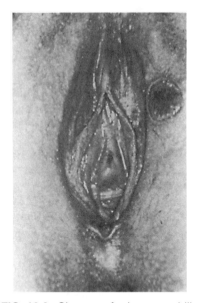

FIG. 19.8. Chancre of primary syphilis.

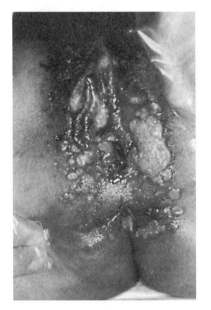

FIG. 19.9. Condylomata lata of secondary syphilis.

Again, with or without treatment, the manifestations of secondary syphilis resolve and the patient enters the latent stage. During this time, although there is serologic evidence of infection, there are no clinical manifestations. Because transmission requires exposure to mucosal or cutaneous lesions, latency is somewhat arbitrarily divided into early latency (less than 1 year from onset of infection) and late latency, on the basis of the time when untreated patients are most likely to develop spontaneous mucocutaneous infectious relapses.

Occurring at times up to 30 years after onset of infection, the signs and symptoms of tertiary syphilis involve the bones, soft tissues, various visceral organs, cardiovascular system (aneurysm, aortic insufficiency), and central nervous system (paresis, tabes dorsalis). These account for the majority of the morbidity and mortality of the disease.

At each stage of syphilis, the clinical presentation is extremely variable, and "atypical" manifestations are common. This is especially true of patients who are coinfected with HIV (209).

Diagnosis

Dark-field microscopic examination of exudate from the surface of a chancre or condyloma lata, or aspirate from an involved lymph node, can provide the earliest and most direct means of diagnosis of early syphilis. False-negative tests may occur when there are too few organisms to identify, the lesion is healing, or topical or systemic treatment has been initiated. When similar specimens are obtained but cannot be examined immediately or a dark-field microscope is not available, direct fluorescent antibody testing is a reliable alternative.

When lesions are not present and the tests mentioned are not available, serologic tests are used to provide presumptive evidence of syphilis. Generally, a test such as the Venereal Disease Research Laboratory (VDRL) test, rapid plasma reagin (RPR) test, or serologic test for syphilis (STS) is used initially to screen for syphilis by detecting a heterogeneous and nonspecific group of antibodies elevated in syphilis. If this is reactive, a test (e.g., microhemagglutination assay for antibodies to T. pallidum [MHA-TP] and fluorescent treponemal antibody-absorption [FTA-ABS] test) detecting specific antibodies to *T. pallidum* confirms the diagnosis. The sensitivity of these tests approaches 100% in secondary syphilis (210). Biologic false-positives occasionally occur with immunizations, intravenous drug use, febrile illness, or collagen vascular disease, but usually they are of low titer (211,212).

Treatment

The treatment of choice for all stages of syphilis remains intramuscular penicillin G in patients who are not allergic. Parenteral penicillin G is the only therapy with documented effectiveness for treatment of neurosyphilis or for the treatment of syphilis during pregnancy. Specific treatment schedules and alternatives for nonpregnant or penicillin allergic patients recommended by the CDC are noted in Table 19.4. Examination of cerebrospinal fluid to exclude neurosyphilis should be performed if neurologic or ophthalmologic signs or symptoms are present; with symptomatic late syphilis (e.g., gumma, cardiovascular

TABLE 19.4. *1998 Centers for Disease Control and Prevention treatment guidelines for syphilis*

Early syphilis: primary, secondary, latent syphilis
    <1 yr
    Benzathine penicillin G 2.4 million units IM
    Alternative
        Doxycycline 100 mg PO bid × 2 wks
        or
        Tetracycline 500 mg PO qid × 2 wks
Late syphilis: latent syphilis >1 yr, tertiary
        (excluding neurosyphilis)
    Benzathine penicillin G 2.4 million units IM given
        1 wk apart × 3 consecutive wks
    Alternative
        Doxycycline 100 mg PO bid × 4 wks
        or
        Tetracycline 500 mg PO qid × 4 wks

manifestations); with late latent or syphilis of unknown duration in HIV-infected women; and with treatment failure. Lumbar puncture should be considered with the use of a non-penicillin regimen (103).

After treatment, the patient should be followed with examination and RPR, or other quantitative nontreponemal test (same test should be used in sequential testing follow-up) at 6, 12, and 24 months to detect treatment failure or reinfection. If clinical signs persist or recur, or if the titer rises, remains high, or fails to decline appropriately, retreatment is indicated. For patients with early syphilis, all sexual partners within the previous 3 months should be treated presumptively (103).

ECTOPARASITES

Pediculosis Pubis (Pubic Lice)

Epidemiology

Phthirus pubis, the crab louse, is an ectoparasite that generally infests in the pubic area. Sexual contact is the most common, but not the only, means of transmission. Incidence of pubic lice infestation is highest in single persons 15 to 25 years of age (213).

Clinical Presentations

The louse is dependent on human blood, and symptoms occur largely with sensitization after bites. The primary symptom is itching; scratching leads to erythema with further irritation and inflammation. Small blue spots may be seen in the skin, occasionally as a result of bites. After many bites over a short period of time, the individual may have mild fever, malaise, and irritability.

Diagnosis

Diagnosis depends on identification of the adult lice (1 mm long) or their nits (eggs 0.8 mm long) with the naked eye or microscope. At first glance, pubic lice may appear as scabs over papular areas of irritation.

Treatment

Treatment involves administration topically of a medication that will kill both the adult lice and their eggs. Permethrin 1% cream rinse applied to the affected area and washed off after 10 minutes or lindane 1% shampoo applied for 4 minutes and washed off appear equally effective, although failure rates as high as 40% have been reported and require retreatment for definitive cure (214). Over-the-counter liquid or shampoo preparations containing pyrethrins and piperonyl butoxide (e.g., Rid, Triplex) also are effective. Lindane is contraindicated in pregnant women. Sexual contacts should be treated similarly, and the patient's clothing and other fomites should be disinfected by laundering in hot water or dry cleaning. A mild antipruritic/antiinflammatory cream may be helpful for treating pruritus, which often persists after treatment of the infestation itself because of residual irritation or allergic reaction (103,213).

Scabies

Epidemiology

Scabies, a cutaneous infestation caused by the mite *Sarcoptes scabiei,* has been a common disease for at least 3,000 years and occurs in small local outbreaks, as well as large epidemics. In most areas of the world, the highest incidence has been found in children and young adults. Transmission of the mites requires close bodily contact, including but not limited to sexual contact.

Clinical Presentation

Clinical symptoms generally are caused when the mites burrow into the skin to lay eggs. Several weeks later, with sensitization, an erythematous papular rash usually develops, and itching, often exacerbated at night or after a hot bath, is intense and persistent. The mite is quite mobile and likes to gravitate to some favorite places; typical burrows are most commonly found on the hands and wrists. The burrow appears as a short, wavy, "dirty" line that often crosses skin lines.

Diagnosis

Definitive diagnosis requires identification of one of the following: classic burrows, the mite at any stage of development, or its eggs or fecal pellets (215). One technique in wide use involves application of mineral oil to lesions followed by vigorous scraping with a sterile scalpel blade to remove the top of the burrow or papule. The oil and scraped material then are transferred to a glass slide for microscopic examination.

Treatment

The recommended treatment regimen for adolescents is application of 30 g of permethrin 5% cream thinly to all areas of the body from the neck down. This should be washed off after 12 hours. Lindane 1% lotion or cream is an alternative treatment but is less effective than permethrin and potentially neurotoxic. Oral ivermectin is a promising new therapeutic regimen, although it has yet to be compared with current recommended therapies. Both household and sexual partners should be treated simultaneously, and clothes and bed linens be disinfected (216).

FUNGAL INFECTIONS

Vulvovaginal Candidiasis

Epidemiology

It is estimated that three fourths of all women in the United States will have at least one episode of vulvovaginal candidiasis. A total of 80% to 90% of infections are due to *Candida albicans,* but the remainder result from other candidal species that may be more resistant to conventional therapy (217).

Approximately 20% of women have asymptomatic vaginal colonization with candida (218). It remains poorly understood just what factors play a role in the development of symptomatic infection, although it has been noted that germination enhances both colonization and tissue invasion (219). It also has been shown that candidal species undergo high-frequency genetic switching, which may influence transformation from asymptomatic colonization to symptomatic infection and may provide the capacity to invade different sites of the body or change patterns of resistance to antifungal medications (220).

Predisposing factors for vulvovaginal candidiasis include pregnancy (221); oral contraceptive use (222); broad-spectrum antibiotics (223); allergic or hypersensitivity responses to local irritants (douches, spermicides) (224); tight, occlusive, or poorly ventilated clothing (225); and immunosuppression [HIV infection (226,227), diabetes, steroid use].

The gastrointestinal tract is though to be the source of initial vaginal colonization with candida organisms. The role of sexual transmission in the development of vaginal candidiasis is controversial. In a 1987 study, Horowitz et al. (228) evaluated 33 women with recurrent vulvovaginal candidiasis (more than three culture positive episodes per year) and their sexual partners. They found a high correlation between partners with positive cultures involving the same candidal strains. The oral cavity was the site most often colonized, and 15% of ejaculates also were positive for candidal species. Recurrent vaginal infections were eliminated with systemic antifungal treatment, oral clotrimazole troches, and restriction of oral-genital contact between partners.

Clinical Presentation

Pruritus is the most common clinical symptom, present in approximately 90% of women. Other irritative symptoms frequently seen include dyspareunia and vulvar dysuria, often with reflex urgency and frequency. The discharge is classically white and curdy, and it may be adherent to the vaginal walls. Vaginal and vulvar erythema are not uncommonly found.

Diagnosis

In patients with candidiasis, vaginal pH usually is within the normal range. Both wet mount and examination of vaginal secretions in 10% to 20% KOH reveal spores and pseudo-

hyphae in 65% to 85% of cases with *C. albicans* (229), lactobacillus predominance, and a relative paucity of white blood cells. Culture with Sabouraud or Nickerson media may be needed to help confirm the diagnosis in vaginitis of unsure etiology or for species identification in chronically recurrent candidiasis.

Treatment

A variety of topical azole compounds in various formulations including creams, vaginal tablets, and vaginal suppositories are effective for treatment of vulvovaginal candidiasis, with relief of symptoms and negative fungal cultures in 80% to 90% of women who complete therapy (229). Duration of recommended treatment ranges from 1 to 14 days. Several preparations now are available over the counter. Currently available topical agents are oil based and may weaken latex condoms or diaphragms. Intercourse should be deferred during treatment.

Fluconazole, an oral azole compound, is currently the only FDA-approved oral therapy for vulvovaginal candidiasis. It appears to have similar cure rates and is generally well tolerated. These features, plus its ease of administration, single dose, and no mess, are advantages over topical therapies and may result in greater patient acceptance. Disadvantages of oral treatment include the 1- to 2-day delay in symptom relief and potential for systemic toxicity, which is rare with a single dose of fluconazole. Other oral azole agents (ketoconazole and itraconazole) have activity in vulvovaginal candidiasis but are not currently approved by the FDA for this condition. Ketoconazole also has been associated with greater potential hepatotoxicity (230).

Patients who have "uncomplicated" vulvovaginal candidiasis (mild to moderate in severity, sporadic, nonrecurrent disease in a normal host, with normally susceptible *C. albicans*) respond well to short-term (less than 7 days) and single-dose therapies, which will decrease cost and increase adherence. On the other hand, women with severe, recurrent episodes, infections caused by less susceptible nonalbican species, or women who have underlying disorders that impact on immune function (e.g., uncontrolled diabetes, HIV) generally should have a 10- to 14-day course of therapy (103).

Treatment of male sexual partners is not indicated for the routine management of vulvovaginal candidiasis, but it may be considered with chronically recurrent or refractory cases.

PROTOZOAN INFECTIONS

Trichomonas

Epidemiology

Trichomonas vaginalis is a flagellated protozoan that infects at least five million women and their sexual partners each year in the United States (1). Prevalence reported in adolescent populations has ranged from 5% to 16% (231). Transmission is by sexual contact; nonsexual transmission is theoretically possible, but in reality is thought to be a rare event. Up to 60% of male partners of infected women are found to harbor the organism (231), 70% if examined within 48 hours after sexual contact (232). Vaginal trichomoniasis has been associated with adverse pregnancy outcomes, including preterm delivery and premature rupture of membranes (233–236).

Clinical Presentation

Up to 50% of women are asymptomatic, but one third of these women will develop symptoms within 6 months if the condition is left untreated (237). Abnormal vaginal discharge is the most common symptom and is classically described as profuse, purulent, frothy, and foul smelling, although this composite description is found in a minority of women. Irritative symptoms are common, including pruritus, burning, dyspareunia, and vulvar dysuria. Punctate hemorrhagic lesions of the vagina or cervix ("strawberry spots") are another classic, but infrequent, finding (238). Vulvar and vaginal erythema also may be seen (239).

Diagnosis

Vaginal pH usually is elevated to greater than 4.5 with vaginal trichomoniasis. The most common way to confirm the diagnosis is with direct observation of motile organisms on wet mount, which has a sensitivity of 50% to 70% (231). A significant inflammatory component is usual, manifested by excess numbers of white blood cells. Culture on modified Diamond or Kupferberg medium is considered the most sensitive means of making the diagnosis and can be especially useful when low numbers of organisms are present, but requires 2 to 7 days for results. Antigen detection immunoassays and nucleic acid hybridization or amplification tests offer promise as rapid, sensitive, and specific alternatives to culture.

Treatment

Vaginal trichomoniasis is treated with oral metronidazole given to both partners. Both the single 2-g dose and more extended 7-day regimen of 500 mg b.i.d. are effective, with cure rates of 90% to 95% (103,231). Sexual activity should be avoided until completion of treatment and resolution of symptoms. Topical metronidazole is considerably less effective and should not be used for treatment of trichomoniasis. Trichomoniasis should alert the health care provider to the possible presence of other STDs.

PREVENTION

The topic of prevention alone could fill several chapters. However, a few brief comments must suffice. All adolescents should have access to care that is safe, nonjudgmental, confidential, and inexpensive. A sexual history should be elicited from every adolescent in a sensitive and thorough fashion. Each exposure of the individual to the health care system should be seen as an opportunity to discuss sexual issues, including STIs. This should include education about warning signals, complications of STIs, and means of prevention, including alteration of sexual behavior to minimize the number of sexual partners and the use of barrier methods, such as the male or female condom. Because of the link among drug use, sexual behavior, and STDs, each adolescent's education should include information about drug use, abuse, and resources available for aid.

Although each interaction with an adolescent should be considered confidential, a major thrust of the health care provider should be to enlist the parents' support for the adolescent. This may provide the impetus for better understanding and closer interaction in the future.

REFERENCES

1. Cates W, Jr. Estimates of the incidence and prevalence of sexually trasmitted diseases in the United States. American Social Health Association Panel. *Sex Transm Dis* 1996;26:S2–S7.
2. Eng TR, Butler WT, eds. Institute of Medicine Committee on Prevention and Control of Sexually Transmitted Diseases. *The hidden epidemic: confronting sexually transmitted diseases.* Washington: National Academy Press, 1997.
3. Centers for Disease Control and Prevention. Ten leading nationally notifiable diseases—United States, 1995. *MMWR* 1996;45:883–884.
4. Wasserheit JN, Holmes KK. Reproductive tract infections: challenges for international health policy, programs, and research. In: Germain A, Holmes KK, Piot P, et al, eds. *Reproductive tract infections: global impact and priorities for women's reproductive health.* New York: Plenum Press, 1992:7.
5. Bolan G, Ehrhardt AA, Jwasserheit JN. Gender perspectives and STDs. In: Holmes KK, Sparling PF, Mardh PA, et al, eds. *Sexually transmitted diseases,* 3rd ed. New York: McGraw-Hill, 1999:117.
6. Tanner JM. *Foetus into man: physical growth from conception to maturation.* Cambridge, MA: Harvard University Press, 1978:152.
7. Vihko R, Apter D. The role of androgens in adolescent cycles. *J Steroid Biochem* 1980;12:369.
8. Berman SM, Hein K. Adolescents and STDs. In: Holmes KK, Sparling PF, Mardh PA, et al, eds. *Sexually transmitted diseases,* 3rd ed. New York: McGraw-Hill, 1999:129.
9. Rahm VA, Odlind V, Pettersson R. Chlamydia trachomatis in sexually active teenage girls. Factors related to genital chlamydial infection: a prospective study. *Genitourin Med* 1991;67:317.
10. Moss GB, Clemetson D, D'Costa L, et al. Association of cervical ectopy with heterosexual transmission of human immunodeficiency virus: results of a study of couples in Nairobi, Kenya. *J Infect Dis* 1991;165:588.
11. CDC. Trends in sexual risk behaviors among high school students—United States, 1991–1997. *MMWR* 1998;47:749–752.
12. Centers for Disease Control and Prevention, Division of STD Prevention. *Sexually transmitted disease surveillance—1997.* Atlanta: U.S. Department of Health and Human Services, Public Health Service, September 1998.
13. CDC. State-specific pregnancy rates among adolescents—United States, 1992–1995. *MMWR* 1998;47:497–504.
14. Zelnik M, Kantner JF. Sexual and contraceptive experience of young unmarried women in the United States, 1976 and 1971. *Fam Plann Perspect* 1977;9:55.
15. Zabin LS, Hirsch MB, Smith EA, et al. Adolescent sexual attitudes and behavior: are they consistent? *Fam Plann Perspect* 1984;16:181.
16. Sorensen RE. *Adolescent sexuality in contemporary America: personal values and sexual behavior, ages thirteen to nineteen.* New York: World Publishing, 1973:122.
17. Piccinino LJ, Mosher WD. Trends in contraceptive use in the United States: 1982–1995. *Fam Plann Perspect* 1998;30:4–10.
18. Louv WC, Austin H, Perlman J, et al. Oral contraceptive use and the risk of chlamydial and gonococcal infections. *Am J Obstet Gynecol* 1989;160:396.
19. Roye CF. Condom use by Hispanic and African-American adolescent girls who use hormonal contraception. *J Adolesc Health* 1998;23:205–211.
20. Sonenstein FL, Pleck JH, Ku LC. Sexual activity, condom use, and AIDS awareness among adolescent males. *Fam Plann Perspect* 1989;21:152.
21. Binson D, Dolcini MM, Pollack LM, et al. Data from the National AIDS Behavioral Surveys IV: multiple sexual partners among young adults in high-risk cities. *Fam Plann Perspect* 1993;25:268.
22. Shah F, Zelnik M. Parent and peer influence on sexual behavior, contraceptive use, and pregnancy experience of young women. *J Marriage Fam* 1981;43:339.
23. Nathanson CA, Becker MH. Family and peer influence on obtaining a method of contraception. *J Marriage Fam* 1986;48:513.
24. Smith EA, Udry JR. Coital and non-coital sexual behaviors of white and black adolescents. *Am J Public Health* 1985;75:1200.
25. Darrow WW, Redford MH, Duncan GW, Prager DJ. Attitudes towards condom use and the acceptance of venereal disease prophylactics. In: Redford MH, et al., eds. *The condom: increasing utilization in the United States.* San Francisco, CA: San Francisco Press, 1974:173.
26. Reiss IL. Human sexuality in sociological perspective. In: Holmes KK, Mardh P-A, Sparling PF, et al, eds. *Sexually transmitted diseases.* New York: McGraw-Hill, 1984:39.
27. Strasberger VC, ed. Sex, drugs, rock n' roll—understanding common teenage behavior. *Pediatrics* 1985;76[Suppl]:659.
28. Strasburger VC. Television and adolescents. *Pediatr Ann* 1985;14:814.
29. American School Health Association. *The National Adolescent Student Health Survey.* Oakland, CA: Third Party Publishing, 1989.
30. Malus M, LaChance PA, Lamy L, et al. Priorities in adolescent health care: the teenager's viewpoint. *J Fam Pract* 1987;25:159.
31. Joffe A, Radius S, Gall M. Health counseling for ado-

lescents: what they want, what they get, and who gives it. *Pediatrics* 1988:82:481.

32. Holder AR. Minor's rights to consent to medical care. *JAMA* 1987;257:3400.

33. Lih IF, Cuskey WR. Compliance with medical regimens during adolescence. *Pediatr Clin North Am* 1980; 27:3.

34. Centers for Disease Control and Prevention. *HIV/AIDS surveillance report.* 1998;10:1–42.

35. Centers for Disease Control and Prevention. First 500,000 AIDS cases—United States, 1995. *MMWR* 1995;44:849.

36. Rosenberg PS, Biggar RJ, Goedert JJ. Declining age at HIV infection in the Untied States. *N Engl J Med* 1994;330:89.

37. Rosenberg PS, Biggar RJ. Trends in HIV incidence among young adults in the United States. *JAMA* 1998; 29:1894.

38. Wasserheit JN. Epidemiological synergy. Inter-relationships between human immunodeficiency virus infection and other sexually transmitted diseases. *Sex Transm Dis* 1992;19:61–77.

39. Centers for Disease Control and Prevention. Youth risk behavior surveillance—United States, 1995. In: CDC Surveillance Summaries, September 27, 1996. *MMWR* 1996;45[SS-4]:1–85.

40. Sande M. HIV infection and AIDS—editorial overview. *Curr Opin Infect Dis* 1990;3:67.

41. Sterk C. Cocaine and HIV seropositivity. *Lancet* 1988; 2:2052.

42. Hahn JRA, Onorato IM, Jones TS, et al. Prevalence of HIV infection among intravenous drug users in the United States. *JAMA* 1989;261:2677–2684.

43. Quinn T, Glasses D, Cannon R, et al. Human immunodeficiency virus infection among patients attending clinics for sexually transmitted diseases. *N Engl J Med* 1988;318:197.

44. Clark SJ, Saag MS, Decker WD, et al. High titers of cytopathic virus in plasma of patients with symptomatic primary HIV-1 infection. *N Engl J Med* 1991; 324:954–960.

45. Schacker T, Collier AC, Hughes J, et al. Clinical and epidemiologic features of primary HIV infection. *Ann Intern Med* 1996;125:257–264.

46. Fischl MA. Introduction to the clinical spectrum of AIDS. In: Merigan TC Jr, Bartlett JG, Bolognesi D, eds. *Textbook of AIDS medicine,* 2nd ed. Baltimore: Williams & Wilkins, 1999:139.

47. Bartlett JG. *1998 medical management of HIV infection.* Baltimore: Port City Press, 1998:41.

48. Redfield RR, Blattner WA, Gallo RC. HIV/AIDS at the millennium. In: Merigan TC Jr, Bartlett JG, Bolognesi D, eds. *Textbook of AIDS medicine,* 2nd ed. Baltimore: Williams & Wilkins, 1999:3.

49. Gurtler L. Difficulties and strategies of HIV diagnosis. *Lancet* 1996;348:176–179.

50. Update: serologic testing for HIV-1 antibody—United States, 1988 and 1989. *MMWR* 1990;39:380.

51. Bartlett JG. *1998 medical management of HIV infection.* Baltimore: Port City Press, 1998:1.

52. Morens DM. Serological screening tests for antibody to human immunodeficiency virus—the search for perfection in an imperfect world. *Clin Infect Dis* 1997;25:101.

53a. Belshe RB, Clements ML, Keefer MC, et al. Interpreting HIV serodiagnostic test results in the 1990's. Social risks of HIV vaccine studies in uninfected volunteers. NIAID AIDS Vaccine Clinical Trial Group. *Ann Intern Med* 1995;121:584.

53b. Celum CL, Coombs RW, Jones M, et al. Risk factors for repeatedly reactive HIV-1 EIA and indeterminate western blots. A population-based case-control study. *Arch Intern Med* 1994;154:1129–1137.

54. Bartlett JG. *1998 medical management of HIV infection.* Baltimore: Port City Press, 1998:17.

55. Gallo D, George JR, Fitchen JH, et al. Evaluation of a system using oral mucosal transudate for HIV-1 antibody screening and confirmatory testing. OraSure HIV Clinical Trials Group. *JAMA* 1997;277:254.

56. Hein K. Annotation: adolescent HIV testing—who says who signs? *Am J Public Health* 1997;87:1277–1278.

57. Meehan TM, Hansen H, Klein WC. The impact of parental consent on the HIV testing of minors. *Am J Public Health* 1997;87:1338–1341.

58. Rhoads J, Wright C, Redfield R, et al. Chronic vaginal candidiasis in women with human immunodeficiency virus infection. *JAMA* 1987;257:3105.

59. Imam N, Carpenter CC, Mayer KH, et al. Hierarchical pattern of mucosal candida infections in HIV-seropositive women. *Am J Med* 1990;89:142.

60. Maier J, Bergman A, Rose M. Acquired immunodeficiency syndrome manifested by chronic primary genital herpes. *Am J Obstet Gynecol* 1986;155:756.

61. Feingold A, Vermund S, Burk R, et al. Cervical cytologic abnormalities and human immunodeficiency virus. *J Acquir Immune Defic Syndr* 1990;3:896.

62. Maiman M, Fruchter RG, Serar E, et al. Human immunodeficiency virus infection and cervical neoplasia. *Gynecol Oncol* 1990;38:377.

63. Centers for Disease Control and Prevention. Update: mortality attribute to HIV infection among persons aged 25–44 years—United States, 1994. *MMWR* 1996; 45:121–125.

64. Centers for Disease Control and Prevention Mortality and HIV/AIDS. *http://www.cdc.gov/nchstp/hiv_aids/ graphics/mortalit.htm* (updated March 11, 1999).

65. Palella FJ, Delaney KM, Moorman AC, et al. Declining morbidity and mortality among patients with advanced human immunodeficiency virus infection. *N Engl J Med* 1998;338:853–860.

66. Panel on Clinical Practices for Treatment of HIV Infection. Guidelines for the use of antiretroviral agents in HIV-infected adults and adolescents. *MMWR* 1998; 47[RR-30]:38–78 (updated regularly at *http://www. hivatis.org*).

67. Moscicki A-B. Genital HPV infection children and adolescents. *Obstet Gynecol Clin North Am* 1996;23: 675–697.

68. Rosenfeld WD, Vermund SH, Wentz SJ, et al. High prevalence of human papillomavirus infection and association with abnormal Papanicolaou smears in sexually active adolescents. *Am J Dis Child* 1989;143: 1443.

69. Ho GY, Bierman R, Beardsley L, et al. Natural history of cervicovaginal papillomavirus infection in young women. *N Engl J Med* 1998;338:423–428.

70. Burk RD, Ho GY, Beardsley L, et al. Sexual behavior and partner characteristics are the predominant risk factors for genital human papillomavirus infection in young women. *J Infect Dis* 1996;174:679–689.

71. Baur HM, Ting Y, Greer CE, et al. Genital human papillomavirus infection in female university students as determined by a PCR-based method. *JAMA* 1991; 265:472–477.

72. Spitzer M, Krumholz BA, Seltzer VL. Multicentric nature of disease related to human papillomavirus infection of the female lower genital tract. *Obstet Gynecol* 1989;73:303.

73. McNicol PJ, Guijon FB, Paraskevas M, et al. Comparison of filter in situ deoxyribonucleic acid hybridization with cytologic, colposcopic, and histopathologic examination for detection of human papillomavirus infection in women with cervical intraepithelial neoplasia. *Am J Obstet Gynecol* 1989;160:265.

74. Beutner KR, Wiley DJ, Douglas JM, et al. Genital warts and their treatment. *Clin Infect Dis* 1999;28: S37–S56.

75. Broker TR, Botchan M. Papillomaviruses: retrospectives and prospectives. *Cancer Cells* 1986;4:17.

76. Syrjanen KJ. Papillomaviruses and cancer. In: Syrjanen KJ, Gissman L, Koss L, eds. *Papillomaviruses and human disease.* Berlin: Springer Verlag, 1987:468.

77. Bosch FX, Manos MM, Munoz N, et al. Prevalence of human papillomavirus in cervical cancer: a worldwide perspective. *J Natl Cancer Inst* 1995;87:796–802.

78. Shah KV. Human papillomaviruses and genital cancers. *N Engl J Med* 1997;337:1386–1388.

79. Koutsky LA, Kivat NB. Genital human papillomavirus. In: Holmes KK, Sparling PF, Mardh PA, et al, eds. *Sexually transmitted diseases,* 3rd ed. New York: McGraw-Hill, 1999:347.

80. Schiffman MH, Haley NJ, Felton JS, et al. Biochemical epidemiology of cervical neoplasia: measuring cigarette smoke constituents in the cervix. *Cancer Res* 1987;47:3886.

81. Vessey MP. Epidemiology of cervical cancer: role of hormonal factors, cigarette smoking and occupation. In: Peto R, ZurHausen H, eds. *Viral etiology of cervical cancer.* New York: Cold Spring Harbor Laboratory, 1985:29.

82. Schneider V, Kay S, Lee LM. Immunosuppression as a high-risk factor in the development of condyloma acuminatum and squamous neoplasia. *Acta Cytol* 1983;27:220.

83. Wright TC, Sun XW. Anogenital papillomavirus infection and neoplasia in immunodeficient women. *Obstet Gynecol Clin North Am* 1996;23:861–893.

84. Fleming OT, McQuillan GM, Johnson RE, et al. Herpes simplex virus type 2 in the United States 1976 to 1994. *N Engl J Med* 1997;337:1105–1111.

85. Rosenthal SL, Stanberry LR, Biro FM, et al. Seroprevalence of herpes simplex virus types 1 and 2 and cytomegalovirus in adolescents. *Clin Infect Dis* 1997; 24:135–139.

86. Gibson JJ, Hornung CA, Alexander GR, et al. A cross-sectional study of herpes simplex virus types 1 and 2 in college students: occurrence and determinants of infection. *J Infect Dis* 1990;162:306–312.

87. Nahmias AJ, Lee FK, Beckman-Nahmias S. Sero-epidemiological and sociological patterns of herpes simplex virus infection in the world. *Scand J Infect Dis* 1990;69[Suppl]:19–36.

88. Cunningham AL, Lee FK, Ho DWT, et al. Herpes simplex virus type 2 antibody in patients attending antenatal or STD clinics. *Med J Aust* 1993;158:525–528.

89. Corey L, Wald A. Genital herpes. In: Holmes KK, Sparling PF, Mardh PA, et al, eds. *Sexually transmitted diseases,* 3rd ed. New York: McGraw-Hill, 1999:285.

90. Christenson B, Bottiger M, Svensson A, et al. A 15 year surveillance study of antibodies to herpes simplex virus types 1 and 2 in a cohort of young girls. *J Infect Dis* 1992;25:147–154.

91. Mertz GJ, Benedetti J, Ashley R, et al. Risk factors for the sexual transmission of genital herpes. *Ann Intern Med* 1992;116:197–202.

92. Corey L, Adams HG, Brown ZA, et al. Genital herpes simplex complications. *Ann Intern Med* 1983;98:958.

93. Benedetti J, Corey L, Ashley R, et al. Recurrence rates in genital herpes after symptomatic first episode infection. *Ann Intern Med* 1994;121:847–854.

94. Reeves WC, Corey L, Adams HG, et al. Risk of recurrence after first episodes of genital herpes: relation to HSV type and antibody response. *N Engl J Med* 1981; 305:315.

95. Zweerink HJ, Corey L. Virus specific antibodies for HSV-2 in sera from patients with genital herpes simplex virus infection. *Infect Immunol* 1982;37:413–421.

96. Maier J, Bergman A, Rose M. Acquired immunodeficiency syndrome manifested by chronic primary genital herpes. *Am J Obstet Gynecol* 1986;155:756.

97. Siegel FP, Loopez C, Hammer GS, et al. Severe acquired immunodeficiency in male homosexuals manifested by chronic perianal ulcerative herpes simplex lesions. *N Engl J Med* 1988;305:1439.

98. Augenbraum M, Feldman J, Chirgwin K, et al. Increased genital shedding of herpes simplex virus type 2 in HIV-seropositive women. *Ann Intern Med* 1995;123:845–847.

99. Nahmias AJ, Remington JS, Klein JO. Herpes simplex. In: Remington JS, Klein JO, eds. *Infectious diseases of the fetus and newborn infant.* Philadelphia: WB Saunders, 1983:636.

100. Whitley RJ, Nahmias AJ, Visintine AM, et al. The natural history of herpes simplex virus infection of mother and newborn. *Pediatrics* 1980;66:489.

101. Corey L, Spear PG. Infections with herpes simplex viruses. *N Engl J Med* 1986;314:749.

102. Wald A. New therapies and prevention strategies for genital herpes. *Clin Infect Dis* 1999;28:S4–S13.

103. Centers for Disease Control and Prevention. 1998 guidelines for treatment of sexually transmitted diseases. *MMWR* 1998;47[RR-1]:1–118.

104. Reichman RC, Badger GJ, Mertz GJ, et al. Treatment of recurrent genital herpes simplex infections with oral acyclovir: a controlled trial. *JAMA* 1984;251:2103.

105. Centers for Disease Control and Prevention. Recommendations for prevention and control of hepatitis C virus (HCV) infection and HCV-related chronic disease. *MMWR* 1998;47[RR-19]:1–39.

106. Alter MJ, Gerety RJ, Smallwood L, et al. Sporadic non A, non-B hepatitis: frequency and epidemiology in an urban United States population. *J Infect Dis* 1982;145: 886–893.

107. Alter MJ, Coleman PJ, Alexander WJ, et al. Importance of heterosexual activity in the transmission of hepatitis B and non-A, non-B hepatitis. *JAMA* 1989; 262:1201–1205.

108. Thomas DL, Zenilman JM, Alter HJ, et al. Sexual transmission of hepatitis C virus among patients attending sexually transmitted diseases clinics in Bal-

timore—an analysis of 309 sex partnerships. *J Infect Dis* 1995;171:768–775.

109. Coleman PJ, McQuillan GM, Moyer LA, et al. Incidence of hepatitis B virus infection in the United States, 1976–1994: estimates from the National Health and Nutrition Examination Surveys. *J Infect Dis* 1998; 178:954–959.

110. Centers for Disease Control and Prevention. Tracking the hidden epidemics—trends in the STD epidemics. National Center for HIV, STD and TB Prevention. Division of Sexually Transmitted Diseases (*http://www. cdc.gov/nchstp/dstd/Stats_Trends/Stats_and_Trends.htm*), 1998.

111. McQuillan GM, Coleman PJ, Kruszon-Moran D, et al. Prevalence of hepatitis B virus infection in the United States: the National Health and Nutrition Examination Surveys, 1976 through 1994. *Am J Public Health* 1999; 89:14–18.

112. Centers for Disease Control, Immunization Practices Advisory Committee. Protection against viral hepatitis. *MMWR* 1990;39[S-2]:1.

113. Centers for Disease Control and Prevention. Hepatitis B virus: a comprehensive strategy for eliminating transmission in the United States through universal childhood vaccination: Recommendations of the Immunization Practices Advisory Committee (ACIP). *MMWR* 1991;40[RR-13]:1–25.

114. Centers for Disease Control and Prevention. Prevention of hepatitis A through active or passive immunization: Recommendations of the Advisory Committee on Immunization Practices (ACIP). *MMWR* 1996; 45[RR-15]:1–30.

115. Weller TH, Hanshaw JB. Virologic and clinical observations on cytomegalic inclusion disease. *N Engl J Med* 1962;266:1233.

116. Wilkin JK. Molluscum contagiosum venereum in a women's outpatient clinic: a venereally transmitted disease. *Am J Obstet Gynecol* 1977;128:531.

117. Postlethwaite R. Molluscum contagiosum: a review. *Arch Environ Health* 1970;21:432.

118. Douglas JM. Molluscum contagiosum. In: Holmes KK, Sparling PF, Mardh PA, et al, eds. *Sexually transmitted diseases,* 3rd ed. New York: McGraw-Hill, 1999:385.

119. Groseclose SL, Zaidi AA, DeLisle SJ, et al. An approach to estimation of chlamydia incidence and prevalence in the United States. International Congress of Sexually Transmitted Diseases, October 19–22, Seville, Spain, 1997, abstract 0158.

120. Gaydos CA, Howell MR, Pare B, et al. Chlamydia trachomatis infections in female military recruits. *N Engl J Med* 1998;339:739–741.

121. Cohen DA, Nsuami M, Bedimo Etame R, et al. A school-based chlamydia control program using DNA amplification technology. *Pediatrics* 1998;101:E1.

122. Beck-Sague CM, Farshy CE, Jackson TK, et al. Detection of chlamydia trachomatis cervical infection by urine tests among adolescent clinics. *J Adolesc Health* 1998;22:197–204.

123. Barnes RC, Holmes KK. Epidemiology of gonorrhea: current perspectives. *Epidemiol Rev* 1984;6:1.

124. Harrison HR, Constin M, Meder JB, et al. Cervical Chlamydia trachomatis infection in university women: relationship to history, contraception, ectopy and cervicitis. *Am J Obstet Gynecol* 1985;153:244.

125. Stamm WE. Chlamydia trachomatis infections of the adult. In: Holmes KK, Sparling PF, Mardh PA, et al, eds. *Sexually transmitted diseases,* 3rd ed. New York: McGraw-Hill, 1999:407.

126. Paavonen J. Chlamydia trachomatis-induced urethritis in female partners of men with non-gonococcal urethritis. *Sex Transm Dis* 1979;6:69.

127. Paavonen J, Kiviat N, Brunham RC, et al. Prevalence and manifestations of endometritis among women with cervicitis. *Am J Obstet Gynecol* 1985;152:280.

128. Gaydos CA, Howell MR, Quinn TC, et al. Use of ligase chain reaction with urine versus cervical culture for detection of chlamydia trachomatis in an asymptomatic military population of pregnant and nonpregnant females attending Papanicolaou smear clinics. *J Clin Microbiol* 1998;36:1300–1304.

129. Schepetiuk S, Kok T, Martin L, et al. Detection of chlamydia trachomatis in urine samples by nucleic acid tests: comparison with culture and enzyme immunoassay of genital swab specimens. *J Clin Microbiol* 1997;35:3355–3357.

130. Carroll KC, Aldeen WE, Morrison M, et al. Evaluation of the Abbott Lcx ligase chain reaction assay for detection of Chlamydia trachomatis and Neisseria gonorrhoeae in urine and genital swab specimens from a sexually transmitted disease clinic population. *J Clin Microbiol* 1998;36:1630–1633.

131. Puolakkainen M, Hiltunen-Back E, Reunala T, et al. Comparison of performances of two commercially available tests, a PCR assay and a ligase chain reaction test, in detection of urogenital Chlamydia trachomatis infection. *J Clin Microbiol* 1998;36:1489–1493.

132. Davis JD, Riley PK, Peters CW, et al. A comparison of ligase chain reaction to polymerase chain reaction in the detection of chlamydia trachomatis endocervical infections. *Infect Dis Obstet Gynecol* 1998;6:57–60.

133. Centers for Disease Control and Prevention, Division of STD Prevention. *Sexually transmitted disease surveillance–1997.* Atlanta: U.S. Department of Health and Human Services, Public Health Service, Atlanta, September 1998.

134. Hook EW III, Handsfield HH. Gonococcal infections in the adult. In: Holmes KK, Mardh PA, Sparling PF, et al, eds. *Sexually transmitted diseases.* New York: McGraw-Hill, 1990:771.

135. Holmes KK, Johnson DW, Trostle HJ. An estimate of the risk of men acquiring gonorrhea by sexual contact with infected females. *Am J Epidemiol* 1970;91:170.

136. Hooper RR, Reynolds GH, Jones OG, et al. Cohort study of venereal disease: I. The risk of gonorrhea transmission from infected women to men. *Am J Epidemiol* 1978;108:136.

137. Thin RN, Shaw EJ. Diagnosis of gonorrhea in women. *Br J Vener Dis* 1979;55:10.

138. Barlow D, Philips I. Gonorrhea in women: diagnostic, clinical, and laboratory aspects. *Lancet* 1978;1:761.

139. Hook EW III, Handsfield HH. Gonococcal infections in the adult. In: Holmes KK, Sparling PF, Mardh PA, et al, eds. *Sexually transmitted diseases,* 3rd ed. New York: McGraw-Hill, 1999:451.

140. Wiesner PJ, Tronca E, Bonin P, et al. Clinical spectrum of pharyngeal gonococcal infections. *N Engl J Med* 1973;288:181.

141. Tice W, Rodriguez VL. Pharyngeal gonorrhea. *JAMA* 1981;246:2717.

142. Hutt DM, Judson FN. Epidemiology and treatment of oro-pharyngeal gonorrhea. *Ann Intern Med* 1986;104:655.

143. Holmes KK, Counts GW, Beaty HN. Disseminated gonococcal infection. *Ann Intern Med* 1971;74:979.

144. Schink JC, Keith LG. Problems in the culture diagnosis of gonorrhea. *J Reprod Med* 1985;30[Suppl]:244.

145. Ching S, Lee H, Hook EW 3rd, et al. Ligase chain reaction for detection of Neisseria gonorrhoeae in urogenital swabs. *J Clin Microbiol* 1995;33:311.

146. Smith KR, Ching S, Lee H, et al. Evaluation of ligase chain reaction for use with urine for identification of Neisseria gonorrhoeae in females attending a sexually transmitted disease clinic. *J Clin Microbiol* 1995;33:455.

147. Sweet RL. Role of bacterial vaginosis in pelvic inflammatory disease. *Clin Infect Dis* 1995;20[Suppl 2]:S271–S275.

148. Burnakis TG, Hildebrandt NB. Pelvic inflammatory disease: a review with emphasis on antimicrobial therapy. *Rev Infect Dis* 1986;8:86–116.

149. Shafer MA, Sweet RL. Pelvic inflammatory disease in adolescent females. *Pediatr Clin North Am* 1989;36:513.

150. Westrom L. Incidence, prevalence, and trends of acute pelvic inflammatory disease and its consequences in industrialized countries. *Am J Obstet Gynecol* 1980;138:880–892.

151. Hillis SD, Owens LM, Marchbanks PA, et al. Recurrent chlamydial infections increase the risks of hospitalization for ectopic pregnancy and pelvic inflammatory disease. *Am J Obstet Gynecol* 1997;176:103–107.

152. Aral SO, Wasserheit JN. Social and behavioral correlates of pelvic inflammatory disease. *Sex Transm Dis* 1998;25:378–385.

153. Spence MR, Adler J, McLellan R. Pelvic inflammatory disease in the adolescent. *J Adolesc Health Care* 1990;11:304–309.

154. Westrom L, Eschenbach D. Pelvic inflammatory disease. In: Holmes KK, Sparling PF, Mardh PA, et al, eds. *Sexually transmitted diseases,* 3rd ed. New York: McGraw-Hill, 1999:783.

155. Westrom L, Wolner-Hanssen P. Pathogenesis of pelvic inflammatory disease. *Genitourin Med* 1993;69:9.

156. Hillier SL, Kiviat NB, Hawes SE, et al. Role of bacterial vaginosis-associated microorganisms in endometriosis. *Am J Obstet Gynecol* 1996;175:435–441.

157. Peipert JF, Montagno AB, Cooper AS, et al. Bacterial vaginosis as a risk factor for upper genital tract infection. *Am J Obstet Gynecol* 1997;177:1184–1187.

158. Safrin S, Dattel BJ, Hauer L, et al. Seroprevalence and epidemiologic correlates of human immunodeficiency virus infections in women with acute pelvic inflammatory disease. *Obstet Gynecol* 1990;75:666.

159. Sperling RS, Friedman F, Jr., Joyner M, et al. Seroprevalence of human immunodeficiency virus in women admitted to the hospital with pelvic inflammatory disease. *J Reprod Med* 1991;36:122.

160. Barbosa C, Macasaet M, Brockmann S, et al. Pelvic inflammatory disease and human immunodeficiency virus infection. *Obstet Gynecol* 1997;89:65–70.

161. Kamenga MC, DeCock KM, St. Louis ME, et al. The impact of human immunodeficiency virus infection on pelvic inflammatory disease: a case-control study in Abidjan, Ivory Coast. *Am J Obstet Gynecol* 1995;172:919–925.

162. Cohen CR, Sinei S, Reilly M, et al. Effect of human immunodeficiency virus type 1 infection upon acute salpingitis: a laparoscopic study. *J Infect Dis* 1998;178:1352–1358.

163. Jacobson L, Westrom L. Objectivized diagnosis of acute pelvic inflammatory disease. *Am J Obstet Gynecol* 1969.

164. Jones RB, Ardery BR, Hui SL, et al. Correlation between serum antichlamydial antibodies and tubal factors as a cause of infertility. *Fertil Steril* 1982;38:553.

165. Brunham RC, Maclean IW, Binns B, et al. *Chlamydia trachomatis: its role in tubal infertility. J Infect Dis* 1985;152:127.

166. Tjiam KH, Zeilmaker GH, Alberda AT, et al. Prevalence of antibodies to *Chlamydia trachomatis, Neisseria gonorrhoeae,* and *Mycoplasma hominis* infertile women. *Genitourin Med* 1985;61:175.

167. Katzman DK, Friedman IM, McDonald CA, et al. *Chlamydia trachomatis* Fitz-Hugh-Curtis syndrome without salpingitis in female adolescents. *Am J Dis Child* 1988;142:996.

168. Lehtinen M, Laine S, Heinonen PK, et al. Serum C-reactive protein determinations in acute pelvic inflammatory disease. *Am J Obstet Gynecol* 1986;154:158.

169. Landers DV, Sweet RL. Tubo-ovarian abscess. Contemporary approach to management. *Rev Infect Dis* 1983;5:876.

170. Cacciatore B, Leminen A, Ingman-Friberg S, et al. Transvaginal sonographic findings in ambulatory patients with suspected pelvic inflammatory disease. *Obstet Gynecol* 1992;80:912.

171. Paavonen J, Aine R, Teisala K, et al. Comparison of endometrial biopsy and peritoneal fluid cytology with laparoscopy in the diagnosis of acute pelvic inflammatory disease. *Am J Obstet Gynecol* 1986;154:645.

172. Hager WD, Eschenbach PA, Spence MR, et al. Criteria for diagnosis and grading of salpingitis. *Obstet Gynecol* 1983;61:113.

173. Hedberg E, Anberg A. Gonorrheal salpingitis: views on treatment and prognosis. *Fertil Steril* 1965;16:125.

174. Walker CK, Kahn JG, Washington AE, et al. Pelvic inflammatory disease: metaanalysis of antimicrobial regimen efficacy. *J Infect Dis* 1993;168:969.

175. Eschenbach DA. Epidemiology and diagnosis of acute pelvic inflammatory disease. *Obstet Gynecol* 1980;55:1425.

176. Handsfield HH, Lipman TO, Harnisch JP, et al. Asymptomatic gonorrhea in men: diagnosis, natural course, prevalence and significance. *N Engl J Med* 1974;290:117.

177. Schwartz SL, Krauss J. Persistent urethral leukocytosis and asymptomatic chlamydial urethritis. *J Infect Dis* 1979;140:614.

178. Stamm WE, Koutsky LA, Benedetti J, et al. *Chlamydia trachomatis* urethral infections in men. Prevalence, risk factors, and clinical manifestations. *Ann Intern Med* 1984;100:47.

179. Washington AE, Weisner PJ. The silent clap. *JAMA* 1981;245:609.

180. Gerzof SG, Robbins AH, Johnson WC, et al. Percutaneous catheter drainage of abdominal abscesses: a five-year experience. *N Engl J Med* 1981;305:653.

181. Henry-Suchet J, Soler A, Loffredo V. Laparoscopic treatment of tubo-ovarian abscesses. *J Reprod Med* 1984;29:579.
182. Westrom L. Effect of pelvic inflammatory disease on fertility. *Am J Obstet Gynecol* 1975;121:707.
183. Kresch AJ, Seifer DB, Sachs LB, et al. Laparoscopy in 100 women with pelvic pain. *Obstet Gynecol* 1984;64: 672.
184. Svenson L, Mardh PA, Ahlgren M, et al. Ectopic pregnancy and antibodies to *Chlamydia trachomatis*. *Fertil Steril* 1985;44:313.
185. Brunham RC, Binns B, McDowell J, et al. *Chlamydia trachomatis* infection in women with ectopic pregnancy. *Obstet Gynecol* 1986;67:722.
186. Centers for Disease Control. Ectopic pregnancies—United States 1987. *MMWR* 1990;39:401–404.
187. Westrom L. Impact of sexually transmitted diseases on human reproduction: Swedish studies of infertility and ectopic pregnancy. In: *Sexually transmitted diseases, status report, NIAID study group.* Washington, DC: NIH Publication 81–2213, 1980:43.
188. Westrom L. Effect of pelvic inflammatory disease on fertility. *Am J Obstet Gynecol* 1975;121:707.
189. Pedowitz P, Bloomfield RD. Ruptured adnexal abscess with generalized peritonitis. *Am J Obstet Gynecol* 1964;88:721.
190. Rivlin ME, Hunt JA. Ruptured tubo-ovarian abscess: is hysterectomy necessary? *Obstet Gynecol* 1977;50 [Suppl]:518.
191. Spiegel CA, Amsel R, Eschenbach DA, et al. Anaerobic bacteria in nonspecific vaginitis. *N Engl J Med* 1980; 303:601.
192. Amsel R, Totten PA, Spiegel CA, et al. Nonspecific vaginitis: diagnostic criteria and microbial and epidemiologic associations. *Am J Med* 1983;74:14.
193. Gardner HL, Dukes CD. *Haemophilus vaginalis* vaginitis. A newly defined specific infection previously classified "nonspecific" vaginitis. *Am J Obstet Gynecol* 1955;69:962.
194. Pheifer TA, Forsyth PS, Durfee MA, et al. Non-specific vaginitis. Role of *Haemophilus vaginalis* and treatment with metronidazole. *N Engl J Med* 1978;298:1429.
195. Bump RC, Buesching WJ. Bacterial vaginosis in virginal and sexually active adolescent females: evidence against exclusive sexual transmission. *Obstet Gynecol* 1988;158:935.
196. Spiegel CA, Amsel R, Holmes KK. Diagnosis of bacterial vaginosis by direct gram stain of vaginal fluid. *J Clin Microbiol* 1983;18:170.
197. McDonald HM, O'Loughlin JA, Vigneswaran R, et al. Impact of metronidazole therapy on preterm birth in women with bacterial vaginosis flora (Gardnerella vaginalis): a randomized, placebo controlled trial. *Br J Obstet Gynaecol* 1997;104:1391–1397.
198. Morales WJ, Schorr S, Albritton J, et al. Effect of metronidazole in patients with preterm birth in preceding pregnancy and bacterial vaginosis: A placebo-controlled, double-blind study. *Am J Obstet Gynecol* 1994;171:345.
199. Caro-Paton T, Carvajal A, Martin deDiego I, et al. Is metronidazole teratogenic? A meta-analysis. *Br J Clin Pharmacol* 1997;44:179–182.
200. Wilcox RR. Importance of the so-called "other" sexually transmitted diseases. *Br J Vener Dis* 1986;5:735.
201. D'Aunoy R, Von Haam E. Venereal lymphogranuloma. *Arch Pathol* 1939;27:1032.
202. Coutts WE. Lymphogranuloma venereum: a general review. *Bull WHO* 1950;2:545.
203. Schulte JM, Martich FA, Schmid GP. Chancroid in the United States, 1981–1990: evidence of underreporting of cases. *MMWR* 1992;41[SS-3]:57–61.
204. Morse SA. Chancroid detected by polymerase chain reaction: Jackson, Mississippi, 1994–1995. *MMWR* 1995;44:567–574.
205. Ronald AR, Albritton W. Chancroid and Haemophilus ducreyi. In: Holmes KK, Sparling PF, Mardh PA, et al, eds. *Sexually transmitted diseases,* 3rd ed. New York: McGraw-Hill, 1999:515.
206. Wysoki RS, Majmudar B, Willis D. Granuloma inguinale (Donovanosis) in women. *J Reprod Med* 1988;33: 709.
207. Kuberski TM. Granuloma inguinale (Donovanosis). *Sex Transm Dis* 1980;7:29.
208. Goldberg J. Studies on granuloma inguinale: VIII. Some epidemiological considerations of the disease. *Br J Vener Dis* 1964;40:140.
209. Hook EW III. Syphilis and HIV infection. *J Infect Dis* 1989;160:530.
210. Chernesky MA. Laboratory services for sexually transmitted diseases: overview and recent developments. In: Holmes KK, Sparling PF, Mardh PA, et al, eds. *Sexually transmitted diseases,* 3rd ed. New York: McGraw-Hill, 1999:1281.
211. Moore JE, Mohr CF. Biologically false positive serologic tests for syphilis: type, incidence, and cause. *JAMA* 1952;150:467.
212. Tuffanellie DL, Wuepper KD, Bradford LL, et al. Fluorescent treponemal antibody-absorption tests: studies of false positive reactions to tests for syphilis. *N Engl J Med* 1967;276:258.
213. Billstein SA. Public lice. In: Holmes KK, Sparling PF, Mardh PA, et al, eds. *Sexually transmitted diseases,* 3rd ed. New York: McGraw-Hill, 1999:641.
214. Kalter DC, Sparber J, Rosen T, et al. Treatment of pediculosis pubis. Clinical comparison of efficacy and tolerance of 1% lindane shampoo vs 1% permethrin creme rinse. *Arch Dermatol* 1987;123:1315.
215. Green MS. Epidemiology of scabies. *Epidemiol Rev* 1989;11:126.
216. Platts-Mills TA, Rein MF. Scabies. In: Holmes KK, Sparling PF, Mardh PA, et al, eds. *Sexually transmitted diseases,* 3rd ed. New York: McGraw-Hill, 1999: 645.
217. Sobel JD. Pathophysiology of vulvovaginal candidiasis. *J Reprod Med* 1989;34:572.
218. Drake TE, Mailbach HI. Candida and candidiasis: cultural conditions, epidemiology and pathogenesis. *Postgrad Med* 1973;53:83.
219. Sobel JD, Myers PG, Kaye D, et al. C. albicans adherence to vaginal epithelial cells. *J Infect Dis* 1981;143: 76.
220. Soll DR, Gakask R, Schmid J, et al. Genetic dissimilarity of commensal strains of *Candida spp.* carried in different anatomical locations of the same healthy women. *J Clin Microbiol* 1991;29(8):1702.
221. Morton RS, Rashid S. Candidal vaginitis: natural history, predisposing factors and prevention. *Proc R Soc Med* 1977;70[Suppl 4]:3.

222. Odds FC. *Candida and candidosis.* Baltimore: University Park Press, 1979.

223. Oriel JD, Waterworth PM. Effect of minocycline and tetracycline on the vaginal yeast flora. *J Clin Pathol* 1975;28:403.

224. Witkin SS, Jeremias J, Ledger WJ. A localized vaginal allergic response in women with recurrent vaginitis. *J Allergy Clin Immunol* 1988;81:412.

225. Fleury FJ. Adult vaginitis. *Clin Obstet Gynecol* 1981; 24:407.

226. Imam N, Carpenter CC, Mayer KH, et al. Hierarchical pattern of mucosal candida infections in HIV seropositive women. *Am J Med* 1990;89:142.

227. Duerr A, Sierra MF, Feldman J, et al. Immune compromise and prevalence of candida vulvovaginitis in human immunodeficiency virus-infected women. *Obstet Gynecol* 1997;90:252–256.

228. Horowitz BJ, Edelstein SW, Lippman L. Sexual transmission of Candida. *Obstet Gynecol* 1987;69:883.

229. Sobel JD. Vulvovaginal candidiasis. In: Holmes KK, Sparling PF, Mardh PA, et al, eds. *Sexually transmitted diseases,* 3rd ed. New York: McGraw-Hill, 1999:629.

230. Lewis JH, Zimmerman HJ, Benson GD, et al. Hepatic injury associated with ketoconazole therapy: analysis of 33 cases. *Gastroenterology* 1984;86:503.

231. Krieger JN, Alderete JF. Trichomonas vaginalis and trichomoniasis. In: Holmes KK, Sparling PF, Mardh PA, et al, eds. *Sexually transmitted diseases,* 3rd ed. New York: McGraw-Hill, 1999:587.

232. Weston TET, Nicol CS. Natural history of trichomonal infection in males. *Br J Vener Dis* 1963;39:251.

233. Minkoff H, Grunebaum AN, Schwartz RH, et al. Risk factors for prematurity and premature rupture of membranes: a prospective study of vaginal flora in pregnancy. *Am J Obstet Gynecol* 1984;150:965–972.

234. McGregor JA, French JI, Parker R, et al. Prevention of premature birth by screening and treatment for common genital tract infections: results of prospective controlled evaluation. *Am J Obstet Gynecol* 1995;173: 157–167.

235. Meis PJ, Goldenberg RL, Mercer B, et al. The preterm prediction study: significance of vaginal infections. *Am J Obstet Gynecol* 1995;173:1231–1235.

236. Cotch MF, Pastorek JG, Nugent RP, et al. Trichomonas vaginalis associated with low birth weight and preterm delivery. *Sex Transm Dis* 1997;24:1–8.

237. Thomason JL, Gelbart SM. Trichomonas vaginalis. *Obstet Gynecol* 1989;74:539.

238. Fouts AC, Kraus SJ. Trichomonas vaginalis: re-evaluation of its clinical presentation and laboratory diagnosis. *J Infect Dis* 1980;141:137.

239. Wolner-Hanssen P, Krieger JN, Steven CE. Clinical manifestations of vaginal trichomoniasis. *JAMA* 1989; 261:571.

20

Uterovaginal Anomalies

Mark A. Damario and John A. Rock

UTEROVAGINAL DEVELOPMENT

During early embryonic development, both the wolffian (mesonephric) and the müllerian (paramesonephric) duct primordia coexist during the ambisexual period before gonadal differentiation (1). The mesonephric ducts drain the mesonephric kidneys that function briefly, if at all, in human embryos. The paramesonephric ducts develop on each side of the urogenital ridge from invaginations of coelomic epithelium lateral and ventral to the mesonephric ducts. The site of origin of the invaginations remains open and ultimately forms the fimbriated ends of the fallopian tubes. The paramesonephric ducts elongate in a caudomedial direction and cross ventrally to the mesonephric ducts. In the midline, the two paramesonephric ducts come in close contact with one another and fuse to form the uterovaginal primordium. The fused paramesonephric ducts eventually give rise to the corpus and cervix of the uterus. The caudal tip of the combined ducts projects into the posterior wall of the urogenital sinus, where it causes a small swelling, known as the paramesonephric or müllerian tubercle. The mesonephric ducts enters the uterogenital sinus on each side of this tubercle. Shortly after the solid tip of the paramesonephric ducts has reached the urogenital sinus, two solid evaginations grow out from the pelvic part of the sinus. These evaginations, known as the sinovaginal bulbs, proliferate and form a solid mass called the vaginal plate, the center of which ultimately cavitates to form the vaginal canal. Distally, the vaginal canal is separated from the uro-

genital sinus by the hymen until late in fetal life, at which time the hymen usually ruptures, thus affording external communication for the vaginal canal.

In normal females, the mesonephric ducts regress and the paramesonephric ducts develop into the female genital tract. The cranial or unfused portions of the ducts form the fallopian tubes. The caudal portion (or fused portion of the ducts) gives rise to the epithelium and the glands of the uterus, whereas the underlying stroma and myometrium are derived from surrounding mesenchyme.

The uterus therefore develops from the paired müllerian ducts and surrounding mesenchyme. Three well-defined developmental phases are recognized: (a) contact of the müllerian ducts in the midline, (b) fusion of the duct walls, and (c) involution of the dividing septum. Ducts of unequal size or growth rates may result in a unicornuate uterus. A lateral fusion defect may result in a didelphic or bicornuate uterus. Defects in the involution process may result in a persistent midline uterine septum.

The uterine cervix is formed about week 20 of embryonic life. The cervix arises from a condensation of mesenchymal cells around a specific site of the fused müllerian ducts.

According to recent views, the upper third of the vagina is formed from the müllerian tubercle, whereas the lower two thirds develop from the vaginal plate of the urogenital sinus (2). Recent studies suggest that the vaginal canal is actually open and connected to a patent uterus and tubes, even in early embryonic life, and that the vagina does not form and later become canalized from an epithelial cord of squamous cells growing upward from the urogenital sinus. Most investigators now suggest that the vagina develops under the influence of the müllerian ducts and estrogenic stimulation. Failure in development of the müllerian ducts at any time from their origin at 5 weeks to their fusion with the urogenital sinus at 8 weeks may lead to partial or complete vaginal agenesis.

The entirely separate origin of the gonads from the genital ridges explains the infrequent association of uterovaginal anomalies and ovarian anomalies. The close developmental relationships of the mesonephric and paramesonephric ducts, however, does explain the frequency with which anomalies of the urinary tract are seen in accompaniment to anomalies of the female genital system. Failure of development of a paramesonephric (müllerian) duct likewise is associated with failure of development of a ureteric bud from the caudal end of the mesonephric duct. Thus, the entire kidney can be absent on the side ipsilateral to the agenesis of the müllerian duct (3). According to Thompson and Lynn (4), 40% of female patients with congenital absence of the kidney also have associated genital anomalies.

CLASSIFICATION OF UTEROVAGINAL ANOMALIES

Classifications of uterovaginal anomalies originally were organized based on clinical findings. Improved understanding of embryologic development has enabled further categorizations on this basis. The 1988 American Fertility Society (AFS) classification of müllerian anomalies (Table 20.1) offers a system of classification based on the degree of failure of normal uterine development (5). Anomalies are grouped according to similarities of clinical manifestations, treatment, and prognosis. However, this system does not include associated vaginal anomalies, although the scheme allows the user to describe other associated anomalies of the vagina, fallopian tubes, and urinary tract as associated malformations.

We offer a modified classification that comprises four groups based on embryologic considerations (Table 20.2).

Class I: Dysgenesis of the Müllerian Ducts

Dygenesis of the müllerian ducts or agenesis of the uterus and vagina, the Mayer-Rokitansky-Küster-Hauser syndrome, is characterized by the absence of the vagina with or without vestigial uterine structures.

Class II: Disorders of Vertical Fusion of the Müllerian Ducts

Disorders of vertical fusion can be considered to represent faults in the junction between the down-growing müllerian ducts (müllerian tubercle) and the up-growing derivatives of the urogenital sinus. Typically, these disorders are characterized by an atretic portion of the vagina that can be quite thick,

TABLE 20.1. *American Fertility Society classification of müllerian anomalies (1988)*

Classification	Anomaly
Class I	Segmental, müllerian agenesis-hypoplasia A. Vaginal B. Cervical C. Fundal D. Tubal E. Combined anomalies
Class II	Unicornuate A. Communicating B. Noncommunicating C. No cavity D. No horn
Class III	Didelphus
Class IV	Bicornuate A. Complete (division down to internal os) B. Partial
Class V	Septate A. Complete (septum to internal os) B. Partial
Class VI	Arcuate
Class VII	Diethylstilbestrol related

This classification allows the user to indicate the malformation type and provides additional findings to describe associated variations involving the vagina, cervix, fallopian tubes, and kidneys.

Adapted from the American Fertility Society. Classification of müllerian anomalies. *Fertil Steril* 1988;49:944.

TABLE 20.2. *Proposed classification of uterovaginal anomalies*

Classification	Anomaly
Class I	Dysgenesis of the müllerian ducts
Class II	Disorders of vertical fusion of the müllerian ducts
	A. Transverse vaginal septum
	1. Obstructed
	2. Unobstructed
	B. Cervical agenesis or dysgenesis
Class III	Disorders of lateral fusion of the müllerian ducts
	A. Asymmetric obstructed disorder of the uterus or vagina, usually associated with ipsilateral renal agenesis
	1. Unicornuate uterus with a noncommunicating rudimentary horn
	2. Unilateral obstruction of a cavity of a double uterus
	3. Unilateral vaginal obstruction associated with double uterus
	B. Symmetric unobstructed
	1. Didelphic uterus
	a. Complete longitudinal vaginal septum
	b. Partial longitudinal vaginal septum
	c. No longitudinal vaginal septum
	2. Septate uterus
	a. Complete
	i. Complete longitudinal vaginal septum
	ii. Partial longitudinal vaginal septum
	iii. No longitudinal vaginal septum
	b. Partial
	i. Complete longitudinal vaginal septum
	ii. Partial longitudinal vaginal septum
	iii. No longitudinal vaginal septum
	3. Bicornuate uterus
	a. Complete
	i. Complete longitudinal vaginal septum
	ii. Partial longitudinal vaginal septum
	iii. No longitudinal vaginal septum
	b. Partial
	i. Complete longitudinal vaginal septum
	ii. Partial longitudinal vaginal septum
	iii. No longitudinal vaginal septum
	4. T-shaped uterine cavity (diethylstilbestrol related)
	5. Unicornuate uterus
	a. With a rudimentary horn
	i. With endometrial cavity
	A. Communicating
	B. Noncommunicating
	ii. Without endometrial cavity
	b. Without a rudimentary horn
Class IV	Unusual configurations of vertical-lateral fusion defects

Adapted from Rock JA. Surgery for anomalies of the Müllerian ducts. In: *TeLinde's operative gynecology,* 8th ed, Rock JA, Thompson JD, eds. Philadelphia: Lippincott–Raven Publishers, 1997:687–729.

extending over more than half of the distance of the vagina, or it can be quite thin and limited to a small obstructing membrane.

Regardless of the length of the septum, a disorder of vertical fusion should be regarded as a transverse vaginal septum and classified as either obstructed or unobstructed. The term "partial vaginal atresia with uterus and cervix present" probably is a misnomer and invariably would be describing a thick transverse vaginal septum with a large segment of atretic vagina. Cervical agenesis and dysgenesis are included in this group of disorders of vertical fusion.

Class III: Disorders of Lateral Fusion of the Müllerian Ducts

Disorders of lateral fusion of the müllerian ducts may be symmetric or asymmetric and may be obstructed or unobstructed. An example of a symmetric unobstructed defect would be the double uterus (bicornuate, septate, didelphic). Examples of asymmetric obstructed defects include unilateral vaginal obstructions associated with double uteri and noncommunicating rudimentary uterine horns. Obstructed lesions associated with disorders of lateral fusion are particularly noteworthy in that obstruction is unilateral and almost invariably associated with absence of the kidney on the side of the obstruction. It is believed that bilateral obstructive defects are not seen presumably because they would be associated with bilateral renal agenesis, which is incompatible with life.

Of the symmetric unobstructed disorders of lateral fusion there are five groups of disorders: (a) didelphic uterus, (b) bicornuate uterus, (c) septate uterus, (d) T-shaped uterus (often diethylstilbestrol [DES] related), and (e) unicornuate uterus with or without a rudimentary horn.

Uterine septa may be either partial or complete. A complete uterine septum extends throughout the uterine body and cervix, such that two cervical openings are seen on examination. Complete uterine septa almost always are associated with longitudinal vaginal septa, which may extend either to the introitus or partially down the vagina. The bicornuate uterus also can have a partial or almost complete separation of the uterine cavities. The term "arcuate" uterus is used primarily by radiologists to refer to a slight septum in the uterine fundus that forms no clear separation of the uterine cavities. This type of uterus usually is included in the category of partial septate uterus.

The unicornuate uterus may have an attached horn with a cavity that communicates with the main uterine body. Alternatively, there may be a contralateral noncommunicating uterine horn with or without functional endometrium.

Class IV: Unusual Configurations of Vertical/Lateral Fusion Defects

This category includes configurations of combined lateral and vertical fusion defects that do not fit into other categories. For instance, Singh and co-workers (6) described a patient who was noted to have a persistent hymen and a longitudinal vaginal septum with a didelphic uterus. This patient also was noted to have associated urinary anomalies (double urethra and bladder and left renal agenesis). Another unusual müllerian anomaly that would be classified in this category is the recent report of a bifid cervix and septate vagina in the presence of a normal uterine corpus (7).

CLINICAL MANIFESTATIONS OF CLASS I ANOMALIES: DYSGENESIS OF THE MÜLLERIAN DUCTS

The disorders of müllerian dysgenesis include congenital absence of the uterus and vagina. The commonly used term, vaginal agenesis, is somewhat of a misnomer, as the lower portion of the vagina often is present in these patients. In addition, despite lacking a normal midline uterine body, bilateral rudimentary uterine primordia (uterine anlagen) are found in approximately 90% of patients. The fallopian tubes and ovaries usually are normal. This syndrome often is referred to as Mayer-Rokitansky-Küster-Hauser syndrome. This syndrome is probably a heterogeneous group of disorders with various genetic, endocrine, and metabolic manifestations as well as other associated anomalies. The incidence of Mayer-Rokitansky-Küster-Hauser syndrome was reported to be one in 4,000 admissions at the Mayo Clinic (8). Evans (9) reported the incidence as one in 10,588 female births in Michigan from 1963 to 1967.

Patients with an absent vagina and the classic Mayer-Rokitansky-Küster-Hauser syndrome usually are brought to medical attention at around the age of 14 to 15 years, when the absence of menses is of concern. These young women have normal ovaries and secondary sexual characteristics, including external genitalia. Menstruation does not appear because the uterus is absent. Ovulation, however, does occur regularly. Karyotype analysis usually reveals a normal chromosomal constituency (46,XX).

Patients with müllerian agenesis have a high incidence of renal and other associated anomalies. Fore and associates (10) reported that 47% of patients in whom evaluation of the urinary tract was performed had associated urologic anomalies. In other studies, at least one third of patients with müllerian agenesis were noted to have significant urinary anomalies, such as unilateral renal agenesis, unilateral or bilateral pelvic kidney, horseshoe kidney, hydronephrosis, hydroureter, and various patterns of ureteral duplication. In a review of 574 reported cases, Griffin and associates (11) found a 12% incidence of skeletal abnormalities. Most of these involved the spine (wedge vertebrae, fusions, rudimentary vertebral bodies, supernumerary vertebrae), but the limbs and ribs also were involved in some cases. Other anomalies associated with Mayer-Rokitansky-Küster-Hauser syndrome include syndactyly, absence of a digit, congenital heart disease, and inguinal hernias.

A few patients with müllerian agenesis may have associated abnormalities of the upper müllerian ducts. As stated earlier, the uterus in this syndrome is represented by bilateral rudimentary bulbs that are connected by a connective tissue band. These rudimentary uterine bulbs (anlagen) usually are connected to small fallopian tubes and are located on the lateral pelvic side wall adjacent to normal ovaries. They may vary in size, and they may contain a cavity lined by endometrial tissue (Fig. 20.1). If present, the endometrial tissue may appear immature or, rarely, respond cyclically to ovarian hormones. Often the endometrial cavity does not communicate with the peritoneal cavity because the tube may not be patent at the point of juncture between the tube and the rudimentary anlagen. In rare cases, active endometrium may exist within the uterine anlagen and communicate with the peritoneal cavity, increasing the chance for endometriosis from retrograde seeding. If not communicating with the peritoneal cavity, active endometrium within a uterine anlagen may become trapped and a large hematometra result. Several reports have described patients with functioning endometrial tissue in one or both rudimentary uterine anlagen (12). Cyclic abdominal pain, in this circumstance, is relieved by excision of the active uterine anlagen. Some investigators attempted to use the rudimentary uterine bulbs to reconstruct a midline uterus, connecting it to a newly constructed vagina (13). Although allowing cyc-

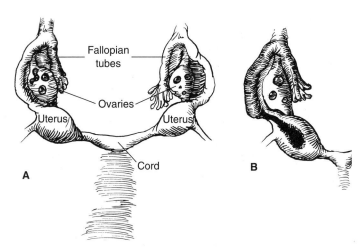

FIG. 20.1. Variations of development seen in patients with congenital absence of the vagina. **A:** Bilateral rudimentary bulbs without endometrium. **B:** Bilateral rudimentary uterine bulbs containing a cavity lined with functioning endometrial tissue. (From Rock JA. Surgery for anomalies of the Mullerian ducts. In: Rock JA, Thompson, JD, eds. *TeLinde's operative gynecology,* 8th ed. Philadelphia: Lippincott–Raven Publishers, 1997:687–729, with permission.)

lic menstruation in some patients, recurrent stenosis and obstruction of the rudimentary horns were common outcomes of these types of efforts.

Etiology

The etiology of congenital absence of the uterus and vagina is not known. Almost all patients have a 46,XX karyotype, although a few chromosomal abnormalities have been reported in patients with this condition (14). Several family aggregates of patients with affected siblings have suggested an autosomal inheritance. However, because monozygotic twins discordant for the condition are known to exist, it is unlikely that every case has an easily explainable genetic cause. Shokeir (15) evaluated 16 Saskatchewan families affected by congenital absence of the uterus and vagina. Ten of the probands had affected siblings or affected paternal relatives, suggesting a autosomal dominant inheritance pattern. A survey of 23 American women with congenital absence of the uterus and vagina, however, failed to identify any affected siblings (16). Further evidence against an autosomal dominant form of inheritance is the lack of identified anomalies (except one male child with a middle ear defect and hearing loss) in 34 liveborn children from patients with Mayer-Rokitansky-Küster-Hauser syndrome who underwent *in vitro* fertilization with subsequent transfer of the embryos to a surrogate carrier (17). Other investigators point to the variety of associated anomalies as support for the etiologic concept of variable expression of a genetic defect possibly precipitated by teratogenic exposure between gestational days 37 and 41, the time during which the vagina is formed. Others have suggested that inappropriate production of antimüllerian hormone ("gain of function mutation") by the female embryonic gonad may be responsible (18). A problem with this latter theory is that approximately 85% of patients with müllerian agenesis have normal fallopian tubes, thereby making a proposed mutation an unlikely cause of this syndrome unless the cranial por-

tions of the müllerian ducts are less sensitive to antimüllerian hormone-mediated regression than are the caudal portions of the ducts. Proposed mutations resulting in inappropriate production of antimüllerian hormone also do not explain the frequent association of nongenital tract anomalies (renal, skeletal) seen in these patients.

Laboratory and Diagnostic Testing

Chromosomal analysis to rule out androgen insensitivity should be done. An intravenous pyelogram is mandatory to define the urinary system and to rule out anomalies. These radiographs may be used to evaluate the lower spine for skeletal anomalies. If symptoms suggest an active uterine anlagen or if a pelvic mass is present, appropriate studies such as ultrasonography or magnetic resonance imaging (MRI) help differentiate between hematometra, hematocolpos, or other abnormalities. Diagnostic laparoscopy is not absolutely essential in patients with a typical presentation of congenital absence of the uterus and vagina; however, it should be considered with atypical presentations.

Timing of Treatment

Most patients present around the age of 15 or 16 years with primary amenorrhea. Psychological counseling is extremely important in the management of these patients. David et al. (19) reported a 15% incidence of psychiatric problems in these patients and suggested that psychiatric intervention be initiated before therapy. The psychological adjustment of the patient to her anomaly appears to be a critical factor in determining the success of therapy, both nonsurgical and surgical.

Formerly, it was customary to advise surgical correction at the time just before marriage. More recently, the procedure is being performed between the ages of 17 and 20 years when the patient is emotionally mature and intellectually capable of understanding the operative procedure and partaking in her postoperative care, which is an extremely important variable in terms of outcome.

If functional endometrial tissue is present, symptoms from cryptomenorrhea may begin soon after secondary sexual characteristics start to develop. Surgical therapy to remove the uterine anlagen should not be delayed, as prompt surgical extirpation will afford complete relief of symptoms and avoid the development or progression of endometriosis if the anlagen is communicating with the peritoneal cavity. In cases where surgical therapy is required to remove a functioning uterine anlagen in a younger patient, it may be best to defer surgical therapy to form a neovagina until a later date when the patient is more mature.

Methods of Creating a Vagina

Both surgical and nonsurgical methods for creating a vagina have been described and successfully used.

Nonsurgical methods focus on progressive dilation techniques. The first method was described by Robert Frank (20) in 1938. This method involved active manipulation by the patient to dilate the neovaginal space. The initial report revealed satisfactory results in eight patients, with permanent depth and caliber of the vagina maintained even in patients who had neglected dilatation for more than 1 year. The chief disadvantage to the Frank technique of active dilatation is that it requires a high level of patient motivation over a prolonged period of time to achieve satisfactory results. In a teenager, such manipulation is difficult even with careful instruction and counseling. Due to these disadvantages, Ingram (21) described a new method of dilatation using a passive technique. With this latter approach, the patient is not required to actively press dilators against the vaginal pouch. Instead, the patient uses specially designed Lucite vaginal dilators (Fig. 20.2) and applies pressure to the vaginal pouch by sitting on a bicycle seat stool. In the initial report, Ingram reported achieving satisfactory results in ten of 12 cases of vaginal agenesis and 32 of 40 cases of various types of vaginal stenosis.

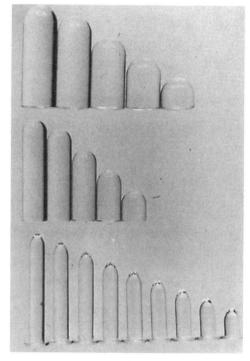

FIG. 20.2. Vaginal dilators used in the Ingram passive dilatation technique.

With the Ingram method, the patient is first instructed with the use of a mirror how to place a dilator against the introital dimple. Precautions should be given to try to avoid inadvertently dilating the urethral meatus. Usually the smallest, narrowest dilator is appropriate at the onset and may be held in place with a light girdle. The patient then is shown how to sit on a racing-type bicycle seat that is placed on a stool 24 inches above the floor. The appropriate bicycle seat apparatus is simple to assemble and is preferable to a stationary exercise bicycle, as the patient would not want to peddle a bicycle while dilating due to the risk of injury. The patient is instructed to sit leaning slightly forward with the dilator in place for at least 2 hours per day at intervals of 15 to 30 minutes. She is followed usually at monthly intervals and can be expected to graduate to the next size larger dilator about every month. An attempt at sexual intercourse may be suggested after the use of the largest dilator for 1 or 2 months. Continued dilatation is recommended if intercourse subsequently is infrequent. In our experience, the functional success rate of passive dilatation approaches 80% (22). Passive dilation may, therefore, be suggested as an initial therapy for vaginal creation if the patient appears appropriately motivated and a vaginal dimple or small pouch is present. Surgical therapy is indicated if dilatation therapy is either inappropriate or fails.

During the past 3 decades, experience has proved the Abbe-Wharton-McIndoe procedure (more popularly called the McIndoe opera-

tion) to be the superior procedure for neovaginal creation in patients with müllerian agenesis (Fig. 20.3) (23). Under special circumstances, the vulvovaginal pouch of Williams or the sigmoid pouch of Pratt may be indicated (24,25).

Three important principles outlined by McIndoe still are emphasized today in operations for vaginal agenesis: (a) dissection of an adequate space between the rectum and bladder, (b) use of an inlay split-thickness skin graft, and (c) the cardinal principle of continuous and prolonged dilatation during the con-

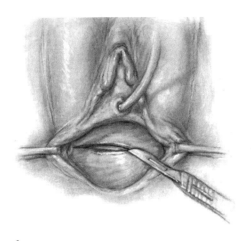

A

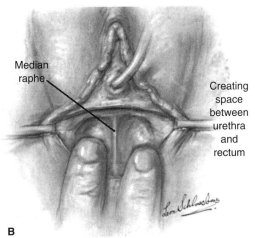

Median raphe

Creating space between urethra and rectum

B

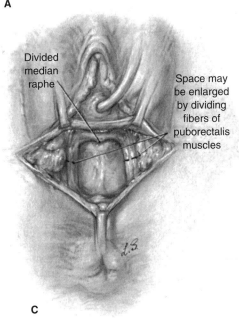

Divided median raphe

Space may be enlarged by dividing fibers of puborectalis muscles

C

FIG. 20.3. McIndoe procedure. **A:** A transverse incision is made in the apex of the vaginal dimple. **B:** A channel usually can be dissected on each side of the median raphe. **C:** A space between the urethra and bladder anteriorly and rectum posteriorly is dissected until peritoneum is reached. (From Rock JA. Surgery for anomalies of the Mullerian ducts. In: Rock JA, Thompson JD, eds. *TeLinde's operative gynecology,* 8th ed. Philadelphia: Lippincott–Raven Publishers, 1997:687–729, with permission.)

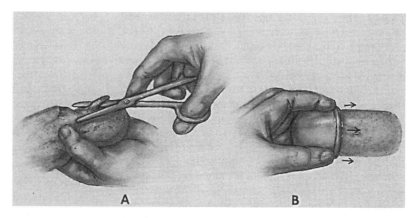

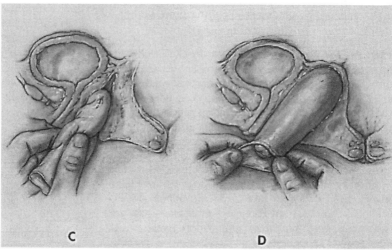

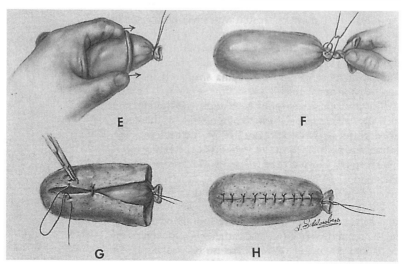

FIG. 20.4. Counsellor-Flor modification of the McIndoe procedure. **A:** A form is cut from a sterile foam rubber block. **B:** A condom is placed over the form. **C:** The form is compressed and placed in the neovagina. **D:** The foam expands and accommodates to the neovaginal space, after which time the condom is closed and the form removed. **E,F:** A second condom is placed over the form and tied securely. **G:** The graft is sewn over the form. **H:** The graft and vaginal form is ready for insertion into the neovagina. (From Rock JA. Surgery for anomalies of the Mullerian ducts. In: Rock JA, Thompson JD, eds. *TeLinde's operative gynecology*, 8th ed. Philadelphia: Lippincott–Raven Publishers, 1997: 687–729, with permission.)

tractile phase of healing. Although other tissues such as peritoneum and human amnion have been used to line the neovaginal space, these tissues generally have had less consistent results. We have favored harvesting the donor skin graft from one of the buttocks. The Padgett electrodermatome appears to be the most satisfactory instrument for taking the graft. The instrument is set to take a graft approximately 0.018 inch thick, 8 to 9 cm wide, and 16 to 20 cm in length. After surgical creation of the neovaginal space, we have used the Counsellor-Flor modification of the McIndoe procedure (Fig. 20.4) (26). This technique uses, instead of a rigid balsa wood form, a foam rubber mold tailored for the vaginal cavity and covered with a condom.

The split-thickness skin graft is carefully sutured over the form such that its undersurface is exteriorized. The form is replaced into the neovaginal cavity and the edges of the graft sutured to the skin edges. The patient is placed on strict bed rest for a period of 7 to 10 days, at which time the vaginal form is removed and the vaginal cavity inspected. The patient continues to wear the foam rubber form continuously for 6 weeks. After 6 weeks, a new form is molded out of neoprene, which is easier to remove and clean. The patient is instructed to use this form during the night for the next 12 months. If there has been no change in the caliber of the vagina by that time, then insertion of the form may continue intermittently until coitus is a frequent occurrence.

The results of the McIndoe operation have improved significantly since the balsa vaginal form was replaced by the foam rubber form. Satisfactory results are seen in 80% to 100% of patients. Of 94 patients operated on at the Johns Hopkins Hospital over a 39-year period, 83% had a 100% take of the graft; significant graft failure occurred in only three patients (2). Serious complications that may still occur include anesthesia morbidity, infection, hemorrhage, graft failure, and postoperative granulation tissue formation. Fistulas from the lower urinary tract or rectum into the neovagina have been reported to occur in approx-

imately 4% of patients (2). Malignancies have been reported to occur in the neovagina (27).

There has been some recent renewed interest in the Vecchietti operation for creation of a neovagina (28). With this technique, continuous progressive pressure is exerted by an acrylic olive applied to the vaginal dimple. Two threads are attached to the olive, passed through the neovaginal space and the abdominal wall, and connected to a traction device that gradually draws the olive upwards. One of the disadvantages of this technique is that it requires a laparotomy for retrieval and manipulation of the threads. Several groups, however, recently reported a modified technique using laparoscopy to retrieve the threads through the cul de sac of Douglas (29,30). Although these limited reports have been encouraging, it is not known at this time whether complication rates will be as low as is presently seen with the McIndoe operation.

CLINICAL MANIFESTATIONS OF CLASS II ANOMALIES: VERTICAL FUSION DEFECTS

The reported incidence of transverse vaginal septum varies from one in 2,100 to one in 72,000 (2). It is probably less common than congenital absence of the uterus and vagina. Its etiology is unknown, although McKusick et al. (31) suggested that it may result from a female-sex limited autosomal recessive inheritance pattern. It represents a developmental defect of incomplete fusion between the müllerian duct component and the urogenital sinus component of the vagina. This incomplete vertical fusion results in a transverse vaginal septum of variable thickness. Lodi (32) reported that 46% occur in the upper vagina, 40% in the midvagina, and 14% in the lower vagina. Rock and associates (33) noted septa in the upper, middle, and lower thirds of the vagina in 46%, 35%, and 19% of patients, respectively. In general, the thicker septa have been noted more commonly closer to the uterine cervix (Fig. 20.5). In contrast to congenital absence of the müllerian ducts, the trans-

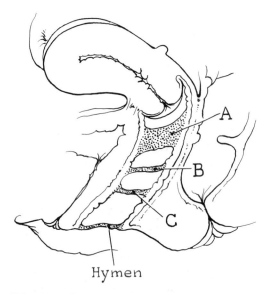

Hymen

FIG. 20.5. Positions of septa responsible for complete vaginal obstruction. **A:** High transverse vaginal septum (most commonly thicker than the septum of the middle or lower vagina). **B:** Transverse vaginal septum of the middle third of the vagina. **C:** Transverse vaginal septum of the lower third of the vagina. (From Rock JA, Zacur HA, Dlugi AM, et al. Pregnancy success following surgical correction of imperforate hymen and complete transverse vaginal septum. *Obstet Gynecol* 1982;59:448–451, with permission.)

verse vaginal septum has been associated with few urologic or other anomalies.

In neonates and young infants, an imperforate transverse vaginal septum with obstruction may lead to serious and life-threatening problems (34). Fluid may accumulate from endocervical glands and müllerian glandular epithelium in the upper vagina that have been stimulated by maternal estrogens. The distended upper vagina creates a large pelvic and lower abdominal mass that may displace the bladder anteriorly, displace the ureters laterally with hydroureter and hydronephrosis, and compress the rectum with associated obstipation and even intestinal obstruction. The mass also may limit diaphragmatic excursion, compress the vena cava, and produce cardiorespiratory failure. Fatalities have been reported. The hydrometrocolpos develops along the axis of the upper vagina and, therefore, may not

cause the vaginal outlet or perineum to bulge on abdominal compression. After appropriate preoperative radiologic and endoscopic investigation, the surgeon should remove the septum through a perineal approach. Because of a subsequent tendency for vaginal stenosis and reaccumulation of fluid in the upper vagina, follow-up studies to assess for recurrence of obstruction are indicated.

In some patients, symptoms may not develop until puberty. Patients with a developing hematocolpos present with cyclic lower abdominal pain without any visible menstrual discharge. Subsequently, a central lower abdominal and pelvic mass develops. Sometimes a small tract will open in the septum, allowing some menstrual blood to escape periodically. Cyclic hematuria may occur if a communication between the bladder and upper vagina exists.

The reported experience at the Johns Hopkins Hospital among 26 patients with complete transverse vaginal septum indicates that, although vaginal patency and coital function were successfully established in all patients, only seven of 19 patients attempting pregnancy eventually had children (33). This is in contrast with other conditions of genital tract obstruction, such as imperforate hymen, in which 86% of patients attempting pregnancy were noted to subsequently deliver (Table 20.3). The incidence of endometriosis and spontaneous abortion is high in patients with transverse vaginal septa. A lowered pregnancy potential and more extensive endometriosis often is present when the transverse septum is located high in the vagina, suggesting that retrograde flow through the uterus and fallopian tubes occurs earlier in these patients (Table 20.4).

Surgical therapy involves incising a transverse septum, but the specific therapy depends on the extent and location of the septum. Therapy for complete obstructing transverse vaginal septum in the lower and middle thirds of the vagina simply involves excising the septum, followed by an anastomosis of the upper and lower vaginal segments (Fig. 20.6). The high transverse septum often poses a more dif-

TABLE 20.3. *Pregnancy success after surgical correction of an intact hymen versus correction of a complete transverse vaginal septum*

	Hymen	Transverse septum	Total
Patients	22	26	48
Adequate follow-up	18	22	40
Patients attempting pregnancy	15	19	34
Patients pregnant[a]	13 (86%)	9 (47%)	22 (65%)
Patients with a living child	20 (66%)	7 (36%)	17 (50%)
Total pregnancies	20	18	38
Term	16	8	24
Premature	1	1	2
Abortion	3	9	12

[a]$p < 0.05$ ($\times^2$ analysis).

TABLE 20.4. *Pregnancy success after surgical correction of complete transverse vaginal septum*

	Lower third	Middle third	Upper third	Total
Patients	5	9	12	26
Adequate follow-up	5	8	9	22 (84%)
Patients attempting pregnancy	4	7	8	19 (73%)
Patients pregnant	4	3	2	9 (47%)
Patients with a living child	4	2	1	7 (36%)
Total pregnancies	6	4	8	18
Term	5	2	1	8
Premature	0	1	0	1
Abortion	1	1	7	9

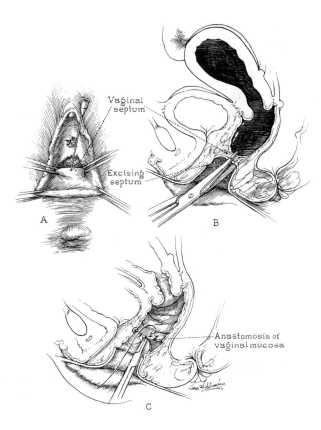

FIG. 20.6. Repair of a transverse vaginal septum of the middle third of the vagina. **A:** The wall of the septum is grasped with Allis clamps. A 14-gauge needle is placed into the vaginal septum, revealing the trapped blood and providing a plane for incision. **B:** The septum is incised with scissors. The septal remnants are excised. **C:** The upper and lower portions of the vagina are anastomosed. (From Rock JA. Anomalous development of the vagina. *Semin Reprod Endocrinol* 1986;4:13–31, with permission.)

ficult surgical problem in that anastomoses of the upper and lower segments may not be feasible. In such cases, a space is created between the rectum and bladder to permit identification of the obstructed upper vagina. Laparotomy may be required when it is not possible to delineate the rectum from the bladder or the mass. A sound may be passed transfundally through the uterus and cervix to tent the vaginal septum and aid in the placement of an appropriate incision and dissection plane (Fig. 20.7). In cases where the mass is readily elucidated by digital examination, an aspirating needle could be used to assure its proper location, over which the septum can be incised with a scalpel. Because the distance between the upper and lower segments frequently is too great to permit a primary anastomosis, an indwelling Lucite form consisting of a bulbous end and a central channel through which menstrual blood may efflux is placed in the vagina.

This form may be anchored in place with a retaining harness. The harness can be removed a few days later, after which time the bulbous end of the Lucite form usually will retain its position in the vagina. This form is left in place for approximately 6 months. An additional several month vaginal dilatation program often is used to prevent constrictive scarring and stenosis.

Congenital Absence or Dysgenesis of the Cervix

Congenital cervical abnormalities are rare, with less than 50 reported cases in the world literature. These rare abnormalities have several different presentations. Some patients have no identifiable cervix (cervical agenesis), whereas others demonstrate differing degrees of incomplete development of the cervix (cervical dysgenesis). When these anomalies

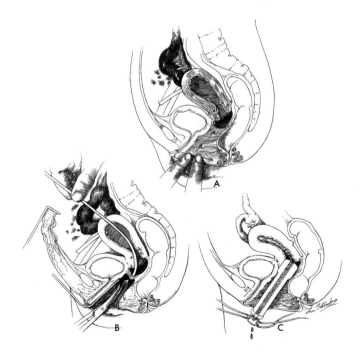

FIG. 20.7. Surgical management of a high transverse vaginal septum. **A:** A large portion of atretic vagina is palpated with two fingers. **B:** If unable to safely enter from below, a sound may be passed through the uterine fundus to tent the upper vagina. **C:** A hollow acrylic resin (Lucite) form may be placed in the neovagina, permitting menstrual egress and preventing stricture. (From Rock JA. Surgery for anomalies of the Mullerian ducts. In: Rock JA, Thompson JD, eds. *TeLinde's operative gynecology,* 8th ed. Philadelphia: Lippincott–Raven Publishers, 1997:687–729, with permission.)

occur, there often is associated absence of a portion or all of the vagina. In many cases, retention of menstrual blood initiates symptoms of cyclic lower abdominal pain without menstrual flow. Often, the diagnosis is difficult before surgery. However, with the help of newer diagnostic methods, such as MRI, the possibility of diagnosis before surgery may exist (35).

Complete cervical agenesis is characterized by narrowing of the lower uterine segment to a terminal point in a peritoneal sleeve at a point well above the normal communication with the vaginal apex. Cervical dysgenesis has had four described subtypes: (a) intact cervical body with obstruction of the cervical os (the cervix is well formed, but a portion of the endocervical lumen is obliterated); (b) a cervical body consisting of a fibrous band of variable length and diameter (endocervical glands may be noted on pathologic examination); (c) stricture of the midportion of the cervix (which is hypoplastic with a bulbous tip and no identifiable cervical lumen); and (d) fragmentation of the cervix (with portions that can be palpated below the fundus that are not connected to the lower uterine segment).

When both the vagina and cervix are absent and a functioning uterine corpus is present, it is quite difficult to obtain a satisfactory fistulous tract through which menstruation can occur. Many methods have been tried, most of them involving creation of a passage through the dense fibrous tissue between the uterine cavity and the vagina and placement of a stent to keep the tract open. Occasional successes in maintaining an open passageway and normal cyclic menstruation have been reported (36,37), but endocervical glands do not develop, and there is no way to compensate for the absence of the cervical mucus, which plays an important role in sperm transport (making pregnancy less likely). Often the uterovaginal fistulous tract closes from fibrous tissue constriction. Endometriosis either can develop along the tract or can occur in the pelvis as a result of retrograde seeding. Recurrent and severe pelvic infections have been seen in some of these cases, requiring hysterectomy and bilateral salpingo-oopho-

rectomy. For these reasons, many authors have recommended hysterectomy as an initial procedure for patients with congenital absence of the cervix and vagina (38,39). If the hysterectomy is performed soon enough, it may be possible to conserve the ovaries. Cannulization procedures may be worthwhile in a few carefully selected cases of cervical dysgenesis in which there is adequate stroma to allow for a cervicovaginal anastomosis or grafting technique.

CLINICAL MANIFESTATIONS OF CLASS III ANOMALIES: LATERAL FUSION DEFECTS

Defects of lateral fusion can be divided into two groups: (a) those with obstruction and (b) those without obstruction.

Unobstructed lateral fusion disorders include bicornuate, septate, or didelphic uterus (Fig. 20.8). Complete failure of midline fusion may result in complete duplication of the vagina, cervix, and uterus. Partial failure of midline fusion can result in a single vagina with a single or duplicate cervix and complete or partial

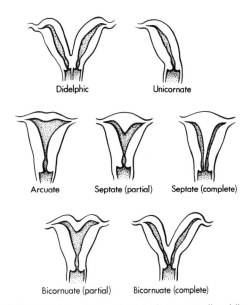

FIG. 20.8. Nonobstructive uterine anomalies (disorders of lateral fusion). (From Rock JA. Diagnosing and repairing uterine anomalies. *Contemp Obstet Gynecol* 1981;17:44, with permission.)

duplication of the uterine corpus. A failure of absorption of the uterine septum between the fused müllerian ducts results in a persistent internal uterine septum, whereas the external contour of the uterus appears normal. The uterine septum may be complete and divide both the uterine cavity and endocervical canal into two components. More often, incomplete disappearance of the septum leaves only the upper cavities of the uterus divided. Each of these and a variety of other forms of double uteri will have their own individual clinical features. In the absence of obstruction, surgical reconstruction is considered in certain cases primarily because of difficulties (or potential difficulties) with reproduction.

Although some uterine anomalies can cause infertility, most patients with uterine anomalies are able to conceive without difficulty. There is no question that uterine anomalies can be associated with a perfectly normal reproductive history. Overall, however, the incidences of spontaneous abortion, premature birth, fetal loss, fetal malpresentation, and cesarean section are clearly increased when a uterine anomaly is present. Unfortunately, it is impossible to predict which patients with uterine anomalies will experience these types of problems.

The true incidence of uterine anomalies in the general and in the infertile population is not accurately known. Reports in the literature are confounded by sampling from selected populations, incomplete data, inaccurate diagnostic methods, and variability in either interpretation or classification of anomalies. Nevertheless, a large study conducted in Spain suggests that müllerian anomalies are not rare in fertile women (40). These investigators evaluated 1,289 patients undergoing tubal sterilization procedures by laparoscopy or laparotomy combined with hysterosalpingography 5 months postoperatively to ensure that sterilization was complete. Müllerian anomalies were noted in 3.8% of patients in this group (including arcuate uterus). This rate was similar to infertile patients evaluated using similar methods (4.0%), although women with history of recurrent spontaneous pregnancy abortions (two or more) were noted to have a significantly higher incidence (6.3%). Other investigators reported that after a history of three or more episodes of spontaneous abortion, the incidence of uterine anomalies is approximately 10% (2). Among chronic second-trimester aborters, the incidence may be even higher. As the etiology of recurrent spontaneous abortion often is complex, most authorities advise a complete workup be carried out even when an anomalous uterus is found. Genetic, hormonal, infectious, and other structural causes (leiomyomas) should be excluded. Repairing other factors first may correct the problem associated with reproductive loss without uterine surgery (41).

The etiology of reproductive failure in patients with uterine anomalies remains unclear. It is hypothesized that the presence of a uterine septum can lead to abortion either due to diminished intrauterine space or the inadequacy of a poorly vascularized septum. Cervical incompetence and luteal phase insufficiency also seem to be more common in patients with uterine anomalies, each of which may contribute to pregnancy wastage.

If a uterine anomaly is associated with obstruction of menstrual flow, then it will cause symptoms that will come to the attention of a gynecologist shortly after menarche. Unobstructed uterine anomalies are diagnosed later in a variety of circumstances (Table 20.5). Young girls may notice difficulty in using tampons or later experience coital difficulty if a longitudinal vaginal septum is pres-

TABLE 20.5. *Observations leading to diagnosis of an anomalous uterus*

Difficulty using tampons
Difficulty with intercourse
Urinary tract anomaly noted on intravenous pyelogram
Dysmenorrhea
Menorrhagia
Abnormality noted at dilation and curettage
Palpable mass
Abnormal ultrasound
Abnormal uterine contour noted during pregnancy
Fetal malpresentation
Pregnancy despite presence of an intrauterine device *in situ*

ent. A patient with an anomalous upper urinary tract on intravenous pyelogram may be found to have a gynecologic anomaly. A uterine anomaly occasionally is found when a patient complains of dysmenorrhea or menorrhagia or when a dilatation and curettage is performed for abortion or some other reason. Semmens (42) pointed out that the diagnosis of a uterine anomaly can be made by the astute observation of an abnormal uterine contour during pregnancy, either in the antepartum period or at the time of abdominal or vaginal delivery. Sometimes the diagnosis is made as an incidental finding at the time of laparoscopy or laparotomy. However, most uterine anomalies presently are diagnosed after hys-

terosalpingography performed during either an infertility or recurrent miscarriage evaluation. Whereas hysterosalpingography is the established testing modality, there are several other promising new diagnostic methods (MRI, high-resolution and three-dimensional ultrasound, sonohysterography) that are continuing to evolve and may play a role in the evaluation of patients with uterine anomalies (43,44).

Hysterosalpingography is best done under fluoroscopy. It is important to remember that the distinction between a septate and bicornuate uterus cannot be established with a hysterosalpingogram (Fig. 20.9). The configuration of the external contour of the uterine

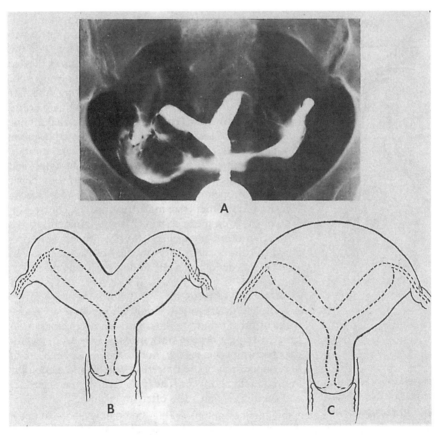

FIG. 20.9. A: Hysterosalpingogram of a double uterus. **B:** Bicornuate uterus. **C:** Septate uterus. Bicornuate and septate uteri cannot be differentiated without visualization of the uterine fundus. (From Rock JA. Surgery for anomalies of the Mullerian ducts. In: Rock JA, Thompson JD, eds. *TeLinde's operative gynecology,* 8th ed. Philadelphia: Lippincott–Raven Publishers, 1997:687–729, with permission.)

fundus can only be made definitively by direct visualization. All patients with müllerian anomalies also should have an intravenous pyelogram, due to the high incidence of associated urinary tract anomalies.

The obstetric outcome of patients with various types of double uteri in unselected series of women who have not been operated on is not known. For all types combined, the incidence of full-term pregnancies is probably about 25%. In patients selected for operation, the rate of full-term pregnancies probably increases from approximately 5% to 10% to approximately 80% to 90% (2). Patients with uncorrected bicornuate and didelphic uteri probably have better fetal survival than patients with uncorrected septate uteri, although this is somewhat controversial (45,46).

Traditionally, the treatment of the double uterus has been a metroplasty performed through the open abdomen using either the Jones, Tompkins, or Strassman technique (2). More recently, hysteroscopic procedures for correction of septate uteri have received much attention, with reported success rates comparable to those of abdominal metroplasty (47–50). However, although hysteroscopic techniques may be used to correct septate uteri, the only feasible approach to uterine unification for patients with bicornuate and didelphic uteri remains the abdominal approach (Strassman procedure).

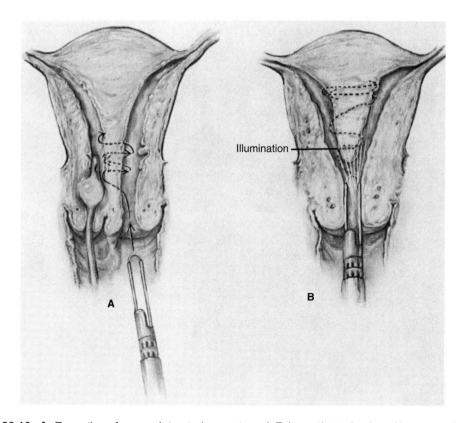

FIG. 20.10. A: Resection of a complete uterine septum. A Foley catheter is placed in one cavity and the resectoscope is placed in the other cavity. The septum is incised initially at a level above the internal os and then carried superiorly to the fundus. **B:** Resection of a partial uterine septum. The septum can be incised with the straight loupe of the resectoscope or by various other methodologies. (From Rock JA. Surgery for anomalies of the Mullerian ducts. In: Rock JA, Thompson JD, eds. *TeLinde's operative gynecology,* 8th ed. Philadelphia: Lippincott–Raven Publishers, 1997:687–729, with permission.)

Hysteroscopic procedures are performed transcervically using either a scissors, resectoscope, or laser (Fig. 20.10). Patients often are prepared with a regimen of danazol or a gonadotropin-releasing hormone agonist for 2 months preoperatively to reduce the amount of endometrium that can obscure the surgeon's view during the procedure. The hysteroscopic lysis of the uterine septum often is carried out in conjunction with laparoscopy to assess the external contour of the uterine fundus and limit the risks of uterine perforation. Careful monitoring of fluid administration is undertaken intraoperatively. As the uterine septum is incised, there often is little bleeding. The incision is continued until both tubal ostia are visualized and there is no appreciable septum remaining. After transcervical lysis of a uterine septum, a 2-month delay before attempting pregnancy is suggested to allow complete resorption of the septum and endometrial regeneration. A hysterosalpingogram often is used to document the postoperative condition of the uterine cavity.

Transcervical lysis can be performed to repair a complete septate uterus (i.e., a single fundus with two cavities and two cervices) (51). In this instance, we insert a no. 8 Foley catheter into one cervix and insert the resectoscope into the other cavity (Fig. 20.10B). The septum is electrosurgically incised at a point above the internal cervical os until the Foley catheter is visualized. The remainder of the septum is incised in a superior direction until complete resection of the fundal portion is complete. The objective of this technique is to remove the portion of the uterine septum within the corpus of the uterus while preserving the portion within the cervix to deter the development of postoperative cervical incompetence.

Advantages of the hysteroscopic approach include lessened morbidity and shorter operative time. Patients can deliver vaginally, whereas patients undergoing abdominal metroplasty are advised to undergo cesarean section. Some patients, however, may exhibit a particularly large or broad uterine septum that cannot be easily incised with a hysteroscopic approach. Such patients may still require an abdominal metroplasty approach, such as the Jones or Tompkins procedure.

Exposure of the female fetus to DES *in utero* can lead to anomalous development of the uterus (52). The T-shaped uterus is the most common anomaly associated with DES. This anomaly is associated with an increased rate of spontaneous abortions, premature deliveries, and ectopic pregnancies.

Nagel and Malo (53) examined the feasibility of correcting the uterine malformation seen in DES-exposed women through operative hysteroscopy. Their goal was to achieve a smooth, straight line from the lower uterine cavity to the tubal ostia by incising lateral constriction rings and septa. Their results in eight patients suggest that hysteroscopic metroplasty may decrease pregnancy loss but does not appear to enhance fertility. The efficacy of such corrective procedures presently is difficult to judge in the absence of larger clinical trials.

A unicornuate uterus can be present alone or with a rudimentary horn or bulb on the opposite side (uterine anlagen). The uterine anlagen may contain a cavity with active endometrium. O'Leary and O'Leary (54) reported that 90% of rudimentary horns are noncommunicating. Surgical intervention is not indicated unless the patient is symptomatic from the anlagen, at which time a hemihysterectomy is indicated.

Some authors suggested that the unicornuate uterus has the poorest fetal survival of all uterine anomalies, whereas other authors did not report a worsened reproductive performance in comparison to other anomalies (45,55). Unfortunately, very little can be done to improve the reproductive performance of patients with a unicornuate uterus. The physician should observe closely for cervical incompetence and perform cerclage as indicated. Although some authors reported that removal of the contralateral rudimentary horn improves the chances for pregnancy, this experience is too small to make a definitive recommendation (56). Cases of asymmetric development of the unicornuate uterus with an opposing rudimentary uterine horn are not amenable to unification.

There is danger of pregnancy in the rudimentary horn of a unicornuate uterus through transperitoneal migration of sperm or ova from the opposite side. Signs and symptoms of an ectopic pregnancy will develop with eventual rupture of the horn if the pregnancy is not detected early. Rupture through the wall of the vascular rudimentary horn has been associated with sudden and severe intraperitoneal hemorrhage, shock, and death in some instances.

Patients with a longitudinal vaginal septum may experience dyspareunia or difficulty in using tampons. It is generally advisable to excise a longitudinal vaginal septum for these reasons.

Lateral Fusion Defects with Asymmetric Obstruction

Patients with asymmetric obstruction of the uterus (i.e., a unicornuate uterus with a noncommunicating rudimentary horn with functioning endometrium) may present with dysmenorrhea or cyclic abdominal pain from cryptomenorrhea. The presence of normal menstrual flow increases the diagnostic challenge of patients with this rare condition. Endometriosis from retrograde menstruation also may be present. Removal of the obstructed horn is the procedure of choice and should alleviate the symptoms. Removal of an obstructed uterine horn through laparoscopic techniques was described recently (57).

Another rarely seen entity is the double uterus with an obstructed hemivagina and ipsilateral renal agenesis (3). These patients can be divided into three diagnostic groups: (a) complete unilateral vaginal obstruction without uterine communication, (b) incomplete unilateral vaginal obstruction without uterine communication, and (c) complete vaginal obstruction with lateral uterine communication (Fig. 20.11). This diagnosis can be difficult. MRI is an extremely useful tool to make the appropriate diagnosis (Fig. 20.12). The kidney on the side of vaginal obstruction usually is absent. Treatment consists of surgical excision of the vaginal septum. Abdominal exploration is unnecessary, and uterine reconstruction is not indicated. Reproductive performance is ultimately related to the type of double uterus present, unless a delay in diagnosis resulted in significant pelvic endometriosis.

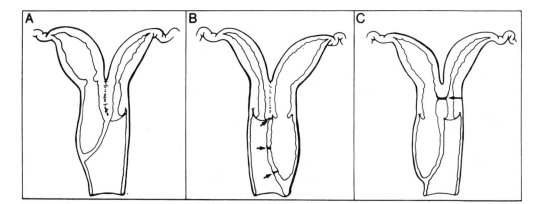

FIG. 20.11. Double uterus, complete or incomplete vaginal obstruction, and ipsilateral renal agenesis. **A:** Complete vaginal obstruction. **B:** Incomplete vaginal obstruction. **C:** Complete vaginal obstruction with a lateral communicating double uterus. (From Rock JA, Jones HW. The double uterus associated with an obstructed hemivagina and ipsilateral renal agenesis. *Am J Obstet Gynecol* 1980; 138:339–342, with permission.)

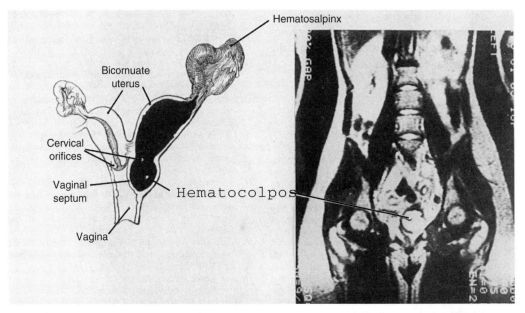

FIG. 20.12. Magnetic resonance imaging demonstrates absence of a kidney on the side of the vaginal obstruction. A double uterus is noted. (From Rock JA. Surgery for anomalies of the Mullerian ducts. In: Rock JA, Thompson JD, eds. *TeLinde's operative gynecology,* 8th ed. Philadelphia: Lippincott–Raven Publishers, 1997:687–729, with permission.)

CLINICAL MANIFESTATIONS OF CLASS IV ANOMALIES: UNUSUAL DEFECTS OF LATERAL AND VERTICAL FUSION

Unusual combinations of lateral and vertical müllerian fusion defects are rare and may require an individualized therapeutic approach. Müllerian duct anomalies have been reported in association with a variety of other problems. For instance, in a series of 70 patients with bladder exstrophy, Stanton (58) reported that 30 (43%) had reproductive tract abnormalities, including congenital absence of the uterus and vagina, and unicornuate, bicornuate, and didelphic uteri. Müllerian duct anomalies also are seen with the McKusick-Kaufman syndrome, an autosomal recessive disorder. Other clinical findings of this syndrome include postaxial polydactyly, syndactyly, congenital heart disease, intravaginal displacement of the urethral meatus, and anorectal anomalies (59).

SUMMARY

Uterovaginal anomalies occur in various forms, although each anomaly is distinct and some generalizations can be made. Classification of uterovaginal anomalies based on certain anatomic findings may be useful in organizing the type of malformation, although there usually are exceptions to each rule. A sound embryologic foundation is necessary to fully comprehend, evaluate, and treat patients with uterovaginal anomalies. An embryologic perspective will remind the physician of other anatomic defects frequently associated with uterovaginal anomalies (i.e., renal anomalies associated with the Mayer-Rokitansky-Küster-Hauser syndrome). The patient with a uterovaginal anomaly often relies on her physician to clarify the reproductive consequences associated with her diagnosis. The physician will allay anxiety by prompt evaluation and accurate description of the reproductive implications or the obstetric consequences of a particular uterovaginal anomaly. However, it must be remembered that, in some cases, the anomaly may not be finally established until the time of surgical correction.

REFERENCES

1. Langman J. The urogenital system. In: *Medical embryology*, 4th ed. Baltimore: Williams & Wilkins, 1981: 234–267.
2. Rock JA. Surgery for anomalies of the Mullerian ducts. In: Rock JA, Thompson, JD, eds. *TeLinde's operative gynecology*, 8th ed. Philadelphia: Lippincott–Raven Publishers, 1997:687–729.
3. Rock JA, Jones HW. The double uterus associated with an obstructed hemivagina and ipsilateral renal agenesis. *Am J Obstet Gynecol* 1980;138:339–342.
4. Thompson DP, Lynn HB. Genital anomalies associated with solitary kidney. *Mayo Clin Proc* 1966;41:538–548.
5. American Fertility Society. The American Fertility Society classifications of adnexal adhesions, distal tubal occlusion, tubal occlusion secondary to tubal ligation, tubal pregnancies, Mullerian anomalies and intrauterine adhesions. *Fertil Steril* 1988;49:944–955.
6. Singh M, Gearhart JP, Rock JA. Double urethra, double bladder, left renal agenesis, persistent hymen, double vagina and uterus didelphys. *Adolesc Pediatr Gynecol* 1993;6:99–101.
7. Goldberg JM, Falcone T. Double cervix and vagina with a normal uterus: an unusual Mullerian anomaly. *Hum Reprod* 1996;11:1350–1351.
8. Counsellor VS. Congenital absence of the vagina. *JAMA* 1948;136:861–866.
9. Evans TN, Poland ML, Boving RL. Vaginal malformations. *Am J Obstet Gynecol* 1981;141:910–920.
10. Fore SR, Hammond CB, Parker RT, et al. Urologic and genital anomalies in patients with congenital absence of the vagina. *Obstet Gynecol* 1975;46:410–416.
11. Griffin JE, Edwards C, Madden JD, et al. Congenital absence of the vagina. *Ann Intern Med* 1976;85:244–236.
12. Murphy AA, Krall A, Rock JA. Bilateral functioning uterine anlagen with the Rokitansky-Mayer-Kuster-Hauser syndrome. *Int J Fertil* 1987;32:316–319.
13. Singh KJ, Devi L. Hysteroplasty and vaginoplasty for reconstruction of the uterus. *Int J Gynecol Obstet* 1980; 17:457–459.
14. Kucheria K, Taneja N, Kinra G. Autosomal translocation of chromosomes 12q and 14q in mullerian duct failure. *Indian J Med Res* 1988;87:290–292.
15. Shokier MHK. Aplasia of the mullerian system: evidence for probably sex-limited autosomal dominant inheritance. *Birth Defects* 1978;14:37–54.
16. Carson SA, Simpson JL, Malinak LR, et al. Heritable aspects of uterine anomalies. II. Genetic analysis of mullerian aplasia. *Fertil Steril* 1983;40:86–90.
17. Petrozza JC, Gray MR, Davis AJ, et al. Congenital absence of the uterus and vagina is not commonly transmitted as a dominant genetic trait: outcomes of surrogate pregnancies. *Fertil Steril* 1997;67:387–389.
18. Lindenman E, Shepard MK, Pescovitz OH. Mullerian agenesis: an update. *Obstet Gynecol* 1997;90:307–312.
19. David A, Carmil D, Bar-David E, et al. Congenital absence of the vagina: clinical and psychological aspects. *Obstet Gynecol* 1975;47:407–409.
20. Frank RT. The formation of an artificial vagina without operation. *Am J Obstet Gynecol* 1938;35:1053–1055.
21. Ingram JM. The bicycle seat stool in the treatment of vaginal agenesis and stenosis: a preliminary report. *Am J Obstet Gynecol* 1981;140:867–873.
22. Rock JA. Congenital outflow tract obstruction. In: Adashi EY, Rock JA, Rosenwaks Z, eds. *Reproductive endocrinology, surgery, and technology*. Philadelphia: Lippincott-Raven Publishers, 1996:1446–1474.
23. McIndoe AH, Banister JB. Operation for cure of congenital absence of vagina. *J Obstet Gynaecol Br Emp* 1938;45:490–494.
24. Williams EA. Congenital absence of the vagina, a simple operation for its relief. *J Obstet Gynaecol Br Commonwealth* 1964;71:511–512.
25. Pratt JH. Vaginal atresia corrected by use of small and large bowel. *Clin Obstet Gynecol* 1972;15:639–649.
26. Counsellor VS, Flor FS. Congenital absence of the vagina: further results of treatment and a new technique. *Surg Clin North Am* 1957;37:1107–1118.
27. Rotmensch J, Rosenshein N, Dillon M, et al. Carcinoma arising in the neovagina: case report and review of the literature. *Obstet Gynecol* 1983;61:534–536.
28. Vecchietti G. Neovagina nella sindrome di Rokitansky-Kuster-Hauser. *Attual Ostet Ginecol* 1965;11:131–147.
29. Fedele L, Bianchi S, Tozzi L, et al. A new laparoscopic procedure for creation of a neovagina in Mayer-Rokitansky-Kuster-Hauser syndrome. *Fertil Steril* 1996;66: 854–857.
30. Veronikis DK, McClure GB, Nichols DH. The Vecchieti operation for constructing a neovagina: indications, instrumentation, and techniques. *Obstet Gynecol* 1997; 90:301–304.
31. McKusick VA, Weilbaccher RG, Gragg GW. Recessive inheritance of a congenital malformation syndrome. *JAMA* 1968;204:111–116.
32. Lodi A. Contributo clinico statistico sulle malformazione della vagina osservate nell clinica Obstetrica e Ginecologica di Milano dal 1906 al 1950. *Ann Obstet Ginecol Med Perinatol* 1951;73:1246–1251.
33. Rock JA, Zacur HA, Dlugi AM, et al. Pregnancy success following surgical correction of imperforate hymen and complete transverse vaginal septum. *Obstet Gynecol* 1982;59:448–451.
34. Mandell J, Stevens PS, Lucey DT. Diagnosis and management of hydrometrocolpos in infancy. *J Urol* 1978; 12:262–265.
35. Markham SM, Parmley TH, Murphy AA, et al. Cervical agenesis combined with vaginal agenesis diagnosed by magnetic resonance imaging. *Fertil Steril* 1987;48: 143–145.
36. Zarou GS, Esposito JM, Zarou DM. Pregnancy following the surgical correction of congenital atresia of the cervix. *Int J Gynecol Obstet* 1973;11:143–146.
37. Farber M, Marchant DM. Reconstructive surgery for congenital atresia of the uterine cervix. *Fertil Steril* 1976;27:1277–1282.
38. Dillon WP, Mudaliar NA, Wingate NB. Congenital atresia of the cervix. *Obstet Gynecol* 1979;54:126–129.
39. Rock JA, Schlaff WD, Zacur HA, et al. The clinical management of congenital absence of the uterine cervix. *Int J Gynecol Obstet* 1984;22:231–235.

40. Raga F, Bauset C, Remohi J, et al. Reproductive impact of congenital Mullerian anomalies. *Hum Reprod* 1997; 12:2277–2281.

41. Rock JA, Jones HW. The clinical management of the double uterus. *Fertil Steril* 1977;28:798–806.

42. Semmens JP. Abdominal contour in the third trimester: an aid to diagnosis of uterine anomalies. *Obstet Gynecol* 1965;25:779–786.

43. Letterie GS, Haggerty M, Lindee G. A comparison of pelvic ultrasound and magnetic resonance imaging as diagnostic studies for mullerian tract abnormalies. *Int J Fertil* 1995;40:34–38.

44. Raga F, Bonilla-Musoles F, Blanes J, et al. Congenital Mullerian anomalies: diagnostic accuracy of three-dimensional ultrasound. *Fertil Steril* 1996;65:523–528.

45. Heinonen PK, Saarikoski S, Pystynen P. Reproductive performance of women with uterine anomalies. *Acta Obstet Gynecol Scand* 1982;61:157–162.

46 Rock JA, Schlaff WD. The obstetric consequences of uterovaginal anomalies. *Fertil Steril* 1985;43:681–692.

47. Daly DC, Walters CA, Soto-Albers CE, et al. Hysteroscopic metroplasty: surgical technique and obstetric outcome. *Fertil Steril* 1983;39:623–628.

48. DeCherney AH, Russell JB, Graebe RA, et al. Resectoscopic management of Mullerian fusion defects. *Fertil Steril* 1986;39:623–628.

49. Valle RF, Sciarra JJ. Hysteroscopic treatment of the septate uterus. *Obstet Gynecol* 1986;67:253–257.

50. Donnez J, Nisolle M. Endoscopic laser treatment of uterine malformations. *Hum Reprod* 1997;12:1381–1387.

51. Rock JA, Murphy AA, Cooper WH. Resectoscopic techniques for the lysis of a class V: complete uterine septum. *Fertil Steril* 1987;48:496–496.

52. Haney AF, Hammond CB, Soules MR, et al. Diethystilbestrol-induced upper genital tract abnormalities. *Fertil Steril* 1979;31:142–146.

53. Nagel TC, Malo JW. Hysteroscopic metroplasty in the diethylstilbestrol-exposed uterus and similar nonfusion anomalies: effects on subsequent reproductive performance, a preliminary report. *Fertil Steril* 1993;59: 502–506.

54. O'Leary JL, O'Leary JA. Rudimentary horn pregnancy. *Obstet Gynecol* 1963;22:371–375.

55. Moutos DM, Damewood MD, Schlaff WD, et al. A comparison of the reproductive outcome between women with a unicornuate uterus and women with a didelphic uterus. *Fertil Steril* 1992;58:88–93.

56. Andrews MC, Jones HW. Impaired reproductive performance of the unicornuate uterus: intrauterine growth retardation, infertility, and recurrent abortion in five cases. *Am J Obstet Gynecol* 1982;144:173–176.

57. Kadir RA, Hart J, Nagele F, et al. Laparoscopic excision of a noncommunicating uterine horn. *Br J Obstet Gynaecol* 1996;103:371–372.

58. Stanton SL. Gynecologic complications of epispadias and bladder exstrophy. *Am J Obstet Gynecol* 1974;119: 749–754.

59. Jabs EW, Leonard CO, Phillips JA. New features of the McKusick-Kaufman syndrome. *Birth Defects* 1982;18: 161–166.

21

Adolescent Sexuality

Melinda B. Stein, Peter J. Fagan, and Sue Ellen Koehler Carpenter

Adolescent sexual development is the basis for further adult sexuality (1,2). How the adolescent sexually changes, adapts, and matures will provide him or her with the foundation of future intimate relationships (1,3). Adolescent sexuality evolves through the interface of biologic, familial, social, academic and cognitive issues (4). In this chapter, we discuss the various emotional and behavioral changes, phases, and risks that occur during adolescent sexual development.

ADOLESCENT DEVELOPMENT: IDENTITY AND INTIMACY

Erikson (1) theorized that the adolescent is faced with the development of identity in which a stable sense of self is achieved. This is followed by the young adult task of developing intimacy, which allows for openness, sharing, mutual trust, self-abandon, and commitment to another. This stepwise developmental progression was challenged by Gilligan (5), who suggests that identity development in adolescent girls involves relationship components. In any case, it is likely that the developing identity in both genders involves some attempts to develop intimate relationships.

As a result of physical, cognitive, and social changes (6), adolescents experiment with sexual relationships and explore sexual roles in their dating and social interaction. Their affectionate and sexual involvement in relationships helps to consolidate sexual identity (7). It is in the managing of the conflict between sexual drives and the emotional, interpersonal,

and biologic results of sexual behavior that the adolescent struggles to achieve adult sexual maturity (8).

SEXUAL DEVELOPMENTAL TASKS

Sexual identity is established on the foundation of gender identity. Gender identity is the sense of maleness or femaleness that the individual predicates to his or her self, e.g., "I am a man" or "I am a woman." It is a profound psychological development typically achieved in the first 2 years of life, detectable in an infant before the end of the first year. In adolescence, gender identity becomes firmly established as sexuality is experienced and integrated into the adolescent's identity.

Sexual identity/role is awareness of self as a sexual person who can be sexually in relationship to persons of the same gender, opposite gender, or both. In one sense, it is the eroticization of gender identity, i.e., the erotic expression of self as a young man or young woman.

Biologic and psychosocial factors are involved in the initiation of sexual activity for both male and female adolescents. However, for males, interpersonal sexual activity appears to be facilitated primarily by the release of free testosterone (9), whereas for females it is the influence of peer groups that is related to sexual activity with others (10). On the other hand, in a 1996 survey of junior high students, females felt more peer support for delaying sexual activity than boys and more often believed that sexual urges could be controlled (11).

The age-specific sexual behavior of early adolescence is masturbation; of older adolescence it is sexual experimentation (including intercourse) with another (2). In masturbation, the adolescent learns to integrate sexual pleasure with the fantasy of relatedness with another. Both somatic autoeroticism (self-pleasuring) and cognitive alloeroticism (erotic relatedness to other) processes are developing in tandem. The central or core masturbatory fantasy of the adolescent often is indicative of the main themes, e.g., object and conflicts, of the individual's sexual relatedness (12). The masturbatory fantasy may not be expressed autoerotically in some adolescents, but the cognitive aspects nevertheless can develop, e.g., in hero worship of sport or performing arts figures.

The autoeroticism of masturbation develops into the sex play with another in the developing adolescents as the central fantasy seeks alloerotic expression. The adolescent "practices" his or her sexual identity in sexual roles that are significantly determined by social and peer group factors (13). The 1988 National Survey of Family Growth reported that 27% of 15-year-old girls had experienced sexual intercourse. The 1997 CDC Youth Risk Behavior Survey found that 48% of high school students had experienced intercourse and that 14% of them had four or more lifetime partners (14).

COGNITION AND MORAL DEVELOPMENT

Sexuality and its meaning to the adolescent seems contingent on the interaction between adolescents and the world around them (15). Turmoil or conflicts are necessary for working through adolescent tasks, including the task of figuring out what should or should not be done sexually. The cognitive development of formal operations (abstract thinking) characteristic of most 11- to 12-year-olds (16) indicates that when the adolescent begins to move from concrete to more abstract thought processes, he or she is able to engage in responsible sexual decision making. Concrete

thinking does not allow for complete understanding of the risks involved in sexual behavior (16). Concrete thought processes are marked by unidimensional and unilateral problem solving. A "relationship" is an abstract concept that requires logical, systematic, and deductive decision making to deal with myriad possibilities and consequences. Although abstract reasoning ability does not ensure appropriate problem solving, it will afford an individual the capacity for responsible sexual judgments.

Transition from elementary to middle school is a difficult time for most youngsters. Lower academic performance, as well as lower educational aspirations, correlates with premature adolescent sexual involvement (17). Many youngsters may not reach formal operations or abstract thinking until later adolescence, making these transitions more difficult.

Sexual intimacy includes a blending of sensuality, abstract thinking, emotional closeness, mutual caring, commitment, and trust. Adolescents who have sex before achieving intimacy in their relationships are at risk for undesirable consequences of their sexual actions. Moreover, an adolescent's level of intimacy and cognitive development may influence his or her determination of appropriate sexual initiation, sexually transmitted disease (STD) protection, and contraceptive practices (18,19).

More intelligent adolescents are less reliant on external moral values for directing sexual decision making (15). Further, more religious adolescents are more oriented toward societal sexual norms. An internal focus of control or self-identity also influences better practical judgment for males in sexual relationships (15).

Sexual behavior is highly influenced by social forces, as indicated by the variety of sexual mores reported in different cultures as well as the differences between generations in the same culture. Although sexuality is at base a biologically motivated behavior, the meaning attributed to sexual expression is largely a social construction. Ethical debates about sexual behavior usually concern whether the meaning of sexual behavior is totally constructed by the situation and the participants, e.g., mutual consenting partners, or whether there is a predetermined meaning in sexual behavior, e.g., for procreation and love in marriage.

FAMILY INFLUENCES

Although adolescence marks the transition from dependence on the family to establishing an independent identity, the sexual behavior of adolescents is affected by parents' attitudes in the home environment (17,19–21). Adolescents who have a close relationship with their mothers are more likely to share their mother's sexual attitudes and behavior (22). Parents who have permissive attitudes toward sexual behavior tend to have adolescents who are both more likely to be sexually active and more likely to use contraception (23,24). The effect of societal messages (such as exposure to sexual messages in music videos) also may be greater for girls from permissive environments (25). Among single-parent households, adolescents whose mothers remarry are more likely to be sexually active than adolescents whose mothers divorce and do not remarry (26).

Increased parental supervision is correlated to decreased sexual risk taking. This includes direct supervision, supervision of children when they are at home with their peers, and indirect supervision (monitoring their activities when away from home) (27). Parenting styles have an impact on an adolescent's preparedness for confronting sexual issues. Authoritarian parents who place a high value on obedience and conformity, discourage independence, and practice punitive and forceful discipline tend to produce dependent, passive children who are less socially adept and less self-assured. Indulgent parents who practice passive discipline and allow a high degree of freedom tend to produce less mature, more irresponsible teens who are likely to conform to their peers. Indifferent parents, who offer little supervision and structure their children's lives around the adults'

needs, engender impulsive adolescents who experiment earlier with substances and sexuality. Authoritative parents, who are warm but firm, set developmentally appropriate limits, and allow independent thought are most likely to produce psychosocially competent adolescents. Health care providers can help parents to modify their parenting style, provide supervision, and understand the implications of their own behavior.

It has been shown that parents need information about sexual development to be able to inform their children and reinforce information they learn in school (28). Teens want to receive sexual information from their parents, and teens who have conversations about sexual initiation with their parents cite parents rather than peers as their best source of advice (29).

SOCIETAL INFLUENCES

An adolescent's social environment plays a significant role in determining sexual attitudes and behavior. The sexual content of television has increased and become more explicit. Adolescents who rely heavily on television for information about sexuality will have unrealistic standards of female beauty and will be more likely to believe that premarital and extramarital intercourse with multiple partners in acceptable (30). The assertion of conservative religious values can help delay sexual initiation (31). This is particularly true if the adolescent's friends attend the same church (32). Commitment to, and involvement in, conventional social activities decreases risk behaviors (33). Using the presence of others is an effective means for girls to avoid engaging in sexual activities (27). Ingestion of alcohol and drugs is consistently correlated with increased sexual risk (32,34,35).

SEXUAL ACTIVITY

Societal messages to girls generally focus on coital behaviors to the exclusion of noncoital behaviors, the "control of sexuality" rather than its healthy expression. Sexuality is unfortunately associated with primarily negative outcomes. Teens need reinforcement for developmentally appropriate relationships and behaviors.

Although less thoroughly evaluated than rates of sexual intercourse, adolescents report a range of noncoital sexual behaviors. Twenty-five to forty percent of adolescent girls are reported to engage in self-masturbation, the majority before age 13 years. A survey of adolescents ages 12 to 15 years in a large southern city self-reported the following incidence of behaviors over the past year: necked 70%, felt breast through clothes 60%, felt breasts directly 45%, felt sex organs directly 42%, felt penis directly 30%, intercourse 25%, none 26% (36).

Healthy female adolescent sexual development will allow girls to develop positive attitudes about their bodies and their sexual feelings. Their goal should be to involve themselves in relationships that are safe and mutually satisfying where partners take responsibility for their own behavior and consider each person's feeling, needs, and desires.

SEXUAL ABUSE

Adolescents with histories of sexual abuse may have more difficulty with identity formation and establishing and maintaining healthy relationships with others (1,2). The abused adolescent may engage in premature sexual behavior in an attempt to achieve pseudointimacy. The latter may temporarily recapitulate or derive for the adolescent feelings of nurturance and gratification of unmet dependency needs, which he or she wishes from the family (2). For example, a male or female adolescent may become sexually involved with an older or female individual to attain an adequate parent figure. Depressive, personality, and conduct disorders frequently are associated with disturbed identity and sexual development (2,4).

Sexually abused children and adolescents frequently are overstimulated and seek immediate release of sexual tension. These youngsters are vulnerable to promiscuity, are highly suggestible, and act without sufficient thought or deliberations. Hence, they are at high risk for pregnancy and STD.

CONTRACEPTION

The United States exceeds the level of teen pregnancies over most other industrialized nations (37). The latter is in part due to poor contraceptive practices among American teenagers. Younger adolescents are poor users of contraception (4,37). It appears that knowledge alone does not determine effective contraceptive use (4). Positive sexual self-concept is associated with frequent contraceptive use during intercourse (38). Further, sexual self-concept seems to improve with age. Parental support increases contraceptive use (39). Contraceptive use was negatively associated with lower socioeconomic status, low educational achievement, low self-esteem, and poor family relationships (40,41).

PREGNANCY

Pregnancy can compromise an adolescent's ability to lead a productive and healthy life (18). A pregnant female adolescent is characteristically under 16 years old and from a divorced, single-parent home where the mother conceived out of wedlock (42). Adolescent birth lowers a female's likelihood of economic success and increases the likelihood of having a large family (43). Pregnant females are at risk of jeopardizing their academic success by dropping out of school (43).

Zabin et al. (44) studied 360 adolescents seeking pregnancy tests. A 2-year follow-up revealed that the adolescents who aborted their pregnancies were more likely to graduate high school and generally were more secure economically. Additionally, the adolescents who obtained abortions had a lower occurrence of another pregnancy within the 2-year follow-up period. The abortion group also showed a more positive psychological profile, including lower anxiety, higher self-esteem, and internal control. The postponement of childbearing appears to improve the social, psychological, academic, and economic outcome of an adolescent's life.

In-depth interviews with young pregnant teens indicate that the girls' sexual decision making centered on several key factors: their attempt to establish a relationship based in trust, a belief in their lack of vulnerability to become pregnant, family structure, and their beliefs about alternatives available once a pregnancy was confirmed (45).

PROBLEMS IN GENDER AND SEXUAL IDENTITY/ROLE

Problems of gender identity in a female adolescent present as rejection of menarche and secondary sexual characteristics. She may resent the loss of buddy relationships with young male adolescents. Gender dysphoric female adolescents typically are homosexual in sexual orientation. Among male adolescents, cross-dressing is one of the manifestations of a potential gender dysphoria in later years. During preadolescence, both genders tend to engage in cross-gender behavior, e.g., tomboy play for girls, effeminacy for boys (46,47). Female family members, e.g., older sisters, mother, grandmother, frequently played an etiologic role in the cross-dressing behaviors of male adolescents by having dressed them as girls (even if only "in play") when younger.

Problems of sexual identity/role in adolescents tend to group around the extremes of near total repression of sexuality or health/life-threatening promiscuity (48). Repression of sexuality may be present under the guise of religious, political, academic, or other ideologic rationale in the mind of the adolescent. It is marked by severe emotional discomfort with sexual pleasure and the avoidance of situations in which sexual role behavior might be appropriate, e.g., school dances and parties. In some cases, it is part of a psychiatric disorder such as anorexia nervosa or major affective illness. When the sexual dysphoria is part of a psychiatric disorder, referral should be made to a mental health professional who has expertise in treating adolescents with the psychiatric disorder in question.

Care must be taken to ensure that the label "sexual promiscuity" is not simply the imposition of an older generation's mores on the younger or applied differentially to each gender, e.g., girls are "promiscuous," whereas boys are "sowing their oats." If, however, the frequency and variety of sexual partners risks physical or psychological health, then the sexual behavior in question usually is an indication of poor integration of sexual identity/role in the adolescent. The adolescent is using promiscuous sexual behavior for purposes for which sexual behavior by itself is ill suited, e.g., security in gender and sexual identity/role, acceptance by others, and status in the peer group. It does little good to criticize the promiscuous sexual behavior of the adolescent without first addressing the psychosexual and psychosocial conflicts that the behavior is attempting to mollify.

PRECOCIOUS AND DELAYED PUBERTY

John Money's longitudinal research and case studies of children with hormonal disorders provided important data on the effects of precocious or delayed puberty on the sexual behavior of the adolescent. He concludes (49), "Pubertally precocious children do not become erotosexually wild and delinquent (50,51), and pubertally delayed teenagers are not inevitably erotosexually inert, though they tend to be neglected by their pubertally developed agemates, except in nonromantic comradeships (52–54)." This conclusion was supported in a study of female adolescents who experienced idiopathic precocious puberty (55). The subjects experienced sexual milestones (first holding hands to first intercourse) about 1 year before their controls. First masturbation occurred approximately 5 years earlier (9.2 years). Later adolescent sexual behavior was not different between the idiopathic precocious puberty adolescents and their controls.

Although a review of the question of general psychological reaction to delayed or precocious puberty is beyond the scope of this chapter, a recent study found that, among a sample of more normally developing adolescents, self-esteem did not vary significantly with pubertal development (measured with Tanner stage-like self-reports) in either males or females (56). There was a modest correlation between self-esteem and the timing of pubertal events in males but not in females. Thus, adolescent boys experienced increased self-esteem with an early (but not precocious) puberty. For adolescent girls, pubertal development was but one of many unspecified factors affecting self-esteem.

Pubertal development may be arrested by environmental stressors or by an intrapsychic condition such as an eating disorder in both female and male adolescents. In the former, intervention should be directed at alleviating the cause of the stress (57). Although the etiology of eating disorders typically is multifactorial, one of the possible factors in both genders is difficulty in integrating the sexual identity role of a young adult (58). Amenorrhea, loss of secondary sex characteristics, and lowered testosterone remove the eating disordered adolescent from some of the normal stress of assuming responsibility for sexual desire and behaviors. It would be a mistake, however, to consider eating disordered adolescents as being sexually naive. Preliminary studies have shown that general sexual attitudes and behaviors of eating disordered females are not significantly different from standardized norms (59). Male eating disordered adolescents in an inpatient setting have been reported to have a 25% incidence of homosexual orientation—approximately twice that of the general population (58).

SEXUAL ORIENTATION

For the majority of adolescents, sexual fantasies and sexual activity with others are exclusively heterosexual (with the possible exception of some same-sex play in early adolescence). The heterosexual orientation of sexual identity and sexual role is taken for granted by themselves, their parents, and their peers. There may be occasional distress that he or she is not as ideal a sexual young man or young woman as the culture demands ("Will I get invited to the prom? How will I do when I do IT for the first time?"), but there is no distress that one is qualitatively different from the ideal.

The same cannot be said for the adolescent who is primarily attracted to others of the same sex. For the homosexual adolescent, the clash between erotic fantasies and behaviors on the one hand and the cultural expectation of heterosexuality on the other frequently make for notable distress. As the sense of homosexual orientation emerges during adolescence both for the young men or women (60), the primary developmental task for the homosexual adolescent is adjustment to a socially stigmatized sexual role (61).

The etiology of homosexual orientation is highly controverted (62–66). At this point in our knowledge, the question of causality might best be framed as an inquiry into the etiologies of homosexualities. There may be genetic, physiologic, and environmental determinants that converge in a multifactorial fashion in the individual. Hypothetically, these may affect the degrees of homosexual and heterosexual orientation in the individual adolescent.

When a clinician is asked about sexual orientation by an adolescent or her parents, the question is usually a dichotomous one: "Am I lesbian? Is he homosexual?" It is not a question that often lends itself to a simple categorical answer. Sexual orientation, especially in a developing adolescent, is a far more subtle and complex reality. As so aptly stated by Kinsey et al. (67):

> The world is not divided into sheep and goats. Not all are black nor all things white. It is fundamental of taxonomy that nature rarely deals with discrete categories and tries to force facts into separated pigeon holes. The living world is a continuum in each and every one of its aspects. The sooner we learn this concerning human sexual behavior the sooner we shall reach a sounder understanding of the realities of sex.

To measure the continuous degrees of both homosexuality and heterosexuality in an individual, Kinsey et al. (67) used sexual fantasy and sexual behavior as the two determining factors on which subjects would be rated from 0 to 6. Exclusive heterosexuality was represented by 0 and exclusive homosexuality by 6. Today, most who write about the assessment of sexual orientation add to erotic fantasy and sexual behavior other determinants involving sexual identity and sexual social role.

Additional determinants of sexual orientation are sexual attraction, sexual behavior, sexual fantasies, emotional preference, social preference, self-identification, and hetero/gay lifestyle (68–70). The Klein Sexual Orientation Grid (KSOG) uses the Kinsey seven-point ratings on past, present, and ideal dimensions of these seven determinants of sexual orientation (70). The resultant dimensional profiles can provide a description of the variations in the sexual orientation of the subjects. For the clinician choosing not to use such an instrument, the KSOG offers a temporal and topical structure that can be used in the exploration of sexual orientation with the adolescent.

It is typically the mental health professional who has the professional time and expertise to assist the adolescent who is conflicted or ambiguous about his or her sexual orientation. As a lengthy review of the literature concludes, attempts to change the homosexual adult's sexual orientation have a poor prognosis (79). The work of therapy with such an adolescent whose sexual identity/role is still developing involves primarily a nonjudgmental exploration into the adolescent's experience of his or her sexual identity/role. Anxiety will be patent as bisexual attractions are dealt with. Premature closure by "deciding" on one orientation simply to bind the anxiety should be avoided. Encouragement to explore the desired sexual orientation will be evident in the therapist by her willingness to process the reactions of the adolescent to this exploration.

If the work of therapy or the self-awareness of the adolescent indicates that there is a clearly homosexual orientation, then the adolescent should be assisted to integrate this sexual orientation into his or her sexual identity/ role. Therapy will address not only the negative reactions of family members to an emerging homosexual orientation in their child but also the negative self-judgments that the adolescent has internalized as a member of a culture that is predominantly homophobic. This is facilitated if suitable role models are available to the adolescent in a therapeutic setting, e.g., group therapy, or identified to the youth as public persons who are homosexual.

Parents and Friends of Lesbians and Gays (PFLAG) is a nationwide organization whose purpose is to assist parents of homosexual children through information and group support. The national address is: Federation PFLAG, P.O. Box 27605, Washington, DC 20038. Nearby university or college student services also might be contacted for the local chapter's meeting place and time.

TALKING ABOUT SEX

Sexually active adolescents have described themselves as being quite ready to receive information on pregnancy and the prevention of venereal disease (71). The importance of talking about sexuality with adolescents and taking a careful sexual history have obviously increased since the pandemic of acquired immunodeficiency syndrome. To the previous aims of reproduction education (72) and the diagnosis and treatment of STDs (73) is added the protection of life itself. It is not merely the homosexual male and the intravenous drug user who is at risk for human immunodeficiency virus (HIV) transmission. For example, a recent national survey of 5,514 first-year Canadian college students (mean age 19.7 years) reported a distressing incidence of high-risk STD-HIV behavior among this population (74). Of the 74% of sexually active men, 14% had participated in anal intercourse and only 25% always used a condom. Of the 69% of sexually active women, 19% had participated in anal intercourse and a mere 16% always used a condom. Nearly 6% of both genders reported a previous STD.

MacDonald et al. (74) suggested three components in effective STD/HIV risk reduction education that should guide clinical conversation about sex with the adolescent. First, the adolescents must be given relevant information that allows them to make an accurate assessment of the risks they are taking in their sexual practices. With this information, they can determine the changes that they can make to reduce risks in their particular social and sexual environment. This requires inquiry into the number of partners, the incidence of oral-anal, oral-genital, anal, and vaginal intercourse, and the use of condoms. Concurrent use of alcohol and drugs should be seen as an increased risk factor.

The second component involves assisting the adolescents to develop successful techniques for practicing safer sex. This is largely the young person's development of interpersonal skills, e.g., how to abstain from intercourse and how to be assertive enough to demand the use of a condom from a partner. The third component is assisting adolescents to be sufficiently motivated to act on their knowledge of STD/HIV risk behavior with interpersonal effectiveness even when this is counter to prevailing social norms. The latter two components suggested by MacDonald et al. (74) generally will entail public health programs beyond the clinical interview and sexual history.

A competent sexual history will occur in the atmosphere of supportive and nonjudgmental rapport with the adolescent. The clinician's first task is to create an environment that is permissive for the adolescent to discuss sexual matters. Sexual orientation should never be presumed because the adolescent appears to conform to sexual stereotypes. The confidentiality of the doctor-patient relationship needs to be conveyed, especially relative to any limitations that may be mandated by law, e.g., parental notification of abortion. To discuss embarrassing or emotionally conflicted sexual issues, the adolescent must be able to trust that what is said will remain confidential.

When a clinician takes a sexual history, she is not merely obtaining quantitative data about behavior, attitudes, and medical conditions. She also is immersing herself in the cultural milieu of the adolescent. At times, the prejudices of the clinician may affect the interaction. For example, physicians assessing abdominal pain in an emergency room setting asked black and Hispanic girls about sexual history more frequently than white girls (75).

Taking the sexual history of homosexual males who are sexually active requires a comprehensive evaluation of the risk factors for possible HIV transmission. A 1986 survey of nonclinical male homosexual teenagers found that the average number of sex partners was seven; the partners averaged 7 years older; two thirds of the initial encounters originated in bars or public places; one third exchanged no personal identification information; nearly half had a history of STD; and the majority met criteria for substance abuse (76). Sexually active gay adolescents should be periodically evaluated for STD, with special attention given to disorders of the urethra, pharynx, proctorectal region, and skin (73).

Last, the more comfortable the clinician is talking about sex, the more at ease the respondent will be. There is no easy way to learn how to talk seriously about sex with another adult. With adolescents, generational and cultural differences make it more difficult. Psychodynamic theory suggests that the adult's own repressed adolescent sexuality issues are brought into (pre)consciousness when talking about sex with an adolescent. This can make conversation about sex emotionally difficult for the adult and secondarily for the adolescent. Desensitization usually is necessary by repeated exposure to the anxiety-provoking stimulus in the *in vivo* situation. The only way to be at ease talking about sex with adolescents is to do it—repeatedly.

CONCLUSION

Adolescent sexual development is a multifaceted process. It includes the interface of biologic, familial, psychological, cognitive, economic, and academic determinants. As sexual identity, orientation and intimacy develop, the adolescent is faced with a myriad of choices and decisions. Pregnancy and STD are major challenges and pitfalls for the adolescent. Clinicians can provide a supportive, sensitive, and instructive environment to assist adolescents through their sexual development.

REFERENCES

1. Erikson EH. *Identity, youth and crisis.* New York: Norton, 1968.
2. Scharff DE. *The sexual relationship: an object relations view of sex and the family.* Boston: Routledge & Kegan Paul, 1982.
3. Sullivan HS. *The interpersonal theory of psychology.* New York: Norton, 1953.
4. Brooks-Gunn J, Furstenberg F. Adolescent sexual behavior. *Am Psychol* 1989;44:249–257.
5. Gilligan C. *In a different voice: psychological theory and women's development.* Cambridge, MA: Harvard University Press, 1982.
6. Berndt T. The features and effects of friendship in early adolescence. *Child Dev* 1982;53:1447–1460.
7. McCabe MP. Toward a theory of adolescent dating. *Adolescence* 1984;19:160–169.
8. Steinberg L. *Adolescence.* New York: Knopf, 1985.
9. Udry JR, Billy JO, Morris NM, et al. Serum androgenic hormones motivate sexual behavior in adolescent boys. *Fertil Steril* 1985;43:90–94.
10. Udry JR, Talbert L, Morris NM. Biosocial foundations for adolescent female sexuality. *Demography* 1986;23:217–229.
11. DeGaston JF, Weed S, Jensen L. Understanding gender differences in adolescent sexuality. *Adolescence* 1996;31:217–231.
12. Laufer M, Laufer ME. *Adolescence and developmental breakdown: a psychoanalytic view.* New Haven: Yale University, 1984.
13. Gagnon JH, Simon W. *Sexual conduct: the social sources of human sexuality.* Chicago: Aldine de Gruyter, 1973.
14. Kann L, Kinchen SA, Williams BI, et al. Youth risk behavior surveillance–United States, 1997. *MMWR* 1998;47:1–92.
15. Juhasz A, Schneider M. Adolescent sexuality: values, morality and decision making. *Adolescence* 1987;87:579–589.
16. Piaget J. Intellectual evolution from adolescence to adulthood. *Hum Dev* 1972;15:1.
17. Hayes CD, ed. *Risking the future: adolescent sexuality, pregnancy and childbearing, vol. I.* Washington, DC: National Academy Press, 1987.
18. Grant LM, Demetriou E. Adolescent sexuality. *Pediatr Clin North Am* 1988;35:1271–1289.
19. Sarrel LJ, Sarrel PM. Sexual unfolding. *J Adolesc Health Care* 1981;2:93.
20. Furstenberg FF Jr. Implicating the family: teenage parenthood and kinship involvement. In: *Teenage pregnancy in a family context.* Ooms T, ed. Philadelphia: Temple University Press, 1981.
21. Herceg-Baron R, Furstenberg FF Jr. Adolescent contraception use: the impact of family support systems. In:
The childbearing decision: fertility attitudes and behavior, Fox G, ed. Beverly Hills: Sage, 1982.
22. Weinstein M, Thornton A. Mother-child relation and adolescent sexual attitude and behavior. *Demography* 1989;26:563–577.
23. Thornton A, Camburn D. The influence of the family on premarital sexual attitudes and behavior. *Demography* 1987;24:323–340.
24. Baker SA, Thalberg SP, Morrison OM. Parents' behavioral norms as predictors of adolescent sexual activity and contraceptive use. *Adolescence* 1988;23:265–281.
25. Strouse JS, Buerkel-Rothfuss N, Long EC. Gender and family as moderators of the relationship between music video exposure and adolescent sexual permissiveness. *Adolescence* 1995;30:505–521.
26. Newcome S, Udley JR. Parental mental status effects on adolescent sexual behavior. *J Marriage Fam* 1987;49:235–240.
27. Rosenthal SL, Lewis LM, Cohen SS. Issues related to the sexual decision-making of inner-city adolescent girls. *Adolescence* 1996;31:731–739.
28. Hockenberry-Eaton M, Richman MJ, Dilorio C, et al. Mother and adolescent knowledge of sexual development: the effects of gender, age, and sexual experience. *Adolescence* 1996;31:35–47.
29. Whitaker DJ, Miller KS. Parent-adolescent discussions about sexual initiation: reducing the impact on peer norms on early sexual initiation. *Int Conf AIDS* 1998;12:210.
30. Brown JD, Childers KW, Waszak CS. Television and adolescent sexuality. *J Adolesc Health Care* 1990;11:62–70.
31. Cooksey EC, Rindfuss RR, Guilkey DK. The initiation of adolescent sexual and contraceptive behavior during changing times. *J Health Soc Behav* 1996;25:61–66.
32. Mott FL, Fondell MM, Hu PN, et al. The determinants of first sex by age 14 in a high-risk adolescent population. *Fam Plann Perspect* 1996;28:13–18.
33. McBride CM, Curry SJ, Cheadle A, et al. School-level application of a social bonding model to adolescent risk-taking behavior. *J Sch Health* 1995;65:63–68.
34. Traaen B, Lewin B. Adolescent sexual experiences in Norway. *Int Cong AIDS* 1991;7:420.
35. Strunin L, Hingson R. Alcohol, drugs, and adolescent sexual behavior. *Int J Addict* 1992;27:129–146.
36. Smith, et al. *Am J Public Health* 1985;75:1200.
37. Jones E, Forrest JD, Goldman N, et al. Teenage pregnancy in developed countries: Determinants and policy implications. *Fam Plann Perspect* 1985;17:53–63.
38. Winter L. The role of sexual self-concept in the use of contraceptives. *Fam Plann Perspect* 1988;20:123–127.
39. Jay MS, DuRant RH, Lih IF. Female adolescents' compliance with contraceptive regimens. *Pediatr Clin North Am* 1989;36:731–745.
40. Chilman CS. Some psychosocial aspects of adolescent sexual and contraceptive behavior in a changing American Society. In: Lancaster JB, Hamburg BA, eds. *School-age pregnancy and parenthood biosocial dimensions.* New York: Aldine de Gruyter, 1986:191–217.
41. Morrison DM. Adolescent contraceptive behavior, a review. *Psychol Bull* 1985;98:538–568.
42. Curtis HA, Lanerence CJ, Tripp JH. Teenage sexual intercourse and pregnancy. *Arch Dis Child* 1988;63:373–379.

43. Furstenberg FF Jr, Brooks-Gunn J, Morgan SP. Adolescent mothers and their children in later life. *Fam Plann Perspect* 1987;19:142–151.

44. Zabin L, Hirsch M, Emerson M. When urban adolescents choose abortion: effects on education, psychological status and subsequent pregnancy. *Fam Plann Perspect* 1989; 21:248–255.

45. Pete JM, DeSantis L. Sexual decision making in young black adolescent females. *Adolescence* 1990;25:183–204.

46. Green R. The *"sissy boy syndrome" and the development of homosexuality*. New Haven: Yale University, 1987.

47. Steiner BW, ed. *Gender dysphoria: development, research and management*. New York: Plenum, 1985.

48. Fagan PJ, Meyer JK, Schmidt CW Jr. Sexual dysfunction within an adult developmental perspective. *J Sex Marital Ther* 1986;12:1–12.

49. Money J. *Venuses penuses: sexology, sexosophy and exigency theory*. Buffalo: Prometheus Books, 1986.

50. Money J, Alexander D. Psychosexual development and absence of homosexuality in males with precocious puberty: review of 18 cases. *J Nerv Ment Dis* 1969;148: 111–123.

51. Money J, Walker P. Psychosexual development, maternalism, nonpromiscuity and body image in 15 females with precocious puberty. *Arch Sex Behav* 1971;1:45–60.

52. Money J, Clopper R. Postpubertal psychosexual function in postsurgical male hypopituitarism. *J Sex Res* 1975;11:25–38.

53. Clopper R, Adelson JM, Money J. Postpubertal psychosexual function in male hypopituitarism without hypogonadotropinism after growth hormone therapy. *J Sex Res* 1976;12:14–32.

54. Money J, Clopper R, Menefee J. Psychosexual development in postpubertal males with idiopathic panhypopituitarism. *J Sex Res* 1980;16:212–225.

55. Ehrhardt AA, Meyer-Bahlburg HF. Idiopathic precocious puberty in girls: long-term effects on adolescent behavior. *Acta Endocrinol Suppl* 1986;279:247–253.

56. Brack CJ, Orr DP, Ingersoll S. Pubertal maturation and self-esteem. *J Adolesc Health Care* 1988;9:280–285.

57. Eisenstein TD, Gerson MJ. Psychosocial growth retardation in adolescence. A reversible condition secondary to severe stress. *J Adolesc Health Care* 1988;9:436–440.

58. Fagan PJ, Andersen AE. Sexuality and eating disorders in adolescence. In: Sugar M, ed. *Atypical adolescence and sexuality*. New York: WW Norton, 2000.

59. Rothschild BS, Fagan PJ, Woodall C, et al. Sexual functioning of female eating disordered patients. Abstract presented at the International Conference for Eating Disorders, New York, April 1990.

60. Chapman BE, Brannock JC. Proposed model of lesbian identity development: an empirical examination. *J Homosex* 1987;14:69–80.

61. Hetrick ES, Martin AD. Developmental issues and their resolution for gay and lesbian adolescents. *J Homosex* 1987;14:25–43.

62. DeCecco JP. Homosexuality's brief recovery: from sickness to health and back again. *J Sex Res* 1987;23: 106–114.

63. DeCecco JP. The two views of Meyer-Bahlburg: a rejoinder. *J Sex Res* 1987;23:123–127.

64. Meyer-Bahlburg HF. Psychoendocrine research and the societal status of homosexuals: a reply to DeCecco. *J Sex Res* 1987;23:114–120.

65. Gagnon JH. Science and the politics of pathology. *J Sex Res* 1987;23:120–123.

66. Perper T. Enough is enough: reflections on the views of DeCecco and Meyer-Bahlburg. *J Sex Res* 1987;23: 127–129.

67. Kinsey AC, Pomeroy WB, Martin CE. *Sexual behavior in the human male*. Philadelphia: WB Saunders, 1948.

68. Klein F. *The bisexual option*. New York: Arbor House, 1978.

69. Klein F. Are you sure you're heterosexual? or homosexual? or bisexual? *Forum Magazine* 1980;December: 41–45.

70. Klein F, Sepekoff B, Wolf TJ. Sexual orientation: a multivariate dynamic process. *J Homosex* 1985;9:35–49.

71. Acosta FX. Etiology and treatment of homosexuality: a review. *Arch Sex Behav* 1975;4:9–29.

72. Amann-Gainotti M. Sexual socialization during early adolescence: the menarche. *Adolescence* 1986;21: 703–710.

73. Zenilman J. Sexually transmitted diseases in homosexual adolescents. *J Adolesc Health Care* 1988;9:129–138.

74. MacDonald NE, Wells GA, Fisher WA, et al. High-risk STD/HIV behavior among college students. *JAMA* 1990;263:3155–3159.

75. Hunt AD, Litt IF, Loebner M. Obtaining a sexual history from adolescent girls. *J Adolesc Health Care* 1988;9: 52–54.

76. Ramefedi GJ. Adolescent homosexuality; psychosocial and medical implications. *Pediatrics* 1987;79:331–337.

22

Adolescent Contraception and Abortion

Vanessa E. Cullins and George R. Huggins

Because the scope of this text is adolescent gynecology, this chapter will emphasize the provider's relationship with the female adolescent patient. There is no intention to deemphasize the importance of the male partner within all contexts of heterosexuality.

Despite slight reductions in birth rates, increasing contraceptive prevalence, and condom use among adolescents (1), approximately one million adolescent girls ages 12 to 19 years in the United States become pregnant each year. The median age at first intercourse of 16 years (2) is comparable to the age of coital initiation in industrialized countries such as Canada, Great Britain, France, The Netherlands, and Sweden, yet the birth, pregnancy, and abortion rates are significantly higher among U.S. adolescents (3–5). The categorical distinction between U.S. teens and teens of other nations is contraceptive use. Teens in the United States, like older U.S. women, are poor contraceptors compared with women of similarly industrialized countries (4). Recent declines in U.S. pregnancy and birth rates are attributed to increasing use of condoms and adolescent use of longer-acting methods such as levonorgestrel implant (Norplant) or medroxyprogesterone acetate (Depo-Provera) (1). Although these trends are encouraging, they should not lull U.S. society into complacency regarding adolescent pregnancy prevention.

It is interesting to note that adolescent birth rates have paralleled adult birth rates in the United States (6). Whereas data regarding adolescent pregnancy are shamefully emphasized in American discourse, a similar but overlooked trend is that American adolescents tend to model adult sexual behavior and birth rates. This information becomes important in the provider's approach to adolescents. The "independent" decisions of teenagers follow the patterns of adults of similar racial or socioeconomic class (6). It appears, therefore, that many of the same cultural, economic, and social factors that influence adult sexual behavior also influence teen behavior. The same nonjudgmental attitudes, tact, and confidentiality (7) recommended for adult clients should be applied to adolescents who, like adults, will make decisions based on a variety of factors that will be incompletely known to the provider.

A plethora of factors may influence an individual's decision regarding contraception. These factors include cultural and religious beliefs; family values; partner attitudes and values; previous contraceptive experiences; previous sexual experiences; career aspirations; desire for pregnancy; perceived risks associated with contraception; cost, convenience, and ease of method use; method effectiveness; and individual risk for sexually transmitted diseases (STDs). Considering the time constraints imposed on typical medical visits, it is impossible for all these issues to be explored in one or two visits. The dialogue about family planning and sexual responsibility will need to be ongoing between the health care team and the teen. The provider can hope to bring attention to social/sexual behaviors that may have an impact on the adolescent's future plans; the provider can play a special role in the teen's life as an impartial adviser.

It is hoped that, at certain stages of this dialogue and with teen consent, the adults with significant influence in the teen's life will be brought into the discussion and influence the process.

Inquiry and counseling responsibilities of an adolescent's primary care provider include the following:

1. Questions about who the adults who influence the adolescent are, and whether the adolescent feels comfortable discussing sexual/contraceptive issues with that person or persons.
2. Explanations by the provider about the importance of family planning, i.e., the importance of deciding (a) whether or not to become pregnant, at this time in life, and (b) how to prevent pregnancy when pregnancy is undesired (abstinence vs. contraception).
3. Questions about current and past sexual activities and behaviors, i.e., presence, absence, and number of sexual partners; use of protection against STDs; whether the sexual activity was and is consensual.
4. Questions about the sexual partner's childbearing intentions, sexual behaviors, attitudes, and career intentions; questions about peer-group sexual behavior and her career intentions.
5. Questions about past use of contraceptives, including condoms, and experience with these preventive methods; questions about acceptability of these methods to the current partner.
6. Questions about the patient or partner's need for more information about family planning, contraception, and STD prevention.

Whereas the optimal approach from a service delivery standpoint is to approach these issues as a health care team, this team approach may prove unacceptable to an adolescent who is seeking secrecy regarding her sexual behavior. Assurance of confidentiality may become believable only if made by one individual. If more than one individual on the health care team can be involved, questions 1,

2, 4, 5, and 6, can be assessed by the nurse or medical office assistant with the aid of a questionnaire. The physician then can be freed to discuss family planning and STD prevention issues that have been identified as being of most concern to the patient (8).

MORE REGARDING APPROACH TO THE ADOLESCENT

Adolescent coitus is a well-documented phenomenon. Sexual contact after puberty is considered normal in traditional cultures. This fact is implicit in rituals that mark transition through puberty, as well as in societal traditions that either acknowledge that contact will occur (early marriage) or attempt to place cultural/societal restrictions to prevent this contact (5,9). Despite common misperceptions, worldwide, the age of sexual intercourse initiation has not dropped substantially. The social convention that has changed is age at first marriage. Worldwide, the trend seen as women become more educated and the economics of their home country advances is that median age at first marriage and median age at first intended pregnancy tends to become delayed (10). In the United States and other similarly industrialized countries, there has been an increasing gap between age of puberty and the ability of youth to be economically independent, i.e., the ability to take on the responsibilities of marriage and parenthood (5,9–13). Despite dominant cultural norms that attempt to impose restrictions on early coitus, the United States continues to exhibit increasing prevalence of early coitus. Other factors purportedly responsible for early coital experience include a decline of institutional influences, such as church and family, and the surge of media exploitation of sex appeal and sex without consequences (11–13). These factors tend to affect all of societal youth and adults. In fact, prevalence of sexual activity initiation is similar across socioeconomic strata. It is the prevalence of adolescent nonmarital childbearing that differs among socioeconomic strata: middle- and upper-class youth are less likely to bear children during adolescence (11–14). Abrahamse et al. (15) found that teens most likely to consider single parenthood tend to exhibit problem behaviors such as school disciplinary problems and nonconforming behavior. Additionally, they found adolescents with the most to lose educationally, economically, and socially are least likely to consider early childbearing.

The consequences of unprotected adolescent intercourse reverberate through U.S. society in the form of rising maternal/perinatal morbidity, rising STD rates, increased private and public expenditures, and the often arrested educational and financial growth of the affected teen, her consort, and her immediate extended family.

The cultural diversity found within the United States contributes to this nation's inability to develop a cohesive strategy to combat teen childbearing. Regardless of personal convictions, health professionals caring for adolescents must be prepared to discuss all aspects of sexual responsibility, including abstinence, contraception, and prevention of STDs. Decisions made by the adolescent should be periodically reassessed for their applicability to the adolescent's immediate and long-range intentions. This is no different from the approach to an adult's family planning and STD prevention decisions.

Constant change is the only invariable feature of adolescence. During this transition from childhood to adulthood, all teens experience varying degrees of physiologic, psychological, and behavioral growth. This period is punctuated by adolescent attempts toward independent behavior, often contrary to childhood upbringing and parental advice. If proper rapport is developed, the primary care physician is in a unique position to provide sensitive guidance to teens during this often confusing, transitional time. The tone of dialogue with teens must be nonjudgmental; the setting must be private. Confidentiality is a must (7). The goal is to help the teen clarify her own set of values and to provide her with the tools to live according to values that she might modify as she grows older. To approach

the sensitive and anxiety-provoking subject of adolescent sexuality, the clinician must first determine the adolescent's behavior, attitudes, and concerns about sexuality. This may be approached by asking the young woman (a) how she feels about teenagers having sex, (b) if any of her friends are engaging in sexual intercourse, (c) if she has had sexual intercourse, and (d) how she feels about her sexual behavior.

Throughout the conversation, the adolescent should be treated as an independent decision maker. She should be helped to see the long-term commitment of raising a child. Often teens define sexual activity in terms of frequency. They often equate infrequent sex with not being "sexually active" and with no risk of pregnancy. The adolescent patient should be helped to acknowledge that one voluntary sexual act makes her a sexually active individual and that with sexual activity comes responsibility to self, i.e., protection against pregnancy and STDs. With time, most will understand that taking charge of sexuality and life does not preclude love and spontaneity. Help the patient understand the nature of relationships, that they are dynamic and sometimes short lived. The role of the clinician and other members of the health care team is one of motivator/reinforcer of all positive aspects of the teen's life, including postponement of intercourse and/or maintenance of sexual health. As motivators and reinforcers, members of the health care team can offer additional perspectives to the teen's life experiences. Listening to and exploring the patient's motivations and experiences often can achieve this (8).

One overriding goal in professional dialogue is to emphasize the educational, economic, and social costs of early childbearing. To be relevant, the conversation should be personalized. This can be accomplished by incorporating a discussion of each teen's future aspirations and by developing a general plan for the accomplishment of these goals. This translates into an active discussion of abstinence for the virgin and contraception for the sexually active teen. This position can be reinforced in subsequent visits by reference to progress toward previously mentioned educational, social, and economic goals.

CONTRACEPTIVE METHODS

As the word implies, contraception is designed to prevent conception. For heterosexual adolescents and adults who do not desire pregnancy and who practice any mode of interpersonal sexuality except lifetime monogamy, the ideal method would perform the dual role of preventing conception and preventing STDs. Only barrier methods provide simultaneous protection against pregnancy and STDs. The barrier method that provides the most protection against bacterial and viral pathogens is the male condom. The dilemma associated with condom use is its typically fair rate of protection against conception compared with other contraceptive methods.

One fourth of the estimated 15 million new STD cases that occur annually in the United States occur in adolescents (16). Given the impermanence of most adolescent relationships and the high probability of multiple, sequential sexual partners before marriage (13,17), the condom is the single best contraceptive choice for most adolescents. Ideally, adolescents and adults who are simultaneously trying to protect themselves against STDs and pregnancy will practice dual protection, i.e., the condom plus another method that has a superior typical-use failure rate for pregnancy prevention. Another approach to optimal protection, aside from abstinence, is condom use with intentions and ability to use emergency contraception in the event of condom accident (slippage, breakage, failure to use) (see section on Emergency Contraception).

Barrier Methods

Barrier methods available in the United States include spermicidal foams, jellies, creams, and suppositories; male condom; female condom; diaphragm; and cervical cap. These methods prevent pregnancy through provision of a physical and/or chemical barrier to sperm. Depending on the product, the method also may be spermicidal, bactericidal, and/or viricidal. Contraceptive effectiveness varies, with pregnancy rates of 4% to 30% in the first year of use (18–21). For barrier methods, both the theoretical effective rate and the use effective rate are best for the male condom, approaching 2% in highly motivated adult couples (21,22). For all barrier methods, use effectiveness tends to increase with increasing age. The older and more motivated the user, the more consistent the use of the barrier method and the lower the failure rate. Theoretically, barrier contraception, especially the male condom, is an ideal method for teens because barrier methods provide excellent dual protection against pregnancy and STDs when used correctly. However, failure rates of the barrier method are high in teens. Even when used correctly, barrier-method continuation rates are low in younger patients. One-year continuation rates for adolescents have ranged from approximately 20% to 80% (22–25).

The major disadvantage of barrier methods is that they are coital related and require comfort/familiarity with the patient's own genitalia or, in the case of the male condom, comfort with the partner's genitalia. In addition, self-assurance is needed to purchase condoms over the counter. The cost of barrier methods can be prohibitive unless the teen gives the need for the method a high priority, i.e., considers barrier-method cost as a necessary expense, just as a new article of clothing may be considered necessary for the next date.

A barrier method may be an excellent choice for adolescents who engage in infrequent intercourse or are poor pill takers. The condom is a must for teens with multiple sexual partners or those who are intimate with others who have multiple partners. Male condoms, female condoms, diaphragms, and chemical barriers are available over the counter. Cervical caps and diaphragms must be fitted and prescribed by a health care provider. Only condoms made of latex or polyurethane are effective against STDs (26). When used with a chemical barrier, condoms, diaphragms, and cervical caps probably are more protective against STDs (27–32).

Comfort with tampon insertion is a good initial indicator of whether a teen is a good candidate for a female barrier method. A teen who is not comfortable inserting or removing a tampon cannot be expected to effectively use a barrier method. As alluded to before, the teen's acknowledgment of sexuality and assertiveness should be gauged before recommending sole use of a barrier method.

As with any contraceptive method, the adolescent should be given detailed instructions on the contraceptive's use. The teen must know exactly what to buy, how to use it, and how to care for any multiple-use device.

All first-time users of barrier methods should have an annual pelvic examination, cervical cytology, and screening for bacterial and viral STDs. Compliance may be optimized if follow-up is scheduled 1 to 3 months after initiation of use. At that time, assess satisfaction with the method. Based on this assessment, future follow-up can be determined. Experienced barrier users should undergo yearly examinations for health maintenance. As with adults using contraception, the adolescent should be advised that no method may be appropriate for a lifetime. As she experiences changes in her lifestyle, relationship(s), and childbearing intentions, she may find another method more convenient or appropriate. The annual examination is an ideal opportunity to reinforce the need for condom use for STD prevention and review family planning decisions.

Male Condom

Male condoms are nonprescription, single-use, contraceptives that serve as a mechanical barrier to sperm, bacteria, and viruses. Only latex, and probably polyurethane, condoms are effective against conception *and* STDs (26,33, 34). Latex condoms have been shown to prevent the transmission of chlamydia, trichomonas, gonorrhea, herpes, human immunodeficiency virus, cytomegalovirus, hepatitis B virus, and probably human papilloma virus

(35–41). For the well-motivated couple, condoms also are an effective safeguard against pregnancy. The first-year failure rate for the condom can be as low as 1% to 4% (42). Among typical users, failure rates are 10% to 20% (18,20,21). Adolescents should be instructed on both the type and correct use of the condom. Natural-membrane condoms do not afford effective protection against STDs, so a latex or polyurethane condom should always be recommended for use with each sexual act. The male condom should be placed on the erect penis and rolled from the glans to the base. If a condom without a reservoir tip is used, a reservoir for semen should be created by gently pinching a half-inch tip at the top of the condom as the condom is placed on the penis. This reservoir will prevent breakage. The rim of the condom must be held when the penis is withdrawn from the vagina. Only a water-based lubricant should be used. The teen should be advised to use intravaginal spermicide and seek emergency contraception (see details later) if the condom breaks. The teen should be advised that the most effective protection against STD transmission, short of abstinence, probably is the combination of condom and spermicidal agent. Suggest that a spermicide be used in place of a lubricant.

Diaphragm

Diaphragms are shallow, flexible domes of rubber that are placed high in the vagina to cover the cervix. There are three types of diaphragms, categorized by the type of spring located in the rim: arcing spring, coil spring, and flat spring. Adolescent patients tend to fare best with either an arcing- or coil-spring diaphragm; both of these diaphragms are easier to compress and insert correctly than the flat-spring diaphragm. The arcing-spring diaphragm forms an arc when compressed. This enables the diaphragm to be inserted easily and correctly in patients with marked anteversion or retroversion. The coil-ring diaphragm is fitted easily in women with normal pelvic anatomy without marked uterine anteversion or retroversion. All three diaphragm types are produced in diameter sizes ranging from 50 to 105 mm. To receive the proper size and type of diaphragm, the patient must be fitted by a knowledgeable health professional. The largest size that will maximize coverage of the cervix yet cause no discomfort is selected. The diaphragm is used with a spermicidal jelly or cream. It should be inserted at least 30 minutes before and up to 6 hours before intercourse. For continued efficacy, the diaphragm must be left in place for at least 6 hours after the last act of intercourse. Additional spermicide must be inserted for each repeat coital act. Although the pregnancy rate can be as low as 1.1 per 100 women per year for a highly motivated couple, typical pregnancy rates are 10% to 20% (18,20,21). Failure rates and discontinuation rates are much higher for new users and younger women. For adolescents, the 1-year continuation rate may be as low as 23% (23).

Side effects from diaphragm use include potential allergy to the spermicide and/or rubber and increased risk of urinary tract infections (43–47). Disadvantages of the diaphragm are that it is a coital-related method and therefore interferes with the spontaneity of sex; preparation and insertion may be messy; insertion of additional spermicide often is inconvenient; and it must be fitted and prescribed by a health professional.

When fitted for a diaphragm, the patient should receive extensive instruction on its use. In the office, she should both remove and replace the diaphragm. She should be seen again in 1 to 2 weeks for a recheck of her placement and removal technique. In addition to routine instructions on use, she should be warned that she will experience a greater chance of diaphragm displacement in female-superior positions. She must be instructed that the diaphragm will need to be refitted after pregnancy and after any change in weight greater than 10 lb. Instruct her on inspection of the diaphragm for holes or tears and on the soap and water cleansing after each diaphragm use. She must be instructed never to leave the diaphragm in place for more than 24 hours to avoid toxic shock syndrome (46,48).

Cervical Cap

The cervical cap is a thimble-shaped dome of rubber that is used with a spermicide and applied over the cervix. Fitting the cap to the cervix is more difficult than fitting a diaphragm. Caps available in the United States are manufactured in four different sizes. Because of the limitation in sizes, approximately 6% of women cannot be fitted (49). The cervical cap is considered as efficacious as the diaphragm (22). Although considered less messy than a diaphragm, its insertion and removal tends to be more difficult. However, it is not necessary to use additional spermicide if repeat intercourse occurs less than 6 hours after placement of the first application of the intracap spermicide. If intercourse occurs later than 6 hours after initial placement of the cap, additional spermicide should be placed intravaginally. An advantage of the cap is that it may be left in place for up to 48 hours. Changing and storage are analogous to diaphragm cleaning and storage. In general, the cervical cap is not a good method for adolescents because of the difficulty involved in placement and removal (49).

Vaginal Contraceptive Sponge

The vaginal contraceptive sponge became available again to U.S. consumers in late 1999. This over-the-counter product was voluntarily withdrawn from the market after the Food and Drug Administration (FDA) cited problems within the manufacturing plant. The original manufacturer believed it was less expensive to cease production than to correct the problems. Allendale Pharmaceuticals, Inc., purchased the rights to the sponge with the intent of correcting the flaws in the manufacturing process.

The vaginal contraceptive sponge is a spermicide-containing polyurethane barrier designed to fit over the cervical os. This single-use device, which contains 1 g of nonoxynol 9, is available in one size and is purchased over the counter. It is moistened with water before insertion and can be inserted any time up to 24 hours before intercourse. Contraceptive action lasts for 24 hours. The sponge may be left in place for a total of 30 hours. No additional spermicide is needed for additional acts of intercourse within the 24-hour period. For the nulliparous, the first-year failure rate of the sponge is similar to that of the diaphragm. The failure rate can rise to 40% for parous women (18,50). As with the diaphragm and cervical cap, adolescents need to be given detailed instructions on sponge use. They should be warned of the potential for dislodgement. Although the occurrence of toxic shock syndrome is rare, the adolescent should be made aware of the relationship between prolonged sponge exposure and this illness. It is prudent to instruct the adolescent on sponge usage as one would instruct for the diaphragm or cervical cap, i.e., have the adolescent insert and remove the sponge in the office.

Spermicides

Nonprescription spermicides (jellies, creams, foams suppositories, tablets, and films) are widely available and may be used independently or in conjunction with the condom, cervical cap, or diaphragm (jellies and creams only for the cervical cap and the diaphragm). The active ingredient found in spermicides available in the United States is either nonoxynol 9 or octoxynol. Contraceptive efficacy is a result of the surfactant's action on sperm. Additionally, these spermicides are bactericidal and probably inactivate most sexually transmissible viruses (20,21,27,30–32, 51–56). Because it is a compliance-dependent method, the failure rate of spermicides used independently of other barrier methods is approximately 26% during the first year of use (50). This contrasts with the theoretical failure rate of 3% to 6% (20,21,50). As with other barrier methods, spermicides are perceived by adolescents as messy and inconvenient. Not only must the spermicide be introduced intravaginally before intercourse, but repeat applications are necessary for additional coital acts. Spermicides are inserted intravaginally 10 to 30 minutes before inter-

course and may remain effective for up to 6 to 8 hours after intercourse. Because of the variety inherent in different products, users should be instructed to carefully follow package directions. Compared with other barrier methods, adolescents may achieve better compliance with spermicidal agents delivered through tubular vaginal applicators, as the insertion mechanism is similar to that of a tampon or medicinal vaginal cream. Even though applicator-inserted spermicides are potentially easier and quicker to use than other barrier methods, consistent use and continuation rates are low.

Emergency Contraception

Emergency contraception refers to methods designed to prevent pregnancy after unprotected intercourse. Methods that have been shown to be effective as emergency contraception include a regimen of high-dose combined oral contraceptive (COC) pills, a regimen of high-dose progestin, intrauterine device (IUD) insertion, and mifepristone.

The most commonly prescribed regimen of emergency contraception was described by Yuzpe in 1974. The regimen requires use within 72 hours of unprotected intercourse to achieve the 75% reduction in expected pregnancies (57–59). The Yuzpe regimen requires the use of COC pills that contain ethinyl estradiol and levonorgestrel or norgestrel. Such pills include Ovral (Wyeth-Ayerst, Philadelphia, PA), Lo-Ovral (Wyeth-Ayerst), Levlen (Berlex, Wayne, NJ), Triphasil (Wyeth-Ayerst), and Tri-Levlen (Berlex). When using low-dose 30 to 35 mm ethinyl estradiol pills, four pills are ingested as soon as possible, but not more than 72 hours after unprotected intercourse. The four-pill dose is repeated 12 hours after the first dose. If a 20-mg pill such as Alesse (Wyeth-Ayerst) is used, five pills are necessary for each dose. If Ovral is used, two pills are taken as soon as possible, but not more than 72 hours after unprotected intercourse. The two-pill dose is repeated 12 hours after the first dose. Preven (Gynetics, Inc. Belle Mead, New Jersey), recently approved by the U.S. FDA, is a prepackaged course of emergency contraception that can be prescribed instead of using standard COC packages.

The Preven emergency contraception kit contains (a) ethinyl estradiol 50 µg with levonorgestrel 250 µg, four pills total; (b) a pregnancy test to rule out pregnancy existing before the unprotected act of intercourse that has prompted emergency contraceptive use; and (c) patient instructions.

The most common side effect associated with the Yuzpe regimen is nausea and vomiting. The dose should be repeated if vomiting occurs within 2 hours of either dose ingestion. Antiemetics can be effective if taken prophylactically. Dimenhydrinate (Dramamine), promethazine hydrochloride (Phenergan), or prochlorperazine (Compazine), given orally or rectally, can be used. The Yuzpe and other methods are not abortifacients. The Yuzpe method works by inhibiting or delaying ovulation (60–63) and may act by inducing endometrial changes that prevent implantation (64). The only contraindication to emergency contraception is known, preexisting pregnancy, yet the adolescent, her partner, and her parents can be reassured that if a pregnancy has been achieved (implantation), there is no evidence of teratogenicity associated with oral contraceptive use (65–67).

Evidence is accumulating that indicates the levonorgestrel (progestin) method of emergency contraception is superior to the Yuzpe method in side effect profile and ability to prevent pregnancy (68,69). The progestin-only emergency contraceptive method requires levonorgestrel 1.5 mg or norgestrel 3.0 mg taken in two divided doses 12 hours apart. This dose translates into 20 Ovrette (Wyeth-Ayerst) for each dose, for a total of 40 pills for the entire regimen. In July 1999, the FDA approved Plan B (Women's Capital Corporation, Kalamazoo, Michigan) which consists of *two* 0.75-mg tablets of levonorgestrel. The first pill is taken within 72 hours of unprotected intercourse, followed by the second pill 12 hours later. As with use of COC pills, the sooner the regimen is started after unprotected intercourse, the more

effective it is for preventing pregnancy (67). The mechanism of action for progestin-only emergency contraception is most likely arrest of follicular growth through suppression of the luteinizing hormone surge or, after ovulation, impairment of corpus luteum function (62). As with the Yuzpe regimen, the only contraindication is known, preexisting pregnancy.

Other forms of emergency contraception include the copper IUD and mifepristone (RU-486) (70,71). Mifepristone currently is not commercially available in the United States. If inserted within 5 days of unprotected intercourse, the IUD is an effective form of emergency contraception. Because it is contraindicated in individuals at risk for STDs, the IUD (see later) is not an appropriate emergency contraceptive for most adolescents.

Oral Contraception

COC pills that contain both an estrogen and a progestin are the most popular reversible form of contraception in the United States (72,73).

Today's low-dose COCs are highly effective (99%, with perfect use) (20,21,74). When used correctly, low-dose pills prevent pregnancy by (a) preventing ovulation, (b) thickening cervical mucus, (c) inducing atrophy of the endometrium, and (d) altering tubal motility (20,21,75,76). Pills containing less than 50 µg of ethinyl estradiol are considered low-dose pills. Most currently available, *low*-dose pills contain from 20 to 35 µg of ethinyl estradiol (Table 22.1). The increase in cervical mucus viscosity also reduces the risk of upper genital tract STD (12).

There are few absolute contraindications to COC use. These contraindications include being at risk for or having active thrombophlebitis or thromboembolic disease; history of or suspected breast cancer; known or suspected pregnancy; undiagnosed, abnormal genital bleeding; current coronary artery disease; current or history of angina, congestive heart failure, myocardial infarction, or cerebrovascular attack; current or history of benign or malignant liver tumors; and at least 35 years old and a smoker. Hypertension, diabetes mellitus,

TABLE 22.1. *Combined oral contraceptives available in the United States*

Trade name	Pharmaceutical company	Estrogen	(µg)	Progestin	(mg)
New progestins/Low-dose estrogen					
Mircette[b]	Organon	Ethinyl estradiol	20/10	Desogestrel	0.150
Desogen	Organon	Ethinyl estradiol	30	Desogestrel	0.150
Ortho-Cyclen	Ortho	Ethinyl estradiol	35	Norgestimate	0.250
Ortho-Tri-cyclen	Ortho	Ethinyl estradiol	35	Norgestimate	0.180/0.215/0.25
Ortho-Cept	Ortho	Ethinyl estradiol	30	Desogestrel	0.150
Older progestins/low-dose estrogen					
Alesse	Wyeth	Ethinyl estradiol	20	Levonorgestrel	0.10
Levlite	Berlex	Ethinyl estradiol	20	Levonorgestrel	0.1
Estrostep	Parke-Davis	Ethinyl estradiol	20/30/35	Norethindrone	1.0
Estrostep Fe	Parke-Davis	Ethinyl estradiol	20/30/35	Norethindrone	1.0
Demulen 1/35	Searle	Ethinyl estradiol	35	Ethyndiol diacetate	1.0
Lo/Ovral	Wyeth	Ethinyl estradiol	30	Norgestrel	0.3
Nordette	Wyeth	Ethinyl estradiol	30	Levonorgestrel	0.15
Norinyl 1/35	Syntex	Ethinyl estradiol	35	Norethindrone	1.0
Ortho-Novum 1/35	Ortho	Ethinyl estradiol	35	Norethindrone	1.0
Ortho-Novum 10/11	Ortho	Ethinyl estradiol	35	Norethindrone	0.5/1.0
Ortho-Novum 7/7/7	Ortho	Ethinyl estradiol	35	Norethindrone	0.5/0.75/1.0
Tri-Norinyl	Syntex	Ethinyl estradiol	35	Norethindrone	0.5/1.00/0.5
Levelen	Berlex	Ethinyl estradiol	30	Levonorgestrel	0.150
Tri-Levelen	Berlex	Ethinyl estradiol	30/40/30	Levonorgestrel	0.05/.075/0.125
Triphasil	Wyeth	Ethinyl estradiol	30/40/30	Levonorgestrel	0.05/0.75/0.125
Nelova 10/11	Warner-Chilcott	Ethinyl estradiol	35	Norethindrone	0.5/1 mg
Nelova 1/35	Warner-Chilcott	Ethinyl estradiol	35	Norethindrone	1 mg
Jenest	Organon	Ethinyl estradiol	35	Norethindrone	0.5 mg
Brevicon	Syntex	Ethinyl estradiol	35	Norethindrone	0.5 mg
Loestrin 1/20	Parke-Davis	Ethinyl estradiol	20	Norethindrone acetate	1.0
Loestrin 1.5/30	Parke-Davis	Ethinyl estradiol	30	Norethindrone acetate	1.5
Modicon	Ortho	Ethinyl estradiol	35	Norethindrone	0.5
Ovcon-35	Mead Johnson	Ethinyl estradiol	35	Norethindrone	0.4
High-dose estrogen oral contraceptives—do not routinely use for contraception[a]					
Demulen	Searle	Ethinyl estradiol	50	Ethynodoil diacetate	1.0
Enovoid-E	Searle	Mestranol	100	Norethynodrel	2.5
Enovoid-5	Searle	Mestranol	75	Norethynodrel	5.0
Enovoid-10	Searle	Mestranol	150	Norethynodrel	9.85
Norinyl 1/50	Syntex	Mestranol	50	Norethindrone	1.0
Norinyl 1/80	Syntex	Mestranol	80	Norethindrone	1.0
Norinyl-2	Syntex	Mestranol	100	Norethindrone	2.0
Noriestrin 1/50	Parke-Davis	Ethinyl estradiol	50	Norethindrone acetate	1.0
Noriestrin 2.5/50	Parke-Davis	Ethinyl estradiol	50	Norethindrone acetate	2.5
Ortho-Novum 1/50	Ortho	Mestranol	50	Norethindrone acetate	1.0
Ortho-Novum 1.80	Ortho	Mestranol	80	Norethindrone acetate	1.0
Ortho-Novum-2	Ortho	Mestranol	100	Norethindrone	1.0
Ovcon-50	Mead-Johnson	Ethinyl estradiol	50	Norethindrone	1.0
Ovral	Wyeth	Ethinyl estradiol	50	Norgstrel	0.5
Ovulen	Searle	Mestranol	100	Ethynodiol diacetate	1.0

[a]May be used for sporadic, emergency, postcoital contraception.
[b]Twenty micrograms of ethyinyl estradiol for 21 d; 10 µg of ethyinyl estradiol for the last 5 d of a 28-pill pack.
Adapted from *The Medical Letter of Drugs and Therapeutics,* Vol. 37, Issue 941, New York, The Medical Letter, Inc., 1995; and Hatcher RA, Trussell J, Stewart F, et al. *Contraceptive technology,* 16th ed. New York: Irvington Publishers, Inc., 1994.

connective tissue disorders, migraine headaches, seizure disorders, gallbladder disease, and cholestatic jaundice of pregnancy are not contraindications to low-dose pills (77–90). The chronic disease should be optimally managed so that the teen is able to use the contraceptive of her choice.

For the healthy teen, prescribe any low-dose pill. Medications that enhance liver metabolism, such as phenytoin, carbamazepine, rifampin, and barbiturates, reduce the contraceptive efficacy of very-low-dose pills. Adolescents taking these medications should consider alternative contraception. If the teen insists on oral contraception, a pill formulation of at least 35 µg of ethinyl estradiol should be prescribed, and the teen should again be counseled about a possible slight reduction in contraceptive efficacy compared with an individual not taking a liver-enzyme-inducing medication (Tables 22.2 and 22.3).

COCs containing less than 50 mg of estrogen have a low incidence of serious side effects, such as venous and arterial thromboembolism (91–93). The original data on the relationship between COCs and pulmonary emboli relate to older, high-dose pills (91,94,

95). Recent data indicate that risk for venous thromboembolism among users of COCs containing desogestrel or gestodene may be higher than the risk associated with low-dose pills containing first- or second-generation progestins (96–99). Much of this excess risk has been attributed to prescribing bias, i.e., the tendency to prescribe the lowest dose and newer pills to individuals with familial risk for venous thromboembolic disease. Even if the excess risk is real with third-generation progestins, the *absolute* risk for venous thromboembolic disease is low (100,101); pills con-

TABLE 22.2. *Combined (estrogen/progestin) contraceptives: interactions with other drugs*

Commonly used or prescribed drugs	Adverse effects	Comments and recommendations
Analgesics Acetaminophen (Tylenol)	Possible decreased pain-relieving effect (increased drug excretion)	Monitor pain-relieving response
Antibiotics (griseofulvin* and rifampin) (no documented clinical effect or significance has been established for penicillins, tetracyclines, cephalosporins, and other commonly used antibiotics. Hormonal methods may be used and no backup method is routinely necessary with these antibiotics.)	Decreased contraceptive effect with low-dose COCs	Help client chose another method or use higher estrogen pill (50 µg EE) or backup method (e.g., condoms)*
Antidepressants (Elavil, Norpramin, Tofranil, and others)	Possible increased antidepressant effect	Use with caution. Low COC doses are probably safe. Monitor antidepressant levels and effects
Antihypertensives (Aldomet and others)	Possible increased antihypertensive effect	Use COCs and monitor BP
Antiseizure Barbiturates (phenobarbitol and others) Carbamazepine (Tegretol) Phenytoin (Dilatin) Primidone (Mysoline)	Decreased contraceptive effect with COCs Possible increase phenytoin effect	Help client choose another method or use higher dose (at least 35 µg EE) or backup method .
Beta blockers (Cogard, Inderal, Lopressor, Tenormin)	Possible increased beta-blocker effect	Monitor cardiovascular status
Bronchodilators Theophylline (Bronkotabs, Primatene, Theo-Dur, and others)	Increased theophylline effect	Monitor for symptoms of theophylline overdose
Hypoglycemia (Diabinese, Orinase, Tolbutamide, Tolinase)	Possible decreased hypoglycemic effect	Monitor blood glucose as for any diabetic patient
Tranquilizers Benzodiazepine (Ativan, Librium, Serax, Tranxene, Xanax, and others)	Possible increase or decreased tranquilizer effects including psychomotor impairment	Use with caution. Commonly prescribed dosages are unlikely to result in significant effects.

*Because griseofulvin usually is used only for a short period of time (2–4 wk), women taking it for fungal infections can continue to use combined oral contraceptives (COCs) with a backup method.

Adapted from Rizack MA. *The medical letter handbook of adverse drug interactions.* New Rochelle, NY; *The Medical Letter*, 1995; and Blumenthal PD, McIntosh N. In: Oliveras E, Riseborough PA, Davis C (eds). *Pocketguide for family planning service providers.* Baltimore, MD: JHPIEGO Corp., 1995:112–113.

TABLE 22.3. *Caution!*

	Explanations/management issues
History of thrombophlebitis associated with IV drug use, immobilization, or trauma	Estrogen promoted thromboembolic phenomenon. COCs are only contraindicated in individuals at risk for future thromboembolic phenomenon.
Elevated liver function enzymes; history of cholestatic jaundice of pregnancy	COCs are metabolized by the liver and affect liver function. Once the liver function tests have stabilized—Ex. Chronic hepatitis with history of elevated liver function tests: COCs can be prescribed.
Migraine headaches; hypertension Diabetes mellitus	Prescribe the COC. Adjust diabetic, antihypertensive and antimigraine medication to control these medical disorders.
Sickle cell disease	Progestins stabilize the red blood cell membrane and thereby decrease the sickling. Risk of thrombosis over the patient's baseline is theoretical.
Lactation	Estrogen can decrease the quantity of breast milk if lactation is not well established. The amount of hormones received by the infant has *not* been shown to adversely affect infant growth and development.
Gallbladder disease	Estrogen may worsen the symptoms of women with gallbladder disease.
Taking rifampin or antiseizure medication except valproic acid	These medications increase metabolism of COCs and thereby may decrease contraceptive efficacy.

Adapted from Hatcher RA, Tressel J, Stewart GK, et al. *Contraceptive technology*, 16th ed. Irvington Publishers, Inc, New York; 1994 and Blumenthal PD, McIntosh N. 1995; In: Oliveras E, Riseborough PA, Davis C, eds. *Pocket-guide for family planning service providers*. Baltimore, MD: JHPIEGO Corp., 1995:92–101.

taining gestodene or desogestrel may be prescribed if the teen does not have a history or risk factors for thromboembolic disease.

COC pills containing gestodene (not available in the United States), desogestrel, or norgestimate were designed to minimize the androgenic side effects (muscular weight gain, acne, oiliness of the skin, adverse effects on the lipid profile, and carbohydrate tolerance) seen with earlier progestins such as levonorgestrel, norethindrone, or ethynodiol diacetate. Progestins found in oral contraceptives are derived from 19-nortestosterone. The first- and second-generation progestins tend to retain more androgenic effects than the third-generation progestins. Current data indicate that pill formulations containing norgestimate, desogestrel, or gestodene are associated with less oiliness of the skin and improved acne (102). The data are less convincing with respect to clinical improvement of carbohydrate tolerance and lipid profile (103–107). Data indicate that even

with the older progestins, there is little adverse *clinical* outcome with respect to lipid and carbohydrate profile, as long as the chronic disease is controlled (107–114).

Even low-dose pills continue to be associated with nuisance side effects such as weight gain, nausea, breast tenderness, acne, mood changes, and breakthrough bleeding (Table 22.4). The adolescent should be warned about side effects. She should be reassured that these side effects usually will subside within the first 3 months of use. Assure her that her pill formulation will be changed if she has continued problems after approximately 3 months of continuous use (Fig. 22.1). Considering that an estimated 50% of pill discontinuations occur because of side effects (4,20,21, 115), it is important to inquire about side effects and to carefully consider side effect impact on user satisfaction. The particular pill formulation should be tailored to the teen as much as possible, if bothersome side effects

TABLE 22.4. *Common side effect concerns*

Estrogen-related side effects
  Nausea
  Breast growth
  Leukorrhea
  Breast tenderness
  Fluid retention/bloating
  Headaches
Progestin-related side effects
  Headaches
  Breast tenderness
  Increased appetite
  Decreased libido
  Acne/oily skin[a]
  Hirsutism[a]

[a]These androgenic side effects may be minimized by prescribing a pill containing either desogestrel, norgestimate, or gestodene.

are encountered (Table 22.5). For example, a low-dose pill containing a less androgenic progestin, such as desogestrel or norgestrel, should be prescribed if acne is a problem. A monophasic pill should be prescribed if the teen occasionally misses pills (115,116). Teens who miss pills should be informed about emergency contraception (see section on Emergency Contraception).

The noncontraceptive benefit of oral contraceptive use should be stressed. These include reduced risk of ovarian cancer, endometrial cancer, anemia, menorrhagia, dysmenorrhea, functional ovarian cysts, benign breast disease, and pelvic inflammatory disease (117–121). These noncontraceptive health benefits form the basis for therapeutic

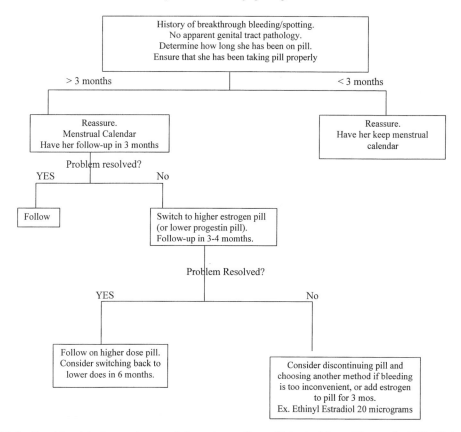

Management of Bleeding/Spotting on COCs

FIG. 22.1. Combined (estrogen/progestin) contraceptives. (Adapted from Blumenthal PD, McIntosh N. In: Oliveras E, Riseborough PA, Davis C, eds. *Pocket Guide for Family Planning Service Providers.* Baltimore, MD: JHPIEGO Corp., 1995:114.)

TABLE 22.5. *Combined oral contraceptives: management of side effects and health problems*

Side effect or problem (may or may not be pill related)	Assessment	Management
Missed pills	1. Has the client missed only one pill?	No action necessary. Take two pills at next scheduled time and complete pack as usual.
	2. Has client missed two consecutive pills?	Instruct her to take two pills on the day she remembers that two pills have been missed, two pills the next day, then one pill every day afterwards (28-d pack). Use backup method for the remainder of the cycle.
	3. Has client missed more than two consecutive pills?	Instruct her to stop taking her pills and wait for withdrawal bleed. If she does not bleed, rule out pregnancy. If she bleeds, she should begin a new pack of pills on the Sunday after the bleed begins (Sunday start). Revise the start day if you or your client desires a day 1 or day 5 start.
		Instruct her to use a backup method for the first pack of pills.
High blood pressure	Recheck blood pressure on three visits, 1 week apart.	If blood pressure remains consistently elevated, treat the elevated blood pressure or discontinue the COCs and help the client choose a nonhormonal method.
Nausea/dizziness/vomiting (usually improves during the first 3 mos)	1. Find out if pills are taken in the morning or on an empty stomach. 2. Exclude pregnancy. 3. None of the above?	Take with evening meal or before bedtime. If pregnant, manage as "amenorrhea" section. Counsel that the symptom(s) will probably decrease with time or switch to a lower estrogen pill or a progestin-only method.
Amenorrhea (absence or bleeding or spotting)	1. Ask how she has been taking her pills. Has she missed any pills in the cycle?	Missed pills or pills taken late increase risk of pregnancy. Obtain a pregnancy test, if this has been the case. Clients on 21-d packets may forget to leave a pill-free week for menses. If pills are taken continuously, amenorrhea may result. This is not harmful.
	2. Rule out pregnancy by symptoms, physical examination and pregnancy test	If intrauterine pregnancy is confirmed, counsel client regarding options. If client elects to continue the pregnancy, stop COCs and assure her that the small dose of estrogen and progestin in the COCs to which she was exposed will have no harmful effect on the fetus.
	3. Is she using a low-estrogen pill (20–35 μg or less of ethinyl estradiol)?	If the client is taking COCs correctly, reassure. Explain that absent menses is most likely due to lack of buildup of uterine lining; no menstrual blood is present. If the client is unsatisfied, try a 50-μg estrogen pill if there are no conditions requiring caution. Alternatively, choose a pill with the same estrogen dose but lower progestin dose.
	4. Has she stopped taking the pill?	If she is not pregnant, explain that if her periods were irregular before beginning COCs, they usually will become irregular when COCs are stopped and may take some months to return. If she goes back on COCs, her periods will become regular and remain regular as long as her endometrium does not become atrophic.
Spotting or bleeding between periods (common during the first 3 months after starting the pill)	1. Has the client recently begun COCs?	Reassure. Spotting and bleeding decrease markedly in most women by the fourth month of use.
	2. Ask if she has missed one or more pills or if she takes pills at different times every day.	If yes, instruct according to "Missed Pills" and advise to take pill at the same time each day. If no, switch to a higher estrogen pill (50 μg of ethinyl estradiol) for several cycles until spotting resolves. Then, return to lower dose pill (see Fig. 1, "Management of Bleeding/Spotting on COCs)."

(continued)

TABLE 22.5. *Continued*

Side effect or problem (may or may not be pill related)	Assessment	Management
	3. Exclude gynecologic problems, e.g., tumor, pregnancy, abortion, pelvic inflammatory disease, vaginitis.	If gynecologic problems are present, refer or manage according to clinic practice.
	4. Is client taking new medicine (e.g., rifampin)?	She may require a higher dose COC. Use higher dose pill (EE, 50 µg), switch to injectable (Depo-Provera) or nonhormonal method, or use backup method (e.g., condoms).
Headaches	1. Are the headaches severe, frequent, or associated with nausea? Has she had loss of speech, numbness, weakness, tingling, or visual changes associated with the headaches?	Refer if "yes" answer is associated with any of these symptoms. Discontinue COC; help client make informed choice of a progestin-only or nonhormonal method. If not severe, frequent, or associated with nausea, reassure, and treat with a nonsteroidal anti-inflammatory drug.
	2. Has she ever had high blood pressure?	Regardless of history, check the blood pressure. If elevated, see "High Blood Pressure" section.
	3. Have the headaches become worse since she began the pill?	If worse on COCs, switch to progestin-only or nonhormonal contraceptive method. If no worse or better, explore the cause of headaches. COCs can be continued unless neurologic symptoms or signs develop, or headaches worsen on COCs.
	Does she have nasal drip or tenderness in area of sinuses?	Treat for sinusitis. Continue pill.
Breast fullness or tenderness (usually improves within three mos of starting COCs)	1. Determine whether client is pregnant by history, pelvic examination, and/or pregnancy test.	If pregnant, manage as in "Amenorrhea" section.
	2. Determine whether the woman has breast lumps or nipple discharge suspicious for cancer.	If physical examination shows a lump or a discharge suspicious for cancer, refer to appropriate source for diagnosis. If malignancy is discovered, help her make an informed choice of another method.
	3. If she is breastfeeding and breasts are tender, examine for breast infection.	If breasts are not infected, recommend appropriate clothing for support. If breast infection is present, prescribe warm compresses. Prescribe antibiotics. Advise to continue breastfeeding.
	4. Ask whether the client notices this only at a certain time of the month.	Decrease estrogen in pill if not already on lowest estrogen COC. Advise client to avoid caffeine and chocolate. If the lowest does pill is unacceptable and symptomatic management not helpful, assist client to make an informed choice of progestin-only or other method.
Depression	Ask about causes (e.g., family, job, financial, or social problems).	Counsel, treat, or refer as appropriate. Work with the provide treating the depression to get the depression under control. If depression worsens on COCs, help client make informed choice of a nonhormonal method. If COC has not caused depression to worsen, the pills can be continued.

COC, combined oral contraceptive.
Adapted from Blumenthal PD, McIntosh N. In: Oliveras E, Riseborough PA, Davis C, eds. Baltimore, MD: JHPIEGO Corp., 1995:104–111.

uses of oral contraceptives in instances of dysfunctional uterine bleeding, iron deficiency anemia associated with menorrhagia, hypothalamic amenorrhea with associated osteoporosis, dysmenorrhea, mittelschmerz, polycystic ovarian syndrome, acne, recurrent functional cysts, and family history of ovarian cancer (20,21,122,123). Another advantage of the COC is that it is not a coitally related method. COC pills also can be used to delay menses (Table 22.6). Levonorgestrel-containing pills can be used as emergency contraception (see section on Emergency Contraception).

Data regarding the relationship between oral contraceptive use and cervical cancer have been contradictory. Detection bias and inappropriate comparison groups confounded earlier cervical cancer studies. Recent studies show there may be a slight increase in risk (67,124,125). If the risk for cervical cancer is increased, the absolute magnitude of the increase is small (67). Presence or history of cervical dysplasia is not a contraindication to oral contraceptive use. Overall risk of breast cancer (occurring at all ages) is not increased among current or former users of oral contraceptives (67,126–128). Subgroup analysis of breast cancer data shows that oral contraceptive users are at a slightly increased risk (odds ratio of 1.4; 95% confidence interval 1.0 to 2.1) of breast cancer that occurs before age 45 years (67,128–131). Because breast cancer is very rare in those under age 45 years, the absolute risk is minimal.

Disadvantages for the adolescent are that the pill must be taken every day, preferably at the same time each day; the cost of the pills can be prohibitive to the teen unless she is covered by a prescription plan, has a substantial source of income, or is a patient in a federally subsidized family planning program; and lack of protection against STDs. Although there is evidence that the pill provides protection against upper genital tract disease (pelvic inflammatory disease) (121), this does not lessen the need for condom use to prevent STDs.

For teens, it is prudent to prescribe a 28-day rather than a 21-day pill-pack. Taking a pill every day tends to encourage pill compliance and prevent extension of the progestin-free interval beyond the recommended 7 days. Recommendations to begin the first pack of pills on the first day, fifth day, or Sunday after menses begins are designed to minimize starting the pill in someone who is already pregnant. The pill may be begun at any time as long as pregnancy is ruled out. This becomes an important principle for those switching from other hormonal methods who may be experiencing amenorrhea. If the pill is accidentally begun during the first trimester of pregnancy, the teen can be reassured that first-trimester pill use does not increase teratogenic risk (65–67). Return of fertility usually occurs within 3 months of pill discontinuation (66–67).

In a normally menstruating adolescent who is contemplating intercourse, the pill may be

TABLE 22.6. *Combined oral contraceptives*

How to prescribe combined oral contraceptives
 New start—never been on COCs before
  Prescribe any low-dose COC (<50 µg ethinyl estradiol)
 New start—history of COCs in the past
  If no problems with a previously prescribed low-dose pill, prescribe the previous COC.
  If problems (bothersome side effects) prescribe a combination pill, which should minimize the
   bothersome side effect (see Tables 5 and 6 for guidance).
 Switcher—problems with current COCs
  Prescribe a combination pill, which should minimize the bothersome side effects
How to delay bleeding (vacation or other inopportune time for bleeding)
 Advise the woman to not take hormone-free pills or adhere to the pill-free interval. She should immediately
  begin a new pack of pills on the day 22 of a 28-d pack. If using a 21-day pack, she begins a new pack
  without waiting for 7 d to elapse.

begun without performing a pelvic examination. In these situations, the pelvic examination usually is deferred until after intercourse has occurred. The usual time period of deferment is 3 months. Remember, the purpose of the pelvic examination is to rule out gynecologic abnormalities, which are unlikely if she is menstruating normally and has not been exposed to sexual intercourse. The adolescent should be advised of the need for an annual pelvic examination, with screening for cervical cancer and other STDs. Counseling for oral contraceptives should include failure rate, side effects, noncontraceptive health benefits, mechanism of action, how to take the pill, what to do if a pill(s) is missed, and safety, reversibility, and need for condom use for STD protection. Depending on the teen and her circumstances, this information should be tailored and timed to the teen's needs.

The progestin-only "mini-pill" generally is reserved for lactating patients or patients who are unable to take estrogen. Very few teens will be medically unable to take estrogen. In addition to decreased effectiveness, progestin-only pills have the disadvantage of more frequent and persistent, irregular bleeding episodes. Whereas the efficacy of COCs is approximately 24 hours per pill, the efficacy of progestin-only pills is approximately 20 to 24 hours. The mini-pill is less forgiving of missed pills; the pregnancy rate associated with missed pills among mini-pill users is quite high. Because of the high incidence of irregular bleeding and higher pregnancy rates, mini-pills are not well suited for teens.

Depo-Provera

Medroxyprogesterone acetate (Depo-Provera) is a first-generation, long-acting injectable progestin contraceptive. Depo-Provera 150 mg via deep intramuscular injection provides contraceptive efficacy for 3 months. Depo-Provera produces consistent and complete ovulatory inhibition, increases cervical mucus viscosity, and causes endometrial atrophy (132–135). The 1-year failure rate is 0.3% (134). Although Depo-Provera is available in formulations of 150 and 400 mg/dL, only the 150-mg formulation should be used for contraception. The 150-mg formulation has greater bioavailability and is associated with the low failure rate cited. Usual administration is in the deltoid or gluteal muscle, using a 1.5-inch needle to ensure deep injection. The injected site should not be massaged, as efficacy depends on the concentration of the drug within the area of injection. Ideally, the initial injection of Depo-Provera is given within 5 days of onset of normal menses, immediately postpartum in the adolescent who is not breastfeeding, or immediately postabortion. Current guidelines recommend beginning this method 6 weeks postpartum in the lactating individual (136). When administered during time periods other than those described, pregnancy should be ruled out before injection, and a backup form of contraception should be used for the first 2 weeks after initial injection. If injection inadvertently occurs during early pregnancy, the adolescent, her partner, and her parents can be reassured that Depo-Provera is not a teratogen (132,135). Although efficacy can last as long as 14 weeks, repeat injections generally are scheduled every 11 to 12 weeks to enhance compliance. If the adolescent returns more than 14 weeks after the last injection, pregnancy must be ruled out (e.g., sensitive human chorionic gonadotropin test after an appropriate interval of abstinence, usually 2 weeks from last intercourse).

The most common side effect of Depo-Provera is menstrual irregularities. Nearly all users will experience a change in menstrual pattern. Users should be educated and reassured about this, as irregular bleeding constitutes the most common reason for discontinuation. As with Norplant, this bleeding is unpredictable and eventually may result in amenorrhea. With Depo-Provera, approximately 50% of consistent users are amenorrheic at the end of the first year of use (128, 135,137). Other side effects include those related to any progestin-containing compound: headache, dizziness, abdominal bloating, mood changes, nervousness, nausea,

TABLE 22.7. *Management of Depo-Provero side effects*

Bleeding: Over time, Depo-Provera causes more complete endometrial suppression than Norplant or oral contraceptives. Traditionally, bleeding associated with Depo-Provera has been managed with estrogen:
  Premarin: 1.25 mg daily for approximately 14 d
  Ethinyl estradiol: 50 µg daily for approximately 14 d
  (135A)

For management of other side effects, refer to "Management of Norplant® Side Effects."

weight gain, acne, mastalgia, hirsutism, and hair loss. As with other forms of hormonal contraception, most of these nonmenstrual side effects are short lived. Side effects may be managed symptomatically, according to recommendations listed for management of Depo-Provera side effects (Table 22.7).

Depo-Provera is not the ideal choice for anyone who desires pregnancy within the next 1 to 2 years, because as many as 30% of users may fail to conceive within the first 12 months after discontinuation. Return to fertility may be delayed as long as 18 months in some users (132–135). Adolescents at risk for osteoporosis (e.g., chronic steroid users, amenorrheic athletes) should consider another contraceptive. Recent studies document reversible loss in bone density among Depo-Provera users (138–140); however, none of these studies showed an increase in clinical fractures (141–143).

Although side effects and contraindications related to the estrogenic content of oral contraceptives are not relevant to Depo-Provera, the package insert of Depo-Provera contains almost identical contraindications as those stated for COCs (Table 22.8) (136). Contra-

TABLE 22.8. *Depo-Provera absolute contraindications*

1. *Active* thrombophlebitis, thromboembolic disorder, or past history of thrombophlebetic disorder or cerebrovascular disease
2. Undiagnosed, abnormal genital bleeding
3. Known or suspected pregnancy
4. Acute liver disease: benign or malignant liver tumors
5. Known or suspected malignancy of the breast

indications that are stated for Depo-Provera, yet have been shown to be related to estrogen, include active thrombophlebitis, or current or past history of thromboembolic disorders or cerebral vascular disease.

The noncontraceptive health benefits of Depo-Provera include protection against endometrial cancer (144,145), reduced incidence of iron deficiency anemia, dysmenorrhea, mittelschmerz, and ovarian cysts (146,147). In women with sickle cell anemia, Depo-Provera has been shown to increase hematocrit and to be associated with fewer crises (148,149). Depo-Provera may be the hormonal contraceptive of choice for women with seizure disorders, because contraceptive efficacy is not compromised by antiseizure medication, and some studies indicate that Depo-Provera may increase seizure threshold (150–152). Although Depo-Provera appears to protect against upper genital tract STDs (132,146, 147), it does not protect against lower genital tract diseases. At-risk users should use condoms for STD protection.

Counseling points for Depo-Provera include failure rate, side effects, mechanism of action, safety, reversibility, noncontraceptive benefits, and lack of protection against acquired lower genital tract STDs. Users should be encouraged to return at least every 3 months for reinjection and on an annual basis for gynecologic examination, including, as indicated, cervical cancer screening and STD screening.

Norplant

Approved by the FDA in December 1990, Norplant is the only implantable contraceptive method available in the United States. Norplant is a long-acting, levonorgestrel-containing contraceptive designed to be implanted subdermally in the upper arm. Each of the six matchstick-sized capsules is 34 mm long and 2.4 mm in diameter and contains 36 mg of levonorgestrel. Once steady-state serum levels are obtained, approximately 30 µg of levonorgestrel is released per day (153). The failure rate is 0.2% in the first year of use (154). Contraceptive efficacy lasts for 5 years (153,154).

Although Norplant's serum levonorgestrel concentrations vary according to body weight and individual clearance rate, there are no weight restrictions to Norplant use. Earlier studies using capsules not available in the United States revealed that the lowest failure rates occurred in patients weighing less than 50 kg. The 5-year cumulative failure rate for patients weighing less than 50 kg was 0.2 per 100 users. The failure rate rose to 8.5 for patients weighing 70 kg or more (154). It should be noted, however, that a 5-year cumulative pregnancy rate of 8.5 per 100 users is still less than the cumulative 5-year pregnancy rate for typical users of oral contraceptives (21).

Norplant capsules used in the United States are a modification of the original Silastic capsules used in early testing (155). Current data show that diffusion of hormone from these new capsules is improved (155); failure rates are consistent across weight classes. Heavier adolescents and women should not be denied access to Norplant because of weight greater than 50 kg.

Norplant prevents pregnancy primarily through thickening of the cervical mucus and atrophic effects on the endometrial lining (153). Because serum levels of levonorgestrel are low, ovulation is inconsistently inhibited. The steady, low levels of levonorgestrel also result in this method's primary side effect, irregular bleeding. Menstrual irregularities may include prolonged bleeding during the first months of use, unexpected bleeding, spotting between periods, or amenorrhea (156,157). Varying degrees of these cycle changes may last a year or more. Although frequency of bleeding may be increased, blood loss usually is less than that of normal menses (153). Hemoglobin levels tend to rise among Norplant users (153,155,158). Other side effects are those common to progestin-containing compounds, including headache, nervousness, nausea, dizziness, acne, change in appetite, weight gain, mastalgia, hirsutism, and hair loss. With the exception of change in

menstrual pattern, these side effects tend to be short lived. None can be predicted based on user profile or experience with other hormonal methods. Although not medically serious, these side effects may account for a substantial percentage of discontinuations. For the user who likes the method but dislikes the side effects, attempts can be made to symptomatically treat the side effects (Table 22.9). Clinical research indicates that users who were properly counseled about side effects before Norplant insertion tended to continue the method (159–162). Both adolescents and adults have registered user satisfaction and high continuation rates (159,160).

Because it contains no estrogen, the safety profile of Norplant is better than that of COCs. Contraindications listed on the package label are almost identical to those for oral contraceptives (Table 22.10). As with Depo-Provera, the contraindication regarding thromboembolic disorders has no scientific rationale (see section on Depo-Provera). As with low-dose oral contraceptives, medications that enhance liver metabolism, such as phenytoin, carbamazepine, rifampin, and barbiturates, reduce the contraceptive efficacy of Norplant. Adolescents taking these medications should consider alternative contraception.

There has been no evidence of adverse cardiovascular, respiratory, or central nervous system disorder(s) as a result of Norplant (153). Once the implant system is removed, return to fertility is quite rapid and comparable to rates seen after discontinuation of barrier methods. Because of the cervical mucus effect, a modicum of protection against upper genital tract STDs is expected. This protection, similar to that seen with oral contracep-

TABLE 22.9. *Norplant absolute contraindications*

1. *Active* thrombophlebitic or thromboembolic disorder
2. Undiagnosed, abnormal genital bleeding
3. Known or suspected pregnancy
4. *Acute* liver disease; benign or malignant liver tumors
5. Known or suspected carcinoma of the breast

TABLE 22.10. *Management of Norplant side effects*

Although most Norplant side effects are short lived and can be managed symptomatically, the provider must not force the woman to endure disconcerting side effects. If the woman desires removal, remove the Norplant.

Headaches
   a. Determine preinsertion versus postinsertion headache frequency and characteristics. Determine history of migraine headaches, cluster headache, tension headache, and oral contraceptive-related and/or menstrual-related headaches before insertion.
   b. Physical examination.
      Funduscopic exam for papilledema.
   c. Trial on nonsteroidal antiinflammatory drugs
   d. Neurology consultation, if the patient does not respond to nonsteroidal antiinflammatory drugs.

Alopecia
   a. Determine onset of alopecia with timing of insertion.
   b. Remember postpartum hair loss occurs naturally in some women.
   c. Determine cultural perceptions about hair loss.
   d. Determine the hair treatment products used by individual and whether there has been any change in hair treatment products.
   e. Consider dermatology consultation.

Mastalgia
   a. Supportive bra.
      Discontinue methylzanthines, such as coffee, tea, cola, and caffeine.
      Vitamin E 400 IU bid.
   b. Danazol 200 mg qd or bromocriptine 2.5 mg qd or tamoxifen 20 mg qd.

Weight change
   a. Meal diary, activity diary, and nutritional consultation.

Acne
   a. Antibacterial soap, topical antibiotic (Erycette pads bid), Retin A cream qhs.
   b. Dermatology consultation.

Bloating
   a. Herbal diuretic tea.
   b. Consider diuretic during time period of bloating.

Abdominal pain
   Evaluate as one would evaluate any form of abdominal pain.
   Obtain studies as indicated based on the history and physical examination.

Prolonged or frequent bleeding
   a. Currently, there are few published studies that assesses the treatment of frequent or prolonged bleeding on Norplant (160, 160A, 160B).
   b. The patient with prolonged and/or frequent bleeding needs a history that assesses the patient's bleeding pattern, sexual activity pattern, stress and intercurrent illness, medications, and substance abuse. The physical examination should include a detailed pelvic examination to assess for other causes of bleeding, including vaginitis, genital lesions, and foreign bodies. The laboratory workup should include gonorrhea and chlamydia tests; wet prep and KOH preparation, as indicated. The clinician should *consider* a hemoglobin/hematocrit to *reassure the patient* that the bleeding has not caused a drop in these parameters.
   c. Remember the histologic pattern of the endometrium of patients on the Norplant system is generally that of suppression or a mixed picture. Routine transvaginal sonogram or endometrial biopsy is *not* recommended.
   d. *Treatment regimens*
      1. Ibuprofen 800 mg tid × 5 d.
      2. Any ≤50 µg ethinyl estradiol, preparation of a combined oral contraceptive pill pack.
      3. Ethinyl estradiol 50 µg qd × 20 or 21 d.
   e. The minipill is not predictive of how a patient will react to the Norplant system. Depo-Provera is not predictive of how a patient with react to the Norplant system.

Amenorrhea
   a. Reassurance.
   b. Do not induce bleeding. Obtain a human chorionic gonadotropin level
      1. If the patient is worried about pregnancy
      2. If insertion was not within 5 to 7 d of the last menstrual period, and the patient has persistent amenorrhea
      3. If amenorrhea occurs after the establishment of regular cycles.

tives or Depo-Provera, is incomplete, and adolescents should be advised to use condoms along with the Norplant.

Insertion of Norplant is recommended within 7 days of onset of menses (154). The important issue is whether the adolescent is already pregnant. If pregnancy is ruled out, the Norplant implants can be inserted at any time during the menstrual cycle. Norplant can be inserted immediately postpartum or post-abortion (163). Current recommendations are that breastfeeding mothers wait 6 weeks postpartum before Norplant insertion (154). If Norplant is inadvertently inserted in a pregnant adolescent, the adolescent, her partner, and her parents can be reassured that Norplant is not associated with an increased risk of birth defects (153).

Counseling points for Norplant include failure rate, mechanism of action, safety, reversibility, nonprotection against STDs, and side effects. To assure continued use of this method, the adolescent should be counseled in-depth about the irregular bleeding patterns. She should be reassured that the irregular bleeding and amenorrhea seen with this method are a normal occurrence and do not indicate an abnormal condition. Original recommendations not to attempt hormonal manipulations for prolonged or frequent bleeding episodes have been modified, based on recent publications (156,157,164–166). Options for the individual experiencing bothersome irregular bleeding include ibuprofen 800 mg three times a day for 5 days; ethinyl estradiol 50 µg every day for 20 or 21 days; or any preparation of less than 50 µg ethinyl estradiol in a COC for one pill-pack.

Before prescribing any one of the regimens, the following evaluation should be performed. A history should be taken that assesses the patient's bleeding pattern, sexual activity pattern, stress and intercurrent illness, medications, and substance abuse. The physical examination should include a pelvic examination to assess other causes of bleeding, including vaginitis, genital lesions, and foreign bodies. The laboratory workup should include gonorrhea and chlamydia tests, wet prep, and KOH preparation, as indicated. The clinician should consider a hemoglobin/hematocrit if needed to reassure the patient that the bleeding has not caused anemia. The histologic pattern of the endometrium of individuals using Norplant is generally one of suppression; routine transvaginal sonogram or endometrial biopsy are not recommended. The amenorrheic Norplant user should be reassured. Bleeding should not be induced. Obtain a pregnancy test if the patient is worried about pregnancy, the insertion was not within 5 to 7 days of onset of the last menstrual period, or amenorrhea occurs after the establishment of regular cycles on Norplant.

Norplant users should return on at least an annual basis for routine pelvic examination, including, as indicated, Pap smear and screening for STDs. Initial users may benefit from visits at 3 to 6 months after insertion to assess method satisfaction. A Norplant user who desires removal should be accorded prompt and expert removal, regardless of how long she has had the implants.

This promising contraceptive method enjoyed an initial flurry of demand that abated in a cloud of public relations and legal controversy in the United States. The controversy surrounds three issues: the Silastic content of the capsules, removal difficulties, and known side effects. Even though Silastic has been used safely for more than 40 years in intracorporeal applications (e.g., heart valves, sterilization rings), litigation was brought based on its similarity to silicone, previously used in breast implants. To date, there is no proof that Silastic used for implantable capsules is harmful. Removal difficulties stem from incorrect placement; both removal and insertion require training in a specific, minor surgical technique. When Norplant is inserted as directed, removal problems are rare. The side effects associated with Norplant (discussed in detail earlier) are those that one would expect of a low-dose, progestin-only contraception; they may be bothersome but they are not life threatening. Despite Norplant's safety profile and the satisfaction enjoyed by some users, reduction in demand has resulted in termination of distribution in Great Britain (news article). Norplant continues to be available in the United States.

FUTURE CONTRACEPTIVE METHODS

Given the current political climate and recent experiences with Norplant, it is difficult to predict which contraceptive methods will come to market soon in the United States. Methods that are already available in other parts of the world include injectable microspheres and capsules, vaginal rings, and the levonorgestrel and frameless IUDs (neither IUD would tend to be appropriate for most adolescents, see later). Methods that are now part of the FDA approval process include Lunelle, the monthly injectable that contains both estrogen (estradiol cypionate 5 mg) and progestin (medroxyprogesterone acetate 25 mg); Implanon, the Silastic capsule that contains desogestrel and is effective for 3 years; Norplant II, the two-capsule levonorgestrel-containing system that is effective for at least 3 years; Evra, a weekly estrogen/progestin skin patch; and FemCap and Lea Shield barrier contraceptives. It is anticipated that Lunelle (probably available in 2000) will be the first new method available for general use. The Lunelle injectable is designed to minimize the irregular bleeding associated with progestin-only contraceptives. Users typically can expect regular bleeding episodes, approximately once a month, after several months of continuous use.

Research is also under way for additional synthetic male condom materials. Current research is very active in the area of microbicides, yet most investigators believe that a viable microbicide will not be available for years.

CONTRACEPTIVE METHODS NOT SUITABLE FOR ADOLESCENTS

The two methods least suitable for adolescents include sterilization and the IUD. Because of the increased risk of pelvic inflammatory disease among IUD users exposed to sexually transmissible pathogens, the IUD is an inappropriate method for most adolescents. If the adolescent is in a long-term, mutually monogamous relationship (married and confident about monogamy) and has a child, then she may be a candidate for the IUD. Tubal sterilization should not be considered a reversible procedure and thus should not be performed in teens. Because of their tendency toward irregular menses, anovulatory cycles, poor motivation, and discomfort with methods that require extensive genital manipulation, most teens are poor candidates for natural family planning methods, i.e., rhythm, basal body temperature method, mucus method, or symptothermal method.

PREGNANT ADOLESCENTS

One of the most disconcerting situations a gynecologic health professional faces is the pregnant adolescent. Pregnant teens need to be advised of all options: (a) childbearing with raising the infant, (b) childbearing with adoption, and (c) abortion. The teen should be referred to appropriate counseling and service facilities, pending the chosen option. As much as possible, she should be encouraged to fully contemplate the implications of her decision within the context of her and her own family's future.

ABORTION

Approximately 1.3 million legal abortions are performed each year in the United States (167,168). Approximately 20% of all abortions occur among women younger than age 20 years (168). The percentage of pregnancies terminated by abortions is approximately 45% among adolescents aged 15 to 19 years (13). For adolescents, the recent decrease in unintended pregnancies was reflected in a reduction in the adolescent abortion rate (169). This reduction in unintended pregnancies and in elective abortions is thought to be secondary to increased condom use, increased use of longer-acting contraceptive methods such as injectables and implants, and increased tendency (compared to earlier time periods) of adolescents to give birth.

Recriminalization of abortion would have a tremendous impact on adolescent childbearing. Using statistical modeling, Joyce and Mocan (170) estimate that if legal abortion were banned in New York City, adolescent births would rise by 18.7% among blacks and 14.0% among whites. Most laws restricting adolescent access to fertility control services are levied from the state level; therefore, it is important to know the laws of the state in which the clinician practices.

Abortion continues to be much safer than childbirth overall. The risk of death from an abortion is approximately 0.6 per 100,000 cases (171). The safest abortions are those done in the first trimester. The death rate from an abortion performed at 8 weeks' gestation or less is 0.4 deaths per 100,000 procedures. This rate increases to 6.9 deaths at 16 to 20 weeks' gestation (171).

As of 1997, approximately 163 U.S. medical facilities offered early nonsurgical abortions (167). In 1995, as part of the FDA approval process, experimental protocols with mifepristone and prostaglandin for termination of gestations less than 63 days from the last menstrual period had begun. These protocols did not include adolescents. Successful termination of first-trimester pregnancies up to 9 weeks' estimated gestational age have been reported with oral mifepristone 200 or 600 mg followed approximately 2 days later with oral misoprostol 400, 600, or 800 μg, or intravaginal misoprostol 800 μg (172). Success rates are highest with earlier gestation. In a recent U.S. study by Spitz et al. (173), success was 92% for gestations through 49 days from the last menstrual period; 83% for gestations from 50 through 56 days; and 77% for gestations 57 through 63 days. The regimen used consisted of mifepristone 600 mg followed 2 days later with oral misoprostol 400 μg. Common side effects/experiences include abdominal pain, nausea, vomiting, diarrhea, and vaginal bleeding. Within 24 hours of misoprostol dosing, 75% of women had experienced completion of termination (173).

Median duration of bleeding or spotting was 13 to 15 days, depending on gestational age. A total of 10% of women bled or spotted for 30 to 60 days. Transfusions were performed in 0.2% of participants (four of 2,015) (173). The experience reported by Spitz et al. is consistent with experiences with mifepristone and misoprostol in Europe (174). It is anticipated that the mifepristone method will be available for general use in the United States in 2000.

Delays in approval of mifepristone have led clinical researchers to investigate other regimens for medical abortion. Experimental medical abortion methods that currently are undergoing safety and efficacy trials in the United States include off-label use of methotrexate and misoprostol, and tamoxifen and misoprostol. Methotrexate 50 mg/m^2 via intramuscular injection, followed 7 days later by misoprostol 800 μg intravaginally, has resulted in an 88% successful termination rate among gestations through 56 days (175). This regimen resulted in prolonged time to completion of termination compared with other methods (175). Only 65% of women aborted within 24 hours of the first or second dose of misoprostol. The delay among the remaining 23% of women was 23.5 ± 9.1 days. Side effects/experiences included nausea, vomiting, diarrhea, headache, dizziness, and subjective fever/chills. Average number of bleeding days was 14 ± 7 days in the immediate aborters and 11 ± 9 days among the delayed aborters (175). Creinin's results are similar to those of other studies (176,177).

A small initial study used tamoxifen 20 mg daily for 4 days followed 4 days later with intravaginal placement of four saline-moistened tablets of misoprostol 200 μg. The misoprostol dose was repeated if abortion did not occur within 24 hours. Complete abortion occurred in 92% of participants: 4% after tamoxifen, 85% after one dose of misoprostol, and 3% after a second dose of misoprostol (178). Common side effects/experiences included abdominal pain, bleeding, nausea, vomiting, and diarrhea.

Regardless of the medical abortion technique used, none is 100% effective. The incidence of incomplete termination, no matter how small, requires the backup measure of surgical evacuation for unsuccessful medical abortion termination attempts. Any provider of medical abortion, therefore, must have access to surgical uterine evacuation through personal provision of the service or referral.

First-trimester Abortion

Most first-trimester abortions are performed by suction curettage (synonymous with vacuum curettage and vacuum aspiration). Suction curettage can be accomplished either through the use of an electromechanical suction machine or through a manual vacuum aspirator. Whether using electrical suction aspiration, manual vacuum aspiration, or sharp curettage (not recommended for termination procedures because of the volume of products of conception and the increased risk of perforation), the cervix is dilated and the uterine contents are evacuated. Whereas many providers are familiar with and proficient in the use of electrical vacuum aspiration, few providers in the United States are familiar with and use manual vacuum aspiration. The system involves a 60-cc hand-held syringe vacuum and flexible cannulas of increasing diameter for increasing gestational age (179). For nulliparous patients greater than 10 weeks' gestational age, initial cervical dilation usually is accomplished using a hydroscopic cervical dilator such as a Laminaria stent. The use of these hydroscopic devices minimizes the incidence of cervical trauma possible during rapid operative dilation. Almost all first-trimester procedures are performed using local rather than general anesthesia. The incidence of uterine perforation, intraabdominal hemorrhage, and cervical trauma is less in women receiving local anesthesia (180,181).

The complication rate of first-trimester abortion is low. Complications include hemorrhage (transfusion rate of 0.6 per 100 abortions) (181), hematometra (0.2 to 1 per 100 abortions) (182,183), coagulopathy (8 per 100,000 cases) (184), perforation of the uterus (0.2 per 100 procedures) (181,185), cervical injury (0.18 to 0.96 per 100 abortions) (181,185), retained products of conception (0.61 cases per 100 abortions) (181), and infection (0.75 per 100 procedures) (181). The risk of fatal pulmonary embolus is extremely low for first-trimester abortions (184).

Studies in the United States have not shown a reduction in fertility among patients who have undergone first-trimester abortion (186). Chung et al. (187) did not find an increase in frequency of fetal wastage among women with prior legal abortions. Results have varied as to increased risk of premature deliveries (188).

Second-trimester Abortion

Approximately 25% of abortions performed in adolescents less than age 15 years and approximately 16% of abortions among those ages 15 to 19 years are second-trimester abortions. Second-trimester abortions comprise approximately 11% of the total abortions performed in the United States (168, 180). Second-trimester abortions are attended by higher mortality and morbidity than first-trimester abortions. The risk of major complications is between 5% and 18% (189). This complication rate is significantly lower, however, than that for childbirth (189). Adolescents are not at increased risk for developing major complications (189).

There are many different methods of performing second-trimester abortions. The two most common types of second trimester abortions are (a) dilation and evacuation and (b) labor-induction methods. Dilation and evacuation is performed between 13 and 16 weeks. Between 16 and 20 weeks, dilation and evacuation or a labor-induction method may be used. Both of these two major methods of pregnancy termination require hydroscopic cervical dilators such as Laminaria. In dilation and evacuation, a large suction cannula is used to drain the amniotic fluid and remove remaining placental tissue and clot after most of the uterine contents have been evacuated with long, heavy forceps. There are many different methods and variations of methods for second-trimester labor induction: intravaginal prostaglandin E_2, intramuscular 15-methyl prostaglandin α, high-dose oxytocin (Pitocin), hypertonic saline, intraamniotic urea, or a combination thereof. Complications associated with second-trimester abortions include hemorrhage, infection uterine rupture, disseminated intravascular coagulopathy (hypertonic saline, interamniotic urea, dilation and evacuation) and cervical laceration. Fortunately, major complications are rare (180,189).

The psychological impact of abortion will vary per individual. In 1989, the Surgeon General, C. Everett Koop, concluded after review of more than 250 studies that abortion is not detrimental to a woman's mental health (190).

Counseling before an abortion procedure should include pregnancy options, abortion method options, details of the procedure, expected physical experience and side effects, postabortion contraception, warning signs of postprocedure infection, indications for emergency follow-up visit, and reasons and encouragement for routine follow-up examination after the procedure. Adolescents who opt for first-trimester medical termination of pregnancy should be aware that these methods are currently deemed investigational in the United States as part of a research protocol, and she undoubtedly will need parental consent, even in states where she could give sole consent for other pregnancy-related care. She should be informed that a medical abortion takes a longer time period to complete than a surgical procedure. She should be counseled that in the event the medical procedure is unsuccessful, surgical termination is recommended, as methotrexate is a teratogen and evidence is accumulating that misoprostol also is associated with an increased incidence of fetal abnormalities (191). All adolescents should fully consider and hopefully opt for postprocedure contraception and postprocedure STD protection. Whereas abstinence is theoretically the ideal choice, the teen, her confidant, and family should realistically consider all options for STD and pregnancy prevention.

ADOLESCENT SEXUAL RESPONSIBILITY

Promotion of sexual responsibility should be the charge of all health professionals caring for adolescents. The framework of sexual responsibility includes prevention of pregnancy, STDs, and premature childbearing. Integration of an effective contraceptive method with the desire and maturational state of the adolescent often is difficult. Method or compliance failure must be backed up with childbearing or childraising alternatives.

REFERENCES

1. Olenick I. U.S. teenagers' birthrate and pregnancy rate fall during the mid-1990s. *Fam Plann Perspect* 1998; 30:292.
2. Warren CW, Santelli JS, Everett SA, et al. Sexual behavior among U.S. high school students, 1990–1995. *Fam Plann Perspect* 1998;30:170–172,200.
3. Jones EF, Forrest JD, Henshaw SK, et al. Unintended pregnancy, contraceptive practice and family planning services in developed countries. *Fam Plann Perspect* 1988;20:53–67.
4. Rosoff JI. Not just teenagers. *Fam Plann Perspect* 1988;20:52.
5. Zabin LS. Addressing adolescent sexual behavior and childbearing: self-esteem or social change? Women's Health Issues, Official Publication of the Jacobs Institute of Women's Health. 1994;492.
6. Males M. There's no such thing as "teenage sex." *PSAY Network* 1996;4:1–3.
7. Ford CA, Millstein SG, Halpern-Felsher BL, et al. Influence of physician confidentiality assurances on adolescents' willingness to disclose information and seek future health care. *JAMA* 1997;278:1029.
8. Oakley D, Denyes MJ, O'Connor N. Expanded nursing care for contraceptive use. *Appl Nurs Res* 1989;2: 121–127.
9. Zabin LS. Adolescent pregnancy: the clinician's role in intervention. *J Gen Intern Med* 1990;5:581–588.
10. Meeting the needs of young adults. *Populat Rep* 1995; Series J:3–11.
11. Kirby D. No easy answers. Washington, DC: The National Campaign to Prevent Teen Pregnancy. 1997: 3–9.
12. Moore KA, Miller BC, Sugland BW, et al. *Beginning too soon: adolescent sexual behavior, pregnancy, and parenthood.* Washington, DC: Child's Trends, Inc. 1995.
13. The Alan Guttmacher Institute. *Sex and America's teenagers.* New York: The Alan Guttmacher Institute, 1994:9–29,44–63.
14. Moore KA, Manlove J, Glei DA, et al. Nonmarital school-age motherhood: family, individual, and school characteristics. *J Adolesc Res* 1998;13:433–457.
15. Abrahamse AF, Morrison PA, Waite LJ. Teenagers willing to consider single parenthood: who is at greatest risk? *Fam Plann Perspect* 1988;20:13.
16. American Social Health Association. Sexually trans-

mitted diseases in America: how many cases and at what cost? *Kaiser Family Foundation* 1998:4–9.

17. Santelli JS, Brener ND, Lowry R, et al. Multiple sexual partners among U.S. adolescents and young adults. *Fam Plann Perspect* 1998;30:271.

18. Trussell J, Hatcher RA, Cates W, et al. Contraceptive failure in the United States: an update. *Stud Fam Plann* 1990;21:51.

19. The Alan Guttmacher Institute. Pregnancies occurring during contraceptive use. In: *Preventing pregnancy, protecting health: a new look at birth control choices in the United States.* New York: The Alan Guttmacher Institute, 1991:33.

20. Speroff L, Darney PD. *A clinical guide for contraception*, 2nd ed. Baltimore: Williams & Wilkins, 1996.

21. Hatcher RA, Trussell J, Stewart F, et al. *Contraceptive technology*, 17th rev ed. Ardent Media, Inc., New York 1998.

22. Grimes DA, ed. Which patterns may benefit from alternative contraceptive methods? *Contraceptive Report* 1990;1:7–12.

23. Goldman JA, Dicker D, Feldberg D, et al. Barrier contraception in the teenager: a comparison of four methods in adolescent girls. *Pediatr Adolesc Gynecol* 1985; 3:59.

24. Kulig JW. Adolescent contraception: non-hormonal methods. *Adolesc Gynecol* 1989;36:717.

25. Lane ME, Arceo R, Sobero AJ. Successful use of the diaphragm and jelly by a young population: report of a clinical study. *Fam Plann Perspect* 1976;8:81.

26. Donovan B. Condoms and the prevention of sexually transmissible disease. *Hosp Med* 1996;54:575–578.

27. Cook RL, Rosenberg MJ. Do spermicides containing nonoxynol-9 prevent sexually transmitted infection?: a meta-analysis. *Sex Transm Dis* 1998;25:144–150.

28. Roddy RE, Zekeng L, Ryan KA, et al. A controlled trial of nonoxynol 9 film to reduce male-to-female transmission of sexually transmitted diseases. *N Engl J Med* 1998;339:504–510.

29. Roddy RE, Schulz KF, Cates W. Microbicides, meta-analysis, and the N-9 question: where's the research? [Editorial]. *Sex Transm Dis* 1998;25:151–153.

30. Wittkowski KM, Susser E, Dietz K. The protective effect of condoms and nonoxynol-9 against HIV infection. *Am J Public Health* 1998;88:590.

31. Feldblum PJ, Weir SS, Cates W Jr. The protective effect of condoms and nonoxynol-9 against HIV infection: a response to Wittkowski and colleagues. [Letter]. *Am J Public Health* 1999;89:108

32. Roddy RE, Zekeng L, Ryan KA, et al. A controlled trial of nonoxynol 9 film to reduce male-to-female transmission of sexually transmitted diseases. *N Engl J Med* 1998;339:504.

33. Lytle CD, Routson LB, Seaborn GB, et al. An in vitro evaluation of condoms as barriers to a small virus. *Sex Transm Dis* 1997;24:161–164.

34. Bounds W. Female condoms. *Eur J Contraception Reprod Health Care* 1997;2:113–116.

35. Stone KM, Grimes DA, Magder LS. Personal protection against sexually transmitted diseases. *Am J Obstet Gynecol* 1986;155:180.

36. Conant MA, Spicer DW, Smith CD. Herpes simplex virus transmission: condom studies. *Sex Transm Dis* 1984;11:94.

37. Katznelson S, Drew WL, Mintz L. Efficacy of the condom as a barrier to the transmission of cytomegalovirus. *J Infect Dis* 1984;150:155.

38. Levy JA. Condoms prevent transmission of AID-associated retrovirus. *JAMA* 1986;255:1706.

39. Rielmeijer CA, Krebs JW, Feorino PM, et al. Condoms as physical and chemical barriers against human immunodeficiency virus. *JAMA* 1988;259:1851.

40. de Vincenzi I. A longitudinal study of human immunodeficiency virus transmission by heterosexual partners. European study group on heterosexual transmission of HIV. *N Engl J Med* 1994;11;331:391–392.

41. Richardson AC, Lyon JB. The effect of condom use on squamous cell cervical intraepithelial neoplasia. *Am J Obstet Gynecol* 1981;140:909.

42. Schirm AL, Trussell J, Menken J, et al. Contraceptive failure in the United States: the impact of social, economic and demographic factors. *Fam Plann Perspect* 1982;14:68.

43. Gillespie I. The diaphragm: an accomplice in recurrent urinary tract infections. *Urology* 1984;24:25.

44. Fihn SD, Latham RH, Roberts P, et al. Association between diaphragm use and urinary tract infection. *JAMA* 1985;254:240.

45. Foxman B, Frerichs R. Epidemiology of urinary tract infection: Diaphragm use and sexual intercourse. *Am J Public Health* 1985;75:1308.

46. Jaffe R. Toxic shock syndrome associated with diaphragm use [Letter]. *N Engl J Med* 1981;305:1585.

47. Fihn SD, Latham RH, Roberts P, et al. Association between diaphragm use and urinary tract infection. *JAMA* 1985;254:240–245.

48. Bachler EA, Dillon WP, Cumbo TJ, et al. Prolonged use of a diaphragm and toxic shock syndrome. *Fertil Steril* 1982;38:248.

49. Klitsch M. FDA approval ends cervical cap's marathon. *Fam Plann Perspect* 1988;20:137.

50. Trussell J, Vaughan B. Contraceptive failure, method-related discontinuation and resumption in use: results from the 1995 national survey of family growth. *Fam Plann Perspect* 1999;31:64–72,93.

51. Grimes DA, Cates W Jr. Family planning and sexually transmitted diseases. *Sex Transm Dis* 1990:1087.

52. Stone KM, Grimes DA, Magder LS. Personal protection against sexually transmitted diseases. *Am J Obstet Gynecol* 1986;155:180.

53. Cutler JC, Singh B, Carpenter U, et al. Vaginal contraceptives as prophylaxis against gonorrhea and other sexually transmissible disease. *Adv Plann Parenthood* 1977;12:45.

54. Hicks DR, Martin LS, Getchell JP, et al. Inactivation of HTLV III/LAV infected cultures of normal human lymphocytes by nonoxynol-9 in vitro. *Lancet* 1985;2: 1422.

55. Austin H, Louv WC, Alexander WJ. A case-control study of spermicides and gonorrhea. *JAMA* 1984;251: 2822.

56. Weir SS, Feldblum PJ, Zekeng L, et al. The use of nonoxynol-9 for protection against cervical gonorrhea. *Am J Public Health* 1994;84:890–891.

57. Grou F, Rodriques I. The morning-after pill—how long after? *Am J Obstet Gynecol* 1995;171:1529–1534.

58. Trussell J, Rodriquez G, Ellertson C. New estimates of the effectiveness of the Yuzpe regimen of emergency contraception. *Contraception* 1998;57:363–369.

59. Creinin MD. A reassessment of efficacy of the Yuzpe regimen of emergency contraception. *Hum Reprod* 1997;12:496–498.

60. Yuzpe AA, Lanier WJ. Ethinyl estradiol and dL-norgestrel as a postcoital contraceptive. *Fertil Steril* 1977;28:932–936.

61. American College of Obstetrics and Gynecology. Emergency oral contraception. *ACOG Practice Patterns* 1996;31:1–8.

62. Van Hertzen H, Van Look PFA. Research on new methods of emergency contraception. *Fam Plann Perspect* 1996;28:52–57,88.

63. Swahn ML, Westlund P, Johannison E, et al. Effect of post-coital contraceptive methods on the endometrium and the menstrual cycle. *Acta Obstet Gynecol Scand* 1996;75:738–744.

64. Young DC, Wehle RD, Joshi SG, et al. Emergency contraception alters progesterone associated endometrial protein in serum and uterine luminal fluid. *Obstet Gynecol* 1994;84:266.

65. Linn S, Schoenbaum SC, Monson RR, et al. Lack of association between contraceptive usage and congenital malformations in offspring. *Am J Obstet Gynecol* 1983;147:923–928.

66. Huggins GR, Cullins VE. Fertility after contraception or abortion. *Fertil Steril* 1990;54:4.

67. Hormonal contraception. *ACOG Techn Bull* 1994;October:198.

68. Ho PC, Kwan MS. A prospective randomized comparison of levonorgestrel with the Yuzpe regimen in postcoital contraception. *Hum Reprod* 1993;8:389–392.

69. World Health Organization. Randomized controlled trial of levonorgestrel versus the Yuzpe regimen of combined oral contraceptives for emergency contraception. *Lancet* 1998;352:428–433.

70. Webb AM. Intrauterine contraceptive devices and antigestagens as emergency contraception. *Eur J Contraception Reprod Health Care* 1997;2:243–246.

71. McCann MF, Potter LS. Progestin-only oral contraception: a comprehensive review. *Contraception* 1994;50 [6 Suppl 1]:S1–A195.

72. Piccinino LJ, Mosher WD. Trends in contraceptive use in the United States: 1982–1995. *Fam Plann Perspect* 1998;30:4–10,46.

73. Forrest JD, Fordyce RR. Women's contraceptive attitudes and use in 1992. *Fam Plann Perspect* 1993;25:175–179.

74. Foster DC. Low dose monophasic and multiphasic oral contraceptives: a review of potency, efficacy and side effects. *Semin Reprod Endocrinol* 1989;7:205.

75. Moghissi KS, Syner FN, McBride LC. Contraceptive mechanism of microdose norethindrone. *Obstet Gynecol* 1973;41:585–594.

76. Elstein M, Morris SE, Groom GOV, et al. Studies on low-dose oral contraceptives: cervical mucus and plasma hormone changes in relation to circulating d-norgestrel and 17 ethynyl estradiol concentrations. *Fertil Steril* 1976;27:892–898.

77. Grimes DA, ed. Metabolic effects of oral contraceptives: fact vs. fiction. *Contraception Report* 1996;VI:4–14.

78. Klein B, Moss SE, Klein R. Oral contraceptives in women with diabetes. *Diabetes Care* 1990;13:895–898.

79. Garg SK, Chase HP, Marshall G, et al. Oral contraceptives and renal and retinal complications in young women with insulin-dependent diabetes mellitus. *JAMA* 1994;271:1099–1102.

80. Sullivan JM, Lobo RA. Considerations for contraception in women with cardiovascular disorders. *Am J Obstet Gynecol* 1993;168:2006–2011.

81. Stone SC. Clinical challenge: oral contraceptives and hypertension. *Int J Fertil* 1994;39:143–147.

82. Wild RA. Clinical challenge: the diabetic on OCs. *Int J Fertil* 1994;39(3):148–152.

83. Mestman JH, Schmidt-Sarosi C. Diabetes mellitus and fertility control: contraception management issues. *Am J Obstet Gynecol* 1993;168:2012–2020.

84. Loriaux DL, Wild RA. Contraceptive choices for women with endocrine complications. *Am J Obstet Gynecol* 1993;168:1990–1993.

85. Comp PC, Zacur HA. Contraceptive choices in women with coagulation disorders. *Am J Obstet Gynecol* 1993;168:199–203.

86. Knopp RH, LaRosa JC, Burkman RT Jr. Contraception and dyslipidemia. *Am J Obstet Gynecol* 1993;168:1994–2005.

87. Upton GV. Lipids, cardiovascular disease, and oral contraceptives: a practical perspective. *Fertil Steril* 1990;53:1–12.

88. Breckwoldt M, Wieacker P, Geisthovel F. Oral contraception in disease states. *Am J Obstet Gynecol* 1990;163:2213–2216.

89. Kyos SL, Shoupe D, Douyan S, et al. Effect of low-dose oral contraceptives on carbohydrate and lipid metabolism in women with recent gestational diabetes: results of a controlled, randomized, prospective study. *Am J Obstet Gynecol* 1990;163:1822–1827.

90. Vessey M, Painter R. Oral contraceptive use and benign gallbladder disease; revisited. *Contraception* 1994;50:167–173.

91. Vessey M, Mant D, Smith A, et al. Oral contraceptives and venous thromboembolism: findings in a large prospective study. *Br Med J* 1986;292:526.

92. Grodstein F, Stampfer M, Goldhaber SZ, et al. Prospective study of exogenous hormones and risk of pulmonary embolism in women. *Lancet* 1996;348:983–987.

93. Gerstmann BB, Pip JM, Tomita DK, et al. Oral contraceptive estrogen dose and the risk of deep venous thromboembolic disease. *Am J Epidemiol* 1991;133:32–37.

94. Ramcharan S, Pellegrin FA, Ray RM, et al. A prospective study of the side effects of oral contraceptives. Volume III, an interim report: a comparison of disease occurrence leading to hospitalization or death in users and nonusers of oral contraceptives. *J Reprod Med* 1980;25:345–372.

95. Royal College of General Practitioners' Oral Contraception Study. Further analyses of mortality in oral contraceptive users. *Lancet* 1981;1:541–546.

96. World Health Organization Collaborative Study of Cardiovascular Disease and Steroid Hormone Contraception. Effect of different progestagens in low oestrogen oral contraceptives on venous thromboembolic disease. *Lancet* 1995;346:1582–1588.

97. Jick H, Jick SS, Gurewich V, et al. Risk of idiopathic cardiovascular death and nonfatal venous thromboembolism in women using oral contraceptives with differing progestagen components. *Lancet* 1995;346:1589–1593.

98. World Health Organization Collaborative Study of Cardiovascular Disease and Steroid Hormone Contraception. Venous thromboembolic disease and combined oral contraceptives: results of international multicentre case-control study. *Lancet* 1995;346:1575–1582.

99. Bloemanekamp KWM, Rosendaal FR, Helmerhorst FM, et al. Enhancement by factor V Leiden mutation of risk of deep-vein thrombosis associated with oral contraceptives containing a third-generation progestagen. *Lancet* 1995;346:1593–1596.

100. Farmer RDT, Lawrenson RA, Thompson CR, et al. Population-based study of risk of venous thromboembolism associated with various oral contraceptives. *Lancet* 1997;349:83–88.

101. Farmer RDT, Todd JC, MacRae KD, et al. Oral contraception was not associated with venous thromboembolic disease in recent study. *BMJ* 1998;316: 1090–1091.

102. Palatsi R, Hirvensalo E, Liukko P, et al. Serum total and unbound testosterone and sex hormone binding globulin (SHBG) in female acne patients treated with two different oral contraceptives. *Acta Derm Venereol* 1984;64:517–523.

103. Phillips A, Demarest K, Hahn DW, et al. Progestational and androgenic receptor binding affinities and in vivo activities of norgestimate and other progestins. *Contraception* 1990;41:339–410.

104. Archer DF. Clinical and metabolic features of desogestrel: a new oral contraceptive preparation. *Am J Obstet Gynecol* 1004;170:1550–1555.

105. Gutmann JN, Corson SL. The new progestins: pharmacologic and clinical aspects. *Int J Fertil* 1994;39-[Suppl 3]:163–176.

106. Derman RJ. Oral contraceptives: androgenicity and estrogenicity. *Int J Fertil* 1994;39[Suppl 3]:177–182.

107. Fotherby K, Caldwell ADS. New progestogens in oral contraception. *Contraception* 1994;49:1–32.

108. Krauss RM, Burkman RT, Jr. The metabolic impact of oral contraceptives. *Am J Obstet Gynecol* 1992;167:-1177–1184.

109. Burkman RT, Robinson C, Moran-Kruszon D, et al. Lipid and lipoprotein changes associated with oral contraceptive use: a randomized clinical trial. *Obstet Gynecol* 1988;71:33.

110. Porter JB, Jick H, Walker AM. Mortality among oral contraceptive users. *Obstet Gynecol* 1987;70:29.

111. Porter JB, Hunter JR, Jick H, et al. Oral contraceptives and nonfatal vascular disease. *Obstet Gynecol* 1985; 66:1.

112. Godsland IF, Crook D, Simpson R, et al. The effects of different formulations of oral contraceptive agents on lipid and carbohydrate metabolism. *N Engl J Med* 1990;323:1375–1381.

113. Adams MR, Clarkson TB, Koritnik DR, et al. Contraceptive steroids and coronary artery atherosclerosis in cynomolgus macaques. *Fertil Steril* 1987;47: 1010–1018.

114. Clarkson TB, Shively CA, Morgan TM, et al. Oral contraceptives and coronary artery atherosclerosis of cynomolgus monkeys. *Obstet Gynecol* 1990;75: 217–222.

115. Rosenberg MJ, Waugh MS, Burnhill MS. Compliance, counseling and satisfaction with oral contraceptives: a prospective evaluation. *Fam Plann Perspect* 1998;30: 89–92,104.

116. Grimes DA, ed. OC compliance and contraceptive failure. *Contraception Report* 1990;1:3–6.

117. CDC/NICHD. Oral contraceptives and endometrial cancer: combination oral contraceptive use and the risk of endometrial cancer. *JAMA* 1987;257:6.

118. The Centers for Disease Control Cancer and Steroid Hormone Study. Oral contraceptive use and the risk of endometrial cancer. *JAMA* 1983;249:1600–1604.

119. The Centers for Disease Control Cancer and Steroid Hormone Study. Oral contraceptive use and the risk of ovarian cancer. *JAMA* 1983;249;12:1596–1599.

120. Kost K, Forrest JD, Harlap S. Comparing the health risks and benefits of contraceptive choices. *Fam Plann Perspect* 1991;23:54–61.

121. Mishell DR Jr. Noncontraceptive health benefits of oral steroidal contraceptives. *Am J Obstet Gynecol* 1982;142:809.

122. Andrews WC, Jones KP. Therapeutic uses of oral contraceptives. *Dialogues Contraception* 1991;3:1–8.

123. Jones KP, Ravnikar VA, Tulchinsky D, et al. Comparison of bone density in amenorrheic women due to athletics, weight loss, and premature menopause. *Obstet Gynecol* 1985;66:5.

124. Schlesselman JJ. Cancer of the breast and reproductive tract in relation to use of oral contraceptives. *Contraception* 1989;40:1–38.

125. The New Zealand Contraception and Health Study Group. Risk of cervical dysplasia in users of oral contraceptives, intrauterine devices or depot-medroxyprogesterone acetate. *Contraception* 1994;50:431–441.

126. Harlap S. Oral contraceptives and breast cancer. Cause and effect? *J Reprod Med* 1991;36:374–395.

127. The Cancer and Steroid Hormone Study of the Centers for Disease Control and the National Institute of Child Health and Human Development. Oral-contraceptive use and the risk of breast cancer. *N Engl J Med* 1986; 315:405–411.

128. Wingo PA, Lee NC, Ory HW, et al. Age-specific differences in the relationship between oral contraceptive use and breast cancer. *Obstet Gynecol* 1991;78: 161–170.

129. McGonigle KF, Huggins GR. Oral contraceptives and breast disease. *Fertil Steril* 1991;56:799–819.

130. Wingo PA, Lee NC, Ory HW, et al. Age-specific differences in the relationship between oral contraceptive use and breast cancer. *Cancer* 1993;71[4 Suppl]:1506–1517.

131. Rookus MA, van Leeuwen FE. Oral contraceptives and risk of breast cancer in women aged 20–54 years. *Lancet* 1994;344:844–851.

132. Kaunitz AM. Injectable contraception. *Clin Obstet Gynecol* 1989;32:2.

133. Rosenfield A, Maine D, Rochat R, et al. The Food and Drug Administration and medroxyprogesterone acetate. *JAMA* 1983;249:2922–2928.

134. Kaunitz AM. Long-acting injectable contraception with depot medroxyprogesterone acetate. *Am J Obstet Gynecol* 1994;170:1543–1549.

135. Kaunitz AM, Mishell DR. Progestin-only contraceptives: current perspectives and future directions. *Dialogues Contraception* 1994;4:1–5.

136. Wyeth-Ayerst Laboratories. Depo-Provera. In: *Physicians' desk reference*, 52nd ed. Montvale, NJ: Medical Economics, 1998:2259–2261.

137. Said S, Sadek W, Rocca M, et al. Clinical evaluation of the therapeutic effectiveness of ethinyl oestradiol and

oestrone sulphate on prolonged bleeding in women using depot medroxyprogesterone acetate for contraception. World Health Organization, Special Programme of Research, Development and Research Training in Human Reproduction, Task Force on Long-acting Systemic Agents for Fertility Regulation. *Hum Reprod* 1996;11[Suppl 2]:1–13.

138. Cundy T, Evans M, Roberts H, et al. Bone density in women receiving depot medroxyprogesterone acetate for contraception. *BMJ* 191;303:13–16.

139. Cundy T, Farquhar CM, Cornish J, et al. Short-term effects of high dose oral medroxyprogesterone acetate on bone density in premenopausal women. *J Clin Endocrinol Metab* 1996;81:1014–1017.

140. Cromer BA, Blair JM, Mahan JD, et al. A prospective comparison of bone density in adolescent girls receiving depot medroxyprogesterone acetate (Depo-Provera), levonorgestrel (Norplant), or oral contraceptives. *J Pediatr* 1996;129:671–676.

141. Taneepanichskul S, Intaraprasert S, Theppisai U, et al. Bone mineral density in long-term depot medroxyprogesterone acetate acceptors. *Contraception* 1997;56:1–3.

142. Taneepanichskul S, Intaraprasert S, Theppisai U, et al. Bone mineral density during long-term treatment with Norplant implants and depot medroxyprogesterone acetate. A cross-sectional study of Thai women. *Contraception* 1997;56:153–155.

143. Gbolade B, Willis S, Murby B, et al. Bone density in long term users of depot medroxyprogesterone acetate. *Br J Obstet Gynaecol* 1998;105:790–794.

144. WHO Collaborative Study of Neoplasia and Steroid Contraceptives. Depot medroxyprogesterone acetate (DMPA) and risk of endometrial cancer. *Int J Cancer* 1991;49:186–190.

145. WHO. Depot-medroxyprogesterone acetate (DMPA) and cancer: memorandum from a WHO meeting. *Bull WHO* 1993;71:669–676.

146. Cullins VE. Noncontraceptive benefits and therapeutic uses of depot medroxyprogesterone acetate. *J Reprod Med* 1996;41[5 Suppl]:428–433.

147. Kaunitz AM. Injectable depot medroxyprogesterone acetate contraception: an update for U.S. clinicians. *Int J Fertil Womens Med* 1998;43:73–83.

148. Isaacs WA, Hayhoe FGJ. Steroid hormones in sickle-cell disease. *Nature* 1967;215:1139–1142.

149. DeCeulaer K, Hayes R, Gruber C, et al. Medroxyprogesterone acetate and homozygous sickle-cell disease. *Lancet* 1982;2:229–231.

150. Mattson RH, Cramer JA, Caldwell BV, et al. Treatment of seizures with medroxyprogesterone acetate: preliminary report. *Neurology* 1984;34:1255–1258.

151. Blackham A, Spencer PSJ. Response of female mice to anticonvulsants after pretreatment with sex steroids [Letter]. *J Pharm Pharmacol* 1970;22:304–305.

152. Zimmerman AW, Holden KR, Reiter EO, et al. Medroxyprogesterone acetate in the treatment of seizures associated with menstruation. *J Pediatr* 1973; 83:959–963.

153. Population Council. *Norplant levonorgestrel implants. A summary of scientific data.* New York: Population Council, 1990.

154. Wyeth-Ayerst Laboratories. Norplant. In: *Physicians' desk reference*, 52nd ed. Montvale, NJ: Medical Economics, 1998:3085–3089.

155. Sivin I. International experience with Norplant and Norplant-2 contraceptives. *Stud Fam Plann* 1998:19: 81–94.

156. Alvarez-Sanchez F, Brache V, Thevenin F, et al. Hormonal treatment for bleeding irregularities in Norplant implant users. *Am J Obstet Gynecol* 1996;174: 919–922.

157. Witjaksono J, Lau JM, Affandi B, et al. Oestrogen treatment for increased bleeding in Norplant users: preliminary results. *Hum Reprod* 1996;11:109–114.

158. Injectables and implants. Hormonal contraception: new long-acting methods. *Populat Rep* 1987;Series K:3.

159. Cullins VE, Remsburg RE, Blumenthal PD, et al. Comparison of adolescent and adult experiences with Norplant levonorgestrel contraceptive implants. *Obstet Gynecol* 1994;83:1026–1032.

160. Haugen MM, Evans CB, Kim MH. Patient satisfaction with a levonorgestrel-releasing contraceptive implant. Reasons for and patterns of removal. *J Reprod Med* 1996;4:849–854.

161. Berenson AB, Wiemann CM. Patient satisfaction and side effects with levonorgestrel implant (Norplant) use in adolescents 18 years of age or younger. *Pediatrics* 1993;92:257–260.

162. Klaisle CM, Wysocki S. Innovations in contraception: the Norplant system. *NAACOGS Clin Issues Perinat Womens Health Nurs* 1992;3:267–279.

163. Phemister DA, Laurent S, Harrison FNH Jr. Obstetrics: use of Norplant contraceptive implants in the immediate postpartum period: safety and tolerance. *Am J Obstet Gynecol* 1995;172:175–179.

164. Diaz S, Croxatto HB, Panez M, et al. Clinical assessment of treatments for prolonged bleeding in users of Norplant implants. *Contraception* 1990;42:97–109.

165. Alvarez-Sanchez F, Brache V, Thevenin F, et al. Hormonal treatment for bleeding irregularities in Norplant implant users. *Am J Obstet Gynecol* 1996;174:919–922.

166. Witjaksono J, Lau JM, Affandi B, et al. Oestrogen treatment for increased bleeding in Norplant users: preliminary results. *Hum Reprod* 1996;11:109–114.

167. Henshaw SK. Abortion incidence and services in the United States, 1995–1996. *Fam Plann Perspect* 1998; 30:263–270,287.

168. Koonin LM, Attrash HK, Smith JC, et al. Abortion surveillance. *CDC Surveillance Summaries* 1990;39[SS-2]:23–56.

169. Henshaw ST. Unintended pregnancy in the United States. *Fam Plann Perspect* 1998;30:24–29,46.

170. Joyce TJ, Mocan NH. The impact of legalized abortion on adolescent childbearing in New York City. *Am J Public Health* 1990;80:273.

171. The Alan Guttmacher Institute. Abortion in practice: safe and unsafe conditions for women. In: *Sharing responsibility women society & abortion worldwide.* New York: The Alan Guttmacher Institute, 1999;32.

172. Grimes DA. Medical abortion in early pregnancy: a review of the evidence. *Obstet Gynecol* 1997;89:790.

173. Spitz IM, Bardin CW, Benton L, et al. Early pregnancy termination with mifepristone and misoprostol in the United States. *N Engl J Med* 1998;338:1241.

174. Peyton R, Aubeny E, Targosz V, et al. Early termination of pregnancy with mifepristone (RU486) and the orally active prostaglandin misoprostol. *N Engl J Med* 1993;328:1509–1513.

175. Creinin MD, Vittinghoff E, Keder L, et al. Methotrex-

ate and misoprostol for early abortion: a multicenter trial. I. Safety and efficacy. *Contraception* 1996;53: 321–327.

176. Wiebe ER. Abortion induced with methotrexate and misoprostol: a comparison of various protocols. *Contraception* 1997;55:159–163.

177. Carbonell JLL, Varela L, Valazco A, et al. Oral methotrexate and vaginal misoprostol for early abortion. *Contraception* 1998;57:83–88.

178. Mishell DR Jr, Jain JK, Byrne JD, et al. A medical method of early pregnancy termination using tamoxifen and misoprostol. *Contraception* 1998;58:1–6.

179. International Projects Assistance Services. First trimester abortion menstrual regulation treatment of incomplete abortion. IPAS Product Literature, 1997.

180. Corson SL, Derman RJ, Tyrer LB, eds. *Fertility control*, 2nd ed. Ontario, Canada: Goldin Publishers, 1994: 465–483.

181. Grimes DA, Schulz KF, Cates W Jr, et al. Local versus general anesthesia: which is safer for performing suction curettage abortions? *Am J Obstet Gynecol* 1979; 135:1030.

182. Sands RX, Burnhill MS, Hakim-Elahi F. Postabortal uterine atony. *Obstet Gynecol* 1974;43:595.

183. Nathanson BN. The postabortal pain syndrome: a new entity. *Obstet Gynecol* 1973;41:739.

184. Kaunitz AM, Grimes DA. First-trimester abortion technology. In: Corson SL, Derman RJ, Turer LB, eds. *Fertility control,* 1st ed. Boston: Little, Brown and Company, 1985:63–76.

185. Bozorg N. Statistical analysis of first trimester pregnancy terminations in an ambulatory surgical center. *Am J Obstet Gynecol* 1977;127:763.

186. Daling JR, Sapdoni LR, Emanuel I. Role of induced abortion in secondary infertility. *Obstet Gynecol* 1981; 57:59.

187. Chung CS, Smith RG, Steinhoff PG. Induced abortion and spontaneous fetal loss in subsequent pregnancies. *Am J Public Health* 1982;72:548.

188. Hogue CJR, Cates W Jr, Tietze C. The effect of induced abortion on subsequent reproduction. *Epidemiol Rev* 1982;4:66.

189. Gold RB. *Abortion and women's health: a turning point for America?* New York: The Alan Guttmacher Institute, 1990.

190. Estes EH. Report H (A-92). Induced termination of pregnancy before and after Roe v Wade. Trends in the mortality and morbidity of women. Resolution 17, A-91.

191. Pastuszak AL, Schuler L, Speck-Martins CE, et al. Use of misoprostol during pregnancy and Mobius' syndrome in infants. *N Engl J Med* 1998;338:1881–1885.

23

Tumors of the Vulva

Robert A. Ambros and Robert J. Kurman

Tumors of the vulva are very uncommon in the pediatric age group. The relative frequent occurrence of vulvar neoplasms in adult women compared to children and adolescents most likely is related to the accumulated influence of environmental factors, including exposure to sexually transmitted diseases such as human papillomaviruses (HPVs). Most vulvar growths in children and adolescents do not represent neoplastic growths and require little treatment. Due perhaps to their rarity, when true benign and malignant neoplasms do occur, they can be confused with other conditions such as congenital adrenal hyperplasia and abuse, leading to delays in diagnosis and appropriate treatment. Conversely, neoplasms and other vulvar growths in infancy and childhood can signal other problems such as child abuse or genetic syndromes, underscoring the need for careful evaluation of all vulvar lesions in this age group.

BENIGN TUMORS

Hymenal Tags

Hymenal tags are relatively common and represent small nonneoplastic nodules of fibroconnective tissue at the margin of the hymen. Excision is recommended if the tags are large and cause discomfort, or if there is any doubt as to their nature.

Simple Cysts in the Neonate

Several types of simple cysts can occur in the neonate, all of which are fairly uncommon. They may be lined by cuboidal, columnar, or squamous epithelium and most frequently occur near the urethral meatus and hymen.

Hymenal Cysts

These lesions must be differentiated from an imperforate membrane with hydrocolpos (1). Hymenal cysts have an opening and usually regress spontaneously. They can be treated by incision and drainage. Simple puncture without anesthesia also has been performed successfully (2).

Paraurethral Cysts

These cysts are lined by squamous epithelium and are thought to arise from remnants of the wolffian duct by some (3) and as invaginations from the vagina mucosa by others (4). They either rupture spontaneously or are treated by marsupialization. These cysts can closely simulate ureteroceles. Conversely, a significant percentage of ectopic ureteroceles present initially as paraurethral cysts (5). For this reason, complete urologic examination is necessary after discovery of any neonatal paraurethral cyst (4).

Simple Cysts in Childhood and Adolescence

Epithelial Inclusion Cysts

Epithelial inclusion cysts are uncommon but may occur in the adolescent age group. They develop by invagination of the surface epithelium into the underlying dermis. Histologically, they are lined by squamous epithelium with keratinaceous material filling the lumen. Treatment is simple excision.

Mucous Cysts

Mucous cysts lined by mucus producing columnar epithelium may occur in the vulvar vestibule. They are more common in adults but have been reported in adolescents (6). They usually are small, but they can become symptomatic by obstructing the urethra. They most likely arise by the obstruction of small mucinous glands, which are normal constituents of the vulvar vestibule (6,7).

Hydroceles

Hydroceles, also known as cysts of the canal of Nuck, represent swellings of the blind remnant of the "processus vaginalis" (8). Normally, this remnant regresses, but a cyst develops if the peritoneal protrusion that extends into the labium majus fills with fluid and persists. Like scrotal hydroceles, vulvar hydroceles must be distinguished from true inguinal hernias. The latter can contain bowel or adnexal structures and usually are reducible. Hydroceles are treated by surgical excision.

Urethral Prolapse

Urethral prolapse of the urethral mucosa may produce a painless vulvar mass. In a report of 12 cases by Capraro et al. (9), the mean age was 5 years, with patients presenting either with a vulvar mass or bleeding. Redundancy of the urethral mucosa, increased abdominal pressure, and lack of estrogen have been proposed as predisposing factors. Treatment is simple excision.

Bartholin's Gland Cysts

Bartholin's gland cysts have been reported in adolescents (10). They may develop as a result of occlusion of a main duct or small ductule of Bartholin's gland. They are lined by transitional or mucinous epithelium, depending on their derivation from the main duct or ductule, respectively. Cysts may present as a mass or become secondarily infected to form a painful Bartholin's gland abscess. Bartholin's gland cysts are treated by excision or marsupialization.

Squamous Papillomas and Condylomata

Squamous Papillomas

These (skin tags, acrochordons) are polypoid growths that usually involve the outer aspects of the labia. Microscopically, the lesion is characterized by squamous epithelium overlying a fibroconnective tissue core. Complexity, arborization of the papillae, and koilocytosis as seen in a condyloma acuminatum does not occur in a papilloma.

Condylomata Acuminata

Condylomata acuminata result from infection by a specific type of HPV, most frequently types 6 and 11 (11). Although uncommon, the frequency of genital HPV infection in children is believed to be increasing (12). Transmission is by direct contact. In the pediatric patient, this suggests either transmission during childbirth or sexual abuse. Because the incubation period can be up to 3 months (13), the development of condylomata after this time period is suggestive, but not conclusive evidence, of sexual abuse. Patients range in age from 10 months to adolescence (12, 14–21). In many of the reported cases of vulvar condylomata, sexual abuse was either not admitted or suspected by the parents, and the mode of transmission could not be established. Parents sought medical attention because of the observation of a vulvar mass or bleeding after minor trauma. Condylomata are similar to squamous papillomas on gross and microscopic examination, but they show a more highly arborized pattern of the papillary fronds and often display koilocytosis, a feature pathognomonic of HPV infection. The finding is characterized by nuclear enlargement, wrinkling of the nuclear membrane,

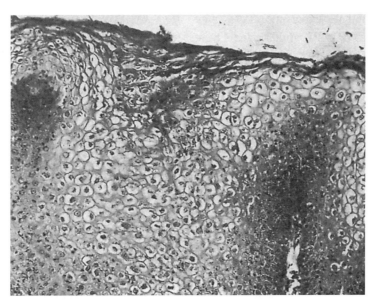

FIG. 23.1. Condyloma in a 16-year-old girl characterized by koilocytotic cells with enlarged nuclei, wrinkled nuclear membranes, and perinuclear halos.

and formation of a perinuclear halo (Fig. 23.1). A diagnosis of vulvar condylomata acuminata mandates the search for other venereally transmitted infections, because they may coexist in these patients (20). In sexually active adolescents, a cervicovaginal smear should be obtained. Treatment includes application of trichloroacetic acid or podophyllin, surgical excision, electrocoagulation, and laser vaporization. Laser therapy is widely believed to produce the least scarring and has been advocated particularly for periurethral lesions (12). Recently, removal by ultrasonic aspiration has been used and found to be preferable to laser (22).

Vascular Lesions

Hemangiomas

Hemangiomas are the most common vascular lesions and are divided into two groups based on their gross and microscopic appearance: capillary and cavernous. Although their appearance usually is characteristic, hemangiomas of the vulva can be confused with other conditions. For example, ulceration of hemangiomas has been confused with burns secondary to child abuse, and clitoral hemangiomas have been confused with phallic structures (23,24). Rarely, vulvar hemangiomas may occur as a component of a syndrome such as vulvar congenital dysplastic angiopathy (Klippel-Trénaunay syndrome) (25). The protean manifestations of vulvar hemangiomas emphasize the need for histologic examination of vulvar growths.

Capillary Hemangiomas

Capillary hemangiomas (strawberry nevi) are flat or slightly elevated neoplasms composed of small blood vessels. On microscopic examination, they are composed of aggregations of thin-walled capillaries in the dermis that may extend with finger-like projections into deeper tissue resembling a malignant tumor.

Cavernous Hemangiomas

Cavernous hemangiomas are composed of large thin-walled vessels and can be more deeply located than capillary hemangiomas.

Cutaneous vascular tumors in the infant can be mixed and show both capillary and cavernous areas. They may be present at birth but commonly develop during the first 2 months. After a period of rapid growth lasting from several months to several years, the vast majority regress. Complete regression by age 5 years is seen in approximately 80% of the patients (26). The percentage of vulvar lesions undergoing spontaneous regression probably is smaller. Treatment is reserved for lesions that fail to regress, are associated with psychological trauma, or develop complications such as bleeding or ulceration (23,27,28). Ulceration is particularly prone to occur in hemangiomas that have a cavernous component. Treatment may be sclerotherapy, cryotherapy, laser therapy, or surgical excision. Radiotherapy is no longer used (29) due to the potential adverse effects on the ovary (28).

Port Wine Nevus

Port wine nevus (nevus flammeus, birthmark) is present from birth and does not represent a true neoplasm. It must be distinguished from a capillary or cavernous nevus. The port wine nevus is variable in size, and it is pink to purple in color. The lesion rarely is limited to the vulva. Microscopically, it is composed of dilated vessels in the dermis. It occasionally may be associated with the Sturge-Weber syndrome and Klippel-Trénaunay-Weber syndrome. Port wine nevi at other sites have been treated for cosmetic purposes but rarely are treated on the vulva.

Angiokeratoma

Angiokeratoma is a form of cavernous hemangioma in which the blood vessels are intimately associated with the overlying epidermis that typically displays acanthosis and hyperkeratosis (Fig. 23.2) (30). The lesions appear as dark red elevations ranging in size from 1 to 10 mm. Angiokeratomas can be localized to the vulva or widely distributed in other sites. In the latter form, they tend to occur on the fingers, toes, and scrotum/vulva (31). Rarely, they are manifestations of a metabolic disorder and may be associated with renal and central nervous system dysfunction, i.e., Fabry's disease (32). Angiokeratomas most frequently occur in adult women but have been reported in adolescents (30,33). They are frequently asymptomatic but can cause discomfort, irritation, and bleeding (31). Treatment, which currently is with the argon laser, is reserved for symptomatic lesions.

Lymphangiomas

Lymphangiomas of the vulva are rare but have been reported in women with congenital

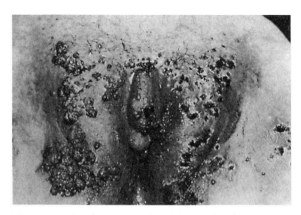

FIG. 23.2. Vulvar angiokeratoma involving the clitoral hood, labia majora, and inner thighs. (From Dotters DJ, Fowler WC, Powers SK, et al. Argon laser therapy of vulvar angiokeratoma. *Obstet Gynecol* 1986;68:56S–59S, with permission.)

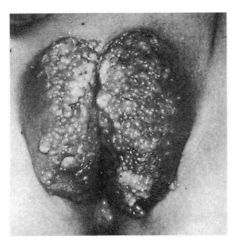

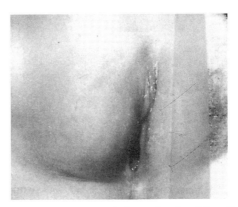

FIG. 23.4. Lipomas of the vulva involving the right labium majus in a young girl. (Courtesy of Dr. C.J. Dewhurst.)

FIG. 23.3. Acquired vulvar lymphangiectasis 6.5 years after radical therapy for rhabdomyosarcomas of the bladder. (From Rabinowitz R, Churchill BM, Alexis ME, et al. Acquired vulvar lymphangiectasis in a child. *Urology* 1977;10: 459–460, with permission.)

lymphedema of the lower extremities (34). More commonly, lymphatic lesions in the vulva are acquired and represent dilatations of existing lymphatic vessels due to disruption of more proximal channels. Lymphangiectasis is a more appropriate term for the latter, as they do not represent true neoplasms. Vulvar lymphangiectasis has been reported in adult women after radiation therapy for cervical carcinoma. A single case has been reported in a 6-year-old child, 4 years after pelvic exenteration for a malignant bladder tumor (Fig. 23.3) (35).

Soft Tissue Tumors

Soft tissue tumors other than vascular lesions are rare but include lipomas and leiomyomas (Fig. 23.4) (1,36).

Neurogenic Tumors

Neurofibromas

Vulvar neurofibromas are very uncommon in children but occasionally can represent the earliest clinical manifestation of neurofibromatosis. Neurofibromatosis is transmitted as

a mendelian dominant disease with variability in gene expression. The origin of this disease recently was traced to a specific gene region on chromosome 17 (37). Approximately 50% of patients have a family history of the disorder. The lesions in the remainder are believed to arise from new mutations. The disorder usually is manifested in young children by the presence of multiple café-au-lait spots. More than six spots are considered to be pathognomonic of the disease. Neurofibromas may appear in late childhood and adolescence. Other manifestations include bone overgrowth, congenital bowing and pseudarthrosis of bone and soft tissue, kyphoscoliosis, focal gigantism, and megalencephaly (38,39). In addition, approximately 10% of children have mild-to-moderate mental retardation. The diagnosis currently is based on physical findings, but in the near future will probably be based on molecular genetic analysis. Neurofibromas are well-circumscribed tumors arising from Schwann cells (Fig. 23.5). Histologically, they are composed of elongated spindle cells forming interlacing bands admixed with nerve fibers. The frequency of malignant neurogenic tumors in patients with neurofibromatosis is higher than in the general population, with rates varying from 5% to 30% (40,41). Malignant transformation, however, is rare in children. Presentation as a solitary vulvar neurofibroma is very unusual but can

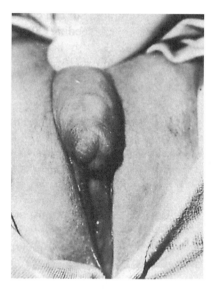

FIG. 23.5. Neurofibromas of the clitoris presenting as phallus-like structure. (From Kaneti J, Liebrman F, Moshe P, et al. A case of ambiguous genitalia owing to neurofibromatosis—review of the literature. *J Urol* 1988;140:584–585, with permission.)

occur and be confused with other conditions. Usually, the neurofibroma is confused with a phallus, leading to a diagnosis of pseudohermaphroditism (42–45). The diagnosis should be suspected in a child with multiple café-au-lait spots. Physical examination and cystoscopy may reveal additional neurofibromas in the vagina and bladder (38).

Granular Cell Tumor

This is a benign neoplasm occurring in the breast and tongue and less commonly in the vulva. Several vulvar lesions have been reported in the pediatric age group (46,47). Based on electron microscopic and immunohistochemical studies, a Schwann cell origin of this neoplasm has been proposed (48). Excision is curative.

Melanocytic Lesions

Nevi

Vulvar nevi are uncommon in the pediatric age group. In a 14-year review of patients

with pigmented vulvar lesions at The Johns Hopkins Hospital, only two of 59 nevi occurred in patients under the age of 20 years (49). In the same review, the frequency of dysplasia was not higher in the vulva compared to nevi in other locations. Vulvar lesions did, however, show greater tendency to display variability in the size and shape of melanocytic nests. Both junctional and intradermal nevi have been described.

MALIGNANT NEOPLASMS

Malignant tumors of the vulva are rare in the pediatric age group but have been sporadically reported since the latter part of the nineteenth century. Our review of the world literature since 1871 revealed 41 cases (50–57). Although it is difficult to determine histologic type in many of these cases, it appears that squamous cell carcinomas, embryonal rhabdomyosarcomas, and endodermal sinus tumors are the most common. The rarity of squamous cell carcinomas in this age group underscores the role of environmental factors in the development of these tumors in adults. Conversely, the occurrence of sarcomas and endodermal sinus tumors in this age group and their virtual absence in the adult population suggest a role of congenital genetic factors in the development of these neoplasms.

Squamous Cell Carcinomas

Although rare, squamous cell carcinomas of the vulva have been reported in adolescents, and some have proved to be fatal (50, 57,58). As in other sites, squamous carcinoma presents as a raised lesion that can be ulcerated and confused with an infectious process (Figs. 23.6–23.7) (58). Biopsy reveals nests of malignant squamous cells in a desmoplastic stroma. Patients have been treated by radical vulvectomy with inguinal node dissection or by radiation therapy. Although precursor lesions have not been well studied in this age group, atypias of the vulvar epithelium have been reported (59,60). The relationship of these lesions to HPV infection has not been studied in these patients.

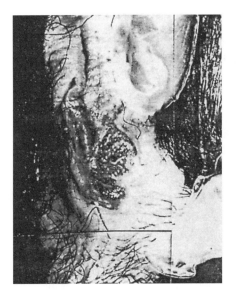

FIG. 23.6. Squamous cell carcinoma of the vulva presenting as an ulcerated lesion with raised margins. The surrounding white area is lichen sclerosus. (From Cario GM, House MJ, Paradinas FJ. Squamous cell carcinoma of the vulva in association with mixed vulvar dystrophy in an 18-year-old girl. Case report. *Br J Obstet Gynaecol* 1984;91:87–90, with permission.)

Sarcoma Botryoides

Sarcoma botryoides (embryonal rhabdomyosarcomas) of the vulva are rare. Almost all patients have been infants who presented with a vulvar mass (61–66). Large lesions may involve both vulva and vagina. Microscopically, the tumor is composed of immature rhabdomyoblasts showing varying degree of differentiation toward skeletal muscle. A condensation of primitive cells designated the "cambium layer" frequently is seen immediately beneath the epithelium and aids in the histologic diagnosis. The stroma frequently is myxoid and on gross examination results in the appearance of a "bunch of grapes," accounting for the term "sarcoma botryoides." Although these tumors are highly aggressive and have a tendency to recur locally (61,63,64), the multimodality approach using surgery, radiation therapy, and chemotherapy has increased survival in genitourinary rhabdomyosarcomas from 18% to 75% (67). A similar aggressive approach has resulted in long-term survival of patients with vulvar sarcoma botryoides (62).

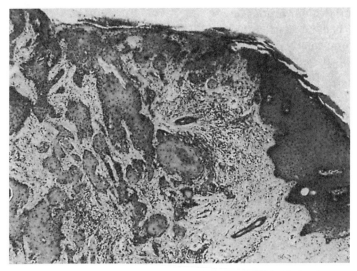

FIG. 23.7. Well-differentiated squamous carcinoma characterized by irregular nests of squamous epithelial infiltrates underlying the stroma. The adjacent epithelium shows squamous hyperplasia but no evidence of carcinoma *in situ* (hematoxylin and eosin stain). (From Cario GM, House MJ, Paradinas FJ. Squamous cell carcinoma of the vulva in association with mixed vulvar dystrophy in an 18-year-old girl. Case report. *Br J Obstet Gynaecol* 1984;91:87–90, with permission.)

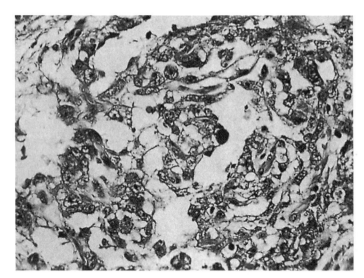

FIG. 23.8. Endodermal sinus tumor of the vulva characterized by a reticular pattern (hematoxylin and eosin stain). (From Dudley AG, Young RH, Lawrence WD, et al. Endodermal sinus tumor of the vulva in an infant. *Obstet Gynecol* 1983;61:76S–79S, with permission.)

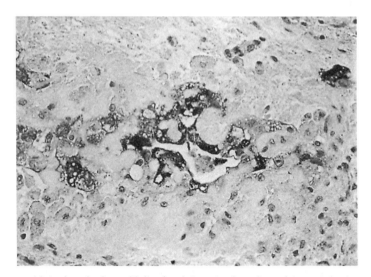

FIG. 23.9. Immunohistochemical positivity for intracytoplasmic α-fetoprotein in an endodermal sinus tumor of the vulva (same case as in Fig. 23.8). (From Dudley AG, Young RH, Lawrence WD, et al. Endodermal sinus tumor of the vulva in an infant. *Obstet Gynecol* 1983;61:76S–79S, with permission.)

Recently, vulvar pediatric rhabdomyosarcomas have been described to be adequately treated by wide excision and chemotherapy alone (68).

Endodermal Sinus Tumor

Three pediatric cases of endodermal sinus tumor involving the vulva have been reported (69–71). Two were young children younger than 3 years of age at presentation, and the third was an adolescent. Histologically, the tumor is composed of nests of primitive cells in a reticular pattern identical to its counterpart in the ovary. Intracytoplasmic inclusions containing α-fetoprotein were common (Figs. 23.8–23.9). Serum α-fetoprotein levels have not been elevated. One of the three cases showed areas of embryonal carcinoma in addition to the endodermal component. These tumors have been highly malignant, with two of the three patients dying of tumor despite radical surgery and adjuvant chemotherapy.

Malignant Melanoma

To our knowledge, only five vulvar cases in the pediatric age group have been reported. Malignant melanoma has been described in both preteen girls and adolescents (52,53,72, 73). The 5-year survival for malignant melanoma of the vulva in the adult age group is approximately 75% for lesions confined to the vulva when treated by radial vulvectomy and lymph node dissection (74).

REFERENCES

1. Dewhurst CJ. Tumors of the genital tract in childhood and adolescence. *Clin Obstet Gynecol* 1977;20:595–606.
2. Lottmann H, Cendron J, Baviera E, et al. Kystes vulvaires a revelation neonatale. *Ann Urol* 1985;19:259–262.
3. Cohen HJ, Klein MD, Laver MB. Cysts of the vagina in the newborn infant. *Am J Dis Child* 1957;94:322.
4. Blaivas JG, Pais VM, Retik AB. Paraurethral cysts in female neonate. *Urology* 1976;7:504–507.
5. Williams DI. Problems in the management of ectopic ureteroceles. *J Urol* 1964;92:635.
6. Friedrich EG, Wilkinson EJ. Mucous cysts of the vulvar vestibule. *Obstet Gynecol* 1972;42:407.
7. Robboy SJ, Ross JS, Prat J, et al. Urogenital sinus origin of mucinous and ciliated cysts of the vulva. *Obstet Gynecol* 1978;51:347.
8. Huffman JW. Tumors of the vulva and vagina during childhood. In: Huffman JW. *The gynecology of childhood and adolescence.* Philadelphia: WB Saunders, 1981:225–259.
9. Capraro VJ, Bayonet-Rivera NP, Magoss I. Vulvar tumor in children due to prolapse of urethral mucosa. *Am J Obstet Gynecol* 1970;108:572–575.
10. Lee YH, Rankin JS, Alpert S, et al. Microbiological investigation of Bartholin's gland abscesses and cysts. *Am J Obstet Gynecol* 1977;129:150–153.
11. Reid R, Greenberg M, Jenson AB, et al. Sexually transmitted papillomaviral infection. *Am J Obstet Gynecol* 1987;156:212–222.
12. Randrup ER, Sangisetty KV. Condyloma acuminatum in children. *Urology* 1985;26:176–177.
13. Powell LC. Condyloma acuminatum: recent advances in development, carcinogenesis and treatment. *Clin Obstet Gynecol* 1978;21:1061–1079.
14. McCoy CR, Applebaum H, Besser AS. Condyloma acuminata: an unusual presentation of child abuse. *J Pediatr Surg* 1982;17:505–507.
15. Seidel J, Zonana J, Totten E. Condylomata acuminata as a sign of sexual abuse in children. *J Pediatr* 1979;95: 553–554.
16. DeJong AR, Weiss JC, Brent RL. Condyloma acuminata in children. *Am J Dis Child* 1982;136:704–706.
17. Sadan O, Koller AB, Adno A, et al. Massive vulvar condyloma acuminata in a 10-month-old child with suspected sexual abuse. Case report. *Br J Obstet Gynaecol* 1985;92:1201–1203.
18. Stumpf PG. Increasing occurrence of condylomata acuminata in premenarchal children. *Obstet Gynecol* 1980; 56:262–264.
19. Grace DA, Ochsner JA, McLain CR, et al. Vulvar condylomata acuminata in prepubertal females. *JAMA* 1967; 201:151–152.
20. Goldman L, Clarke GE. Infectious papilloma (so called condyloma acuminatum) with genital, perineal and lip lesions in a 3 year old girl. *Urol Cutan Rev* 1940;44: 677–678.
21. Eftaiha MS, Amshel AL, Shonberg IL. Condyloma acuminata in an infant and mother: report of a case. *Dis Colon Rectum* 1978;21:369–371.
22. Smith YR, Isacsm C, Namroum AB, et al. Ultrasonic surgical aspiration to treat genital condyloma in children. *J Pediatr Adolesc Gynecol* 1996;9:145–147.
23. Levin AV, Selbst SM. Vulvar hemangioma simulating child abuse. *Clin Pediatr* 1988;27:213–215.
24. Kaufman-Friedman K. Hemangioma of the clitoris confused with adrenogenital syndrome. *Plast Reconstr Surg* 1978;62:452–454.
25. Tjaden BL, Buscema J, Haller JA, et al. Vulvar congenital dysplastic angiopathy. *Obstet Gynecol* 1990;75: 552–554.
26. MacColum DW, Martin LW. Hemangioma in infancy and childhood. A report based on 6479 cases. *Surg Clin North Am* 1957;36:1947.
27. Bellone F, Gloria M, Diani F. Considerazioni cliniche sugli emangiomi della vulva in eta infantile. *Minerv Ginecol* 1985;37:747–750.
28. Urbanowisz W. Naczyniaki sromu u dziewczynek. *Ginekol Pol* 1973;44:687–691.
29. Mobius VW, Krause W. Das Vulvahamagiom biem Saugling und Kleinkind und seine Behandlung. *Zbl Gynak* 1974;96:280–286.
30. Cohen PR, Young AW, Tovell MM. Angiokeratoma of the vulva: diagnosis and review of the literature. *Obstet Gynecol Surg* 1989;44:339–346.

31. Dotters DJ, Fowler WC, Powers SK, et al. Argon laser therapy of vulvar angiokeratoma. *Obstet Gynecol* 1986; 68:56S–59S.

32. Robbins SL, Cotran RS, Kumar V. *Pathologic basis of disease.* Philadelphia: WB Saunders, 1984:152–153.

33. Imperial R, Helwig EB. Angiokeratoma of the vulva. *Obstet Gynecol* 1967;29:307–312.

34. Wilkinson EJ. *Pathology of vulva and vagina.* New York: Churchill Livingston, 1987:211.

35. Rabinowitz R, Churchill BM, Alexis ME, et al. Acquired vulvar lymphangiectasis in a child. *Urology* 1977;10: 459–460.

36. Tavassoli FA, Norris HJ. Smooth muscle tumors of the vulva. *Obstet Gynecol* 1979;53:213–217.

37. Diehl SR, Boehnke M, Erickson RP, et al. A refined genetic map of the region of chromosome 17 surrounding the von Recklinghausen neurofibromatosis (NFI) gene. *Am J Hum Genet* 1987;44:33–37.

38. Rink RC, Mitchell ME. Genitourinary neurofibromatosis in childhood. *J Urol* 1983;130:1176–1179.

39. Vaughan V, McKay RJ, Behrman RE. *Nelson textbook of pediatrics.* Philadelphia: WB Saunders, 1979:1765, 1865–1872.

40. D'Agostina AN, Soule EH, Miller RH. Sarcomas of the peripheral nerves and somatic soft tissues associated with multiple neurofibromatosis (von Recklinghausen's disease). *Cancer* 1963;16:1015.

41. Das Gupta TK, Brasfield RD. Von Recklinghausen's disease. *Cancer* 1971;21:174.

42. Labardini MM, Kallet HA, Cerny JC. Urogenital neurofibromatosis simulating an intersex problem. *J Urol* 1968;98:627–632.

43. Ogawa A, Watanabe K. Genitourinary neurofibromatosis in a child presenting with an enlarged penis and scrotum. *J Urol* 1986;135:755–757.

44. Schepel SJ, Tolhurst DE. Neurofibromata of clitoris and labium majus simulating a penis and testicle. *Br J Plast Surg* 1981;34:221–223.

45. Kaneti J, Liebrman F, Moshe P, et al. A case of ambiguous genitalia owing to neurofibromatosis—review of the literature. *J Urol* 1988;140:584–585.

46. Brooks GG. Granular cell myoblastoma of the vulva in a 6 year old girl. *Am J Obstet Gynecol* 1985;153: 897–898.

47. Hashem M. The pathology and histogenesis of the granular cell myoblastoma. *J Egypt Med Assoc* 1959;42: 239–260.

48. Coates JB, Hales JS. Granular cell myoblastoma of the vulva. *Obstet Gynecol* 1973;41:796.

49. Christensen WN, Friedman KJ, Woodruff JD, et al. Histologic characteristics of vulvar nevocellular nevi. *J Cutan Pathol* 1987;14:87–91.

50. Mesrogli M, Lelle RJ. [Vulvar cancer in a 13-year-old girl]. *Geburtshilfe Frauenheilkd* 1986;46:754–756.

51. Addison A. Adenocarcinoma of Bartholin's gland in a 14-year-old girl: report of a case. *Am J Obstet Gynecol* 1977;127:214–215.

52. Pack GT, Oropeza R. A comparative study of melanomas and epidermoid carcinomas of the vulva: a review of 44 melanomas and 58 epidermoid carcinomas (1930–1965). *Rev Surg* 1967;5:305–324.

53. Chung AF, Woodruff JM, Lewis JL. Malignant melanoma of the vulva: a report of 44 cases. *Obstet Gynecol* 1975;45:631–646.

54. Lister UM, Akinla O. Carcinoma of the vulva in child-

hood. *J Obstet Gynaecol Br Commonwealth* 1972;79: 470–473.

55. Elaraby II, Dent PB, Hunter JDW, et al. Histiocytosis X: late manifestations in a long-term survivor of Letterer-Siwe disease. *J Pediatr* 1976;89:961–962.

56. Egwuatu VE, Ejeckam GC, Okaqro JM. Burkitt's lymphoma of the vulva. Case report. *Br J Obstet Gynaecol* 1980;87:827–830.

57. Emerich J, Konefka T. Inwazyjny Rak Sromu U Szesnastoletniej Chorej. *Ginekol Pol* 1996;67:101–104.

58. Cario GM, House MJ, Paradinas FJ. Squamous cell carcinoma of the vulva in association with mixed vulvar dystrophy in an 18-year-old girl. Case report. *Br J Obstet Gynaecol* 1984;91:87–90.

59. Friedrich EG. Reversible vulvar atypia: a case report. *Obstet Gynecol* 1972;39:173–181.

60. Shafi MI, Luesley DM, Byrne P, et al. Vulval intraepithelial neoplasia—management and outcome. *Br J Obstet Gynaecol* 1989;96:1339–1344.

61. Moonen WA, Janknegt RA, Hoek WD von der. Sarcoma botryoides: radical treatment by pelvic exenteration with 11 years survival. *Arch Chir Neerl* 1970;22:1–6.

62. Piver MS, Rose PG. Long-term follow-up and complications of infants with vulvovaginal embryonal rhabdomyosarcoma treated with surgery, radiation therapy and chemotherapy. *Obstet Gynecol* 1988;71:435–437.

63. Hildebrand HF, Krivosic I, Grandier-Vazeille X, et al. Perineal rhabdomyosarcoma in a newborn child: pathological and biochemical studies with emphasis on contractile proteins. *J Clin Pathol* 1980;33: 823–829.

64. Talerman A. Sarcoma botryoides presenting as a polyp on the labium majus. *Cancer* 1973;32:994–999.

65. James GB, Guthrie W, Buchan A. Embryonic sarcoma of the vulva in an infant. *J Obstet Gynaecol Br Commonwealth* 1969;76:458–461.

66. Piver MS, Barlow JJ, Wang JJ, et al. Combined radical surgery, radiation therapy and chemotherapy in infants with vulvovaginal embryonal rhabdomyosarcoma. *Obstet Gynecol* 1973;42:522–526.

67. Ghavimi F, Herr H, Jereb B, et al. Treatment of genitourinary rhabdomyosarcoma in children. *J Urol* 1984; 132:313.

68. Andrassy RJ, Hays DM, Raney RB, et al. Conservative surgical management of vaginal and vulvar pediatric rhabdomyosarcoma: a report from the Intergroup Rhabdomyosarcoma Study III. *J Pediatr Surg* 1995;30: 1034–1036.

69. Castaldo TW, Petrilli ES, Ballon SC, et al. Endodermal sinus tumor of the clitoris. *Gynecol Oncol* 1980;9: 376–380.

70. Ungerleider RS, Donaldson SS, Warnke RA, et al. Endodermal sinus tumor: the Stanford experience and the first reported case arising in the vulva. *Cancer* 1978; 41:1627–1634.

71. Dudley AG, Young RH, Lawrence WD, et al. Endodermal sinus tumor of the vulva in an infant. *Obstet Gynecol* 1983;61:76S–79S.

72. Friedman RJ, Knopf AW, Jones WB. Malignant melanoma in association with lichen sclerosus on the vulva of a 14 year old. *Am J Dermatopathol* 1984;6:253–256.

73. Egan CA, Bradley RR, Loysdon UK, et al. Vulvar melanoma in childhood. *Arch Dermatol* 1997;133:345–348.

74. Morrow CP, Rutledge FN. Melanoma of the vulva. *Obstet Gynecol* 1972;39:745–752.

24

Malignant Neoplasms of the Vagina and Cervix in the Neonate, Child, and Adolescent

Carol M. Choi, Bhagirath Majmudar, and Ira R. Horowitz

Malignant neoplasms of the vagina and cervix in the neonate, child, and adolescent are extremely rare and unique. In this age group, the most common neoplasm of the lower genital tract is sarcoma botryoides followed by endodermal sinus tumors.

In the 1970s and early 1980s, the incidence of clear cell adenocarcinoma of the vagina and cervix became prominent due to *in utero* exposure to diethylstilbestrol (DES). The significant decline in DES use after 1955, however, should result in decreased incidence of clear cell adenocarcinoma and other sequelae in children and adolescents.

This chapter reviews the presentation, pathology, diagnosis, and management of each of these neoplastic processes.

SARCOMA BOTRYOIDES

Incidence/Epidemiology

Sarcoma botryoides is a form of rhabdomyosarcoma that occurs more commonly in the vagina than in the uterine cervix or corpus of children and adolescents. Rhabdomyosarcomas are the most common soft tissue sarcoma in children and adolescents (1–3) and are the most common malignancy of the head and neck and urogenital area, in that order (1,4,5). It is seen predominantly in children less than 2 years of age (5). Pelvic and genitourinary rhabdomyosarcomas account for approximately 20% of the tumors in this loca-

tion (1–3,6), whereas sarcoma botryoides of the lower genital tract accounts for approximately 3% of all cases of rhabdomyosarcomas (1).

Rhabdomyosarcoma can arise in the perineum, vulva, vagina, uterine cervix, and uterine corpus (1,7). This tumor generally is found in the vagina in infancy and early childhood, in the uterine cervix in the adolescent and reproductive years, and in the uterine corpus in the postmenopausal years (2,3).

This tumor typically invades into the wall of the vagina and soft tissue of the pelvis and readily metastasizes to lymph nodes, lung, liver, and bone. Local recurrence is common (4,5,8).

Pathology: Gross and Microscopic

There are five histologic classifications of rhabdomyosarcomas: embryonal, botryoid, alveolar, pleomorphic, and undifferentiated. Embryonal rhabdomyosarcomas account for more than half of all cases of rhabdomyosarcomas and are found more commonly in the head and neck region, retroperitoneum, and genitourinary system (14% to 45% of all cases) (1,2).

Sarcoma botryoides is the polypoid form of embryonal rhabdomyosarcoma. Its appearance occurs as a result of the rhabdomyosarcoma arising below a mucus membrane producing the typical grape-like, edematous, polypoid appearance (Fig. 24.1) (1,2,4).

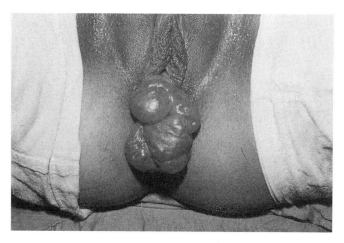

FIG. 24.1. Sarcoma botryoides. Grape-like edematous, polypoid mass extruding from the vagina of a child.

Microscopically, there is a dense cambium layer of tumor cells immediately below the surface epithelium (Fig. 24.2). Below the cambium layer, tumor cells are found in a dense collagenous stroma or loosely myxoid stroma. The cells are small, round to spindle shaped, and have oval nuclei with an open chromatin pattern. Cross-striations may be demonstrated in the cytoplasm representing rhabdomyogenesis (Fig. 24.3) (9).

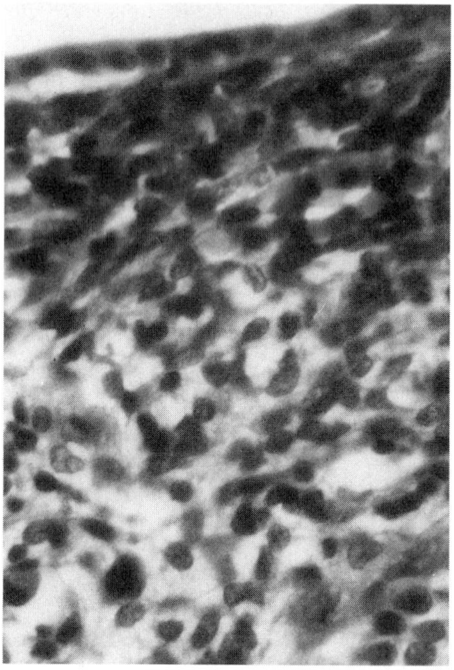

It is thought that embryonal rhabdomyosarcoma originates from abnormal differentiation of primitive embryonal mesenchyme of the urogenital sinus (1,5). There is a theory that one primitive mesenchymal cell is the stem cell of the entire range of soft tissue sarcomas, which would explain the appearance of rhabdomyocytes in locations where they are not normally found (10).

Symptoms/Physical Findings

Sarcoma botryoides is a superficial lesion. Bleeding or blood-tinged discharge is the most common presentation and usually occurs early (4,11).

Sarcoma botryoides frequently arises from the anterior vaginal wall, which is the area of the embryonic vesicovaginal septum or urogenital sinus. The bladder, prostatic utricle, prostate, and lower vagina are structures that arise from the urogenital sinus (12). The tumor may appear as small nodules, papillae, or pedunculated or sessile soft polypoid masses. Larger polypoid masses resembling

FIG. 24.2. Sarcoma botryoides. A dense cambium layer of tumor cells seen underneath mucosa (top layer). Undifferentiated rhabdomyoblasts are seen at the bottom.

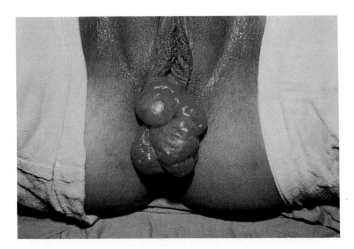

COLOR PLATE 5. Sarcoma botryoides. Grape-like edematous, polypoid mass extruding from the vagina of a child.

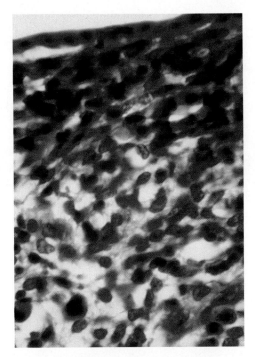

COLOR PLATE 6. Sarcoma botryoides. A dense cambium layer of tumor cells seen underneath mucosa (top layer). Undifferentiated rhabdomyoblasts are seen at the bottom.

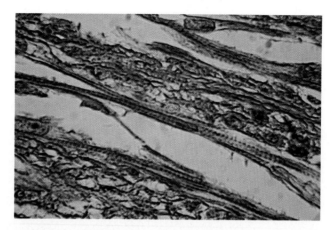

COLOR PLATE 7. Sarcoma botryoides. Cross-striations are seen in the better differentiated tumor cells away from the mucosa.

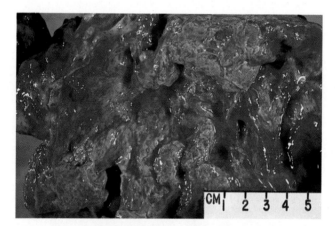

COLOR PLATE 8. Endodermal sinus tumor. A fleshy, necrotic vulvovaginal mass suggests malignancy.

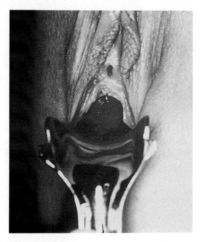

COLOR PLATE 9. Adenosis of vagina appearing as a red patch.

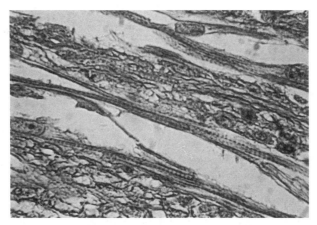

FIG. 24.3. Sarcoma botryoides. Cross-striations are seen in the better differentiated tumor cells away from the mucosa.

grapes may protrude from the vagina. More rarely, patients will present with an abdominopelvic mass (Figs. 24.4–24.5) (7,9). A polypoid mass should raise a suspicion of rhabdomyosarcoma. The differential diagnosis includes endodermal sinus tumor or a benign polyp (5). Diagnosis can be established by generous biopsies, preferably with the patient under anesthesia (4,5). Cytology of the lesion may be helpful (4). Pertinent clinical history provided to the pathologist can enhance the diagnostic procedure.

Diagnosis

The differential diagnosis of vaginal bleeding or a vaginal mass in an infant less than 3 years of age is endodermal sinus tumor (Fig. 24.6), sarcoma botryoides, or a benign polypoid mass such as condyloma (Fig. 24.7) (5).

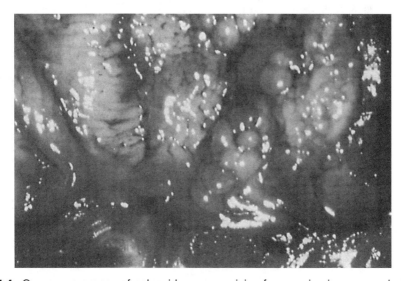

FIG. 24.4. Gross appearance of polypoid masses arising from vagina in sarcoma botryoides.

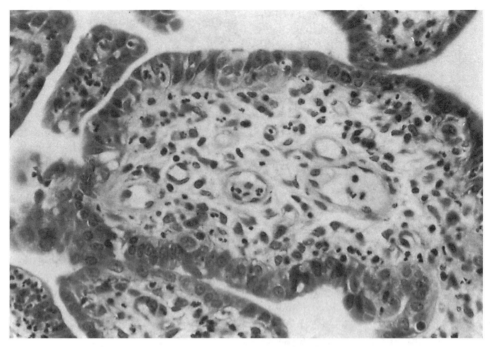

FIG. 24.5. Microscopic appearance of sarcoma botryoides.

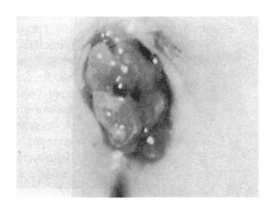

FIG. 24.6. Endodermal sinus tumor arising in infant vagina.

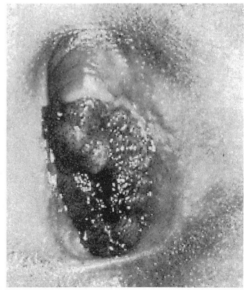

FIG. 24.7. Benign vaginal condylomata acuminata in an infant.

Cystoscopy and proctoscopy can be performed to determine if involvement of the bladder or rectum is present. Although most cases of sarcoma botryoides arise from the anterior vaginal wall and are confined to the pelvis at diagnosis, hematogenous and lymphogenous metastases can occur. The urethra and posterior bladder wall frequently are involved with tumor. Less often, the rectum, vulva, pelvic lymph nodes, lung, liver, and bone can be involved (5). A complete staging workup should, therefore, be performed, including chest x-ray and abdominopelvic computed tomographic scan. An intravenous pyelogram and bone scan may be useful.

Sarcoma botryoides is believed to arise from primitive embryonal mesenchyme in the lamina propria. It spreads beneath the mucous membrane of the vaginal wall or other pelvic structures. Microscopically, the tumor consists of poorly differentiated round or spindle cells. Striated muscle cells may be present.

Staging

There are several staging systems for rhabdomyosarcomas. The Intergroup Rhabdomyosarcoma Study staging system is surgical and based on treatment considerations as opposed to clinical extent of disease (Table 24.1, top) (13).

The simplest staging system was developed by Grosfeld et al. (14) and is based on clinical findings (Table 24.1, bottom).

Treatment

Treatment for rhabdomyosarcomas of the female genital tract has progressed from radical surgery to neoadjuvant chemotherapy followed by surgery and postoperative radiation (15,16). In the past, radical surgery or pelvic exenteration was the only acceptable treatment for genital rhabdomyosarcomas (17). Hilgers et al. (18) reviewed 49 cases of vaginal rhabdomyosarcoma and reported an 18% survival rate. Eight of the nine survivors were treated with radical surgery alone and one with radiation alone (18), supporting the use of radical surgery. Radiation therapy was used once the radiosensitivity of rhabdomyosarcomas was demonstrated. Unfortunately, it was not successful when used as single modality (1,19). In 1972, the Intergroup Rhabdomyosarcoma Study (IRS I) was formed as a cooperative effort of the Children's Cancer Study Group, the Southwest Oncology Group, and the Cancer and Leukemia Group. The results of their study showed excellent survival with early radical surgery followed by postoperative chemotherapy and radiotherapy (10). The surgery, however, was still radical and obviously influenced quality of life.

Kumar et al. (20) reported on the use of preoperative chemotherapy and radiotherapy followed by colpohysterectomy, resulting in a disease-free interval of 3 years. In 1979, Flamant et al. (21) demonstrated the effectiveness of primary chemotherapy and radiotherapy. One patient in their series of eight required a colpo-

TABLE 24.1. *Staging systems for rhabdomyosarcomas*

Intergroup Rhabdomyosarcoma Study	
Group I	Local disease, completely resected, regional lymph nodes not involved
Group Ia	Confined to muscle or organ of origin
Group Ib	Contiguous involvement. Infiltration outside the muscle or organ of origin, as through fascial planes
Group II	Regional disease
Group IIa	Negative nodes, completely resected, microscopic residual
Group IIb	Positive nodes, completely resected, no microscopic residual
Group IIc	Positive nodes, microscopic residual
Group III	Incomplete resection or biopsy, gross residual disease
Group IV	Distant metastasis
Grosfeld et al.	
Stage I	Local disease
Stage II	Regional disease
Stage III	Disseminated disease

hysterectomy. Rivard et al. (22) and Ortega (23) demonstrated that primary chemotherapy followed by less radical surgery had comparable survival to radical surgery and postoperative chemotherapy. Hays (11) conducted a review of the literature on neoadjuvant chemotherapy and/or radiation and found that the majority of rhabdomyosarcomas of the female genital system responded to chemotherapy without radical surgery.

IRS II (1978–1984) was formed to evaluate protocols with the aim of preserving the urinary tract while maintaining high survival rates, as in IRS I (24). In 1984, IRS III gave all patients with group III disease primary chemotherapy and reserved radiation and surgery for cases with residual disease. As of 1995, no recurrences had been documented (12).

Presently, multimodality therapy has allowed for less radical surgical resection with the use of chemotherapy and/or radiation before resection (2,6,25). Balat et al. (26) reported a case of endocervical sarcoma botryoides treated with vincristine, actinomycin D, and cyclophosphamide (VAC) combination chemotherapy followed by simple hysterectomy without evidence of disease for 8 years. Lin et al. (27) also reported a case of cervical sarcoma botryoides treated with cervicectomy and subsequent VAC combination chemotherapy, with a 3-year disease-free interval. Gerbaulet et al. (28) combined exploratory laparotomy with lymph node sampling and ovarian transposition with brachytherapy and chemotherapy in 14 patients with rhabdomyosarcoma of 37 children and adolescents with lower genital tract malignancies in the series. They reported an overall 94% local control rate and 80% long-term survival. The other patients in the series had endodermal sinus tumors of the vagina or cervix (6), clear cell adenocarcinoma of the vagina or cervix (13), sarcoma of the vulva (3), and undifferentiated tumor of the vulva (1).

It is now accepted that treatment for sarcoma botryoides begins with combination chemotherapy (VAC) followed by surgery if there is a response to the chemotherapy. If there is no response, then radiation therapy should be used. With partial response to preoperative chemotherapy or radiation, all gross tumor should be excised with preservation of major organs (bladder, rectum, ovaries, vagina). When there is regional nodal spread or residual microscopic disease, radiation should be added. Chemotherapy should continue in all cases for 18 to 24 months (1,2,4, 5). The only role for radical surgery involves no response to preoperative chemotherapy or radiation (1).

Prognosis

Prognosis for children with rhabdomyosarcoma before 1970 was poor. Survival rates were less than 15% when treated with radical surgery or radiation alone (1,6). With the development of combined modality approach over the years, using surgery, chemotherapy, and radiotherapy, survival has improved, with rates greater than 60% for all stages of any site and up to 90% for localized disease (1,3). Rhabdomyosarcomas of the vagina and vulva have better outcome overall compared to primary uterine rhabdomyosarcomas (11). A recent review of the literature by Zeisler et al. (3) indicated patients with group I disease have good prognosis, and extensive surgery is not necessary to improve survival. Recurrences and metastasis are prognostically unfavorable factors (4).

ENDODERMAL SINUS TUMORS

Incidence/Epidemiology

Endodermal sinus tumors of the vagina and cervix are an extremely rare entity. There are approximately 50 cases reported in the literature worldwide. All cases with histopathologic evidence were diagnosed in children less than 3 years of age (29), although Ishi et al. (30) recently reported a case of endodermal sinus tumor originating in the vagina of a 10-year-old girl.

The etiology of this tumor remains unknown and controversial. Given their midline location, it has been postulated that these tumors may have originated from germ cells that did not

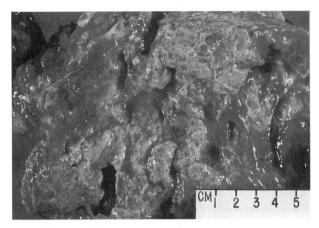

FIG. 24.8. Endodermal sinus tumor. A fleshy, necrotic vulvovaginal mass suggests malignancy.

completely migrate to the gonads from the hindgut. However, other malignant germ cell tumors have not been found in the lower genital tract (31). Although the histology and presence of α-fetoprotein are consistent with germ cell origin of this tumor in the vagina and cervix, again other germ cell elements are not found, as would be expected (29).

Pathology

The gross and histologic features of vaginal endodermal sinus tumors are similar to those tumors of ovarian origin. Typically, they are tan or white soft vaginal masses, polypoid or sessile, and measure 1 to 5 cm in diameter. Hemorrhage and necrosis are evident on gross

examination (Fig. 24.8). The histologic patterns may be microcystic, reticular, papillary, or solid. Schiller-Duval bodies are present and assist in diagnosis (Fig. 24.9). Similarly, extracellular and intracellular periodic-acid–Schiff (PAS)-positive hyaline drops commonly are found. Immunohistochemically, these tumors stain positive for α-fetoprotein and $α_1$-antitrypsin, which distinguishes them from other tumors (31).

Symptoms/Physical Findings

The usual presenting symptom is bloody or blood-tinged vaginal discharge similar to sarcoma botryoides. Physical examination reveals a polypoid, friable lesion arising from

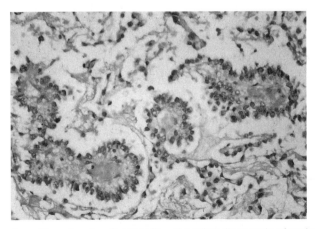

FIG. 24.9. Microscopic section showing Schiller-Duval bodies diagnostic of endodermal sinus tumor.

the vagina or cervix resembling sarcoma botryoides (29,32). As previously mentioned in sarcoma botryoides, an examination with the patient under anesthesia may be required. Biopsy of the lesion is the only definitive way to make the diagnosis.

Diagnosis

The differential diagnosis includes sarcoma botryoides and clear cell adenocarcinoma (32, 33). The histologic difference between sarcoma botryoides and endodermal sinus tumors is clear. It is more difficult, however, to differentiate endodermal sinus tumors from clear cell adenocarcinomas. The difference in age range for the tumors, less than 3 years for endodermal sinus tumors and more than 8 years for clear cell adenocarcinoma, can help clinically. Histopathologically, endodermal sinus tumors of the infant vagina are identical to endodermal sinus tumors of the ovary and may have a tubuloacinar, reticular, or solid pattern. Schiller-Duval bodies, PAS-positive globules, and positive staining for α-fetoprotein should be present (33). The serum α-fetoprotein level that can be measured by radioimmunoassay may be used both for diagnostic purposes and to follow the status of the disease throughout therapy.

Again, an examination with the patient under anesthesia is preferable, which would allow for a thorough examination with biopsies and accurate staging (29).

Treatment

Current treatment for endodermal sinus tumors of the vagina and cervix involves a combination of surgery (radical or simple excision) and chemotherapy. Vawter (34) introduced the use of actinomycin D for treatment of endodermal sinus tumors of the vagina. Young and Scully (32) reported nine cases of vaginal endodermal sinus tumor. The first two patients did not receive chemotherapy and died 6 and 13 months after diagnosis. The third patient was treated with hysterectomy and total vaginectomy. Chemotherapy

was initiated when recurrence was documented 6 months later. The following six cases received VAC chemotherapy and were free of disease. Four of these six patients received preoperative chemotherapy, and three surgical specimens were free of cancer. Copeland et al. (29) reported a series of six patients with endodermal sinus tumor of the vagina or cervix treated with surgery and postoperative chemotherapy with VAC. Four of the six were alive and free of disease at or beyond 2 years. One of the survivors was disease-free for 23 years and another for 10 years. These two patients underwent total pelvic exenteration and radical hysterectomy with vaginectomy, respectively. Another survivor had hysterectomy with partial vaginectomy and was alive and well at 33 months. The other survivor had excisional biopsy and was disease-free for 24 months. Interestingly, they had one patient with pulmonary metastases who had a biopsy for diagnosis only and was treated with VAC, resulting in complete response until recurrence at 11 months (Table 24.2).

Collins et al. (35) reported a patient with vaginal endodermal sinus tumor treated with chemotherapy who was disease-free for 45 months. The chemotherapeutic agents used were vinblastine, bleomycin, and cisplatin, followed by VAC. Andersen et al. (36) treated a patient with preoperative VAC followed by local excision, resulting in a disease-free interval of 50 months.

Although these tumors are radiosensitive (37), radiation may not be necessary for treatment. Ovarian function may be preserved, and possible adverse affects of radiation on the bone growth plates may be avoided with the

TABLE 24.2. *Chemotherapeutic agents useful in therapy of endodermal sinus tumor*

Vincristine
Vinblastine
Actinomycin D
Adriamycin
Cyclophosphamide
Bleomycin
Cisplatinum
Etoposide (VP-16)

combination of surgery and chemotherapy. Likewise, radical surgery may not be essential in the treatment regimen for all patients with endodermal sinus tumors of the vagina and cervix. It is possible to preserve reproductive and sexual function with a combination of conservative surgery and neoadjuvant or adjuvant chemotherapy (29–39).

Recurrent disease remains a problem. There are few cases of recurrence that were treated successfully (38,40). Serum α-fetoprotein levels can be monitored during treatment to follow the course of disease (32). Elevated levels in the treated patients is a sensitive marker indicating recurrence (41).

Prognosis

Prognosis is poor in this group of tumors. Without treatment, patients die within 6 months of presentation (32). Median survival is approximately 11 months. Of these patients, 10% to 15% die within 2 years. Of those who survive 2 years, 10% will have recurrence within 12 months (29). As of 1985, only five patients were reported to have survived 5 years (29,40,42,43). Since then, there have been other patients with at least a 5-year, disease-free interval (39,41), most likely attributable to the newer chemotherapeutic agents.

DIETHYSTILBESTROL-RELATED VAGINAL AND CERVICAL LESIONS

DES is a nonsteroid estrogen that initially was introduced in 1946 and widely used in the early 1950s for various indications, including threatened abortions, recurrent abortions, premature labor, preeclampsia/eclampsia, history of prior stillbirths, and essential hypertension. In 1953, Dieckmann et al. (44) demonstrated no beneficial effects of DES use in pregnancy via double-blind prospective study. However, because no harmful effects were noted with DES use, it continued to be prescribed until the early 1970s. Brackbill et al. (45) reanalyzed the data of Dieckmann et al. and found that DES use actually increased abortions, premature births, and neonatal deaths.

In 1971, Herbst et al. (46) reported eight cases of vaginal adenocarcinoma (both clear cell and endometrial type) occurring over a 4-year time span in New England. Retrospective investigation revealed that the patients were born between 1946 and 1951, and seven of the eight patients were exposed to DES *in utero* during the first trimester. Then in 1974, 170 cases were reported by Herbst et al. (47). The National Cancer Institute commissioned the formation of a national cooperative program, Diethylstilbestrol Adenosis (DESAD), in 1974 to investigate the occurrence of cancer and genital tract abnormalities in women who were exposed to DES *in utero* (48,49).

In utero exposure to DES is associated with vaginal epithelial abnormalities, reproductive tract structural abnormalities, clear cell adenocarcinoma of the vagina and cervix, and increased risk for dysplasia. The most predominant vaginal epithelial change is adenosis or the presence of endocervical glands in the vaginal mucosa (Fig. 24.10). The characteristic columnar epithelium can be found anywhere in the vagina but usually close to

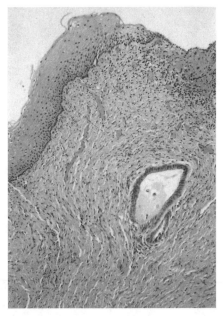

FIG. 24.10. Squamous epithelium of vagina **(top)** overlying a deep focus of vaginal adenosis.

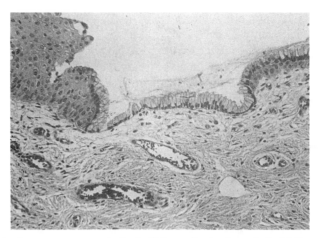

FIG. 24.11. Squamous metaplasia **(left)** in vaginal adenosis **(middle and right)**.

the cervix in the fornices of the vagina, as well as on the cervix itself. Squamous metaplasia then replaces the columnar epithelium with squamous epithelium (Fig. 24.11). Often, submucosal cystic or nodular structures may be visible or palpable in areas of adenosis. Given that adenocarcinomas originate submucosally, evaluation of these lesions with biopsy is important (Figs. 24.12–24.13) (50).

Structural abnormalities include cervical hoods or collars, cervical cockscombs (Fig. 24.14), transverse vaginal ridges, wide cervical ectropions (Fig. 24.15), and cervical hypo-

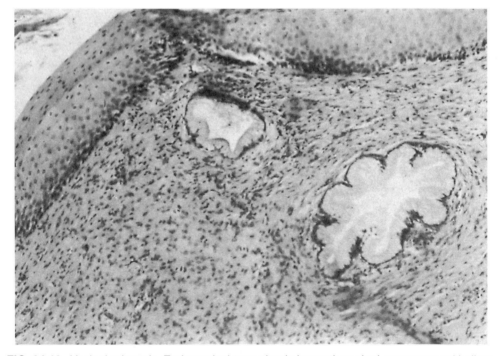

FIG. 24.12. Vaginal adenosis. Endocervical-type glands beneath vaginal squamous epithelium.

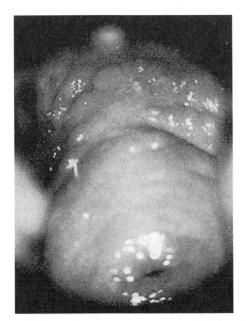

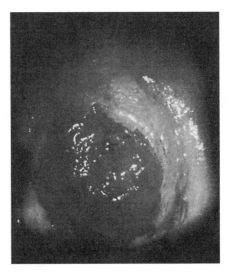

FIG. 24.15. Cervical eversion with darker columnar epithelium extending onto exocervix.

FIG. 24.13. Anterior vaginal wall with manifestations of vaginal adenosis.

plasia (Fig. 24.16). These structural abnormalities tend to disappear progressively, as does vaginal adenosis (51). DES exposure also affects the uterus, resulting in a T-shaped endometrial cavity, constricting bands in the

endometrial cavity, and uterine hypoplasia (50).

DES exposure *in utero* confers a greater risk for development of cervical and vaginal intraepithelial neoplasia, although there is no explanation for this increased risk (52). Current recommendations for women exposed to DES *in utero* are evaluation at age 14 years or menarche. Inspection, palpation, and cytologic sampling of the vagina and cervix are essential, preferably every 6 months (53,54).

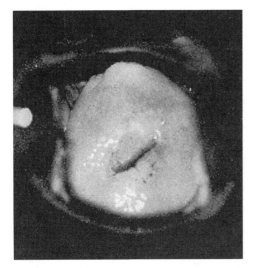

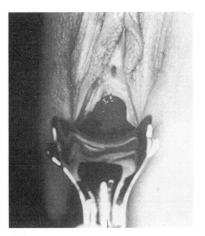

FIG. 24.14. Cockscomb abnormality of anterior cervix.

FIG. 24.16. Adenosis of vagina appearing as a red patch.

CLEAR CELL ADENOCARCINOMAS

Incidence/Epidemiology

Before 1970, clear cell adenocarcinoma of the vagina and cervix was a very rare phenomenon. Carcinoma of the vagina usually affected older women and was mainly of squamous origin (55). The subsequent increase in incidence of clear cell adenocarcinoma of the vagina in the 1970s in younger women led to the discovery of its association with DES exposure *in utero* (46,47). The estimated risk of developing vaginal clear cell adenocarcinoma after *in utero* exposure to DES is one in 1,000 (56). Vaginal adenosis, an epithelial abnormality associated with DES exposure, was almost universally present in all patients with clear cell adenocarcinoma (46,57).

More than 500 cases of vaginal or cervical clear cell adenocarcinoma were reported from 1971 to 1992 in the Registry for Research on Hormonal Transplacental Carcinogenesis (58). This registry was established by Herbst and Scully to investigate clear cell adenocarcinoma of the vagina and cervix in women born after 1940. Approximately two thirds of the cases had a history of exposure to DES, hexestrol, or dienestrol *in utero* during the first trimester. Another 12% were exposed to an unknown medication used for high-risk pregnancies, and 25% had no known maternal hormone ingestion (59,60).

Peak incidence of clear cell adenocarcinoma of the vagina in patients exposed to DES occurs at age 19 years (range 7 to 33 years) (61,62). Clear cell adenocarcinoma usually spreads by direct extension, lymphatic dissemination, and hematogenous dissemination (63). Approximately one sixth of stage I tumors have metastasized to the pelvic lymph nodes on further exploration. Compared with squamous cell cancers, clear cell adenocarcinomas tend to recur late and spread outside the abdominal cavity more frequently (54,64,65).

Symptoms/Physical Findings

Prolonged vaginal bleeding is the most common symptom. Diagnosis can be delayed when the bleeding has been attributed to anovulation in this age group. Vaginal discharge is another symptom usually associated with larger tumors (63). Once awareness of the tumor was established, the tumor was detected at an earlier, asymptomatic stage.

Approximately 60% of clear cell adenocarcinoma lesions are confined to the upper third of the anterior vagina, although any portion of the vagina or cervix may be involved. The site of the tumor corresponds to the common sites of adenosis (63).

Pathology

Grossly, these tumors vary in size from microscopic to large. The larger lesions usually are polypoid and nodular, but they can be flat and ulcerated with an indurated surface. The smaller tumors may not be visible by gross or colposcopic examination if they are confined to the lamina propria and are covered by intact squamous epithelium. They can, however, be palpable. Most clear cell adenocarcinomas of the vagina and cervix are superficial with a few millimeters depth of invasion, although some lesions are more extensive than expected on gross inspection and examination (Fig. 24.17) (63).

Histologically, DES-associated clear cell adenocarcinoma of the vagina or cervix is identical to clear cell adenocarcinoma of the endometrium and the ovary (Fig. 24.18). The tumor can show several histologic patterns. The most characteristic pattern has solid sheets of clear cells. The second most common pattern is tubulocystic, which consists of tubules and cysts lined by hobnails, flat cells, or cells resembling müllerian-type epithelium. Hobnail cells have a bulbous nucleus that protrudes into the lumen. Flat cells appear benign and may make it difficult to differentiate from adenosis (63).

Other less common patterns include a papillary pattern, a tubular pattern similar to endometrial carcinoma, and a pattern of cords of cells with eosinophilic cytoplasm. The cytoplasm in any of these patterns does not contain mucin, although the lumen may have mucin.

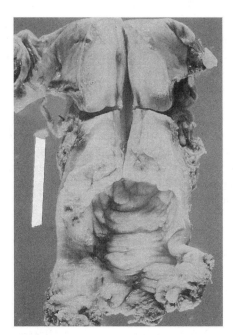

FIG. 24.17. Diffuse involvement of vagina by clear cell carcinoma in a young woman.

Interestingly, atypical adenosis has been found adjacent to most clear cell adenocarcinomas. Atypical adenosis is characterized by nuclear pleomorphism, hyperchromasia, prominent nucleoli, and glands with cellular stratification without any overt changes of malignancy or invasion (63).

Diagnosis

An abnormal Papanicolaou (Pap) smear may lead to the diagnosis, as may an abnormality on routine pelvic examination. Definitive diagnosis is made or biopsy of the lesion, which may arise from any portion of the vagina or cervix, but which most frequently occurs on the anterior wall or the upper vagina. The differential diagnosis includes microglandular hyperplasia and the Arias-Stella reaction. Microglandular hyperplasia is a benign condition associated with oral contraceptive use and occasionally with pregnancy. This lesion can be differentiated from clear cell adenocarcinoma by the presence of clefts lined with mucinous epithelium that courses through metaplastic squamous epithelium. The glands are continuous with the clefts, suggesting that they resulted from budding and arborization of the mucinous epithelium constituting vaginal adenosis (not tuboendometrial type) or the endocervix. Microglandular hyperplasia is reversed once oral contraceptives are discontinued or pregnancy has ended (63).

The Arias-Stella reaction usually is found in the endometrium of pregnant women. It also has been identified in the endocervix and tuboendometrial type vaginal adenosis. Hypersecretory glands are lined with cells with

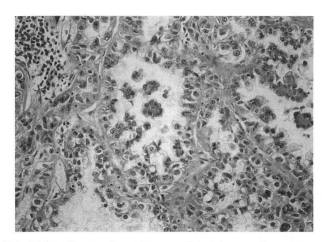

FIG. 24.18. Clear cell carcinoma with a micropapillary pattern.

enlarged nuclei that resemble hobnail cells, usually are smudged, appear degenerative, and have no mitotic activity (63).

Treatment

The challenge of treatment lies in preserving ovarian and vaginal function in younger women who usually have this tumor. For stage I tumors, a combination of wide local excision, retroperitoneal lymphadenectomy, and local irradiation was found to be as successful in terms of survival and recurrence as conventional treatment that involved radical hysterectomy with pelvic lymphadenectomy and partial or total vaginectomy with subsequent split-thickness skin graft (66). However, Jones et al. (54) recommend radical surgery when the tumor is confined to the vagina or cervix.

Frequent follow-up after primary therapy is important given the tendency of the tumor to recur late. Follow-up should include evaluation of the abdomen, lungs, and supraclavicular regions (63,67,68). Jones et al. (69) reported three cases of late recurrence of clear cell adenocarcinoma of the vagina and cervix. One patient underwent wide local excision, staging laparotomy, and pelvic irradiation for vaginal clear cell adenocarcinoma. She remained disease-free for 7 years 3 months, when recurrence was found in the lung. The mass was resected and she received radiation and chemotherapy and has remained free of disease for 13 years. Fishman et al. (70) reported two cases of vaginal clear cell adenocarcinoma with recurrences 17 and 19 years after initial therapy, further emphasizing the need for long-term surveillance.

Prognosis

Overall 5-year survival rate is 78%. Survival is 87% for stage I disease, 76% for stage II disease, and 30% for stage III disease (59,60). When clear cell adenocarcinoma of the vagina or cervix is discovered in asymptomatic patients during examination secondary to history of DES exposure, survival approaches 100%. Factors associated with better prognosis are age older than 19 years and a tubulocystic pattern (59). Recurrence usually occurs within 3 years, and one fifth of patients who have recurrence survive an additional 3 years (63).

Waggoner et al. (71) compared prognosis of vaginal clear cell adenocarcinoma in patients with a history of DES exposure *in utero* versus those without prior exposure and reported a poorer prognosis and higher rate of distant metastasis in patients without DES exposure. The reasons for this difference have yet to be determined.

SQUAMOUS CELL LESIONS

Squamous cell carcinomas of the cervix in patients under 18 years of age are essentially unknown. Likewise, vaginal squamous cell carcinoma in this age group is extraordinarily rare, with only five documented cases between ages 11 and 20 years, as reported by DiDomenico (72). Two of these patients were pregnant at the time of diagnosis. Common symptoms of vaginal squamous carcinoma include vaginal bleeding and/or pelvic pain. Symptoms related to the urinary tract, including hematuria, dysuria, or urgency, may occur. Diagnosis is confirmed by biopsy of the vaginal lesions. Radiation is the mainstay of therapy, although radical hysterectomy can be performed on lesions confined to the upper vagina.

DYSPLASIA

More commonly encountered in the adolescent are premalignant squamous lesions of the cervix or dysplasia. Any sexually active female is at risk for development of dysplasia. Screening should, therefore, begin with the onset of sexual activity or age 20 years, whichever occurs first. Although the frequency of screening is controversial, most clinicians in the United States continue to screen normal sexually active women at yearly intervals and high-risk women, such as those with a past history of dysplasia, more frequently.

Pathologically, cervical dysplasia consists of a proliferation of undifferentiated basal cells with malignant features and a decrease in superficial cell differentiation. Cervical

TABLE 24.3. *Classification of cervical dysplasia*

	Low-grade SIL
	HPV changes
CIN I	Mild dysplasia
	High-grade SIL
CIN II	Moderate dysplasia
CIN III	Severe dysplasia
CIN III	Carcinoma *in situ*

CIN, cervical intraepithelial neoplasia; HPV, human papilloma virus; SIL, squamous intraepithelial lesions.

dysplasia has been divided into three grades (Table 24.3): cervical intraepithelial neoplasia (CIN) I, or mild dysplasia; CIN II, or moderate dysplasia; and CIN III, or severe dysplasia/carcinoma *in situ* based on the degree of proliferation of undifferentiated cells. In CIN I, these cells occupy approximately one third of the epithelium, with the upper two thirds demonstrating some cytoplasmic differentiation. In CIN II, the lower two thirds of the epithelium are occupied by undifferentiated cells. In CIN III, full-thickness changes occur. Mitosis and nuclear pleomorphism are common.

The development of cervical dysplasia is believed to be dependent, at least in part, on infection by HPV. Manifestations of this infection, such as koilocytosis (cells with eccentric nuclei with perinuclear clearing representing the episomal viral particles), often are seen in early dysplastic lesions (Fig. 24.19). As the severity of dysplasia increases, the presence of koilocytes often decreases, as the viral DNA becomes integrated into the host genome (Fig. 24.20) (Table 24.3). For a further discussion of HPV, see Chapter 19.

Recently, a new system for classification of cervical dysplasia has been proposed. The Bethesda System (72) divides cervical dysplasia into low-grade squamous intraepithelial lesions (SIL), including HPV changes and CIN; and high-grade SIL, including CIN II and CIN III. This two-tiered system had not been universally accepted, as the natural history and therapeutic management plan for the categories within each group may differ significantly.

Evaluation of dysplasia in the adolescent is identical to the evaluation performed in an

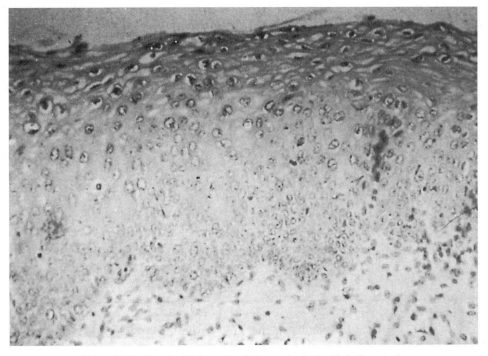

FIG. 24.19. Cervical intraepithelial neoplasia I with koilocytosis.

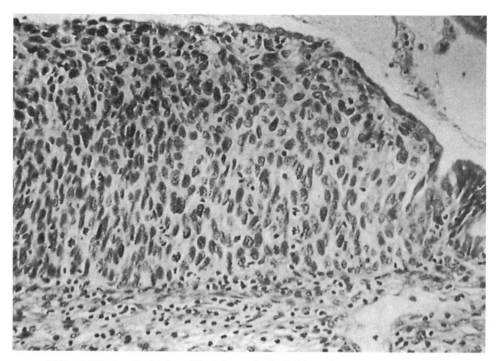

FIG. 24.20. Cervical intraepithelial neoplasia III. Note absence of koilocytosis.

adult. A complete discussion of the evaluation and therapy of dysplasia is beyond the scope of this chapter, and the interested reader is referred to one of the many texts on gynecologic oncology or colposcopy. A synopsis of the diagnosis and management of CIN will be presented.

The diagnosis of cervical dysplasia begins with the abnormal Pap smear. To obtain the highest yield and the lowest false-negative rate, the Pap smear must be performed correctly. Most dysplasia originates in the transformation zone or at the squamocolumnar junction. This area must, therefore, be sampled with the exocervical scrape. In adolescents, a wide eversion may be present, necessitating sampling away from the endocervical canal and near the vaginal fornices. An endocervical sample also should be obtained. The sample should be smeared on the slide uniformly thin and should be fixed immediately to avoid air-drying artifact. Performance of the Pap smear during heavy vaginal bleeding should be avoided, as the blood may obscure the epithelial cells and make evaluation diffi-

cult. A small amount of bleeding usually presents no difficulty.

All abnormal Pap smears should be evaluated with colposcopy and biopsy, if indicated (Table 24.4). This includes Pap smears with persistent atypia that is not of inflammatory origin, glandular atypia, HPV, squamous dysplasia of any degree, or any indication of carcinoma.

Colposcopic evaluation of the cervix is performed after the application of 3% acetic acid. The acetic acid not only serves to remove cervical mucous but also dehydrates the cells, turning those cells with larger nuclei a bright white due to greater reflection of light. The magnification of the colposcope and the use of the green filter, which accentuates vascular patterns, allow identification of abnormal dysplas-

TABLE 24.4. *Indications for colposcopy*

- Persistent squamous atypia (noninflammatory)
- Glandular atypia
- Human papilloma virus changes
- Squamous dysplasia
- Suspicion of carcinoma

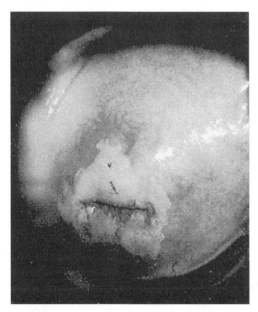

FIG. 24.21. Cervical intraepithelial neoplasia III. Colposcopic view with white epithelium and mosaic pattern at 12 o'clock.

tic tissue. The main patterns seen with dysplasia are white epithelium (Fig. 24.21), mosaicism (Fig. 24.22), and punctation. When squamous metaplasia is present, it appears as a thin white covering over glandular epithelium, which often can be peeled away by a cotton swab. The hallmark of invasive cervical cancer is the presence of abnormal vessels. Abnormal vessels are characterized by their abnormal branching pattern and not by their size, as enlarged but normally branching vessels can be seen overlying nabothian cysts and in inflammatory processes. Any colposcopic abnormality should be biopsied to obtain a definitive diagnosis. Any gross lesion of the cervix should be biopsied regardless of the Pap smear result.

During the colposcopic procedure, a decision must be made regarding the adequacy of the study. An adequate colposcopy is one in which the entire lesion and the entire squamocolumnar junction can be visualized. If the lesion extends into the canal beyond visualization capability, even after the use of an endocervical speculum, or if the entire squamocolumnar junction cannot be seen, further diagnostic procedures such as a cervical conization may be necessary.

Although routine sampling of the endocervix at the time of colposcopy is somewhat controversial, many colposcopists believe that this important step should never be omitted. Endocervical curettage not only allows the detection of squamous lesions in the endocervical canal that may be missed on colposcopic visualization of the cervix, but also aids in the detection of adenocarcinoma of the endocervix, which often is difficult to detect on Pap smear. Certainly, it is absolutely necessary in any patient being evaluated for glandular atypia on Pap smear, which is often the only indication of adenocarcinoma. Endocervical curettage should not be performed during pregnancy.

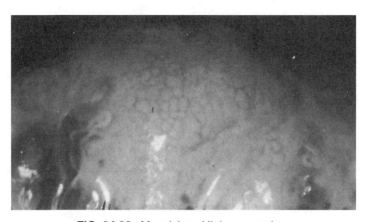

FIG. 24.22. Mosaicism. High-power view.

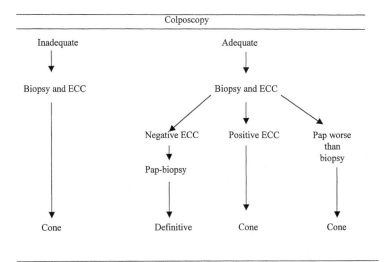

FIG. 24.23. Management of the abnormal Pap smear.

Therapy

After the cervical biopsy is performed, the pathology must be correlated with the Pap smear result (Fig. 24.23). If the biopsy is equal to or more abnormal than the Pap smear (with one degree of latitude) and the colposcopy is adequate, then definitive therapy may be performed. If the biopsy is less abnormal than the Pap smear, if the colposcopy is inadequate, or if the endocervical curettage is positive, then a cervical conization should be performed. If frankly invasive cervical carcinoma is found, definitive therapy may be planned. However, the finding of microinvasive carcinoma without vascular or lymphatic invasion on biopsy necessitates cone biopsy before definitive treatment planning.

When cervical conization is not required for further evaluation, there are several options for the therapy of CIN I, CIN II, and CIN III that have been adequately evaluated and correlated (Table 24.5). These include observation, cryotherapy, laser ablation, loop excision of the transformation zone, conization, and hysterectomy.

Observation alone may be used in patients with subclinical HPV infection only and no evidence of dysplasia. It also may be elected in highly motivated patients with mild dyspla-

sia, as up to 62% (73) of untreated mild dysplasia may regress to normal without therapy. Observation should never be chosen in patients who are noncompliant, and therapy should be instituted immediately if progression of the dysplasia is noted at follow-up visits, which should be performed every 3 to 4 months. Observation alone has some distinct advantages in adolescents whose low-grade dysplasia may purely be a manifestation of infection with HPV. The initiation of ablative therapies at a young age may result in increasingly difficult cervical evaluation should the process recur. This may lead to repetitive and increasingly aggressive procedures for this low-grade abnormality.

Cryotherapy, laser ablation, and loop excision are appropriate therapies for CIN I, CIN II, and small CIN III lesions. Cryotherapy has the advantage of being inexpensive, easily

TABLE 24.5. *Available therapies for cervical dysplasia*

- Observation
- Cryotherapy
- Laser vaporization
- Cold knife conization
- Loop excision
- Hysterectomy

and quickly performed, and readily available. Although few serious side effects are noted from cryotherapy, patients do note a thin watery discharge for approximately 14 days, and the procedure may cause the squamo-columnar junction to migrate into the endo-cervical canal, making further colposcopic evaluation difficult. Laser ablation is more costly, is more difficult and time consuming to perform, and may cause pain and bleeding. Healing after laser therapy, however, is more rapid, and the position of the squamocolum-nar junction on the exocervix often can be preserved, thus facilitating future colposcopic evaluation. The cure rates for cryotherapy and laser therapy for CIN I, CIN II, and small CIN III lesions are identical. Large CIN III lesions have a higher failure rate and often are treated by cervical conization. An approximate 2% incidence of invasive disease is present when cervical conization is performed (74).

Loop excision of the transformation zone is a new procedure that has tremendous poten-tial in the therapy of all grades of CIN (75, 76). This technique has the advantage of be-ing fast, easy, and well tolerated. It has few side effects and provides a tissue specimen for definitive pathologic evaluation. The dia-thermy loop may be used to perform cone biopsies in an office setting (77). The major disadvantage of loop excision is the necessity for injection of local anesthesia with a vaso-constrictor into the cervix for anesthesia and prevention of bleeding. When performed properly, the incidence of bleeding is minimal and healing is rapid. The location of the squa-mocolumnar junction usually is preserved on the exocervix. Although a large body of data has not yet been collected on loop excision of the transformation zone, it seems a very promising new technique.

Hysterectomy as a therapy for cervical dys-plasia has a limited role and should be reserved for those patients with CIN III who have no further childbearing in mind.

Follow-up after therapy for cervical dyspla-sia should be performed 4 months after ther-apy and every 3 to 4 months thereafter. If Pap smears remain normal for 1 year, the patient then may be seen at 6-month intervals. Any recurrence of abnormality on Pap smear should reinitiate the entire evaluation and therapeutic process.

ACKNOWLEDGMENTS

The authors are grateful to the late J. Don-ald Woodruff, M.D., for providing Fig. 24.1 and Figs. 24.4–24.7 and to Michelle Dudzin-ski for the section on squamous lesions pre-sent in the first edition.

REFERENCES

1. Bell J, Averette H, Davis J, et al. Genital rhabdomyosar-coma: current management and review of the literature. *Obstet Gynecol Surv* 1986;41:257–263.
2. Brand E, Berek JS, Nieberg RK, et al. Rhabdomyosar-coma of the uterine cervix: sarcoma botryoides. *Cancer* 1987;60:1552–1560.
3. Zeisler H, Mayerhofer K, Joura A, et al. Embryonal rhabdomyosarcoma of the uterine cervix: case report and review of the literature. *Gynecol Oncol* 1998;69:78–83.
4. Copeland LJ, Gershenson DM, Saul PB, et al. Sarcoma botryoides of the female genital tract. *Obstet Gynecol* 1985;66:262–266.
5. McHenry CR, Reynolds M, Raffensparger JG. Vaginal neoplasms in infancy: the combined role of chemother-apy and conservative surgical resection. *J Pediatr Surg* 1988;23:842–845.
6. Fleming ID, Etcubanas E, Patterson R, et al. The role of surgical resection when combined with chemother-apy and radiation in the management of pelvic rhabdo-myosarcoma. *Ann Surg* 1984;199:509–514.
7. Hicks ML, Piver MS. Conservative surgery plus adjuvant therapy for vulvovaginal rhabdomyosarcoma, diethyl-stilbestrol clear cell adenocarcinoma of the vagina, and unilateral germ cell tumors of the ovary. *Pediatr Adolesc Gynecol* 1992;19:219–233.
8. Maurer HM, Moon T, Donaldson M, et al. The Inter-group Rhabdomyosarcoma Study: a preliminary report. *Cancer* 1977;40:2015–2026.
9. Zaino RJ, Robboy SJ, Bentley R, et al. Diseases of the vagina. In: Kurman RJ, ed. *Blaustein's pathology of the female genital tract,* 4th ed. New York: Springer-Verlag, 1994:168–170.
10. Gaiger AM, Soule EH, Newton WA Jr. Pathology of rhabdomyosarcoma: experience of the Intergroup Rhab-domyosarcoma Study, 1972–1978. *Natl Cancer Inst Monogr* 1981;56:19–27.
11. Hays DM. Pelvic rhabdomyosarcomas in childhood: diagnosis and concepts of management reviewed. *Can-cer* 1980;45:1810–1814.
12. Andrassy RJ, Hays DM, Raney B, et al. Conservative surgical management of vaginal and vulvar pediatric rhabdomyosarcoma: a report from the Intergroup Rhab-domyosarcoma Study III. *J Pediatr Surg* 1995;30:1034–1037.

13. Maurer HM. The Intergroup Rhabdomyosarcoma Study (NIH): objectives and clinical staging classification. *J Pediatr Surg* 1975;10:977–978.

14. Grosfeld JL, Clatworthy W Jr, Newton WA Jr. Combined therapy in childhood rhabdomyosarcoma: an analysis of 42 cases. *J Pediatr Surg* 1969;4:637–645.

15. Hahlin M, Jaworski RC, Wain GV, et al. Integrated multimodality therapy for embryonal rhabdomyosarcoma of the lower genital tract in postpubertal females. *Gynecol Oncol* 1998;70:141–146.

16. Loughlin KR, Retik AB, Weinstein HJ, et al. Genitourinary rhabdomyosarcoma in children. *Cancer* 1989;63: 1600–1606.

17. Rutledge F, Sullivan MP. Sarcoma botryoides. *Ann N Y Acad Sci* 1967;142:694–708.

18. Hilgers RD. Pelvic exenteration for vaginal embryonal rhabdomyosarcoma: a review. *Obstet Gynecol* 1975;45: 175–180.

19. Stobbe GD, Dargeon WH. Embryonal rhabdomyosarcoma of the head and neck in children and adolescents. *Cancer* 1950;3:826–836.

20. Kumar AP, Wrenn EL Jr, Fleming ID, et al. Combined therapy to prevent complete pelvic exenteration for rhabdomyosarcoma of the vagina or uterus. *Cancer* 1976;37: 118–122.

21. Flamant F, Chassagne D, Cosset J, et al. Embryonal rhabdomyosarcoma of the vagina in children: conservative treatment with curietherapy and chemotherapy. *Eur J Cancer* 1979;15:257.

22. Rivard G, Ortega J, Hittle R, et al. Intensive chemotherapy as primary treatment for rhabdomyosarcoma of the pelvis. *Cancer* 1975;36:1593–1597.

23. Ortega JA. A therapeutic approach to childhood pelvic rhabdomyosarcoma without pelvic exenteration. *J Pediatr* 1979;94:205–209.

24. Raney RB Jr, Gehan EA, Hays DM, et al. Primary chemotherapy with or without radiation therapy and/or surgery for children with localized sarcoma of the bladder, prostate, vagina, uterus, and cervix. *Cancer* 1990;66: 2072–2081.

25. Piver MS, Rose PG. Long-term follow-up and complications of infants with vulvovaginal embryonal rhabdomyosarcoma treated with surgery, radiation therapy, and chemotherapy. *Obstet Gynecol* 1988;71:435–437.

26. Balat O, Balat A, Verschraegen C, et al. Sarcoma botryoides of the uterine endocervix: long-term results of conservative surgery. *Eur J Gynecol Oncol* 1996;17: 335–337.

27. Lin J, Lam SK, Cheung TH. Sarcoma botryoides of the cervix treated with limited surgery and chemotherapy to preserve fertility. *Gynecol Oncol* 1995;58:270–273.

28. Gerbaulet AP, Esche BA, Haie CM, et al. Conservative treatment for lower gynecological tract malignancies in children and adolescents: the Institut Gustave-Roussy experience. *Int J Radiat Oncol Biol Phys* 1989;17: 655–658.

29. Copeland LJ, Sneige N, Ordonez NG, et al. Endodermal sinus tumor of the vagina and cervix. *Cancer* 1985;55: 2558–2565.

30. Ishi K, Suzuki F, Saito A, et al. Cytodiagnosis of vaginal endodermal sinus tumor: a case report. *Acta Cytol* 1998; 42:399–402.

31. Zaino RJ, Robboy SJ, Bentley R, et al. Diseases of the vagina. In: Kurman RJ, ed. *Blaustein's pathology of the female genital tract,* 4th ed. New York: Springer-Verlag, 1994:171.

32. Young RH, Scully RE. Endodermal sinus tumor of the vagina: a report of nine cases and review of the literature. *Gynecol Oncol* 1984;18:380–392.

33. Liebhart M. Histopathological diagnosis of vaginal endodermal sinus tumors in infants. *Int J Gynecol Pathol* 1986;5:217–222.

34. Vawter GF. Carcinoma of the vagina in infancy. *Cancer* 1965;18:1479–1484.

35. Collins HS, Burke TW, Heller PB, et al. Endodermal sinus tumor of the infant vagina treated exclusively by chemotherapy. *Obstet Gynecol* 1989;73:507–509.

36. Andersen WA, Sabio H, Durso N, et al. Endodermal sinus tumor of the vagina: the role of primary chemotherapy. *Cancer* 1985;56:1025–1027.

37. Siegel HA, Sagerman R, Berdon WE, et al. Mesonephric adenocarcinoma of the vagina in a 7-month-old infant simulating sarcoma botryoides: successful control with supervoltage radiotherapy. *J Pediatr Surg* 1970;5: 468–470.

38. Hwang EH, Han SJ, Lee MK, et al. Clinical experience with conservative surgery for vaginal endodermal sinus tumor. *J Pediatr Surg* 1996;31:219–222.

39. Kohorn EI, McIntosh S, Lytton B, et al. Endodermal sinus tumor of the infant vagina. *Gynecol Oncol* 1985; 20:196–203.

40. Allyn DL, Silverberg SG, Salzberg AM. Endodermal sinus tumor of the vagina: report of a case with 7-year survival and literature review of so-called "mesonephromas." *Cancer* 1971;27:1231–1238.

41. Davidoff AM, Hebra A, Bunin N, et al. Endodermal sinus tumor in children. *J Pediatr Surg* 1996;31: 1075–1079.

42. Norris HJ, Bagley GP, Taylor HB. Carcinoma of the infant vagina: a distinctive tumor. *Arch Pathol* 1070;90: 473–479.

43. Dewhurst J, Ferreira HP. An endodermal sinus tumour of the vagina in an infant with seven year survival. *Br J Obstet Gynaecol* 1981;88:859–862.

44. Dieckmann WJ, Davis ME, Rynkiewicz LM, et al. Does the administration of diethylstilbestrol during pregnancy have therapeutic value? *Am J Obstet Gynecol* 1953;66: 1062–1081.

45. Brackbill Y, Berendes HW. Dangers of diethylstilbestrol: review of a 1953 paper. *Lancet* 1978;2:520.

46. Herbst AL, Ulfelder H, Poskanzer DC. Adenocarcinoma of the vagina: association of maternal stilbestrol therapy with tumor appearance in young women. *N Engl J Med* 1971;284:878–881.

47. Herbst AL, Robboy SJ, Scully RE, et al. Clear-cell adenocarcinoma of the vagina and cervix in girls: analysis of 170 registry cases. *Am J Obstet Gynecol* 1974;119: 713–724.

48. Robboy SJ, Kaufman RH, Prat J, et al. Pathologic findings in young women enrolled in the National Cooperative Diethylstilbestrol Adenosis (DESAD) Project. *Obstet Gynecol* 1979;53:309–317.

49. O'Brien PC, Noller KL, Robboy SJ, et al. Vaginal epithelial changes in young women enrolled in the National Cooperative Diethylstilbestrol Adenosis (DESAD) Project. *Obstet Gynecol* 1979;53:300–308.

50. Ostergard DR. DES-related vaginal lesions. *Clin Obstet Gynecol* 1981;24:379–394.

51. Antonioli DA, Burke L, Friedman EA. Natural history of diethylstilbestrol associated genital tract lesions: cervical ectopy and cervicovaginal hood. *Am J Obstet Gynecol* 1980;137:847–853.

52. Bornstein J, Adam E, Adler-Stothz K, et al. Development of cervical and vaginal squamous cell neoplasia as a late consequence of in utero exposure to diethylstilbestrol. *Obstet Gynecol Surv* 1988;43:15–21.

53. Berek JS, Hacker NF. *Practical gynecologic oncology,* 2nd ed. Baltimore: Williams & Wilkins, 1994:448–449.

54. Jones WB, Koulos JP, Saigo PE, et al. Clear-cell adenocarcinoma of the lower genital tract: Memorial Hospital 1974–1984. *Obstet Gynecol* 1987;70:573–577.

55. Herbst AL, Scully RE. Adenocarcinoma of the vagina in adolescence: a report of 7 cases including 6 clear-cell carcinomas (so-called mesonephromas). *Cancer* 1970; 25:745–757.

56. Melnick S, Cole P, Anderson D, et al. Rates and risks of diethylstilbestrol-related clear cell adenocarcinoma of the vagina and cervix: an update. *N Engl J Med* 1987; 316:514–516.

57. Herbst AL, Kurman RJ, Scully RE. Vaginal and cervical abnormalities after exposure to stilbestrol in utero. *Obstet Gynecol* 1972;40:287–298.

58. Trimble EL, Rubinstein LV, Menck HR, et al. Vaginal clear cell adenocarcinoma in the United States. *Gynecol Oncol* 1996;61:113–115.

59. Herbst AL, Cole P, Norusis MJ, et al. Epidemiologic aspects and factors related to survival in 384 Registry cases of clear cell adenocarcinoma of the vagina and cervix. *Am J Obstet Gynecol* 1979;135:876–886.

60. Herbst AL. Clear cell adenocarcinoma and the current status of DES-exposed females. *Cancer* 1981;48: 484–488.

61. Carlson JA Jr, Morgan M, Boothby R, et al. Stage II papillary clear cell adenocarcinoma of the vagina during observation in a diethylstilbestrol-exposed daughter. *Gynecol Oncol* 1989;32:86–87.

62. Horwitz RI, Viscoli CM, Merino M, et al. Clear cell adenocarcinoma of the vagina and cervix: incidence, undetected disease, and diethylstilbestrol. *J Clin Epidemiol* 1988;41:593–597.

63. Zaino RJ, Robboy SJ, Bentley R, et al. Diseases of the vagina. In: Kurman RJ, ed. *Blaustein's pathology of the female genital tract,* 4th ed. New York: Springer-Verlag, 1994:162–168.

64. Robboy SJ, Herbst AL, Scully RE. Clear cell adenocarcinoma of the vagina and cervix in young females: analysis of 37 tumors that persisted or recurred after primary therapy. *Cancer* 1974;34:606–614.

65. Herbst AL, Norusis MJ, Rosenow PJ, et al. An analysis of 346 cases of clear cell adenocarcinoma of the vagina and cervix with emphasis on recurrence and survival. *Gynecol Oncol* 1979;7:111–122.

66. Senekjian EK, Frey KW, Anderson D, et al. Local therapy in Stage I clear cell adenocarcinoma of the vagina. *Cancer* 1987;60:1319–1324.

67. Goodman A, Sullinger JC, Rice LW, et al. Clear cell adenocarcinoma of the vagina: a second primary in a diethylstilbestrol-exposed woman? Case report. *Gynecol Oncol* 1991;43:173–177.

68. Burks RT, Schwartz AM, Wheeler JE, et al. Late recurrence of clear cell adenocarcinoma of the cervix: case report. *Obstet Gynecol* 1990;76:525–527.

69. Jones WB, Tan LK, Lewis JL Jr. Late recurrence of clear cell adenocarcinoma of the vagina and cervix: a report of three cases. *Gynecol Oncol* 1993;51:266–271.

70. Fishman DA, Williams S, Small W Jr, et al. Late recurrences of vaginal clear cell adenocarcinoma. *Gynecol Oncol* 1996;62:128–132.

71. Waggoner SE, Mittendorf R, Biney N, et al. Influence of in utero diethylstilbestrol exposure on the prognosis and biologic behavior of vaginal clear-cell adenocarcinoma. *Gynecol Oncol* 1994;55:238–244.

72. National Cancer Institute Workshop. The 1988 Bethesda System for reporting cervical/vaginal cytologic diagnoses. *JAMA* 1989;262:931–934.

73. Nasiell K, Roger V, Nasiell M. Behavior of mild cervical dysplasia during long-term follow-up. *Obstet Gynecol* 1986;67:665–669.

74. McIndoe GA, Robson MS, Tidy JA, et al. Laser excision rather than vaporization: the treatment of choice for cervical intraepithelial neoplasia. *Obstet Gynecol* 1989;74: 165.

75. Prendiville W, Cullimore J, Norman S. Large loop excision of the transformation zone (LLETZ). A new method of management for women with cervical intraepithelial neoplasia. *Br J Obstet Gynaecol* 1989;96: 1054–1060.

76. Whiteley PF, Olah KS. Treatment of cervical intraepithelial neoplasia: experience with the low-voltage diathermy loop. *Am J Obstet Gynecol* 1990;162:1272–1277.

77. Mor-Yosef S, Lopes A, Pearson S, et al. Loop diathermy cone biopsy. *Obstet Gynecol* 1990;75:884–886.

25

Tumors of the Uterine Corpus and Gestational Trophoblastic Disease

Lesley L. Breech and Janet S. Rader

UTERINE CORPUS

Uterine tumors rarely develop in early life. However, when tumors of the uterus are found in children and adolescents, they are likely to be malignant. The clinical presentation of most uterine tumors is vaginal bleeding. Therefore, the possibility of a neoplasm of the genitalia must be seriously considered and explored whenever vaginal bleeding occurs in a child younger than 9 years of age or in any child without secondary sexual development. Difficulties in treatment of genital neoplasms in children frequently arise because of delayed diagnosis. Often, neoplasms are detected only after the tumor has reached an advanced stage or large size. Further difficulties arise in the surgical management of children because of undeveloped genital organs and small pelvis size.

The patient's subsequent sexual and somatic development and future childbearing should be considered in choosing treatment options. Chemotherapeutic treatments that preserve ovarian function rather than radiation or surgical removal of the uterus and ovaries should be selected when possible.

Endometrial Hyperplasia and Cancer

Endometrial adenocarcinoma, the most common malignancy of the adult female genital tract, is the least common malignancy in children. Endometrial cancer is predominately a cancer of obese postmenopausal women. Only a few cases of endometrial cancer have been reported in children or teenagers. The clinical presentation of the patients included a rapidly growing tumor, vaginal bleeding, and no sign of sexual precocity. Most of the patients died within 6 months even with aggressive treatment due to the advanced stage of the disease at the time of diagnosis (1,2).

The predisposing factor for this malignancy and its associated lesion, endometrial hyperplasia, is unopposed estrogen stimulation, either endogenous or exogenous. Unopposed estrogen causes incomplete shedding of the endometrium. The abnormal endometrial proliferations range from various degrees, from glandular crowding and cytologic atypia to invasive cancer. Endometrial hyperplasia can be seen in children with Turner's syndrome given unopposed estrogen therapy or women with polycystic ovarian syndrome where extraglandular aromatization of androgens to estrone occurs (3,4).

The diagnosis usually is made by endometrial curettage when the patient presents with vaginal bleeding. Most cases of endometrial hyperplasia do not progress to invasive cancer (5,6). Therefore, young women with endometrial hyperplasia can be treated medically with progestin therapy and monitored with periodic endometrial sampling (Fig. 25.1). Progestin therapy ensures more complete sloughing of the endometrium, which in turn prevents continued proliferation. Only when patients are unresponsive to progestin therapy

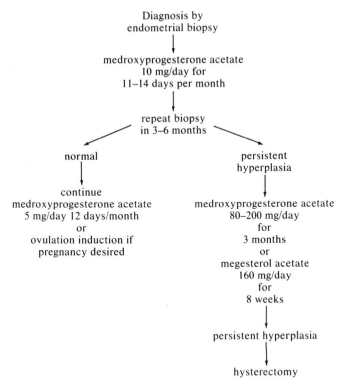

Diagnosis by
endometrial biopsy

medroxyprogesterone acetate
10 mg/day for
11–14 days per month

repeat biopsy
in 3–6 months

normal

persistent
hyperplasia

continue
medroxyprogesterone acetate
5 mg/day 12 days/month
or
ovulation induction if
pregnancy desired

medroxyprogesterone acetate
80–200 mg/day
for
3 months
or
megesterol acetate
160 mg/day
for
8 weeks

persistent hyperplasia

hysterectomy

FIG. 25.1. Management of endometrial hyperplasia.

or progress to endometrial carcinoma is hysterectomy necessary. When an adenocarcinoma of the uterus is present, an abdominal hysterectomy with bilateral salpingo-oophorectomy and intraoperative staging is done. Further radiation therapy can be based on examination of the surgical specimen.

In adolescents who are anovulatory and have irregular bleeding, progesterone should be given to interrupt the steady estrogen stimulation of the uterus. Patients should be given medroxyprogesterone acetate 10 mg for at least 10 days each month to ensure complete withdrawal bleeding and to prevent endometrial hyperplasia. When the patient also is in need of contraception, low-dose combination oral contraception in the usual cyclic fashion can be given in place of progesterone therapy alone (7). Hormonal therapy should be used until the patient establishes normal ovu-

lation or is ready for ovulation induction and childbearing.

Leiomyomas of the Uterus

Leiomyomas are benign tumors composed mainly of smooth muscle cells and various amounts of fibrous connective tissue. A case of uterine leiomyoma in a child 10 years old has been reported, and there are a few reported cases in teenagers. Wiscot et al. (8) described a case in a 13-year-old girl who presented with profuse vaginal bleeding and a lower abdominal mass 8 months after beginning menses. Augensen (9) described a 15-year-old who presented with amenorrhea for 8 weeks, urinary retention, and a lower abdominal mass. Both patients were treated conservatively with myomectomy and did well postoperatively with resumption of normal menses. Farber et al. (10) presented the case of a myoma that developed in a rudimentary muscular bud in a patient with vaginal and uterine agenesis (Rokitansky-Küster-Hauser syndrome). The patient was treated with excision of the leiomyoma from its attachment to the right myometrial bud.

Fields and Neinstein (11) described five cases from their institution as well as three additional cases reported in the literature of patients less than 21 years old with uterine myomas. Four of five of the patients were managed conservatively without surgery, and only one underwent myomectomy. The review emphasizes that, although uncommon in adolescents, myomas should be considered in the adolescent female who presents with a pelvic mass, abdominal pain, and abnormal uterine bleeding. Physical examination and ultrasound may assist in making the diagnosis. Conservative management should be considered using a hormonal regimen with oral contraceptive pills followed by conservative surgery, if necessary, with hysteroscopic or laparoscopic myomectomy. Rarely, a gonadotropin-releasing hormone agonist may be considered only after diagnosis of a benign condition has been established.

Sarcomas of the Uterus

Sarcomatous tumors of the uterus constitute only about 3% of uterine malignancies. There are three distinct histologic types of uterine sarcomas: mixed mesodermal tumors, leiomyosarcomas, and endometrial stromal sarcomas.

Mixed mesodermal tumors have been the most commonly reported sarcomas in adolescents. Mixed mesodermal tumors are a group of neoplasms that arise from malignant epithelial and mesenchymal stromal elements of the uterus. They are classified according to the nature of the sarcomatous component into homologous (tissue normally found in the uterus) or heterologous (tissue not normally found in the uterus, i.e., striated muscle or cartilage). The tumors are firm and sessile, filling the uterine cavity, unlike the grape-like

sarcomas of the vagina. This tumor usually is seen in postmenopausal women, but several mixed müllerian tumors have been reported in children and adolescents ages 4 to 19 years (1,12–14). Patients usually present with vaginal bleeding and a pelvic mass. Treatment of the tumor requires early diagnosis and radical surgery, followed by radiation and chemotherapy tailored to the patient.

One of the types of mixed mesodermal tumors is the adenosarcoma. It is thought to be of low-grade malignancy with a potential for local recurrence. Adenosarcomas have been reported to occur in adolescents. Nine patients less than 20 years of age were reviewed by Andrade et al. (15). Six had primary lesions in the cervix and three presented with initial lesions in the body of the uterus. Abdominal radical hysterectomy was the treatment in those young women. A conservative approach may be an option if the disease can be completely resected by dilatation and curettage or local resection. Close gynecologic follow-up should be emphasized, as adenosarcomas usually recur locally. In the presence of a recurrence, a hysterectomy with complete histologic examination of the uterus is necessary.

Leiomyosarcoma is rare during adolescence and childhood. Lammers and Fowler (16) recently described a 15-year-old girl who presented with acute abdominal pain and a pelvic mass. She underwent an exploratory laparotomy for definitive diagnosis and excision of the mass. A large multilobulated fleshy tumor was found in the posterior uterine fundus. Pathologic analysis of the myomectomy specimen revealed high-grade leiomyosarcoma with severe atypia, extending to the borders of the tumor and invading vascular spaces. She then underwent a total abdominal hysterectomy, bilateral salpingo-oophorectomy, and pelvic and paraaortic lymphadenectomy. The uterus was enlarged, $10 \times 6 \times 5$ cm, with uterine sections showing leiomyosarcoma invading the myometrium. The adnexae were normal. She underwent chemotherapy with doxorubicin, cyclophosphamide, and cisplatinum for six courses. She also received hormone replacement therapy with estrogen patches. No evidence of recurrence was reported for at least 7 months postoperatively.

Endometrial stromal sarcoma (ESS) is extremely rare in adolescent patients; most frequently it is encountered in the 40- to 50-year-old age group. There are three general categories: benign stromal nodule, low-grade stromal sarcoma, and high-grade or poorly differentiated stromal sarcoma. Until 1990, only five cases of ESS in adolescents had been published in the literature (17). Michalas et al. (18) described a case of high-grade malignant ESS arising in a rudimentary uterine horn in a 16-year-old girl. The patient presented with symptoms of an acute abdomen after the uterine horn had ruptured from the growing tumor. The patient underwent a total abdominal hysterectomy, bilateral salpingo-oophorectomy, and an omentectomy. Chemotherapy and radiation were planned; however, the patient died of diffuse metastases within 1 week. Generally, treatment of ESS is surgical. Regardless of the patient's age, preservation of ovarian tissue is not recommended because of the likelihood of ovarian metastases. Also, ESS may have steroid receptors, and estrogen production by the ovaries may stimulate residual disease. A total hysterectomy, bilateral salpingo-oophorectomy, and staging procedure are suggested. Postoperative pelvic radiation may be recommended in adolescent patients because it has been noted to treat residual disease and decrease the likelihood of local recurrences (19).

Rhabdomyosarcoma also may occur in the pelvis. Careful staging of the extent of disease is very important in the treatment and prognosis of children with rhabdomyosarcoma. Pelvic ultrasound and computed tomography can be very useful in evaluating the extent of disease and measuring tumor regression during chemotherapy (20). In a large review of 47 children and adolescents with rhabdomyosarcoma of the female genital tract from 1972 to 1984, Hays et al. (21) noted six patients with uterine disease. The patients ranged in age from 4 to 15 years. Four patients had a single large polyp protruding from the cervix, and two patients

had intramural involvement of the uterus. All patients were treated with chemotherapy. Three of the patients with polypoid lesions had polypectomies, and the last patient underwent a radical hysterectomy. All four patients were disease-free 2.7 to 6.5 years after treatment. Both patients with intramural corpus involvement had intraperitoneal disease. One patient died of sepsis during chemotherapy, and the other patient died of distant disease after radiation and chemotherapy.

Since 1990, several reports of conservative treatment of uterine or cervical rhabdomyosarcoma have been identified in the literature. Hammerman and Runowicz (22) reported a 15-year-old patient who also presented with a polypoid uterine mass without other evidence of disease. This patient and her family declined hysterectomy due to religious beliefs. She was treated with primary chemotherapy of vincristine, etoposide, and ifosamide. After three courses of therapy, a polypectomy was performed with evidence of embryonal rhabdomyosarcoma on pathologic review. She received two additional courses of chemotherapy. Seven months after initial presentation, a follow-up hysteroscopy with multiple biopsies was negative for malignancy. She was followed by physical examination and endovaginal ultrasound every 3 to 4 months. Three years later, she had no evidence of disease. Before the late 1970s, treatment for uterine rhabdomyosarcoma involved radical surgery then chemotherapy and radiation. An article in 1979 by Ortega (23) stimulated a shift to treatment with primary chemotherapy followed by delayed surgery for locally advanced or distantly metastatic uterine rhabdomyosarcoma. Chemotherapy with conservative surgery has been curative in a limited number of anecdotal reports. Limited surgery may, after more extensive investigation, provide an option to conserve bowel and bladder function as well as reproductive potential.

Other Tumors

Other reported uterine tumors include glioma, peripheral primitive neuroectodermal tumor, hemangioendothelioma, non-Hodgkin's lymphoma, and Wilms' tumor (24–29). Corpus uteri cancer in children and adolescents is a rarity. All available information primarily emanates from individual case reports, and treatment consequently has been empirical.

GESTATIONAL TROPHOBLASTIC DISEASE

Gestational trophoblastic diseases (GTDs) are a spectrum of benign and malignant conditions derived from early embryonic tissues of conception. In addition to their malignant potential, molar pregnancies are associated with significant complications, including hemorrhage, intrauterine infection, and toxemia. Because these conditions are associated with pregnancy, they are a particularly threatening disease in young women. According to 1995 statistics, the overall teenage pregnancy rate is 83.6 per 1,000 women aged 15 to 19 years. In 1995, there were 735,751 teenage pregnancies in the United States (30).

GTDs are pathologically divided into four distinct forms. (i) Hydatidiform mole is a local degenerative process with histologic features of hydropic villi and trophoblastic hyperplasia. (ii) Invasive hydatidiform mole is a tumor that invades the uterine myometrium in addition to the presence of placental villous structures and trophoblastic hyperplasia. (iii) Choriocarcinoma is an uncontrolled growth of the cytotrophoblast and syncytiotrophoblast without the presence of villous structures. (iv) Placental site trophoblastic tumor is an uncommon tumor composed of infiltrating intermediate trophoblastic cells resembling cells found at the placental implantation site. Clinically, patients are classified on the basis of high- and low-risk factors and whether the tumor is metastatic or nonmetastatic (31).

Hydatidiform Mole

Molar pregnancy rates in population-based studies range from 0.2 to 1.2 cases per 1,000 pregnancies or births. The incidence in the United States is about one per 1,500 live births (32). A woman's age appears to be a risk factor, with molar pregnancy rates higher at the extremes of reproductive life. Studies have shown pregnancy in women under 20 years and over 35 to 40 years of age is more likely to result in molar gestation and persistent trophoblastic disease (33–37). However, several other authors have not shown an increased risk of disease in the adolescent population (36,38–40). Among very young patients with molar pregnancies, various methods of reporting incidence and relative risk estimates, in addition to small numbers of patients in most series, make comparisons difficult.

Grossly, hydatidiform mole is characterized by a mass of vesicles that partially or completely replace the normal placental architecture. The vesicles are individual villi that have become edematous (hydropic degeneration), varying in size from a few millimeters up to 2 to 3 cm in diameter (Fig. 25.2). Microscopic examination reveals three major features of

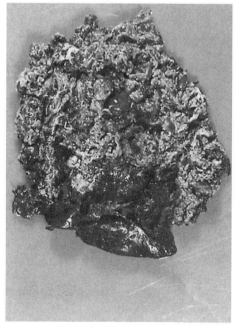

FIG. 25.2. Hydroponic degeneration of a molar pregnancy showing edematous villi varying in size from a few millimeters to 2 cm in diameter.

TABLE 25.1. *Features of complete and partial hydatidiform mole*

	Complete	Partial
Karyotype	46,XX, 46,XY	Triploid
Fetal or embryonic tissue	Absent	Present
Swelling of chorionic villi	Diffuse	Focal
Trophoblastic hyperplasia	Diffuse	Focal
Percent persistent gestational trophoblastic disease	20%	5%

hydatidiform mole: (i) edematous swelling of chronic villi, (ii) proliferation of trophoblast, and (iii) absence of fetal blood vessels in the villi. As a result of cytogenetic studies, hydatidiform mole is divided into two principal forms: partial and complete (Table 25.1) (41,42).

Partial moles are characterized by (a) focal hydropic villi with scalloping, (b) focal mild-to-moderate trophoblastic hyperplasia, and (c) identifiable fetal or embryonic structures. Chromosome analysis reveals a polyploid karyotype, which is most frequently triploid.

Complete moles are characterized by (a) hydropic swelling of all villi, (b) marked hyperplasia and anaplasia of the trophoblast, and (c) complete absence of fetal structures. The karyotype of the complete mole is 46,XX. Chromosomal banding studies found that the chromosomal material of complete hydatidiform moles is completely inherited from the paternal contribution (43). Most fertilizations occur with an egg from which the nucleus has been lost or is inactivated by a sperm. The paternal 23,X chromosomes then duplicate to 46,XX (43–45). In a study of molar pregnancy in Hawaii, Jacobs et al. (46) found an excess of women aged less than 20 years in the group with complete moles compared to partial moles.

About 80% of complete hydatidiform moles will resolve after evacuation of the uterus. The remainder of the patients will develop malignant trophoblastic sequelae (invasive mole or choriocarcinoma). About 15% of the persistent disease will be local uterine invasion and 4% distant spread (47). In contrast, patients with a partial molar preg-nancy are much less likely to develop persistent trophoblastic disease, with a range from 0 to 6.6% (48–51).

Invasive Mole

Invasive mole is characterized by hydropic chorionic villi and trophoblastic hyperplasia within the myometrium and vascular spaces. The tumor may metastasize to the vulva, vagina, and lung. The frequency of invasive mole is difficult to determine because a uterine curettage is unlikely to yield villi invading the myometrium. A pathologic diagnosis is rarely made between invasive mole and choriocarcinoma before treatment. This is made possible by the reliability of human chorionic gonadotropin (hCG) levels as a tumor marker and the effectiveness of chemotherapeutic agents in killing trophoblastic disease with various histologic types and anatomic locations. Therefore, these tumors are treated under the general clinical terms of a gestational trophoblastic tumor and a metastatic trophoblastic tumor (31).

Choriocarcinoma

Choriocarcinoma is a highly malignant tumor derived from trophoblastic epithelium that lacks chorionic villi. The tumor is extremely vascular and prone to blood-borne metastasis. Microscopic examination shows the abundant growth of both cytotrophoblast and syncytiotrophoblast in anaplastic sheets and columns invading uterine muscle. Hemorrhage and necrosis usually are present (52). As with invasive mole, this tumor is very difficult to diagnose in uterine curettings.

Most cases of choriocarcinoma appear to follow a recognizable gestation. About 50% of choriocarcinomas are preceded by a hydatidiform molar pregnancy, 25% occur after a spontaneous abortion, 22.5% after normal pregnancy, and 2.5% after ectopic pregnancy. About one of every 40 molar gestations is followed by choriocarcinoma (53). There are reported cases of choriocarcinoma arising from the trophoblast of an otherwise normal placenta (54). Choriocarcinoma usually occurs shortly after the preceding pregnancy. However, very long latency periods of more than 10 years have been reported (55,56). Some studies showed higher rates of choriocarcinoma for adolescents (57,58), whereas other reports noted lower rates for adolescents than women 20 to 40 years old (59,60).

Abnormal uterine bleeding is the most frequent clinical presentation of choriocarcinoma. Other manifestations of choriocarcinoma usually relate to the location of the metastases. The lungs are the most frequent site of extrauterine spread (61,62), and disease usually is noted on x-ray examination. In addition, the patient may present with hemoptysis, cough, or dyspnea (63,64). Other sites of metastasis, in the order of decreasing frequency, are vagina, brain, liver, kidneys, small intestines, and spleen. The symptoms usually relate to hemorrhage in these areas (61). Thyrotoxicosis may occur with choriocarcinoma (65). This tumor was uniformly fatal before the advent of chemotherapeutic treatment in 1956.

Classification and Staging

Gestational trophoblastic tumors can be classified according to an anatomic staging or clinical prognostic scoring system. The International Federation of Gynecology and Obstetrics (FIGO) staging system is based on clinical examination and radiologic findings (Table 25.2) (66). However, most treatment centers in the United States determine therapy according to good and poor prognostic factors other than just the anatomic location of the tumor. These systems take into account addi-

TABLE 25.2. *Gestational trophoblastic disease according to the FIGO staging system*

Stage	Disease state
I	Disease confined to the uterus
II	Disease confined to the pelvis
III	Disease confined to pelvis and lungs
IV	Metastatic to any other site

FIGO, International Federation of Gynecology and Obstetrics.

TABLE 25.3. *Prognostic group classification*

Nonmetastatic
　Persistent hydatidiform mole
　Invasive mole
　Choriocarcinoma
Metastatic
　Low risk, good prognosis
　　Serum hCG <400,000 mIU/mL
　　Duration of symptoms <4 mo
　　No brain or liver metastasis
　　No prior chemotherapy for GTD
　　Disease after GTD, abortion, or ectopic (not term delivery)
　High risk, poor prognosis
　　Serum hCG >40,000 mIU/mL
　　Duration of symptoms >4 mo
　　Brain or liver metastasis
　　Prior failed chemotherapy
　　Disease after term delivery
　　Recurrent or metastatic placental site trophoblastic tumor

GTD, gestational trophoblastic disease; hCG, human chorionic gonadotropin.

tional information about antecedent pregnancies, laboratory values, and symptoms. Patients are identified in need of initial aggressive multiagent chemotherapy. The gestational trophoblastic tumors are divided into three groups: nonmetastatic, metastatic low-risk, and metastatic high-risk (Table 25.3). The high-risk patients are those who are not likely to be cured with single-agent methotrexate or actinomycin D chemotherapy (31,66,67). Another prognostic scoring system was proposed by Bagshawe based on the patient's age, history of prior chemotherapy, antecedent pregnancy, and number, site, and size of metastasis. A weighted score is applied to each variable and the individual scores added. Patients with a final score of 4 or less are considered low risk, those with a score of 5 to 7 are middle risk, and those with a score of 8 or greater are high risk (Table 25.4) (31,53,68).

Clinical Management

Clinical suspicion of GTD should arise when a pregnancy is accompanied by excessive nausea and vomiting, vaginal bleeding, a uterus large for gestational age, or preeclampsia occurring early in pregnancy.

TABLE 25.4. *Prognostic scoring system*[a]

Prognostic factor	Score			
	0	1	2	4
Age of patient (yr)	≤39	>39		
Preceding pregnancy	Mole	Abortion	Term	
Months since prior pregnancy	<4	4–6	7–12	>12
hCG level (IU/L)	<10³	10³–10⁴	10⁴–10⁵	>10⁵
	A × O			
Largest tumor diameter (cm)		3–5	>5	
Site of metastases		Spleen	GI tract	Brain
Number of metastasis		1–4	4–8	>8
Prior chemotherapy			1 drug	≥2 drugs

[a] Total score: ≤4, low risk; 5–7, middle risk; ≥8, high risk. The total score for a patient is obtained by adding the individual prognostic factors.

GI, gastrointestinal; hCG, human chorionic gonadotropin.

Modified from Gestational trophoblastic disease; World Health Organization Technical Report, Series 692. Geneva: WHO, 1983.

The method of choice for diagnosing a molar pregnancy is ultrasonography, which is an accurate, noninvasive technique. The ultrasonic picture of the mole depends on the gestational age of the patient. In the first trimester, an endometrial cavity filled with an irregular mixed echodense/echospared mass is present similar to that of an incomplete or missed abortion. By the second trimester, the characteristic fluid-filled vesicles are evident. Their size varies from 2 mm at 8.5 weeks' gestation to 10 mm or more at 18.5 weeks' gestation. The sonographic picture reveals multiple echoes in the uterine cavity, which usually is described as a snow storm pattern (Fig. 25.3). This characteristic picture is due to the multiple interfaces between the hydropic chorionic villi (69,70). However, ultrasound cannot always differentiate a mole from a first trimester abortion, degenerating

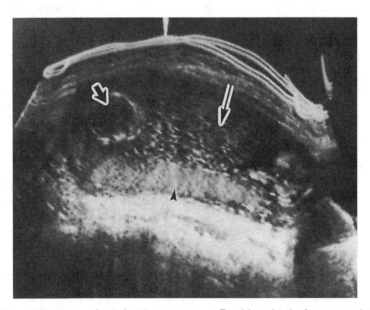

FIG. 25.3. Ultrasonic picture of a twin pregnancy. —> Fetal head twin A; > normal placenta twin A; —-> "snow storm" pattern of hydatiform twin B.

fibroids, or even ovarian dysgerminomas (71,72). Taylor et al. (73) described a technique of assessing blood flow and tissue perfusion of the uterus by duplex Doppler ultrasound. They showed higher systolic and diastolic Doppler shifts in gestational trophoblastic neoplasia compared to a nongravid uterus, first trimester pregnancy, and incomplete abortion.

When the diagnosis of hydatidiform mole is confirmed, the uterus is emptied as soon as possible by suction and sharp curettage, regardless of the uterine size. This allows preservation of fertility in the young patient. Curettage in patients with a uterine size less than 16 weeks has a low complication rate. Patients with a larger uterus are at increased risk of hemorrhage, sepsis, and uterine perforation. Application of oxytocin infusion during evacuation will decrease uterine bleeding and the risk of uterine perforation (74). During evacuation, molar tissue may enter the maternal venous sinuses and invade the lungs. About 2% of patients with molar pregnancy develop pulmonary embolisms and exhibit such symptoms as tachycardia, tachypnea, cyanosis, cough, and chest pain (75).

Preeclampsia has been diagnosed in 27% of patients with a complete mole. Toxemia occurs almost exclusively in patients with markedly elevated hCG levels and excessive uterine size. The syndrome is associated with hypertension, proteinuria, and hyperreflexia. Toxemia occurs in the third trimester of pregnancy, and the diagnosis of molar pregnancy should be considered in any patient who suffers toxemia early in gestation (76).

Antigenic fetal products may enter the maternal circulation after evacuation of the mole, causing sensitization against antigens of the Rh system. These antibodies can be detrimental to an Rh-incompatible fetus of a subsequent pregnancy. Therefore, all unsensitized Rh-negative patients should receive human anti-D-gamma-globulin (Rhogam). The Rhogam should be given intramuscularly within 72 hours after evacuation of the hydatidiform molar pregnancy (77). At the time of molar evacuation, a complete physical examination and chest x-ray are performed to rule out metastatic disease. If disease is confined to the uterus, patients then are followed with serial β-hCG levels. The purpose of following β-hCG levels after evacuation of a hydatidiform mole is to detect continued trophoblastic activity and to begin appropriate chemotherapy. Weekly levels are obtained until three consecutive assays are normal (nondetectable) and then monthly for 1 year. The time for β-hCG levels to return to normal is influenced by the initial preevacuation level and the clearance rate. Most patients with spontaneous regression of trophoblastic disease will have normal levels by 12 weeks postevacuation (31,78). However, it is the trend in β-hCG levels that is important and the most specific prognostic indicator (47). Persistent trophoblastic disease requiring treatment is indicated by β-hCG levels that maintain a plateau over 3 consecutive weeks or increase at any time. The frequency of persistent trophoblastic disease is increased in pregnancies with large-for-dates uterus, ovarian theca lutein cysts larger than 5 cm, and postevacuation uterine bleeding (39,78). Approximately 20% to 25% of patients with hydatidiform mole will require chemotherapy after evacuation (39,47,79).

Pregnancy prevention for 6 months to 2 years after evacuation of a hydatidiform mole is standard practice. In following the patient, the β-hCG assay is unable to differentiate normal pregnancy from other post-molar sequelae. Oral contraceptives usually are given because of their safety and high effectiveness. Stone and Bagshawe (34) and Stone et al. (80) reported a delay in the fall of β-hCG molar evacuation and the need for chemotherapy increased two to three times in patients taking oral contraceptives. However, other studies did not confirm this and have shown no abnormal β-hCG regression time after molar evacuation in oral contraceptive users (81–83). If a patient were to become pregnant shortly after evacuation, the β-hCG can be correlated with serial ultrasonography for accurate diagnosis.

Chemotherapy

Initially, the prophylactic use of chemotherapy at the time of evacuation of the uterus was shown to decrease the development of persistent trophoblastic disease in some studies (84–86). The routine use of prophylactic chemotherapy in all patients with molar pregnancy is no longer considered standard of care, because 80% of patients with hydatidiform mole will experience spontaneous resolution. In addition, if patients are followed closely and treated appropriately, nearly all are curable. The most powerful indicators of persistent GTD by multivariate analysis in women with hydatidiform mole were trophoblastic hyperplasia (relative risk [RR] = 3.56), age (RR = 2.87), and a history of a prior mole (RR = 2.57) (87). The high-risk subset may require close follow-up, but the usefulness of prophylactic chemotherapy has not been confirmed by prospective clinical trials. Therefore, it may only be useful in special situations where the risk of developing a molar pregnancy is very high or where β-hCG levels are unavailable.

Chemotherapy is initiated in trophoblastic disease when either metastatic lesions are identified or β-hCG titers are plateauing or rising. Once either one of these occurrences is noted, the patient is completely reevaluated with x-ray studies to examine the brain, lungs, liver, and pelvis to determine the extent of disease. A repeat uterine curettage for histologic confirmation is not needed, because invasive mole and choriocarcinoma is intramuscular and curettings often are negative.

Patients requiring chemotherapy have a wide spectrum of disease, ranging from a few thousand trophoblastic cells remaining in the uterus to large metastatic lesions. The extent of disease greatly affects a patient's future outcome. Therefore, various prognostic factors have been identified to predict long-term survival or poor outcome. This allows patients at high risk of treatment failure to be recognized and given aggressive combination chemotherapy. After complete reevaluation with physical examination and hematologic and radiographic studies, patients are categorized as having nonmetastatic or metastatic GTD. Patients with metastatic tumors are further classified as being at high risk based on the presence of one or more of the following: (a) pretreatment serum β-hCG of 40,000 mIU/mL, (b) greater than 4 months from an antecedent pregnancy to treatment, (c) metastasis to sites other than the lungs or vagina, (d) antecedent term gestation compared with hydatidiform mole, abortion, or ectopic pregnancy, or (e) prior unsuccessful chemotherapy (Table 25.3) (31,53,88). Chemotherapy is then given according to a patient's prognostic factors.

Approximately 80% of all patients are in the low-risk metastatic and nonmetastatic groups and are treated with single-agent methotrexate or actinomycin D (Table 25.5). The preferred treatment for the low-risk groups with normal renal and hepatic function is methotrexate. Single-agent methotrexate with or without folinic acid rescue has a high remission rate with toxicity compared to that of single-dose actinomycin D. Chemotherapy is changed to actinomycin D if toxicity precludes an adequate dose or frequency of treatment.

Response to chemotherapy can be monitored accurately by the β-hCG level. The patient's response to chemotherapy is monitored by weekly β-hCG levels. A plateau of the β-hCG level over 2 weeks indicates resistance to chemotherapy. Complete remission is diagnosed after three consecutive weekly β-hCG levels are within normal range and there

TABLE 25.5. *Gestational trophoblastic disease single-agent chemotherapy*

Methotrexate
  0.4 mg/kg/d IM or IV for 5 d every 2 weeks
  30–50 mg/M^2 iM every week
Methotrexate and folinic acid
  Methotrexate 1 mg/kg iM on days 1, 3, 5, and 7
  Folinic acid 0.1 mg/kg iM on days 2, 4,
    6, and 8 every 2 weeks
Actinomycin D
  10–12 µg/kg/d IV for 5 d every 2 weeks
  1.25 mg/M^2 IV every 2 weeks

is no clinical or radiologic evidence of disease. An additional two courses of chemotherapy usually are given after the first normal β-hCG level to decrease the incidence of relapse (88).

The most common toxic reactions to these drugs are oropharyngeal ulcerations (stomatitis) and ulceration of the esophagus, stomach, and small and large bowel. Topical anesthetics combined with antibiotics and systemic analgesics will provide some relief from these complications. A reversible elevation of hepatic enzymes may occur in some patients. Less common toxic reactions are skin rash, nausea and vomiting, significant alopecia, and myelotoxicity (89).

Present studies show an 86% to 97% initial complete remission in patients with non-metastatic GTD initially treated with single-agent chemotherapy (90–92). Patients with low-risk metastatic disease can achieve similar cure rates. About 10% to 15% of patients will require combination chemotherapy with or without surgery to achieve complete remission. In one study between 1964 and 1986, 487 patients with GTD were treated with methotrexate and folinic acid. Beginning in 1974, the patients were stratified into prognostic groups, and 99.7% of patients with low-risk disease were cured by the therapy. Although survival was excellent, 69 of 348 low-risk patients had to change therapy because of drug resistance and 23 needed to change treatment because of drug-induced toxicity (76). The 20% first-line failure rate was similar to that found with weekly methotrexate, which has negligible toxicity. Other authors concluded that high-dose methotrexate does not appear to offer any clinical advantage over conventional 5-day methotrexate in low-risk patients (93). Several studies, including two Gynecologic Oncology Group trials, have used weekly intramuscular methotrexate (94–96). The response rates ranged from 60% to 80%, with no cases of major toxicity. The overall response was comparable in efficacy to other first-line agents with the added advantage of convenience, low cost, and low toxicity. Single-dose actinomycin D also has the advantage of convenience and low toxicity. Petrilli et al. (97) reported a 94% response rate when actinomycin D was given intravenously every 14 days. Current information would indicate that both weekly intramuscular methotrexate and intravenous actinomycin D offer safe, effective, and convenient first-line therapy for treatment of low-risk GTD. A review of the efficacy and toxicity of single-agent chemotherapy for low-risk GTD by Roberts et al. (98) described a total of 92 patients. All patients were cured. Only one patient required multiagent chemotherapy. Primary remission was achieved in 62 patients with an initial agent. A second sequential agent was used in 30 patients due to either drug resistance or toxicity. When a young patient with nonmetastatic disease is resistant to single-agent chemotherapy, further treatment is multiagent chemotherapy.

Patients with high-risk metastatic disease initially are treated with aggressive combination chemotherapy with or without adjunctive surgery. The present chemotherapy regimen is EMA-CO (etoposide, methotrexate, actinomycin D, cyclophosphamide, oncovin) (Table 25.6) (68). Studies have shown complete remission rates in high-risk metastatic cancer patients to be 67% to 83% in those treated initially with combination chemotherapy (68,99–103). However, high-risk patients treated with single-agent therapy followed by

TABLE 25.6. *Gestational trophoblastic disease multiagent chemotherapy*

Drug	Regimen
Course 1: EMA	
Day 1	
Actinomycin D	0.5 mg IV bolus
Etoposide	100 mg/m^2 IV
Methotrexate	300 mg/m^2 IV over 12 h
Day 2	
Actinomycin D	0.5 mg IV bolus
Etoposide	100 mg/m^2 IV
Folinic acid	15 mg/m^2 IM or PO every 12 h for four doses
Course 2: CO	
Day 8	
Vincristine	1.0 mg/m^2 IV bolus
Cyclophosphamide	600 mg/m^2 IV

combination treatment had about half the cure rate (67,88,104). EMA-CO offers high response rates, good long-term survival rates, and minimal acute and cumulative toxicity (105,106).

Patients with central nervous system metastases are given whole-brain irradiation in addition to chemotherapy. Additional intrathecal or high-dose (1 g/M²) methotrexate must be used. About 50% of patients can be cured with this aggressive treatment (107–109). Liver metastasis from GTD is particularly ominous. Three of nine patients from the Southeastern Regional Trophoblastic Disease Center and none of six patients from the Brewer Trophoblastic Disease Center survived (88,110). Bakri et al. (111), from the New England Trophoblastic Disease Center, were able to achieve remission in five of eight patients (62.5%) with liver metastases treated with cisplatin, etoposide, and actinomycin D without liver irradiation, compared to their past experience of no survivors using methotrexate, actinomycin D, and cyclophosphamide (MAC) chemotherapy. Grumbine et al. (112) described a technique to control hemorrhage from hepatic metastasis by using silicone balloons to occlude selective hepatic arteries. Chemotherapeutic regimens used in resistant trophoblastic disease include cisplatinum, vinblastine, and bleomycin (VPB) (113) and cisplatinum, vincristine, methotrexate, and bleomycin (POMB) (114,115).

Options in patients with disease resistant to chemotherapy include conservative operative treatment and pelvic arterial infusion chemotherapy. Wilson et al. (116) reported on the local uterine resection of invasive trophoblastic tumors in five patients. All five patients achieved complete sustained remissions with no further treatment, and one patient had two subsequent term pregnancies. Maroulis et al. (117) performed pelvic arterial infusion chemotherapy with methotrexate or actinomycin D in five patients whose disease was resistant to systemic chemotherapy. Two patients were cured. Three other patients subsequently underwent hysterectomy and entered remission.

Reproductive Performance

Treatment of GTD in adolescent girls with cytotoxic drugs leads to concern over their future reproductive performance and the incidence of congenital malformations, pregnancy complications, and recurrent molar pregnancies. It is known that intensive chemotherapy induces amenorrhea and depletion of ovarian germ cells and sterility (118). Ovarian dysfunction and subsequent infertility after chemotherapy has been reported with Hodgkin's disease (119,120). Premature ovarian failure with loss of primordial follicles that is age and dose related has been shown in women treated for Hodgkin's disease with nitrogen mustard, vinblastine, procarbazine, and prenisolone (119). Generally, younger patients are able to tolerate larger cumulative doses before clinical evidence of ovarian dysfunction occurs and have a greater likelihood of resumption of function. Chemotherapy in patients with GTD does not appear to affect subsequent pregnancy rates (121–125). Ovarian dysfunction occurring after the use of etoposide was evaluated in a study of patients with gestational trophoblastic neoplasms (126). After an average cumulative dose of 5 g, seven of 22 patients developed permanent ovarian failure as evidenced by hypergonadotropic, hypoestrogenic amenorrhea. Song et al. (122) reviewed 265 cases of choriocarcinoma and invasive mole in young women treated between 1959 and 1980 at a hospital in Beijing, China. There were 355 pregnancies in the 265 patients. There was no difference in the rate of fetal wastage, malformations, twin pregnancies, and neonatal and infantile deaths than in the normal population. Cytogenetic study of the peripheral lymphocytes of 94 of the children revealed no increase of chromosomal aberrations. Long-term follow-up of the mothers revealed no increase in the rate of recurrence of GTD. Kim et al. (127) reported 70.4% of patients with a history of a molar pregnancy or GTD became pregnant within 1 year of discontinuing contraception and 85.2% within 3 years. Berkowitz et al. (128) reported on the reproductive results of the patients in the New England Trophoblastic Disease Center between June 1, 1965 and December 31, 1996. After partial mole, complete mole, and persistent trophoblastic tumor, the patients had 195, 1,234, and 504 later pregnancies, respectively. These patients had a later pregnancy experience comparable to that of the general population.

In several studies, the incidence of spontaneous abortions has been reported to be higher in patients before and after GTD. More recent reviews do not support an increased rate of spontaneous abortions compared to the general population (127,128). Spontaneous abortions and molar pregnancies may be caused by chromosomal disorders that sometimes led to a halt in development, as in a spontaneous abortion, and other times to abnormal development, as in GTD (123,129,130).

Cytotoxic drugs can be teratogenic when given during pregnancy, but studies of women treated for gestational trophoblastic tumors suggest that they do not have a deleterious effect on later conceptions (131). It has been suggested to delay conception for 1 year after cessation of chemotherapy to allow elimination of damaged ova from exposure to cytotoxic agents (121). In addition, methotrexate has been shown to be retained in mammalian tissues for up to 8 months (132).

The most remarkable obstetric complication noted in gestational trophoblastic patients is an increased risk of placenta accreta (placenta that has invaded the uterine musculature). Van Thiel et al. (133) reviewed 90 pregnancies in 51 women treated for GTD and found four patients with partial placenta accreta complicating the pregnancies, which was higher than the reported incidence in the general population. All four of their patients also had at least one other risk factor for placenta accreta, such as hysterectomy and curettage. Pastorfide et al. (123) discovered eight cases of placenta accreta of 303 deliveries. The adherent placenta may be due to destruction of the endometrium by trophoblastic disease and curettage.

Chemotherapeutic agents are known carcinogens and have been known to cause other malignancies after curing a cancer. There are limited reports of increased incidence of secondary malignancies after being treated with sequential or combination chemotherapy for gestational trophoblastic neoplasms. This increased incidence has appeared with longer follow-up and the introduction of etoposide. Rustin et al. (134) performed a further review of 1,377 long-term survivors treated until 1990. An overall 50% excess of risk (RR = 1.5, p <0.011) was observed with 37 second cancers detected. The risk was significantly elevated for myeloid leukemia (RR = 16.6), colon cancer (RR = 4.6), and breast cancer when the survival exceeded 25 years (RR = 5.8). The risk was not significantly increased among the 554 women who received single-agent therapy (RR = 1.3). Leukemias only developed in patients receiving etoposide in addition to other cytotoxic drugs.

A patient who had a molar pregnancy is at an increased risk of developing repeat trophoblastic disease in subsequent conceptions. The incidence of repeat GTD has been reported to occur in 0.6% to 2.6% of patients (127,128,135). Patients who develop repeat molar pregnancies with subsequent gestations are at an increased risk of having persistent trophoblastic disease with their subsequent molar pregnancies (51,127,128,136). In a review by Berkowitz et al. (128) of the New England Trophoblastic Disease Center results, 29 patients had 26 later conceptions resulting in 14 full-term deliveries (53.8%) and six molar pregnancies (23.1%) after two episodes of molar gestation. Sand et al. (135) reported similar results in their review of 22 patients with repetitive GTD.

Evaluation for GTD should be performed when irregular bleeding or suggestions of metastatic tumor occurs in the adolescent of reproductive age. β-hCG testing and ultrasound examination are essential techniques for obtaining an early diagnosis that can be critical for survival.

ACKNOWLEDGMENT

The authors are grateful to Diana Gray, M.D., for providing Fig. 25.3.

REFERENCES

1. Huffman JW. Tumors of the uterus, uterine tubes, and broad ligaments. In: Huffman JW, Dewhurst CJ, Capraro VJ, eds. *The gynecology of childhood and adolescence.* Philadelphia: WB Saunders, 1981:260–276.

2. Koh KS, Blajer S, Vadas G. Adenocarcinoma of the endometrium in a teenager. *CMAJ* 1975;112:980–981.

3. Carlson JA. Gynecologic neoplasms. In: Lavery JP, Sanfilippo JS, eds. *Pediatric and adolescent obstetrics and gynecology.* New York: Springer-Verlag, 1985: 124–148.

4. Jafari K, Javaheri G, Ruiz G. Endometrial adenocarcinoma and the Stein-Leventhal syndrome. *Obstet Gynecol* 1978;51:97–100.

5. Huang SJ, Amparo EG, Fu YS. Endometrial hyperplasia: histologic clarification and behavior. *Surg Pathol* 1988;1:215–229.

6. Kurman RJ, Kaminski RP, Norris HJ. The behavior of endometrial hyperplasia—a long term study of "untreated" hyperplasia in 170 patients. *Cancer* 1985; 56:403–412.

7. Speroff L, Glass RH, Kase NG. Dysfunctional uterine bleeding. In: Seifer DB, Speroff L, eds. *Clinical gynecologic endocrinology and infertility*, 5th ed. Baltimore: Williams & Wilkins, 1994:531–546.

8. Wiscot AL, Neimand KM, Rosenthal AH. Symptomatic myoma in a 13-year-old girl. *Am J Obstet Gynecol* 1969;105:639–641.

9. Augensen K. Uterine myoma in a 15-year-old girl. *Acta Obstet Gynecol Scand* 1981;60:591.

10. Farber M, Stein A, Adashi E. Rokitansky-Kuster-Hauser syndrome and leiomyoma uteri. *Obstet Gynecol* 1977;51:70s–73s.

11. Fields KR, Neinstein LS. Uterine myomas in adolescents: case reports and a review of the literature. *J Pediatr Adolesc Gynecol* 1996;9:195–198.

12. Chumas JC, Mann WJ, Tseng L. Malignant mixed mullerian tumor of the endometrium in a young woman with polycystic ovaries. *Cancer* 1983;52:1478–1481.

13. Amr SS, Tavassoli FA, Hassan AA, et al. Mixed mesodermal tumor of the uterus in a 4-year-old girl. *Int J Gynecol* 1986;5:371–378.

14. Craig JK. Inversion of the uterus associated with a malignant tumor in a girl of 14 years of age. *J Obstet Gynaecol Br Commonwealth* 1958;65:497–499.

15. Andrade LA, Derchain SF, Vial JS, et al. Mullerian adenosarcoma of the uterus in adolescents. *Int J Gynecol Obstet* 1992;38:119–123.

16. Lammers C, Fowler J. Leiomyosarcoma of the uterus in a 15 year old with acute abdominal pain. *J Adolesc Health* 1998;23:303–306.

17. Bellone F, Nicolo G, Remorgida V. A case of sarcoma originating from the endometrial stroma in a 16-year-old. *Adolesc Pediatr Gynecol* 1990;3:212–216.

18. Michalas S, Creatsas G, Deligeoroglou E, et al. High grade endometrial stromal sarcoma in a 16-year-old girl. *Gynecol Oncol* 1994;54:95–98.

19. Berchuck A, Rubin SC, Hoskins WJ, et al. Treatment of endometrial stromal tumors. *Gynecol Oncol* 1990;36: 60–65.

20. Geoffray A, Covanet D, Montagne JP, et al. Ultrasonography and computed tomography for diagnosis and follow up of pelvic rhabdomyosarcomas in children. *Pediatr Radiol* 1987;17:132–136.

21. Hays DM, Shimada H, Raney RB, et al. Clinical staging and treatment results in rhabdomyosarcoma of the female genital tract among children and adolescents. *Cancer* 1988;61:1893–1903.

22. Hammerman RM, Runowicz CD. Conservative management of uterine rhabdomyosarcoma. *Obstet Gynecol* 1998;92:669–670.

23. Ortega JA. A therapeutic approach to childhood pelvic rhabdomyosarcoma without pelvic exenteration. *J Pediatr* 1979;94:204–209.

24. Young RH, Kleinman GM, Scully RE. Glioma of the uterus. Report of a case with comments on histogenesis. *Am J Surg Pathol* 1981;12:695–699.

25. Rose PG, O'Toole RV, Keyhani-Rofagha S, et al. Malignant peripheral primitive neuroectodermal tumor of the uterus. *J Surg Oncol* 1987;35:165–169.

26. Ehrmann RL, Griffiths CT. Malignant hemangioendothelioma of the uterus. *Gynecol Oncol* 1979;8:376–383.

27. Egwuatu VE. Non-Hodgkin's lymphoma of the uterus in a child. *J Pediatr Surg* 1989;24:220–222.

28. Bittencourt AL, Britto JF, Fonseca LE. Wilm's tumor of the uterus: the first report of the literature. *Cancer* 1981; 47:2496–2499.

29. Wakely PE, Sprague RI, Kornstein MJ. Extrarenal Wilm's tumor: an analysis of four cases. *Hum Pathol* 1989;20:691–695.

30. Centers for Disease Control and Prevention. State-specific birth rates for teenagers-United States, 1990–1996. *MMWR* 1997;46:837–842.

31. Gestational trophoblastic disease. World Health Organization Technical Report Series 692. Geneva: WHO, 1983.

32. Bracken MB. Incidence and etiology of hydatidiform mole and epidemiologic review. *Br J Obstet Gynaecol* 1987;94:1123–1135.

33. Hayashi K, Braken MB, Freeman DH, et al. Hydatiform mole in the United States (1970–1977): a statistical and theoretical analysis. *Am J Epidemiol* 1982;115:67–77.

34. Stone M, Bagshawe KD. An analysis of the influences of maternal age, gestational age, contraception method, and the mode of primary treatment of patients with hydatiform moles on the incidence of subsequent chemotherapy. *Br J Obstet Gynaecol* 1979;86:782–792.

35. Teoh ES, Dawood MY, Ratnam SS. Epidemiology of hydatiform mole in Singapore. *Am J Obstet Gynecol* 1971;110:415–420.

36. Bandy LC, Clarke-Pearson DL, Hammond CB. Malignant potential of gestational trophoblastic disease at the extreme ages of reproductive life. *Obstet Gynecol* 1984;64:395–399.

37. Slocomb JC, Lund CJ. Incidence of trophoblastic disease: increased rate in youngest age group. *Am J Obstet Gynecol* 1969;104:421–423.

38. Marquez-Monter H, de la Vega GA, Robles M, et al. Epidemiology and pathology of hydatiform mole in the General Hospital of Mexico. *Am J Obstet Gynecol* 1963;85:856–864.

39. Curry SL, Hammond CB, Tyrey L, et al. Hydatiform mole: diagnosis, management and long-term follow-up of 347 patients. *Obstet Gynecol* 1975;45:1–8.

40. Franke HR, Risse KJ, Kenemans P, et al. Epidemiologic features of hydatiform mole in the Netherlands. *Obstet Gynecol* 1983;62:613–616.

41. Vassilakos P, Riotton G, Kajii T. Hydatiform mole: two entities. A morphologic and cytogenetic study with

some clinical considerations. *Am J Obstet Gynecol* 1977;127:167–170.

42. Szulman AE, Surti U. The syndromes of hydatiform mole. I. Cytogenetic and morphologic correlations. *Am J Obstet Gynecol* 1978;131:665–671.

43. Kajii T, Ohama K. Androgenetic origin of hydatiform mole. *Nature* 1977;368:633–634.

44. Szulman AE, Surti U. The syndromes of hydatiform mole. II. Morphologic evolution of the complete and partial mole. *Am J Obstet Gynecol* 1978;132:20–27.

45. Jacobs PA, Wilson CM, Sprenkle JA, et al. Mechanism of origin of complete hydatiform mole. *Nature* 1980; 286:714–716.

46. Jacobs PA, Hunt PA, Matsuura JS, et al. Complete and partial hydatiform mole in Hawaii: cytogenetics, morphology and epidemiology. *Br J Obstet Gynaecol* 1982; 89:258–266.

47. Lurain JR, Brewer JI, Torok EE, et al. Natural history of hydatiform mole after primary evacuation. *Am J Obstet Gynecol* 1983;145:591–595.

48. Czernobilsky B, Barash A. Partial moles: a clinicopathologic study of 25 cases. *Obstet Gynecol* 1982;59: 75–77.

49. Stone M, Bagshawe KD. Hydatiform mole: two entities. *Lancet* 1976;1:535–536.

50. Szulman AE, Surti U. The clinicopathologic profile of the partial hydatidiform mole. *Obstet Gynecol* 1982;59: 597–602.

51. Rice LW, Berkowitz RS, Lage JM, et al. Persistent gestational trophoblastic tumor after partial hydatiform mole. *Gynecol Oncol* 1990;36:358–362.

52. Mazur MT, Kurman RJ. Choriocarcinoma and placental site trophoblastic tumor. In: Szulman A, Buchsbaum H, eds. *Gestational trophoblastic disease.* New York: Springer-Verlag, 1987:45–68.

53. Bagshawe KD. Risk and prognostic factors in trophoblastic neoplasia. *Cancer* 1976;38:1373–1385.

54. Tsukamoto N, Kashimura Y, Sano M, et al. Choriocarcinoma occurring within the normal placenta with breast metastasis. *Gynecol Oncol* 1981;11:348–363.

55. Guvener S, Kazancigil A, Erez S. Long latent development of trophoblastic disease. *Am J Obstet Gynecol* 1972;114:679–684.

56. Lathrop J, Wachtel TJ, Meissner GF. Uterine choriocarcinoma fourteen years following bilateral tubal ligation. *Obstet Gynecol* 1978;51:477–482.

57. Aranda JM, Martinez I. Choriocarcinoma in Puerto Rico. *Bol Assoc Med PR* 1972;60:523–535.

58. Teoh ES, Dawood MY, Ratnam SS. Observations on choriocarcinoma in Singapore. *Obstet Gynecol* 1972; 40:519–524.

59. Ringertz N. Hydatiform mole, invasive mole, and choriocarcinoma in Sweden 1958–65. *Acta Obstet Gynecol* 1970;49:195–203.

60. Rolan PA, de Lopez BH. Malignant trophoblastic disease in Paraguay. *J Reprod Med* 1979;23:94–96.

61. Mazur MT, Lurain JR, Brewer JI. Fatal gestational choriocarcinoma. Clinicopathologic study of patients treated at a trophoblastic disease center. *Cancer* 1982; 50:1833–1846.

62. Libshitz HI, Baber CE, Hammond CB. The pulmonary metastases of choriocarcinoma. *Obstet Gynecol* 1977; 49:412–416.

63. Kumar J, Ilancheran A, Ratnam SS. Pulmonary metastasis in gestational trophoblastic disease: a review of 97 cases. *Br J Obstet Gynaecol* 1988;95:70–74.

64. Kelly MP, Rustin GJS, Ivory C, et al. Respiratory failure due to choriocarcinoma: a study of 103 dyspneic patients. *Gynecol Oncol* 1990;38:149–154.

65. Nisula BC, Taliadouros GS. Thyroid function in gestational trophoblastic neoplasia: evidence that the thyrotropic activity of chorionic gonadotropin mediates the thyrotoxicosis of choriocarcinoma. *Am J Obstet Gynecol* 1980;138:77–85.

66. Miller SM, Lurain JR. Classification and staging of gestational trophoblastic tumor. *Obstet Gynecol North Am* 1988;15:477–490.

67. Hammond CB, Borchert LG, Trey L, et al. Treatment of metastatic trophoblastic disease: good and poor prognosis. *Am J Obstet Gynecol* 1973;115:451–457.

68. Bagshawe KD. Treatment of high-risk choriocarcinoma. *J Reprod Med* 1984;29:813–820.

69. Munyer TP, Callen PW, Filly RA, et al. Further observations on the sonographic spectrum of gestational trophoblastic disease. *J Clin Ultrasound* 1981;9: 349–358.

70. Hill LM, Buchsbaum, Kanal E. Radiographic techniques in diagnosis and management. In: Szulman A, Buchsbaum H, eds. *Gestational trophoblastic disease.* New York: Springer-Verlag, 1987:101–111.

71. Roberts DK, Wells MM, Horbelt DV. Dysgerminoma in the differential diagnosis of hydatiform mole. *Obstet Gynecol* 1986;67:92s–94s.

72. Reid MH, McGahan JP, Oi R. Sonographic evaluation of hydatiform mole and its lookalikes. *Am J Radiol* 1983;140:307–311.

73. Taylor KJ, Schwartz PE, Kohorn EI. Gestational trophoblastic neoplasia: diagnosis with Doppler US. *Radiology* 1987;165:445–448.

74. Goldstein DP, Berkowitz RS, Bernstein MR. Management of molar pregnancy. *J Reprod Med* 1981;26: 208–212.

75. Kohorn EI, McGinn RC, Gee BL. Pulmonary embolization of trophoblastic tissue in molar pregnancy. *Obstet Gynecol* 1978;51:16–24.

76. Berkowitz RS, Goldstein DP. Diagnosis and management of the primary hydatidiform mole. *Obstet Gynecol Clin North Am* 1988;15:491–503.

77. McDonald TW, Ruffalo EH. Modern management of gestational trophoblastic disease. *Obstet Gynecol Surv* 1983;38:67–83.

78. Morrow CP, Kletzky OA, DiSaia PJ, et al. Clinical and laboratory correlates of molar pregnancy and trophoblastic disease. *Am J Obstet Gynecol* 1977;128:424–430.

79. Goldstein DP. The chemotherapy of gestational trophoblastic disease: principles of clinical management. *JAMA* 1972;220:209–213.

80. Stone M, Dent J, Kardana A, et al. Relationship of oral contraception to development of trophoblastic tumor after evacuation of a hydatidiform mole. *Br J Obstet Gynaecol* 1976;83:913–916.

81. Berkowitz RS, Goldstein DP, Marean AR, et al. Oral contraceptives and postmolar trophoblastic disease. *Obstet Gynecol* 1981;58:474–477.

82. Morrow P, Nakamura R, Schlaerth J, et al. The influence of oral contraceptives on the postmolar human chorionic gonadotropin curve. *Am J Obstet Gynecol* 1985; 151:906–914.

83. Franke HR, Risse EKJ, Kaneman SP, et al. Plasma human chorionic gonadotropin disappearance in hydatidiform mole: a central registry from the Netherlands. *Obstet Gynecol* 1983;62:467–473.

84. Goldstein DP. Prevention of gestational trophoblastic disease by use of actinomycin-D in molar pregnancies. *Obstet Gynecol* 1974;43:475–479.

85. Fascoli M, Ratti E, Franceschi S, et al. Management of gestational trophoblastic disease: results of a cooperative study. *Obstet Gynecol* 1982;60:205–209.

86. Kashimura Y, Kashimura M, Sugimori H, et al. Prophylactic chemotherapy of hydatidiform mole. Five to 15 years follow-up. *Cancer* 1986;58:624–629.

87. Ayhan A, Tuncer ZS, Halilzade H, et al. Predictors of persistent disease in women with complete hydatidiform mole. *J Reprod Med* 1996;41:591–594.

88. Lurain JR, Brewer JI, Torok EE, et al. Gestational trophoblastic disease. Treatment results at the Brewer Trophoblastic Disease Center. *Obstet Gynecol* 1982; 60:354–360.

89. Lurain JR. Chemotherapy of gestational trophoblastic disease. In: Deppe G, ed. *Chemotherapy of gynecologic cancer.* New York: Wiley-Liss, 1990:273–301.

90. Hammond CB, Hertz R, Ross GT, Lipsett et al. Primary chemotherapy for non-metastatic gestational trophoblastic neoplasms. *Am J Obstet Gynecol* 1967;98:71–78.

91. Hammond CB, Weed JC, Currie JL. The role of operation in the current therapy of gestational trophoblastic disease. *Am J Obstet Gynecol* 1980;136:844–858.

92. Goldstein DP, Berkowitz RS. Nonmetastatic and low-risk metastatic gestational trophoblastic neoplasms. *Semin Oncol* 1982;9:191–197.

93. Elit L, Covens A, Osborne R. High dose methotrexate for gestational trophoblastic disease. *Gynecol Oncol* 1994;54:282–287.

94. Homesley HD, Blessing JA, Rettenmaier M, et al. Weekly intramuscular methotrexate for nonmetastatic gestational trophoblastic disease. *Obstet Gynecol* 1988; 72:413–418.

95. Homesley HD, Blessing JA, Schlaerth J, et al. Rapid escalation of weekly intramuscular methotrexate for nonmetastatic gestational trophoblastic disease: a Gynecologic Oncology Group Study. *Gynecol Oncol* 1990; 39:305–308.

96. Hoffman MS, Fiorica JV, Gleeson NC, et al. A single institution experience with weekly intramuscular methotrexate for nonmetastatic gestational trophoblastic disease. *Gynecol Oncol* 1996;60:292–294.

97. Petrilli ES, Twiggs LB, Blessing JA, et al. Single dose actinomycin-D treatment for nonmetastatic gestational trophoblastic disease: a prospective Phase II trial of the Gynecologic Oncology Group. *Cancer* 1987;60: 2173–2176.

98. Roberts JP, Lurain JR. Treatment of low risk metastatic gestational trophoblastic tumors with single agent chemotherapy. *Am J Obstet Gynecol* 1996;174:1917–1926.

99. Lurain JR, Brewer JI. Treatment of high-risk gestational trophoblastic disease with methotrexate, actinomycin-D, and cyclophosphamide chemotherapy. *Obstet Gynecol* 1985;65:830–636.

100. Schink JC, Singh DK, Rademaker AW, et al. Etoposide, methotrexate, actinomycin-D, cyclophosphamide and vincristine for the treatment of metastatic, high-risk gestational trophoblastic disease. *Obstet Gynecol* 1992; 80:817–820.

101. Soper J, Evans A, Clarke-Pearson D, et al. Alternating weekly chemotherapy with etoposide-methotrexate-actinomycin/cyclophosphamide-vincristine for high risk gestational trophoblastic disease. *Obstet Gynecol* 1994;83:113–117.

102. Quinn M, Murray J, Freidlander M, et al. EMA-CO in high risk gestational trophoblastic disease: the Australian experience. *Aust NZ J Obstet Gynecol* 1994;34: 90–92.

103. Bower M, Newlands ES, Holden L, et al. EMA/CO for high risk gestational trophoblastic tumors: results from a cohort of 272 patients. *J Clin Oncol* 1997;15: 2636–2643.

104. Surwit EA, Childers JM. High-risk metastatic trophoblastic disease: a new dose-intensive multiagent chemotherapeutic regimen. *J Reprod Med* 1991;36:45–48.

105. DuBeshter B, Berkowitz RS, Goldstein DP, et al. Metastatic gestational trophoblastic disease: experience at the New England Trophoblastic Disease Center, 1965–1985. *Obstet Gynecol* 1987;69:390–395.

106. Lurain JR. Management of high-risk gestational trophoblastic disease. *J Reprod Med* 1998;43:44–52.

107. Weed JC, Hammond CB. Cerebral metastatic choriocarcinoma: intensive therapy and prognosis. *Obstet Gynecol* 1980;55:89–94.

108. Athanassiou A, Begent RHJ, Newlands ES, et al. Central nervous system metastases of choriocarcinoma: 23 years' experience at Charing Cross Hospital Center. *Cancer* 1983;52:1728–1735.

109. Small W Jr, Lurain JR, Shetty RM, et al. Gestational trophoblastic disease metastatic to the brain. *Radiology* 1996;200:277–280.

110. Surwit EA, Hammond CB. Treatment of metastatic trophoblastic disease with poor prognosis. *Obstet Gynecol* 1980;55:565–570.

111. Bakri YN, Subhi J, Amer M, et al. Liver metastases of gestational trophoblastic tumor. *Gynecol Oncol* 1993; 48:110–113.

112. Grumbine FC, Rosenshein NB, Berenton HD, et al. Management of liver metastases from gestational trophoblastic disease. *Obstet Gynecol* 1980;137:959–961.

113. Gordon AN, Kavanaugh JJ, Gershenson DM, et al. Cisplatin, vinblastine, and bleomycin combination therapy in resistant gestational trophoblastic disease. *Cancer* 1986;58:1407–1410.

114. Newlands ES, Bagshawe KD. Activity of high dose cisplatinum in combination with vincristine and methotrexate in drug resistant choriocarcinoma. *Br J Cancer* 1979;40:943–945.

115. Newlands ES. New chemotherapeutic agents in the management of gestational trophoblastic disease. *Semin Oncol* 1982;9:239–243.

116. Wilson RB, Beecham CT, Symmonds RE. Conservative surgical management of chorioadenoma destruens. *Obstet Gynecol* 1965;26:814–820.

117. Maroulis GB, Hammond CB, Johnsrude IS, et al. Arteriography and infusional chemotherapy in localized trophoblastic disease. *Obstet Gynecol* 1975;45: 397–406.

118. Damewood MD, Grochow LB. Prospects for fertility after chemotherapy or radiation for neoplastic disease. *Fertil Steril* 1986;45:443–460.

119. Chapman RM, Sutcliffe SB, Malpas JS. Cytotoxic induced ovarian failure in women with Hodgkin's disease: hormone function. *JAMA* 1979;242:1877–1881.

120. Schilsky RL, Lewis BJ, Sherring RJ, et al. Gonadal dysfunction in patients receiving chemotherapy for cancer. *Ann Intern Med* 1980;93:109–114.

121. Walden PAM, Bagshawe KD. Pregnancies after chemotherapy for gestational trophoblastic tumors. *Lancet* 1979;2:1241.

122. Song H, Wu P, Wang Y, et al. Pregnancy outcomes after successful chemotherapy for choriocarcinoma and invasive mole. *Am J Obstet Gynecol* 1988;158: 538–545.

123. Pastorfide GB, Goldstein DP. Pregnancy after hydatidiform mole. *Obstet Gynecol* 1973;42:67–70.

124. Van Thiel DH, Ross GT, Lipsett MD. Pregnancies after chemotherapy of trophoblastic neoplasms. *Science* 1970;169:1326–1327.

125. Rustin GJS, Booth M, Dent J, et al. Pregnancy after cytotoxic chemotherapy for gestational trophoblastic tumours. *Br Med J* 1984;288:103–106.

126. Choo YC, Chan SYW, Wong LC, et al. Ovarian dysfunction in patients with gestational trophoblastic neoplasia treated with short intensive courses of etoposide (VP16-23). *Cancer* 1985;55:2348–2352.

127. Kim JH, Park DC, Bae SN, et al. Subsequent reproductive experience after treatment for gestational trophoblastic disease. *Gynecol Oncol* 1998;71:108–112.

128. Berkowitz RS, Im SS, Bernstein MR, et al. Gestational trophoblastic disease: subsequent pregnancy outcome, including repeat molar pregnancy. *J Reprod Med* 1998; 43:81–86.

129. Meizner I, Leiberman JR, Insler V. Risk factors for gestational trophoblastic neoplasia. *Am J Obstet Gynecol* 1986;155:456–457.

130. Messerli ML, Lilienfeld AM, Parmley T, et al. Risk factors for gestational trophoblastic neoplasia. *Am J Obstet Gynecol* 1985;153:294–300.

131. Ross GT. Congenital anomalies among children born of mothers receiving chemotherapy for gestational trophoblastic neoplasms. *Cancer* 1976;37:1043–1047.

132. Charache S, Condit PT, Humphreys SR. Studies on the folic acid vitamins. IV. The persistent amethopterin in mammalian tissues. *Cancer* 1960;13:236–240.

133. Van Thiel DH, Grodin JM, Ross GT, et al. Partial placenta accreta in pregnancies following chemotherapy for gestational trophoblastic neoplasms. *Am J Obstet Gynecol* 1972;112:54–58.

134. Rustin GJS, Newlands ES, Lutz JM, et al. Combination but not single agent methotrexate chemotherapy for gestational trophoblastic tumors increases the incidence of second tumors. *J Clin Oncol* 1996;14:2769–2773.

135. Sand P, Lurain J, Brewer J. Repeat gestational trophoblastic disease. *Obstet Gynecol* 1984;63:140–144.

136. Parazzini F, Mangili G, Belloni C, et al. The problem of identification of prognostic factors for persistent trophoblastic disease. *Gynecol Oncol* 1988;30:57–62.

26

Benign and Malignant Tumors of the Ovary

Ira R. Horowitz, Ricardo Sainz De La Cuesta, and Bhagirath Majmudar

Evaluation and treatment of a pelvic mass at any age is a traumatic experience. Tumors in childhood and adolescence, although infrequent, are especially devastating to young patients and their families.

Ovarian cancer is the second most common malignancy in women over the age of 35 years. During the first three decades of life, ovarian neoplasms are rare, with less than 5% of ovarian malignancies occurring in children and adolescents. Ovarian tumors in childhood and adolescent females account for approximately 1% of all tumors in these age groups

and 3% of all ovarian neoplasms (1,2). Sixty-five percent of all ovarian tumors are benign, and the remaining 35% have malignant features (Table 26.1). A review by Breen and Mayson (3) of 1,002 ovarian neoplasms in patients less than 20 years of age revealed that germ cell tumors constituted 67.2% of all ovarian neoplasms. Paraovarian and paratubal cysts can account for up to 10% of pelvic masses identified on ultrasound (4). In general, ultrasound has a very low sensitivity and specificity for diagnosis of malignant neoplasms of the ovary in premenopausal

TABLE 26.1. *Ovarian tumors in patients under 20 years of age*

	Tintera and Mitarnum 1990 (2)		Norris and Jensen 1972 (86)		Junaid 1981 (87)	
	n	%	n	%	n	%
Germ cell	28	59.6	205	58	51	30.2 [67.1]
Mature teratoma	11		71		38	
Malignant teratoma	2		28		4	
Dysgerminoma	2		48		7	
Endodermal sinus tumor	8		32		2	
Mixed or choriocarcinoma	5		26		0	
Epithelial	18	38.3	67	19	8	4.7 [10.5]
Cystadenoma and adenofibroma	14		59		4	
Borderline	3		5		1	
Cystadenocarcinoma	1		3		3	
Sex cord stromal	1	2.1	62	18	13	7.7 [17.1]
Fibrothecoma	0		23		4	
Androblastoma	1		14		2	
Granulosa cell tumor	0		12		6	
Nonspecific	0		13		1	
Miscellaneous	0	0	19	5	97	57.4 [5.3]
Lymphoma	0		2		93	
Other	0		17		4	
Total	47	100	353	100	169	100 [100]

Numbers in brackets represent percentages relative to 76 nonlymphoma tumors.
Modified from Tintera H, Mitarnum W. Ovarian neoplasms in childhood and adolescents in Songklanagarind Hospital, February 1983–March 1989. *J Med Assoc Thai* 1990;73:75–80.

patients. Physiologic changes can mimic the ultrasonographic appearance of a malignancy.

FUNCTIONAL CYSTS

Functional cysts are the most frequent cysts present in the human ovary. They can present as follicular, corpus luteum, and theca lutein cysts. All are benign and usually self-limited (Fig. 26.1).

The diameter of these cysts can range up to 8 cm. These cysts usually occur secondary to an abnormality in gonadotropin production and resolve in 4 to 8 weeks. The majority of follicular cysts are an incidental finding on physical examination; however, large cysts may rupture and cause a transient peritonitis. Although peritoneal signs and symptoms are present, they usually resolve in 24 hours. It is imperative that other causes of peritonitis, such as pelvic infections, appendicitis, ruptured viscus including ectopic pregnancy, and hemorrhagic cysts, be ruled out before undergoing a plan of observation. A laparoscopic evaluation should be performed if the etiology of peritonitis is uncertain.

Corpus Luteum Cysts

Corpus luteum cysts, although less common than follicular cysts, are persistently functioning corpora lutea. Corpora lutea are considered corpus luteum cysts when their

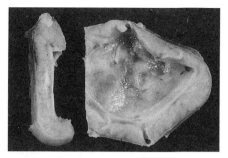

FIG. 26.2. Corpus luteum cyst showing central cystic cavity surrounded by bright yellow zone of luteinization.

diameter is more than 3 cm (Figs. 26.2–26.3). Corpus luteum has normal endocrine function and may express a prolonged progesterone secretion. Haldan (5) described a classic triad of persistently functioning corpus luteum cysts, which includes a normal menses followed by spotting, unilateral pelvic pain, and a slightly enlarged tender adnexal mass (6). The spontaneous rupture and hemorrhage of these cysts may result in a hematoperitoneum requiring operative intervention to control bleeding. Patients on anticoagulation therapy, such as coumarin or heparin, are at greater risk of a hemorrhage from corpus luteum and as such they frequently are treated with oral contraceptives to suppress ovulation. Hallatt et al. (7) reported the most common symptoms identified in 173 patients who required surgical intervention (Tables 26.2–26.3).

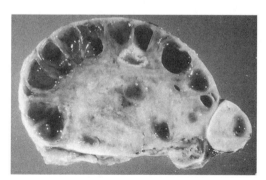

FIG. 26.1. Cut surface of an ovary showing multiple theca lutein cysts.

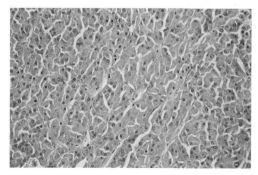

FIG. 26.3. Microscopic section showing luteinized cells characterized by central small nuclei and abundant eosinophilic cytoplasm.

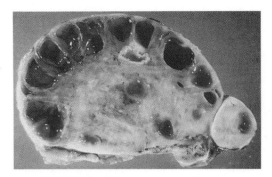

COLOR PLATE 10. Cut surface of an ovary showing multiple theca lutein cysts.

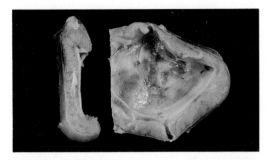

COLOR PLATE 11. Corpus luteum cyst showing central cystic cavity surrounded by bright yellow zone of luteinization.

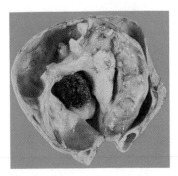

COLOR PLATE 12. Gross photograph of a mature cystic teratoma showing teeth and hair.

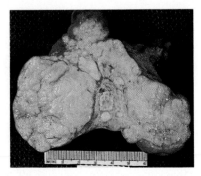

COLOR PLATE 13. Ovarian thecoma showing solid, lobulated, yellow mass.

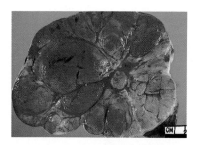

COLOR PLATE 14. Ovarian dysgerminoma showing a solid, lobulated mass.

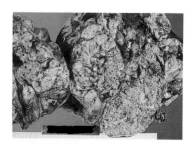

COLOR PLATE 15. Endodermal sinus tumor showing fleshy, necrotic, and hemorrhagic cut surface.

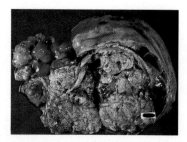

COLOR PLATE 16. Immature teratoma showing partly solid, partly cystic appearance with hemorrhage and necrosis.

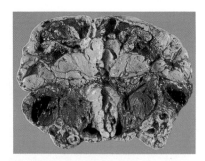

COLOR PLATE 17. Granulosa cell tumor showing a characteristic yellow, lobulated cut surface with areas of hemorrhage.

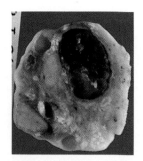

COLOR PLATE 18. Sertoli-Leydig cell tumor showing solid, yellow and white cut surface with hemorrhage. Normal ovarian tissue can be seen on **left** side.

TABLE 26.2. *Clinical features of 173 patients*

	n	%
Age (range 12–52 yr)		
>40 yr	17	10
<20 yr	20	12
Parity		
Nulliparous	66	38
Multiparous	92	53
Unknown	15	9
Prior ovarian cyst operation	9	5
Using intrauterine contraceptive device	19	11
Ovulation induced by clomiphene citrate	2	1.15

From Hallatt JG, Steele CH, Snyder M. Ruptured corpus luteum with hemoperitoneum: a study of 173 surgical cases. *Am J Obstet Gynecol* 1984;149:6, with permission.

Treatment

Treatments for functional cysts and corpus luteum cysts are essentially the same. If left alone, these cysts usually will resolve in 4 to 8 weeks. Spanos (8) reported 80% resolution of cysts up to 4 to 6 cm in size in patients taking oral contraceptives to suppress ovulation. Grimes and Hughes (9) estimated the rate of hospitalization for functional ovarian cysts as 472 to 522 per 100,000 women aged 15 to 44 years who were taking multiphasic oral contraceptives between 1979 and 1986 (Fig. 26.4). Alternative therapies include oral or

TABLE 26.3. *Clinical features of 173 patients*

	n	%
Location		
Right ovary	114	66
Left ovary	56	32
Unknown	3	2
Abdominal pain	173	100
Onset with intercourse	29	17
Right ovary	21	72
Left ovary	8	28
Duration		
Less than 24 h	94	54
1–7 d	40	23
Over 7 d	14	8
Unknown	25	15
Nausea, vomiting, or diarrhea	60	32

From Hallatt JG, Steele CH, Snyder M. Ruptured corpus luteum with hemoperitoneum: a study of 173 surgical cases. *Am J Obstet Gynecol* 1984;149:6, with permission.

intramuscular progesterone. Cysts persisting for more than 4 to 8 weeks require operative intervention. Simple follicular cysts can be drained or excised using operative endoscopy if no evidence suggesting a malignant neoplasm is present. Patients with a ruptured corpus luteal cyst usually present with severe abdominal pain. Differential diagnosis includes ruptured ectopic pregnancy, endometrioma, adnexal torsion, hemorrhage, ruptured spleen, and perforated abdominal viscus. Culdocentesis will only assess for the presence of nonclotting blood. A serum pregnancy test for human chorionic gonadotropin (hCG) should be obtained in all patients with this presentation. If the hematocrit continues to drift downward, a laparoscopy is indicated to make a diagnosis. If bleeding cannot be controlled, an exploratory laparotomy is imperative. Conservative therapy is advocated in the form of a cystectomy and/or cauterization of the bleeding vessels. This is a benign condition and usually does not require an oophorectomy to obtain hemostasis. Hansen et al. (10) identified a 16-year-old adolescent with pelvic pain, galactorrhea, dysfunctional uterine bleeding, and ovarian cysts with primary hypothyroidism. Treatment including bilateral wedge resection and thyroid replacement therapy resulted in resolution of the symptoms.

Theca Lutein Cysts

Theca lutein cysts are the least common of the functional ovarian cysts and usually are bilateral. Approximately 50% of the molar pregnancies and 10% of choriocarcinomas have theca lutein cysts present (6). Multiple gestations, diabetes, and Rh sensitization can result in increased stimulation in the presence of theca lutein cysts. Clomiphene citrate, gonadotropin-releasing hormone analogues, human menopausal gonadotropins, and hCG frequently result in overstimulation of the ovaries and the presence of theca lutein cysts. Theca lutein cysts frequently are large and may reach up to 30 cm in diameter. These polycystic ovaries result in masculinization of the female fetus in approximately 30% of cases.

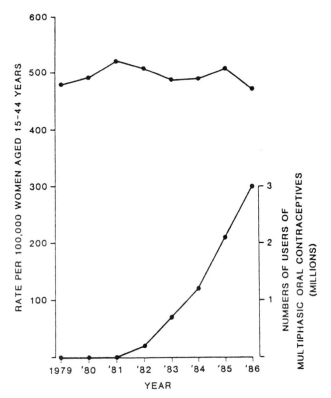

FIG. 26.4. Rates per 100,000 women of hospitalization for functional ovarian cysts among women aged 15 to 44 years and use of multiphasic oral contraceptives, United States, 1979 to 1986. (From Grimes DA, Hughes JM. Use of multiphasic oral contraceptive and hospitalizations of women with functional ovarian cysts in the United States. *Obstet Gynecol* 1989;73:1037–1039, with permission.)

Treatment

Theca lutein cysts regress spontaneously and do not require operative intervention. If the cysts persist or result in torsion, an exploratory laparotomy and resection of the involved cyst or adnexa is suggested. In the presence of an intrauterine pregnancy during the first trimester, consultation with a perinatologist should be obtained for possible treatment with progesterone.

Although benign, functional cysts may persist and result in torsion, requiring operative intervention and a possible adnexectomy.

BENIGN TUMORS

Endometriosis and Endometrioma

Although most frequent in the third and fourth decade of life, endometriosis can be present in childhood and adolescent females. A thorough discussion of endometriosis can be found in Chapter 15.

There are several proposed mechanisms for the etiology of endometriosis, including retrograde menstruation, coelomic metaplasia (11), lymphatic and vascular metastasis, immunologic deficiencies, and genetic predisposition. Endometriosis is found most frequently in menstruating patients. It can present itself as small implants on the peritoneal surface of the ovaries as well as large endometriomas measuring several centimeters. Classic symptoms include severe dysmenorrhea and infertility in older patients. Patients occasionally may present with an adnexal mass, which on evaluation reveals diffuse endometriosis and a large ovarian endometrioma. Serum CA-125 level can be elevated with endometriosis and increased with rupture of the endometrioma (12). This entity is benign and can be treated as described in Chapter 15.

Mature Cystic Teratoma

Benign ovarian teratomas are the most commonly found ovarian tumor, accounting for approximately 11% of all ovarian neoplasms (13,14). The median age of occurrence is 30 years of age (range 2 to 88 years) (13).

Macroscopic

The mature cystic teratoma (dermoid cyst) develops from totipotenital cells and is composed of well-differentiated ectodermal, endodermal, and mesodermal elements. This teratoma is bilateral in 7.9% to 15% of patients. In gross appearance, the tumor can be round, oval, or globular, with a smooth surface. It can measure less than 1 cm to larger than 30 cm in diameter. Cross-section reveals bone, hair, nerve tissue, sebaceous material, and fully developed teeth representing the three germ cell layers. Skin, hair, and sebaceous material are present in the majority of cystic teratomas excised (Figs. 26.5–26.6). Torsion can alter the appearance of the tumor, making it look dark and hemorrhagic.

Microscopic

Microscopic sections of the cyst are composed of ovarian stroma forming an outer wall

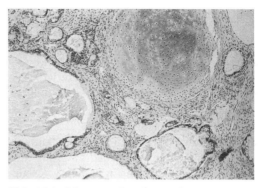

FIG. 26.6. Microscopic section of a mature cystic teratoma showing normal mucus glands and cartilage.

and a cavity lined with squamous epithelium containing sebaceous and sweat glands, glial tissue, and components of various germ cell layers.

Treatment

These tumors are benign; however, their large size predisposes them to undergo torsion and/or rupture, which can result in an acute abdomen. Malignant transformation occurs in 1% to 3% of benign teratomas but usually in postmenopausal patients (15–17).

Abdominal x-ray frequently reveals a soft tissue mass with calcification, occasionally resembling a tooth (Fig. 26.7). Additional studies, such as computed axial tomography (CAT) scan or magnetic resonance imaging

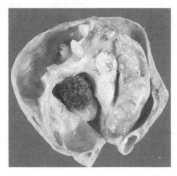

FIG. 26.5. Gross photograph of a mature cystic teratoma showing teeth and hair.

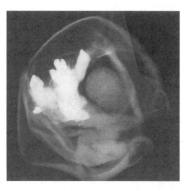

FIG. 26.7. Radiograph of a cystic teratoma showing identifiable teeth.

(MRI) (18), can identify both the calcification and the fat content of dermoid cysts. The treatment of choice for benign cystic teratomas is ovarian cystectomy. Technology is available to perform this procedure with operative endoscopy in the patients with small lesions. Large lesions without normal ovarian tissue identified should be removed through an exploratory laparotomy; oophorectomy or cystectomy can be performed to avoid rupture and spill of the mucin contents. Recurrence after conservative treatment is less than 1% (19). The contralateral ovary should always be evaluated to rule out the possibility of bilateral lesions. The presence of mature unilateral cystic teratomas does not necessitate a wedge resection or bivalving the contralateral ovary.

Functional Teratoma

The presence of thyroid tissue in a benign cystic teratoma occurs in 5% to 20% of benign teratomas (20–23). A diagnosis of struma ovarii is made only when the majority of the solid component is composed of thyroid tissue. Thyrotoxicosis has been associated with struma ovarii (24–26). The diagnosis of struma ovarii is made on excision of the pelvic mass and microscopic evaluation. Most of these lesions are benign, and excision of the tumor usually is adequate.

Carcinoid tumors can be present in benign cystic teratoma. Although an ovarian carcinoid secondary to gastrointestinal metastasis may be present, these lesions usually are bilateral compared to unilateral carcinoids present in mature cystic teratomas. Unlike carcinoids of the intestine, ovarian carcinoids frequently present with the classic carcinoid syndrome of flushes, diarrhea, cardiac valvular lesion, or bronchial constriction (27). This is because the ovarian veins end in systemic venous circulation, bypassing hepatic circulation.

Treatment

Treatment consists of excision of the ovarian lesion.

SEX CORD TUMORS

Thecomas

Thecomas are only rarely seen before puberty and uncommon before the age of 30 years. These tumors frequently are associated with estrogen production and present in the perimenopausal and postmenopausal years (Figs. 26.8–26.9).

Fibromas

Fibromas account for 4% of all ovarian tumors (6,28). Less than 10% of fibromas are encountered in patients under the age of 30 years. These tumors comprise approximately 0.5% to 2% of all ovarian tumors found in infancy and childhood (29–31). Forty percent of patients with fibromas larger than 10 cm present with ascites (32). Patients with ovarian fibromas may present with Meigs' triad, which includes ascites, ipsilateral pleural effusion, and ovarian fibroma.

Microscopic

Microscopically, fibromas are composed of intersecting bundles of spindle cells that produce collagen. Mitotic figures of one to three per high-power field can be present and still be considered a benign neoplasm.

Treatment

In the young adolescent female, conservative resection of the fibroma is recommended.

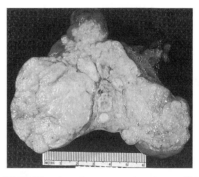

FIG. 26.8. Ovarian thecoma showing solid, lobulated, yellow mass.

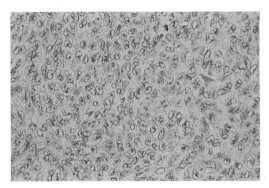

FIG. 26.9. Microscopic section of an ovarian thecoma showing monotonous theca cells with luteinization.

Gonadoblastomas

Originally described by Scully (33), these tumors consist of a germ cell and sex cord stromal elements. These gonads act as a source for germ cell tumors, including dysgerminoma and extraembryonal cell tumors. Patients with gonadoblastomas frequently have a Y chromosome in their karyotype. Patients with gonadal dysgenesis and Y chromosomes are at markedly increased risk for development of a gonadoblastoma and/or malignant germ cell tumor. This is an uncommon tumor, occurring predominantly in young patients under the age of 30 years (34). Patients usually are phenotypic females in a ratio of 4:1 (20–23). Their presentation includes primary amenorrhea, virilization, and/or developmental abnormalities. Thirty-eight percent of the lesions are bilateral.

Macroscopic

Gonadoblastomas can present in size as a microscopic tumor removed in patients with gonadal dysgenesis or as masses up to 8 cm (21,22).

Microscopic

Microscopically, tubules with unencapsulated germ cells and calcified bodies are present. Coexistence with other germ cell components is common (20–23).

Treatment

Treatment for patients with gonadoblastomas includes exploratory laparotomy and bilateral excision of gonads. Regardless of whether or not the lesions are bilateral, the gonads in these patients should be removed. The prognosis is excellent in patients who have gonadectomies. Frequently, a germ cell tumor, such as a dysgerminoma, will be present. These patients, as well as those with an endodermal sinus tumor or immature teratoma, should be treated as outlined in the following sections on germ cell tumors.

MALIGNANT OVARIAN NEOPLASMS

The most common malignant ovarian neoplasms in patients under 20 years of age are germ cell tumors. Seventy percent of ovarian tumors in this age group are of germ cell origin, with approximately 23% being malignant germ cell tumors. Sixty-six percent of ovarian malignances in patients under 20 years of age are of germ cell origin (29,35).

Malignant epithelial tumors of the ovary occur in women older than 40 years of age. Epithelial tumors in patients under age 30 years tend to be of a low malignant potential (30). Epithelial tumors of the ovary in children are exceptionally rare. Because ovarian malignancy of any sort is extremely uncommon in childhood, a thorough histologic and cytologic evaluation should be obtained before radical surgery is undertaken in children.

Clinical Features

Signs and Symptoms

It is difficult to identify abnormal adnexal pathology in the premenarcheal female. Complaints of urinary frequency, dysuria, rectal discomfort, and abdominal fullness with a decrease in appetite are nonspecific and require further evaluation. Although large pelvic masses can be palpated on abdominal examination, the majority of small lesions require radiologic evaluation and/or an examination under anesthesia. In the menarcheal patients, these symptoms as well as menstrual irregularities may be present. As with adults, ascites, abdominal distention, and pleural effusion are indications of advanced disease. The presence of a pelvic mass is the most common finding in more than 90% of cases.

Physical Examination

In the menarcheal female, a thorough physical examination should be performed, with particular note of sexual development including Tanner stages. Germ cell tumors that produce hormones may result in precocious sexual development. A pelvic examination, including a rectal examination, should be performed to identify any adnexal or pelvic pathology.

In the premenarcheal female, it frequently is difficult to perform such an examination, and various imaging techniques should be initiated.

Radiology

Ultrasound, CAT scans, and MRI have all been used to evaluate the pelvic area for ovarian pathology. Ultrasound is the imaging technique of choice secondary to the low cost, minimal complexity, and discomfort to the patient. Imaging techniques afford us an opportunity to identify cystic, solid, and complex components of the adnexal mass. Those masses with complex components have a high probability of being malignant.

CAT scans and MRI technique are superior in evaluating metastatic lesion to the liver, lung, brain, kidney, and lymph nodes compared to ultrasound. When evaluating for pulmonary metastasis, a chest x-ray usually is sufficient to identify large lesions. Further evaluation may require a CAT scan.

TUMOR MARKERS

Monoclonal Antibodies

Monoclonal antibodies that react with antigens associated with various malignancies are extremely useful in the differential diagnosis and subsequent follow-up of ovarian cancers.

Germ cell tumors secrete marker substances that aid in the diagnosis and subsequent evaluation of successful treatment protocols (Fig. 26.10).

CA-125

CA-125 was the first widely available monoclonal antibody against epithelial ovarian cancer (37). The specificity of CA-125 is poor, and it may be elevated with a multitude of intraperitoneal processes such as Crohn's disease, pelvic inflammatory disease, endometriosis, pregnancy, and a host of abdominal malignancies. Although this limits its value, the CA-125 level in premenopausal females can be followed after the diagnosis of a malignancy to assist in determining the level of treatment response. Changes in antigen level correlate with treatment response in approximately 90% of patients (38).

α-Fetoprotein

α-Fetoprotein (AFP) is an oncofetal antigen, a glycoprotein normally expressed by the fetus and reexpressed by endodermal sinus tumors, mixed germ cell tumors, and immature teratomas. It is a reliable marker with a high sensitivity, which permits diagnosis and treatment evaluation of patients with pure endodermal sinus tumors or tumors with endodermal sinus components. Fewer than 10% of epithelial ovarian carcinomas produce AFP (39).

Human Chorionic Gonadotropin

hCG is produced by trophoblastic cells. It is produced by normal human placental tissue as well as hydatidiform moles, placental site trophoblastic tumors, choriocarcinoma, and embryonal ovarian carcinomas with trophoblastic differentiation. Embryonal carcinomas can produce AFP, as previously mentioned.

Carcinoembryonic Antigen

Carcinoembryonic antigen (CEA) has been produced by epithelial and germ cell tumors. CEA may be markedly elevated in patients with colon carcinoma and ovarian mucinous carcinomas. In selected situations, it can be an

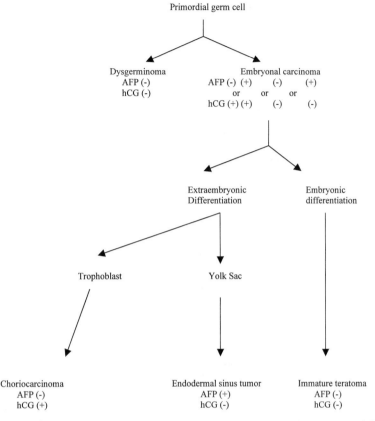

FIG. 26.10. Relationship between examples of pure malignant germ cell tumors and their secreted marker substances. AFP, alpha-fetoprotein; hCG, human chorionic gonadotropin. (From Griffiths CT, Parker L. Cancer of the ovary. In: Knapp RC, Berkowitz RS, eds. *Gynecologic oncology.* New York: MacMillan, 1986:364, with permission.)

additional marker that assesses clinical response to treatment protocols.

SURGICAL STAGING

Ovarian malignancies are surgically staged. Surgical staging is classified according to the International Federation of Gynecology and Obstetrics (FIGO) for primary malignancies of the ovary. A thorough physical examination must be performed. In the premenarcheal female, this may necessitate a twilight or general anesthesia. Before surgical intervention, a complete chemistry profile, including liver function tests and electrolytes, as well as a hemogram should be obtained. Cystoscopic, colonoscopic, and barium enema examinations are performed in those patients in whom blad-der or colon infiltration is suspected. If gross or occult blood is present in the patient's stool, a thorough evaluation of the colon should be performed, including a barium enema and/or colonoscopy. Radiologic evaluation with one of the imaging techniques previously described should be obtained before surgery.

Intravenous pyelography is performed to outline the course of the ureters, their displacement by the pelvic mass, and the presence of a pelvic kidney, abnormal collecting system, or hydronephrosis. Many gynecologic oncologists have replaced this study with a CAT scan using contrast. Although the CAT scan can identify abnormal collection systems, hydronephrosis, and pelvic kidneys, it does not enable the surgeon to follow the course of the ureter through the pelvis with ease.

Evaluation of neoplasms in childhood and adolescence should include CA-125, AFP, β-hCG, and CEA tumor marker levels.

SURGERY

The temptation to enter the abdomen through a transverse incision is to be avoided. A vertical incision that may be extended in a cephalad direction will enable a thorough evaluation and tumor debulking in the upper abdomen. On entering the peritoneal cavity, all ascitic fluid should be aspirated and sent to cytopathology for evaluation. If ascites is not present, abdominal washings from all quadrants should be obtained and sent for cytologic evaluation. A survey of the upper abdomen, including the diaphragm, liver, spleen, colon, pelvic and periaortic lymph nodes, kidneys, adrenals, and small bowel, should be performed to ascertain the spread of tumor. If a large pelvic mass is present, it should be resected and sent to pathology for frozen-section evaluation before examining the upper abdomen. This practice decreases the risk of rupturing the mass and establishes a timely diagnosis, guiding the further course of the surgery. For small lesions, after the abdomen is explored, the ovarian mass should be resected and sent to pathology for immediate frozen-section histologic evaluation. If the ovarian tumor is diagnosed as benign, a thorough evaluation should be made of the contralateral ovary before completing the surgical procedure. Suspicious areas in the peritoneal cavity should be biopsied and sent to pathology for histologic evaluation.

Surgical extirpation and staging of malignant ovarian neoplasms may be less aggressive in the female patient in childhood and adolescence compared to women who have completed childbearing. Early lesions that appear to be confined to a single ovary without excrescences are treated with unilateral adnexectomy. Patients with bulky disease should undergo resection of all visible tumor, infracolic omentectomy, pelvic and periaortic lymph node sampling, total abdominal hysterectomy, and bilateral salpingo-oophorectomy.

GERM CELL TUMORS

Germ cell tumors are the most common ovarian neoplasm in the childhood and adolescent patient. They account for 3% of neoplasms in children. The most common malignant germ cell tumor is endodermal sinus tumor (40). Germ cell tumors arise from a primitive germ cell that can develop into two different tumors: dysgerminomas and embryonal carcinomas. The latter is further classified into extraembryonic and embryonic tumors (Fig. 26.11). A combination of surgery and chemotherapy results in a high cure rate and preserves fertility. Ezzat et al. (41) retrospectively reviewed 67 charts of patients diagnosed with ovarian germ cell tumors. Sixteen children were conceived after therapy and had no congenital abnormalities. Mitchell et al. (42) reported advantages of platinum-based chemotherapy for treatment of nondysgerminomatous ovarian germ cell tumors.

Dysgerminoma

Dysgerminoma is the most common malignant germ cell neoplasm occurring in pure form (35,44). It accounts for approximately 1% to 2% of primary ovarian neoplasms and 2% to 5% of ovarian malignancies (45–48). Ninety percent of patients with dysgerminomas are found in patients younger than 30 years of age (49). Fortunately, the prognosis of these patients is excellent if they are identified promptly and appropriately treated.

Dysgerminomas are bilateral in 10% to 15% of patients. A wedge resection of the contralateral ovary should be performed. The exception to these recommendations are patients with advanced dysgerminomas, who can be treated conservatively to preserve fertility even in the presence of metastatic disease. Unilateral adnexectomy with chemotherapy has enabled conservative surgery and acceptable response rates (Figs. 26.12–26.13). Surgical success rates are in the range from 75% to 90% (50,51).

Macroscopic

Macroscopically, dysgerminoma is a solid tumor, rounded, lobulated, or oval, with a

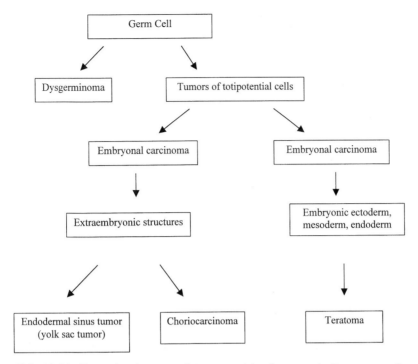

FIG. 26.11. Example of germ cell tumors arising from a primitive germ cell.

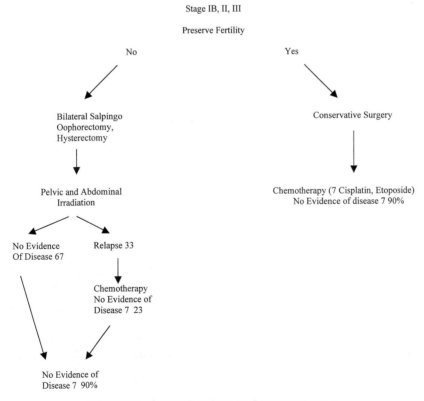

FIG. 26.12. Surgical options and response rates.

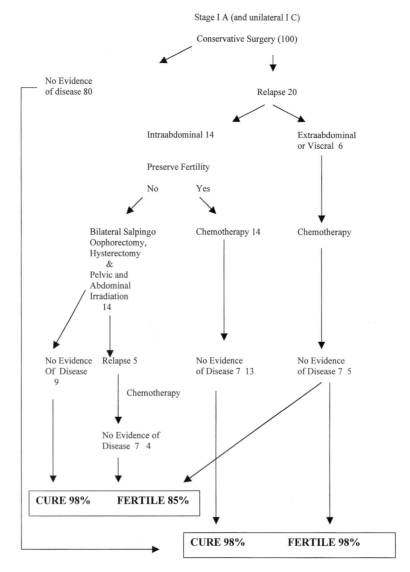

Stage I A (and unilateral I C)

Conservative Surgery (100)

No Evidence
of disease 80

Relapse 20

Intraabdominal 14

Extraabdominal
or Viscral 6

Preserve Fertility

No   Yes

Bilateral Salpingo
Oophorectomy,
Hysterectomy
&
Pelvic and
Abdominal
Irradiation
14

Chemotherapy 14   Chemotherapy

No Evidence   Relapse 5
Of Disease
9

No Evidence
of Disease 7 13

No Evidence
of Disease 7 5

Chemotherapy

No Evidence of
Disease 7 4

CURE 98%   FERTILE 85%

CURE 98%   FERTILE 98%

FIG. 26.13. Conservative surgery resulting in acceptable response rates.

smooth gray-white fibrous capsule (Fig.
26.14). Cystic areas may be present in mixed
germ cell tumors coexisting with immature
teratomas, choriocarcinoma, and endodermal
sinus tumors.

Microscopic

Microscopically, there are aggregates of
large uniform cells with varying amounts of
connective tissue, stroma, and lymphocytic

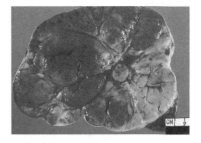

FIG. 26.14. Ovarian dysgerminoma showing a
solid, lobulated mass.

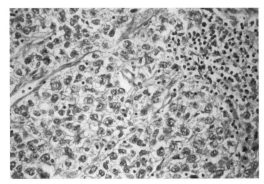

FIG. 26.15. Microscopic section of dysgerminoma showing large, hyperchromatic nuclei, distinct nucleoli, and partially clear cytoplasm. Note the lobular arrangement of cells and lymphocytic infiltrate in the **upper right corner**.

infiltrate (Fig. 26.15). The stromal infiltrate occasionally may form granulomas mimicking tubercles. Moderate pleomorphism and more than ten mitoses per high-power field may be present (52). These tumors have a propensity for lymphatic spread to the periaortic region (51,53,54).

Treatment

Until recently, the primary treatment protocol entailed surgical debulking followed by total abdominal radiation. This approach was based on the highly sensitive nature of the tumor to radiation therapy. The standard therapy advanced by Piver in 1979 for dysgerminomas treated the entire abdomen with 2,000 rad by a moving strip technique with a ^{50}Co unit or open fields using a 25-meV photon beam. A pelvic boost of 1,500 to 2,000 rad then is administered. In patients with periaortic involvement, an additional 1,000 to 1,500 rad was administered, followed by mediastinal and supraclavicular radiation over 3 weeks after a 4-week hiatus status post initial treatment. Until recently, chemotherapy was used when the bulk of the residual disease precluded radiotherapy.

In recent years, chemotherapy has been used as a primary treatment modality for patients with ovarian dysgerminomas (55,56). Dysgerminomas are thought to be equally sensitive to chemotherapy and radiation therapy. This has permitted the preservation of potential fertility and epiphyseal plate growth in premenarcheal patients. The chemotherapy regimens used to treat dysgerminomas and germ cell tumors are outlined in Table 26.4. Bleomycin, etoposide, and cisplatin (BEP) are administered most frequently as a result of the ability of chemotherapeutic agents to preserve future fertility.

TABLE 26.4. *Combination chemotherapy for germ cell tumors of the ovary*

Regimen drugs	Doses and schedule
VAC[a]	
Vincristine	1–1.5 mg/m^2 on day 1 every 4 weeks
Actinomycin D	0.5 mg/d × 5 d every 4 weeks
Cytoxan	150 mg/m^2/d × 5 d every 4 weeks
VBP[a]	
Vinblastine	20 mg/m^2 days 1 and 2 every 3 weeks
Bleomycin	15 U/m^2/week × 5; then on day 1 of course 4
Cisplatin	100 mg/m^2 on day 1 every 3 weeks
BEP[b]	
Bleomycin	10–15 mg on days 1, 2, and 3 every 4 weeks
Etoposide	100 mg/m^2 on days 1, 2, and 3 every 4 weeks
Cisplatin	100 mg/m^2 on day 1 every 4 weeks
EP[a]	
Etoposide	100 mg/m^2/d × 5 d every 3 weeks
Cisplatin	20 mg/m^2/d × 5 d, or 100 mg/m^2/d × 1 d every 3 weeks

[a]Data from Berek JS. Epithelial ovarian cancer. In: Berek JS, Hacker NF, eds. *Practical gynecologic oncology.* Baltimore: Williams & Wilkins, 1989;327–364, and Berek JS, Nonepithelial ovarian and tubal cancer. In: Berek VS, Hacker NF, eds. *Practical gynecologic oncology.* Baltimore: Williams & Wilkins, 1989:365–390.
[b]Data from Kurman RJ, Norns HJ. Endodermal sinus tumor of the ovary. *Cancer* 1976;38:2404.
All doses given intravenously.

It is imperative that patients receiving bleomycin have pulmonary function tests before each course of therapy. A decrease of 25% in diffusing lung capacity or forced expiratory volume (FEV_1) indicates the need for discontinuation of this treatment protocol. These drugs and their toxicity are identified in Table 26.4. The ideal number of chemotherapeutic courses has not been determined.

In patients with no residual disease, the recommendation is four to six courses. A second-look laparotomy is controversial because recurrent tumors can be rapidly growing and documented radiographically within 4 to 6 months. Because this tumor recurs in a short time period after completion of therapy, it is advisable to defer pregnancy for approximately 1 year after chemotherapy. Dysgerminoma has an overall 5-year survival rate of 85% (57).

Endodermal Sinus Tumor

Endodermal sinus tumors were first described by Teilum in 1946. He described the extraembryonal germ cell origin of a tumor that resembled the endodermal sinus of Duval in the yolk sac of the rat placenta and named it "endodermal sinus tumor." This tumor is the second most common germ cell tumor, including mixed forms (58,59). The median age of presentation is 19 years (range 7 to 37 years) (60). Although usually bilateral, 5% of these lesions coexist with a benign cystic teratoma. Only 10% of patients presenting with endodermal sinus tumors are asymptomatic. Ultrasonographic appearance is a large, predominantly cystic, complex abdominal mass (61). The majority of patients present with complaints of abdominal and/or pelvic pain (62). As noted in Fig. 26.10, endodermal sinus tumors produce AFPs. Occasionally, low levels of α_1-antitrypsin may be present. The levels of AFP correlate with the amount of disease and can be used as a tumor marker to track treatment response. Jenderny (63) evaluated seven gonadal yolk sac tumors with chromosome-specific genetic probes. All tumors had an increased number of chromosomal aberrations. Six of seven had gains of chromosome 12. Four of five tumors had a deletion at 1(p36.3). The authors believe that this gene is involved in the pathogenesis of these tumors. These results were confirmed by Stock et al. (64).

Macroscopic

The tumor usually is large, measuring more than 10 cm, and is an encapsulated globular firm mass. The cystic appearance may be secondary to tumor necrosis and/or hemorrhage (Fig. 26.16).

Microscopic

Microscopically, a variety of histologic patterns coexist, including microcystic, endodermal sinus, solid, alveolar-glandular, polyvesicle vitelline, myxomatous, papillary, macrocystic, hepatoid, and intestinal (65). The microcystic pattern is the most frequently encountered. Schiller-Duval bodies are spaces lined by a single layer of fine endothelium protruding as a glomerulus-like tuft with blood vessels in the center (Fig. 26.17). The Schiller-Duval body is present in 68% of the tumors (60). Other components include hyaline bodies and a myxoid stroma. The hyaline bodies strongly stain for AFP.

Treatment

Optimal treatment consists of surgery followed by an aggressive combination of chemotherapy agents. These tumors are aggressive

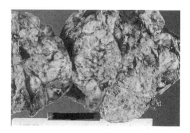

FIG. 26.16. Endodermal sinus tumor showing fleshy, necrotic, and hemorrhagic cut surface.

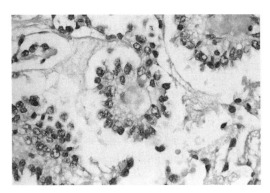

FIG. 26.17. Microscopic section of an endodermal sinus tumor showing pathognomonic Schiller-Duval bodies with a glomeruloid appearance.

and highly malignant, with 33% occurring in the premenarcheal female. The spread of endodermal sinus tumors is primarily intraabdominal and rapid, necessitating immediate surgery and chemotherapy. Vincristine, actinomycin D, and cyclophosphamide (Cytoxan) (VAC), vinblastine, bleomycin, and cisplatin (VBP), and BEP have all been used successfully to treat this lesion (Table 26.4) (66–69). We conclude the best treatment today for an endodermal sinus tumor is a cisplatin base combination. BEP is the recommended first-line therapy because it does not have the neurotoxicity present with vincristine. If a marker is not present, the patient should be treated for four courses. However, if a marker is present, at least one or two courses of therapy should be administered after the marker falls within normal range. The value of a second-look laparotomy has not been established.

Embryonal Carcinoma

The median age of patients presenting with embryonal carcinoma is 14 years (58). These lesions are large, unilateral masses measuring more than 10 to 15 cm (16,17). Embryonal carcinomas can differentiate into embryonic tumors, teratomas, polyembryomas, endodermal sinus tumors, and choriocarcinomas. As a result of the totipotential nature of these tumors, they can present with elevated levels of hCG and AFP (58).

Macroscopic

Macroscopic presentation is usually a large solid tumor with occasional cystic areas secondary to hemorrhage and necrosis.

Microscopic

Microscopically, the tumor consists of pleomorphic epithelial-like cells with markedly hyperchromatic nuclei and eosinophilic cytoplasm. Giant cells or multinucleated cells may be present and can resemble syncytiotrophoblasts.

Treatment

These are aggressive tumors and should receive prompt treatment. Surgical exploration, tumor debulking, and unilateral adnexectomy should be performed before administering chemotherapy. As with all germ cell tumors, it appears that the cisplatin regimen may be superior (70).

Polyembryoma

Polyembryoma is an extremely rare tumor that tends to occur predominantly in premenarcheal patients.

Macroscopic

Macroscopically, this tumor usually is solid with necrotic and hemorrhagic areas.

Microscopic

Microscopically, the tumor is composed of numerous embryoid bodies. The tumor can exhibit signs of early embryonic differentiation including formation of an amniotic cavity, embryonic disc, atypical yolk sac, and extraembryonic mesenchyme (65). Immunoperoxidase stains for hCG are positive in tumor cells.

Treatment

This is a highly aggressive tumor and should be treated with one of the regimens outlined in Table 26.4.

Choriocarcinoma

Nongestational choriocarcinoma is extremely rare. The majority of patients presenting with pure nongestational choriocarcinoma of the ovary usually are less than 20 years of age, with 50% exhibiting signs of isosexual precocity (29).

Macroscopic

Macroscopically, an enlarged adnexal mass, usually unilateral, showing extensive hemorrhage and usually associated with a positive pregnancy test.

Microscopic

Microscopically, diffuse proliferation of trophoblastic cells with extensive hemorrhage and necrosis are seen. Other germ cell tumors are generally a part of it. No chorionic villi are seen to distinguish it from ovarian or tubal pregnancy. Immunohistologic stains for hCG are positive in tumor cells.

Treatment

Patients can be treated with BEP or VBP as outlined in Table 26.4. Alternative therapy would include methotrexate, actinomycin D, and cyclophosphamide triple-therapy protocols used to treat gestational trophoblastic neoplasia. Before instituting chemotherapy, tumor debulking should be performed radically depending on the patient's desire for future fertility. As with gestational trophoblastic disease, β-hCG titers can be followed to determine the effectiveness and response to therapy. The outlook of nongestational choriocarcinoma is far worse than for its gestational counterpart.

Immature Teratomas

Immature teratomas usually present in the first three decades of life, with occurrence at a median age of 21 years (71). These lesions are unilateral, although they may coexist with

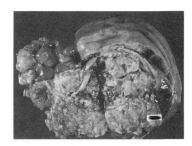

FIG. 26.18. Immature teratoma showing partly solid, partly cystic appearance with hemorrhage and necrosis.

benign cystic teratomas in the contralateral ovary. Immature teratomas are rare and account for 30% of the deaths due to ovarian cancer in the first two decades of life (29). A combined surgical, chemotherapeutic, and radiation approach has greatly improved the prognostic aspect of this tumor. The diagnosis and presentation of these tumors is similar to that of a benign cystic teratoma (Fig. 26.18). A soft tissue mass may be present on physical examination, or an abdominal x-ray will reveal calcification. These tumors rarely produce steroids, and tumor markers are negative unless a mixed germ cell tumor is present.

Microscopic

Microscopically, the tumor is diagnosed by the presence of neuroepithelial rosettes and graded by their quantitative number in the sections (Fig. 26.19).

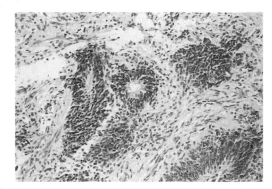

FIG. 26.19. Microscopic section of an immature teratoma showing neuroepithelial rosettes indicating immature brain tissue.

Treatment

Surgical therapy remains the mainstay of treatment for these lesions. In the young patient desiring future fertility, a unilateral salpingo-oophorectomy should be performed if no evidence of metastatic disease is present. For those who have completed childbearing, a total abdominal hysterectomy and a bilateral salpingo-oophorectomy is required. Tumors that do not appear to be confined to the ovary should undergo staging as previously described. VAC, VBP, BEP, and etoposide and cisplatin (EP) are effective chemotherapeutic regimens for treating this lesion. Patients with Stage 1A Grade 1 (1Ag1) lesions do not require chemotherapy. The remaining patients should receive at least four to six courses of the noted therapy. Second-look laparotomy is strongly suggested, especially for those patients who have advanced stage tumors. Patients receiving adjuvant therapy, i.e., stage IA, grades 2 and 3, do not require second-look laparotomy.

SEX CORD STROMAL TUMORS IN CHILDHOOD AND ADOLESCENCE

Sex cord stromal tumors account for 5% to 8% of ovarian malignancies (16,17). Fewer than 10% of all ovarian tumors are of stromal origin; these include tumors containing granulosa, theca, Sertoli, Leydig, and collagen-producing stromal cells or their embryonic precursors. This section concentrates on two malignant tumors: juvenile granulosa cell tumors and Sertoli-Leydig cell tumors. Granulosa cell tumors of childhood constitute less than 7% of all ovarian tumors in the first two decades of life. The majority are of the juvenile type (72–76). Approximately 80% of these patients present with isosexual precocity secondary to hyperestrogenic state produced by the tumor (74). A clinical presentation of precocious puberty and an abdominal mass should arouse the suspicion of granulosa cell tumor. Inhibin levels may be elevated in patients with juvenile granulosa cell tumors (77,78). Although inhibins A and B are uniformly present in granulosa cell tumors, they

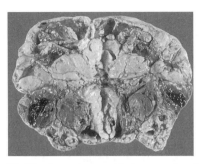

FIG. 26.20. Granulosa cell tumor showing a characteristic yellow, lobulated cut surface with areas of hemorrhage.

also can be present in other germ cell tumors (79,80).

Macroscopic

These tumors can vary in size, although the majority are large and can measure more than 10 cm. The tumors are distinctly yellow, with large areas of hemorrhage and variable number of cysts (Fig. 26.20). These tumors frequently rupture and result in bloody ascites.

Microscopic

Microscopically, the cells have large luteinized cytoplasm occurring in a macrofollicular pattern. Call-Exner bodies are sporadically present in adult granulosa tumors but only rarely in juvenile tumors (Fig. 26.21).

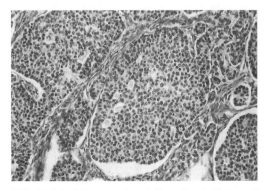

FIG. 26.21. Microscopic section of granulosa cell tumor showing characteristic Call-Exner bodies.

These tumors are considered to be of low-grade malignancy. If the lesion is unilateral without any evidence of spread beyond the capsule, a unilateral salpingo-oophorectomy is appropriate therapy. With extensive or residual disease, combination chemotherapy should be incorporated in the treatment protocol. Zambetti (81) reported a 66% response rate in the treatment of granulosa cell tumors with BEP. The adult granulosa cell tumors have been treated with VAC and with cisplatin, doxorubicin (Adriamycin), and cyclophosphamide (PAC) (16,17). Because the tumor is characterized by recurrence several years after resection, patients should be appropriately followed. Because of its estrogenic activity, the tumor can be associated with endometrial polyp, hyperplasia, or carcinoma.

SERTOLI-LEYDIG CELL TUMORS

Sertoli-Leydig cell tumors account for less than 0.2% of all ovarian neoplasms. They are derived from sex cord and stroma of the embryonic gonad that differentiates in the male direction (29). A typical Sertoli-Leydig cell produces androgens and thereby causes virilization of the female patient (82). Sertoli-Leydig cell tumors usually are of low-grade malignant potential, although well-differentiated tumors can behave innocuously.

Clinical presentation includes signs of virilization, such as acne, hirsutism, clitoromegaly, male pattern baldness, breast atrophy, and voice changes. Serum testosterone and androstenedione usually are elevated, with dehydroepiandrosterone sulfate (DHEAS) being normal or elevated (29).

Macroscopic

Macroscopically, these lesions usually are large and complex in nature, containing both cystic and solid components (Fig. 26.22). Tumors can be 10 to 20 cm and weigh up to 25 lb (16,17).

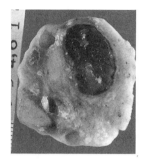

FIG. 26.22. Sertoli-Leydig cell tumor showing solid, yellow and white cut surface with hemorrhage. Normal ovarian tissue can be seen on **left** side.

Microscopic

Microscopically, Sertoli-Leydig cell tumors include the Sertoli tumor with tubules lined with columnar cells and the Leydig cell with their lipid content and Reinke crystals (16,17, 83) (Figs. 26.23–26.24).

Treatment

In light of the benign nature of this lesion and the predominance of low-grade lesions, a unilateral salpingo-oophorectomy with evaluation of the contralateral ovary and of the peritoneal cavity is sufficient treatment. For those patients who have completed childbearing, a total abdominal hysterectomy and bilateral salpingo-oophorectomy should be performed. Radiation and chemotherapy have been used in patients with persistent disease

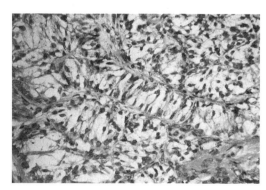

FIG. 26.23. Sertoli cells characterized by tall columnar cells with clear cytoplasm.

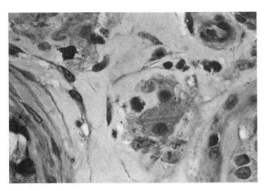

FIG. 26.24. Leydig cells showing crystalloids of Reinke.

(81,84). Gershenson et al. (85) treated poorly differentiated Sertoli-Leydig cell tumors and metastatic sex cord stromal tumors with BEP and had an 83% overall response rate.

EPITHELIAL TUMORS OF THE OVARY

The incidence of epithelial ovarian tumors in young women varies from 4% to 13% (86). Tumors presenting in the first three decades of life are usually of low malignant potential (30). In light of the relative infrequency of these lesions in patients in the first two decades of life, we will not provide further discussion.

SUMMARY

An ovarian tumor can be a catastrophic event to the patient and her family. During the past few decades, treatment has evolved into a conservative approach, with increased emphasis on preserving fertility and contralateral ovarian function. A multitude of chemotherapeutic regimens have been reviewed in this chapter and have proven to be efficacious.

Dysgerminomas, which have been traditionally treated with radiation, now are treated with chemotherapeutic agents, enabling us to decrease early and later radiation toxicity as well as preserve ovarian function and fertility. As research in this area advances and new drugs are identified, the ability to provide therapeutic protocols that result in complete responses and 5-year survival rates above 90% will be enhanced.

REFERENCES

1. Acosta A, Kaplan AL, Kaufman RH. Gynecologic cancer in children. *Am J Obstet Gynecol* 1972;20: 607–625.
2. Tintera H, Mitarnum W. Ovarian neoplasms in childhood and adolescents in Songklanagarind hospital, February 1983–March 1989. *J Med Assoc Thai* 1990; 73:375–380.
3. Breen JL, Mayson WS. Ovarian tumors in children and adolescents. *Clin Obstet Gynecol* 1977;20:607–625.
4. Barloon TJ, Brown BP, Abu-yousef MM, et al. Paraovarian and paratubal cysts: preoperative diagnosis using transabdominal and transvaginal sonography. *J Clin Ultrasound* 1996;24:117–122.
5. Haldan (1915).
6. Droegemueller W. Benign gynecologic lesions. In: Droegemueller W, Herbst AL, Mishell DR Jr, et al, eds. *Comprehensive gynecology.* St. Louis: CV Mosby, 1987:440–492.
7. Hallatt JG, Steele CH, Snyder M. Ruptured corpus luteum with hemoperitoneum: a study of 173 surgical cases. *Am J Obstet Gynecol* 1984;149:6.
8. Spanos WJ. Preoperative hormonal therapy and cystic adnexal masses. *Am J Obstet Gynecol* 1973,116:551.
9. Grimes DA, Hughes JM. Use of multiphasic oral contraceptive and hospitalizations of women with functional ovarian cysts in the United States. *Obstet Gynecol* 1989;73:1037–1039.
10. Hansen KA, Tho SP, Hanley M, et al. Massive ovarian enlargement in primary hypothyroidism. *Fertil Steril* 1997;67:169–171.
11. Matsuura K, Ohtake H, Katabuchi H, et al. Coelomic metaplasia theory of endometriosis: evidence from in vivo studies and an in vitro experimental model. *Gynecol Obstet Invest* 1999;47:18–20.
12. Johansson J, Santala M, Kauppila A. Explosive rise of serum CA125 following the rupture of ovarian endometrioma. *Human Reprod* 1998;13:3503–3504.
13. Surti U, Hoffner L, Chakravariti A, et al. Genetics and biology of human ovarian teratoma. I: Cytogenetic analysis and mechanism of origin. *Am J Hum Genet* 1990; 47:635–643.
14. Gargano G, De Lconardis A, Perrotti P, et al. Ovarian bilateral cystic teratomas: Diagnosis and therapy in a young woman. *Clin Exp Obstet Gynecol* 1990;17(1) 37–42.
15. Woodruff JD, Protos P, Pterson WF. Ovarian teratomas: relationship of histologic and oncogenic factors to prognosis. *Am J Obstet Gynecol* 1968;102:702.
16. Berek JS. Epithelial ovarian cancer. In: Berek JS, Hacker NF, eds. *Practical gynecologic oncology.* Baltimore: Williams & Wilkins, 1989:327–364.
17. Berek JS. Nonepithelial ovarian and tubal cancer. In: Berek JS, Hacker NF, eds. *Practical gynecologic oncology.* Baltimore: Williams & Wilkins, 1989:365–390.
18. Yamashita Y, Hatanaka Y, Torashima M, et al. Mature cystic teratomas of the ovary without fat in the cystic cavity: MR features in 12 cases. *Am J Roentgenol* 1994;163:613–616.

19. Engel T, Greeley DU, Swenney WJ III. Recurrent dermoid cysts of the ovary: report of 2 cases. *Obstet Gynecol* 1965;26:757.

20. Scully RE. Sex cord tumor with annular tubules: a distinctive ovarian tumor of Peutz-Jeghers syndrome. *Cancer* 1970;25:1107.

21. Scully RE. Gonadoblastoma. *Cancer* 1970;25:1340.

22. Scully RE. Recent progress in ovarian cancer. *Hum Pathol* 1970;1:73.

23. Scully RE. Germ cell tumors of the ovary. In: Sturgis SH, Taymore ML, eds. *Progress in gynecology, vol. 5.* New York: Grune & Stratton, 1970:329–348.

24. Grosfeld (1970).

25. Smith FG. Pathology and physiology of stroma ovarii. *Arch Surg* 1946;53:603.

26. Sailers S. Stroma ovarii. *Am J Clin Pathol* 1943;13:271.

27. Oates JA. The carcinoid syndrome. In: Thorn GW, Adams RD, Braunwaid E, et al, eds. *Harrison's principles of internal medicine,* 8th ed. New York: McGraw-Hill, 1977:634–642.

28. Bosch-Banyeras JM, Lucaya X, Bernet M, et al. Calcified ovarian fibroma in prepubertal girls. *Eur J Pediatr* 1989;48:749–750.

29. Scully RE. Tumors of the ovary and maldeveloped gonads. In: *Atlas of tumor pathology. Fascicle 16.* Washington, DC: Armed Forces Institute of Pathology, 1979.

30. Towne BH, Mahour GH, Woolley MM, et al. Ovarian cysts and tumors in infancy and childhood. *J Pediatr Surg* 1975;10:311–320.

31. Charache H. Ovarian tumors in childhood: report of six new cases and a review of the literature. *AMA Arch Surg* 1959;79:573–580.

32. Samanth KK, Black W. Benign ovarian stromal tumors associated with free peritoneal fluid. *Am J Obstet Gynecol* 1970;197;538.

33. Scully (1953).

34. Huffman JW. Ovarian tumors in children and adolescents. In: Huffman JW, Dewhurst CJ, Capraro VJ, eds. *The gynecology of childhood and adolescence.* Philadelphia: WB Saunders, 1981:277–349.

35. Berek JS, Hacker NF, Lagasse LD. Ovarian and fallopian tube cancer. In: Haskell CM, ed. *Cancer treatment,* 2nd ed. Philadelphia: WB Saunders, 1983:409–429.

36. Griffiths CT, Parker L. Cancer of the ovary. In: Knapp RC, Berkowitz RS, eds. *Gynecologic oncology.* New York: MacMillan, 1986:364.

37. Bost RC Jr, Feeney M, Lazarus H, et al. Reactivity of a monoclonal antibody with human ovarian carcinoma. *J Clin Invest* 1981;68:1331.

38. Davis HM, Zurawiski VRJ, Bost RC Jr, et al. Characterization of the CA-125 antigen associated with human epithelial ovarian carcinomas. *Cancer Res* 1986;46:6143.

39. Casper S, Van Nagell S Jr, Powell DF, et al. Immunohistochemical localization of tumor markers in epithelial ovarian cancer. *Am J Obstet Gynecol* 1984;149:154.

40. Davidoff AM, Hebra A, Bunin N, et al. Endodermal sinus tumor in children. *J Pediatr Surg* 1996;31:1075–1078.

41. Ezzat A, Raja M, Bakri Y, et al. Malignant ovarian germ cell tumours—a survival and prognostic analysis. *Acta Oncol* 1999;38:455–460.

42. Mitchell PL, Al-Nasiri N, A'Hern R, et al. Treatment of nondysgerminomatous ovarian germ cell tumors: an analysis of 69 cases. *Cancer* 1999;85:2232–2244.

43. American College of Obstetricians and Gynecologists. *Technical Bulletin* 1991;155:3.

44. DePaolo G, Lattuada A, Kenda R, et al. Germ cell tumors of the ovary: the experience of the National Cancer Institute of Milan. I: Dysgerminoma. *Int J Radiat Oncol Biol Phys* 1987;13:853–860.

45. Boyes DA, Pankratz E, Gailiford BW, et al. Experience with dysgerminomas at Cancer Control Agency of British Columbia. *Gynecol Oncol* 1978;6:123–129.

46. Kreport O, Smith JP, Rutledge F, et al. The treatment for dysgerminoma of the ovary. *Cancer* 1978;41:986–990.

47. Mueller CW, Topkins P, Lapp WA. Dysgerminoma of the ovary: an analysis of 427 cases. *Am J Obstet Gynecol* 1950;60:153.

48. Santesson L. Clinical and pathological survey of ovarian tumors treated at the Radium Hemmet S. Dysgerminoma. *Acta Radiol (Stockh)* 1947;28:643.

49. Mitchell MF, Gershenson DM, Soeters RP, et al. The long term effects of radiation in therapy on patients with ovarian dysgerminoma. *Cancer* 1991;67:1084–1090.

50. Gordon A, Lipton D, Woodruff JD. Dysgerminoma: a review of 58 cases from the Emil Novak Ovarian Tumor Registry. *Obstet Gynecol* 1981;58:497–504.

51. Asadourian A, Taylor HB. Dysgerminoma: an analysis of 105 cases. *Obstet Gynecol* 1969;33:370–379.

52. Bjorkholm E, Lundell M, Gyftodimos A, et al. Dysgerminoma. the Radiumhemmet series 1927–1984. *Cancer* 1990;65:38–44.

53. Santoni P, Cionini L, D'Elia F, et al. Dysgerminomas of the ovary: a report on 29 patients. *Clin Radiol* 1987;38:203–206.

54. DePaolo G, Pilotti S, Kenda R, et al. Natural history of dysgerminoma. *Am J Obstet Gynecol* 1982;143:799–807.

55. Aalders VR, Sicifer JG. Treatment of malignant germ cell tumors of the ovary with cisplatin, vinblastine and bleomycin (PVB). *Can Treat Rep* 1984;68:719.

56. Gershenson DM, Wharton JT, Kline RC, et al. Chemotherapeutic complete remission in patients with metastatic ovarian dysgerminoma. *Cancer* 1986;58:2594.

57. Thomas GM, Dembo AJ, Hacker NF, et al. Current therapy for dysgerminoma of the ovary. *Obstet Gynecol* 1987;70:268–275.

58. Kurman RJ, Norris HJ. Endodermal sinus tumor of the ovary. *Cancer* 1976;38:2404.

59. Kurman RJ, Norris HJ. Malignant mixed germ cell tumors of the ovary. *Hum Pathol* 1977;8:551.

60. Gershenson DM, del Junco G, Herson J, et al. Endodermal sinus tumor of the ovary: the MD Anderson experience. *Obstet Gynecol* 1983;61:194–202.

61. Levitin A, Haller KD, Cohen HL, et al. Endodermal sinus tumor of the ovary: imaging evaluation. *Am J Roentgenol* 1996;167:791–793.

62. Cangir A, Smith J, VanEys J. Improved prognosis in children with ovarian cancers following modified VAC (vincristine sulfate, dactinomycin, and cyclophosphamide) chemotherapy. *Cancer* 1978;42:1234.

63. Jenderny J, Koster E, Meyer A, et al. Detection of chromosome aberrations in paraffin sections of seven gonadal yolk sac tumors of childhood. *Hum Genet* 1995;96:644–650.

64. Stock C, Ambros IM, Lion T, et al. Detection of numerical and structural chromosome abnormalities in pediatric germ cell tumors by means of interphase cytogenetics. *Genes Chromosome Cancer* 1994;11:40–50.

65. Talerman A. Germ cell tumors of the ovary. In: Kurman RJ, ed. *Blaustein's pathology of the female genital tract.* New York: Springer-Verlag, 1987:659–721.

66. Gershenson DM, Morris M, Cangir A, et al. Treatment of malignant germ cell tumors of the ovary with bleomycin, etoposide and cisplatin. *J Clin Oncol* 1990;8: 715–720.

67. Hicks MC, Maxwell SL, Krim W. Management of advanced endodermal sinus tumor of the ovary with preservation of reproductive function. *Henry Ford Hosp Med J* 1990;38:76–78.

68. Curtin JP, Rubin SC, Hoskins WJ, et al. Second-look laparotomy in endodermal sinus tumor: a report of two patients with normal levels of AFP and residual tumor at re-exploration. *Obstet Gynecol* 1989;73:893–895.

69. Athaniker N, Saikia TK, Kamkrishnan G, et al. Aggressive chemotherapy in endodermal sinus tumor. *J Surg Oncol* 1989;40:17–20.

70. Gershenson DM, Wharton JT. Malignant germ cell tumors of the ovary. In: Albert DS, Surwit EA, eds. *Ovarian cancer.* Boston: Martinus Nijhoff, 1985: 227–269.

71. Kouios JP, Hoffman JF, Steinhoff MM. Immature teratoma of the ovary. *Gynecol Oncol* 1989;34:46–49.

72. Roofat F, Ulys H, Rylance G. Juvenile granulosa cell tumor. *Pediatr Pathol* 1990;10:617–623.

73. Fox H. Sex-cord stromal tumors of the ovary. *J Pathol* 1985;145:127–148.

74. Young RH, Dickerson GR, Scully RE. Juvenile granulosa cell tumor of the ovary: a clinico-pathological analysis of 125 cases. *Am J Surg Pathol* 1984;8: 575–596.

75. Young RH, Scully RE. Ovarian sex-cord stromal tumors: recent progress. *Int J Gynecol Pathol* 1982; 101–123.

76. Lack EE, Perez AR, Murthy AS, et al. Granulosa theca cell tumors in premenarchal girls: a clinical and pathological study of ten cases. *Cancer* 1981;48:1846–1854.

77. Nishida M, Jimi S, Haji M, et al. Juvenile granulosa cell tumor in association with a high serum inhibin level. *Gynecol Oncol* 1991;40:90–94.

78. Lappohn RE, Burger HG, Bouma J, et al. Inhibin as a marker for granulosa cell tumors. *N Engl J Med* 1989; 321:790–793.

79. Yamashita K, Yamoto M, Shikone T, et al. Production of inhibin A and inhibin B in human ovarian sex cord stromal tumors. *Am J Obstet Gynecol* 1997;177:1450–1457.

80. Costa MJ, Ames PF, Walls J, et al. Inhibin immunohistochemistry applied to ovarian neoplasms: a novel, effective, diagnostic tool. *Human Pathol* 1997;28: 1247–1254.

81. Zambetti M, Esrobedo A, Pilotti S, et al. Cisplatinum/vinblastine/bleomycin combination chemotherapy in advanced or recurrent granulosa cell tumors of the ovary. *Gynecol Oncol* 1990;36:317–320.

82. Slayton RE. Management of germ cell and stromal tumors of the ovary. *Semin Oncol* 1984;11:299.

83. Woodruff JD. Pathology. In: Berek JS, Hacker NF, eds. *Practical gynecologic oncology.* Baltimore: Williams & Wilkins, 1989:109–166.

84. Slayton RE, Hreshchyshyn MM, Silverberg SC, et al. Treatment of malignant ovarian germ cell tumors: response to vincristine, dactinomycin and cyclophosphamide. *Cancer* 1978;42:390.

85. Gershenson DM, Morris M, Burke TW, et al. Treatment of poor-prognosis sex cord-stromal tumors of the ovary with the combination of bleomycin, etoposide, and cisplatin. *Obstet Gynecol* 1996;87527–531.

86. Smith JP, Day TG. Review of ovarian cancer at the University of Texas Systems Cancer Center, MD Anderson Hospital and Tumor Institute. *Am J Obstet Gynecol* 1979;135:984–993.

SUGGESTED READINGS

87. Norris HJ, Jensen RD. Relative frequency of ovarian neoplasms in children and adolescents. *Cancer* 1972; 30:713.

88. Junaid TA. Ovarian neoplasms in children and adolescents in Ibadan, Nigeria. *Cancer* 1981;47:610–614.

89. Abell MR, Johnson VJ, Holtz F. Ovarian neoplasms in childhood and adolescence. I: Tumors of germ cell origin. *Am J Obstet Gynecol* 1965;92:1059.

90. Abell MR. Ovarian neoplasms in childhood and adolescence. *J Arkansas Med Soc* 1967;63:279.

91. Barber HR, Graber EA. Gynecological tumors in childhood and adolescence. *Obstet Gynecol Surv* 1973;28: 357.

92. Blackwell WJ, Dockerty MB, Masson JC, et al. Dermoid cysts of the ovary: clinical and pathological significance. *Am J Obstet Gynecol* 1946;51:151.

93. Bonazzi C, Columbo N, Lissoni A, et al. Alpha-fetal protein in the management of germ cell tumors of the ovary. *J Nucl Med Allied Sci* 1989;33[Suppl 1]: 53–58.

94. Breen JL, Neubecker RD. Malignant teratoma of the ovary: an analysis of 17 cases. *Obstet Gynecol* 1963; 21:669.

95. Breen JL, Mayson WS, Gregoli CA. Ovarian malignancies in children. In: Sciarra JJ, Bushsloaum HJ, eds. *Obstetrics and gynecology, vol. 4.* Philadelphia: Harper & Row, 1980:1–12.

96. Brody S. Clinical aspects of dysgerminomas of the ovary. *Acta Radiol (Stockh)* 1961;56:209.

97. Carter J, Stkinson K, Coppleson M. A comparative study of proliferating (borderline) and invasive epithelial ovarian tumors in your women. *Aust N Z J Obstet Gynaecol* 1989;29:245.

98. Cheung TH, Wong WSF, Shio W, et al. A new combination chemotherapy for the treatment of endodermal sinus tumor. *Aust N Z Obstet Gynecol* 1989;3:346.

99. Christman JE, Ballon SC. Ovarian fibrosarcoma associated with Maffucci's syndrome. *Gynecol Oncol* 1990; 37:290–291.

100. Creasman WT, Fetter BF, Hammond CB, et al. Germ cell malignancies of the ovary. *Obstet Gynecol* 1979; 53:226.

101. Forney JP. Pregnancy following removal and chemotherapy of ovarian endodermal sinus tumor. *Obstet Gynecol* 1978;52:360–364.

102. Gershenson DM, del Junco G, Copeland LJ, et al. Mixed germ cell tumors of the ovary. *Obstet Gynecol* 1984;64:200.

103. Lucraft HH. A review of thirty-three cases of ovarian dysgerminoma emphasizing the role of radiotherapy. *Clin Radiol* 1979;30:585–9.

104. Herbst AL. Neoplastic diseases of the ovary. In: Droegemueller W, Herbst AL, Mischell DR Jr, et al, eds. *Comprehensive gynecology.* St. Louis: CV Mosby, 1987:833–887.

105. Herson J, Rutledge FN. Endodermal sinus tumor of the ovary: The MD Anderson experience. *Obstet Gynecol* 1983;61:194–202.

106. James P, Lapolla MN, Fiorica JV, et al. Successful therapy of metastatic embryonal carcinoma coexisting with gonadoblastoma in a patient with 46, XY pure gonadal dysgenesis (Swyers syndrome). *Gynecol Oncol* 1990; 37:417–421.

107. Javaheri G, Lifsche ZA, Valle J. Pregnancy following removal of and long-term chemotherapy for ovarian malignant teratoma. *Obstet Gynecol* 1983;61:85–95.

108. Jimerson GK, Woodruff JD. Ovarian extraembryonal teratoma. *Am J Obstet Gynecol* 1977;127:73–79.

109. Jolles CJ, Karayianis S, Smotkin D, et al. Advanced ovarian dysgerminoma with cure of tumor persistent in meninges. *Gynecol Oncol* 1989;33:389–391.

110. Kawai M, Kano T, Furuhashi Y, et al. Prognostic factors in yolk sac tumors of the ovary: a clinicopathologic analysis of 29 cases. *Cancer* 1991;67:184–191.

111. Muram D, Gale CL, Thompson E. Functional ovarian cysts in patients cured of ovarian neoplasms. *Obstet Gynecol* 1990;75:680.

112. Norris HJ, Zirkin HG, Berson WL. Immature (malignant) teratoma of the ovary. *Cancer* 1976;37:2359–2372.

113. Peterson WF, Prevost EC, Edmunds FT, et al. Benign cystic teratomas of the ovary: a clinico-statistical study of 1007 cases with a review of the literature. *Am J Obstet Gynecol* 1955;70:368.

114. Piver MS, Lorain JL. Childhood ovarian cancers: new advances and treatment. *N Y State J Med* 1979;79: 1196.

115. Savage MO, Lowe DG. Gonadal neoplasia and abnormal sexual differentiation. *Clin Endocrinol* 1990;32: 519–533.

116. Schellhas HF, Trujillo JM, Rutledge FN, et al. Germ cell tumors associated with XY gonadal dysgenesis. *Am J Obstet Gynecol* 1971; 109:1197.

117. Scully RE. Gonadoblastoma: a gonadal tumor related to dysgerminoma (seminoma) and capable of sex hormone production. *Cancer* 1983;6:455.

118. Scully RE. World Health Organization classification and nomenclature of ovarian cancer. *Natl Cancer Inst Monogr* 1975;42:5–7.

119. Scully RE. Ovarian tumors. *Am J Pathol* 1977;87: 686–720.

120. Serov SF, Scully RE, Robin LH. Histological typing of ovarian tumors. *International Histological Classification of Tumors 1973, Monograph 9.* Geneva: World Health Organization, 1973.

121. Slayton RE, Park RC, Silverberg SG, et al. Vincristine, dactinomycin, and cyclophosphamide in the treatment of malignant germ cell tumors of the ovary. *Cancer* 1985;56:243–248.

122. Susnerwala SS, Pande SC, Shrivastava SK, et al. Dysgerminoma of the ovary: review of 27 cases. *Surg Oncol* 1991;46:43–47.

123. Swanson SA, Norris HJ, Kelsten ML, et al. DNA content of juvenile granulosa tumors determined by flow cytometry. *Int J Gynecol Pathol* 1990;9:101–1019.

124. Ueda G, Abe Y, Yoshioa M, et al. Embryonal carcinoma of the ovary: a six year survey. *Int J Gynecol Obstet* 1990;31:287–292.

125. Williams SD, Blessing JA, Moore DH, et al. Cisplatin, vinblastine, and bleomycin in advanced and recurrent ovarian germ cell tumors: a trial of the Gynecologic Oncology Group. *Ann Intern Med* 1989; 111:22–27.

126. Young RH, Scully RE. Ovarian Sertoli-Leydig cell tumors: a clinical pathological analysis of 207 cases. *Am J Surg Pathol* 1985;9:543–569.

127. Young RC, Faks Z, Huskins WJ. Cancer of the ovary. In: DeVita VT Jr, Hellman S, Rosenberg SA, eds. *Cancer: principles and practice of oncology,* 3rd ed. Philadelphia: JB Lippincott, 1989;1162–1196.

128. Zalouche KC, Norris JH. Granulosa tumors of the ovary in children: a clinical and pathologic study of 32 cases. *Am J Surg Pathol* 1982;6:503–512.

27

Breast Diseases: Benign and Malignant

Eric A. Wiebke, John E. Niederhuber, and Gary A. Glasser

Pediatric breast disorders represent a varied set of abnormalities best grouped into distinct categories for an ordered method of evaluation and a rational approach to treatment. For example, pediatric disorders of the breast may involve the breast gland or the nipple-areolar complex; and disorders of the gland can be congenital, acquired, developmental, neoplastic, or infectious. A nipple discharge is a frequent problem in the pedi-

atric age group, and such discharges can be endocrine or nonendocrine.

A summary of this algorithm and the various groups to be discussed is presented in Table 27.1. As might be expected, a proportionally large number of breast disorders are classified as congenital or developmental. Therefore, a brief discussion of breast embryology and normal development is presented to serve as an introduction to the congenital and

TABLE 27.1. *Pediatric and adolescent breast disorders*

Congenital	Nipple discharge
Polythelia	Galactorrhea
Polymastia	Neonatal "witch's milk"
Supernumerary breast	Adolescents and children
Amastia	Neurogenic
Nipple inversion	Hypothalamic
Acquired	Pituitary
Amastia	Hormonal/endocrine
Iatrogenic injury	Drug-induced
Irradiation, trauma	Idiopathic
Primary hypoplasia	Nonmilky discharge
Burns and skin contractures	Purulent
Developmental	Serous
Neonatal hypertrophy	Bloody
Premature thelarche	Masses
Precocious puberty	Infections
Idiopathic	Mastitis
Central	Abscess
Peripheral	Cyctic disease
Asymmetry (macromastia)	Simple
Tuberous breast abnormality	Juvenile papillomatosis
Secondary hypoplasia	Fibrocystic changes
Idiopathic	Neoplasms
Delayed puberty	Fibroadenomas
Mastalgia	Phyllodes tumors
Cyclic	Duct ectasia
Noncyclic	Carcinoma
Nonbreast	

developmental problems seen in the pediatric patient population.

BREAST EMBRYOLOGY AND DEVELOPMENT

Embryology

At 4 weeks' gestation, two mammary ridges develop on the ventral body wall of the embryo (Fig. 27.1). These are symmetric thickenings of ectoderm that extend from the inguinal to axillary regions. At 6 weeks' gestation, all but the thoracic component has disappeared, and a downgrowth of epidermis into the underlying mesenchyme occurs. This represents the primary mammary bud. By 16 weeks, the primary bud has grown and branched into multiple secondary buds, which represent early lactiferous ducts. During the last trimester of development, maternal hormones induce a canalization of the primordial ducts. Through the last 8 weeks of gestation, final differentiation occurs, with a large increase in breast mass (1–3).

The nipple-areolar complex develops during the late fetal period. A mammary pit can be seen by week 12 of gestation from continued epidermal downgrowth, and mesenchymal proliferation beneath the developing mammary gland produces a thickening corresponding to the future areola. By 20 to 24 weeks, a pigmented areola is recognizable, but a nipple is not present; it develops later during the perinatal period. At birth, there is no difference between the breasts of males and females. During childhood, the breasts are relatively dormant structures, remaining so until puberty (1,4).

Congenital Anomalies

The most common congenital anomaly in both males and females is the accessory nipple *(polythelia)*. Accessory nipples often are mistaken for moles, often located in the inframammary area. They may be excised, but treatment is not necessary in most instances. Less commonly, accessory breast tissue is found. A distinction is made between *supernumerary breast,* which has a nipple or areola associated with present or atrophic glandular tissue, and *polymastia,* or accessory breast tissue without a nipple or areola (5,6). Supernumerary breasts most commonly are located along the embryologic milk line, but have been reported to be found in such diverse areas as the cheek, neck, shoulder, midline of the chest or abdomen, flank, hip, thigh, and buttock (5,7), whereas polymastia is located near the breast in the axillary, sternal, infraclavicular, or epigastric region (5). These accessory nipples and breast tissue occur in 2% to 6% of women (8). The etiology appears to be failure of appropriate involution of the mammary ridge. Carcinoma has been found in this accessory breast tissue and has been misdiagnosed clinically, necessitating the need for histologic diagnosis of masses around the breast (5). Interestingly, patients with polythelia, along with three or more minor phenotypic abnormalities, are at increased risk for major, yet possibly asymptomatic, urinary tract abnormalities and should be referred for further diagnostic studies (9). An isolated unilateral or bilateral supernumerary nipple does not increase the patient's risk (9).

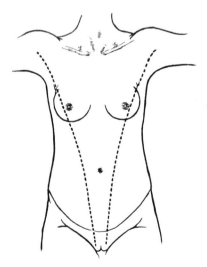

FIG. 27.1. The "milk line" corresponding to the embryologic mammary ridge. Accessory nipples, the most common congenital anomaly, and accessory breast tissue occur along these lines.

In contrast, complete involution of the mammary ridge results in *amastia*. Amastia is a rare abnormality and usually unilateral. Ninety percent of cases of amastia are associated with underlying chest wall deformities. Poland's syndrome is a classic example of this association (absence of pectoralis muscle, chest wall deformity, and amastia) (1,10). Figure 27.2 shows a young woman with Poland's syndrome and marked mammary hypoplasia.

Nipple inversion is common and usually not a significant problem. The nipples generally are inverted at birth but become everted within a few days to weeks postpartum. Nipples that remain inverted in females make a cure difficult, but this is the exception. They pose no other significant problem for nulliparous females other than cosmetic. Rarely, nipple inversion can predispose to infection and breast abscess formation. Nipple inversion can be a difficult anomaly to treat successfully. In general, surgery is avoided. A significant percentage of patients who undergo surgical correction will have recur-

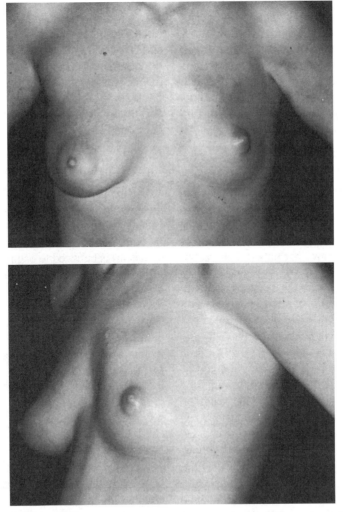

FIG. 27.2. Two views of significant breast asymmetry in a young woman with Poland's syndrome. Note small breast, poorly developed nipple-areolar complex, and lack of pectoral contour on affected side. (Courtesy of Craig Vander Kolk, M.D., Johns Hopkins Hospital.)

rence of the inversion, a poor cosmetic result, or significant damage to the ducts, making nursing difficult or impossible.

Acquired Abnormalities

Injuries to the breast bud occurring during infancy and childhood result in failure of normal breast development. *Iatrogenic injury* often occurs in the neonate or premature infant because of the lack of pigmentation of the areola to serve as a landmark. Biopsy of the hypertrophied breast bud in the neonate and of the preadolescent breast mound are devastating injuries, each requiring reconstructive surgery during late adolescence. Chest wall *irradiation* and *trauma* (burns, tube thoracostomy) can affect normal breast development. *Burns* often result in skin contractures, with an intact breast bud underneath. Contracture release with skin grafts or flaps during early breast growth will allow for near-normal breast development (11).

Development

The onset of breast development (thelarche) occurs early in puberty, followed by adrenarche (the development of secondary sexual characteristics), the growth spurt, and menarche. Recent data show that pubertal characteristics are occurring at younger ages than in previous decades (12). On average, African-American girls begin puberty between years 8 and 9, and white girls begin by year 10 (12). The prevalence of thelarche before age 8, previously thought to be less than 1% (13), is as high as 15% (12). Early puberty is marked by increased secretion of gonadotropin-releasing hormone by the hypothalamus. This results in increased secretion of the gonadotropins by the pituitary and of sex steroids by the ovaries. Estradiol secretion correlates best with breast development, but the gonadotropins and somatomedin appear to be required (14–16). Histologically, growth of the glandular, stromal, and fatty elements of the breast occurs. Glandular tissue accounts for less than 20% of normal breast mass when fully developed (14).

TABLE 27.2. *Tanner stages of breast development during puberty*

Stage	Findings
1	Preadolescent; nipple elevation only
2	Breast bud stage; elevation of breast and nipple as small mound, with enlargement of areola diameter
3	Further enlargement of breast and areola; increased pigmentation of areola
4	Further areola enlargement and pigmentation; nipple and areola now form secondary mound above level of breast
5	Mature stage; smooth contour; projection of nipple only with recession of areola to level of breast

Gross breast development has been characterized in the classic publication by Marshall and Tanner (17). In those studies, normal development is divided into the five Tanner Stages summarized in Table 27.2. These morphologic descriptions have proven useful in describing normal and abnormal adolescent development.

Developmental Abnormalities

Up to 70% of normal newborns develop *neonatal hypertrophy* and nipple discharge, so-called "witch's milk." Small breast enlargement in both newborn males and females (gynecomastia) is believed to occur secondary to the influence of maternal estrogens. Estrogen withdrawal at birth stimulates the pituitary to produce prolactin. This results in nipple discharge. This is usually a self-limited process and requires no intervention. On occasion, continued manipulation of an infant's breast bud in an effort to decompress it of milk by an unsuspecting parent results in continued production of prolactin by the pituitary and, therefore, continued breast enlargement and discharge in the child. Cessation of breast manipulation results in a prompt return to normal.

Developmental abnormalities that occur later in childhood and at puberty include premature thelarche and precocious puberty, breast asymmetry, idiopathic or virginal hypertrophy (gigantomastia), tuberous breast abnormality, and hypoplasia.

Premature thelarche is defined as isolated early breast development, usually before 7 to 8 years, and most commonly is a benign condition. Premature thelarche must be differentiated, however, from true *precocious puberty,* a pathologic disorder resulting in several other developmental abnormalities due to premature estrogen production (18). Table 27.3 lists some of the characteristics that help to differentiate these two entities.

Differentiation of these two entities is very important but sometimes difficult. Premature thelarche requires no treatment and only close follow-up. Studies have shown that thelarche before age 2 years usually regresses completely. After age 2, it persists more frequently, but usually represents the first stage of an early, normal puberty (4,19). Similar findings have been described in other reports (20).

True precocious puberty left untreated results in pubic hair growth, behavioral changes, short stature due to early epiphyseal closure, and accelerated bone maturation, in addition to the early breast development. True precocious puberty is often *idiopathic.* A variety of other conditions, however, can cause precocious puberty, including central nervous system lesions, hypothyroidism *(central precocious puberty)*, ovarian tumors, and adrenal lesions *(peripheral precocious puberty)* (21). A defined structural or endocrinologic abnormality often can be treated successfully. For exam-

ple, thyroid replacement therapy completely reverses the developmental changes associated with hypothyroidism (22,23). Idiopathic precocious puberty must be treated early with hormonal manipulation, most commonly with long-acting gonadotropin-releasing hormone analogues (24–26) (see Chapter 11).

Breast development during puberty can be asymmetric and usually is of no consequence. With time, breast development equilibrates, resulting in nearly symmetric breasts. A small amount of asymmetry in fully developed breasts is normal. An underlying mass, such as a fibroadenoma, accounts for size differences in some cases (27–30). Asymmetry not related to a mass that persists can be corrected surgically if the young woman finds the difference cosmetically unacceptable. Sizes can be normalized by either reduction or augmentation mammoplasty.

Rarely, one or both breasts continue to enlarge in an uncontrolled fashion, resulting in *macromastia* (or, when extremely large, massive virginal hypertrophy or gigantomastia) (Fig. 27.3A). Eighty percent of cases begin in adolescence (31). The definition is difficult to establish, as categorizing breast size by cubic centimeters must be placed in context of the patient's height, weight, and symptoms (31). The cause of macromastia is not clear [even how normal breasts stop growing is unknown (31)], but it may be related to abnormal breast

TABLE 27.3. *Differentiating premature thelarche and precocious puberty*

Premature thelarche	Precocious puberty
Breast development <3 years of age (only to Tanner stage 3)	Breast development, menarche, pubic hair development <8 years of age
LHRH stimulator: FSH-predominant (LH:FSH <1.0)	LHRH stimulator: LH-predominant (LH:FSH >1.0)
No growth spurt	Growth spurt
Normal bone development for age	Advanced bone age
Routine laboratory tests normal	Routine lab tests normal
	Other tests
	Hypothyroidism
	Ultrasound of ovaries for tumor
	Head computed tomography for pituitary hypothalamus tumor
	Elevated urinary steroids
	Body odor
	Vaginal discharge
	Acute

FSH, follicle-stimulating hormone; LH, luteinizing hormone; LHRH, luteinizing hormone, releasing hormone.

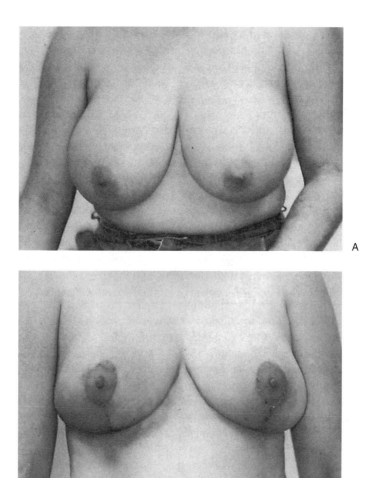

FIG. 27.3. A: Gigantomastia in a teenage girl. **B:** Postoperative appearance after bilateral reduction mammoplasty. (Courtesy of Sheri Slezak, M.D., University of Maryland Hospital.)

tissue sensitivity to normal endocrine signals that promote pubertal breast development or to an abnormal estrogen-to-androgen ratio at the time of thelarche (32–36). Unlike adults who present with clinical features, including discomfort from the weight of the breast, bra grooving in shoulders, back pain, breast pain, and submammary intertrigo, adolescents present with less physical and more psychological complaints, manifesting as socialization problems and altered scholastic and athletic activities (31,37). The growth may occur over months or years (31).

Differential diagnosis includes inflammatory conditions of the breast, phyllodes tumor, fibroadenomas, lymphoma, sarcoma, and car-

cinoma (35). Treatments can include observation until breast development is completed, breast surgery alone, or surgery with postoperative hormonal manipulation (with medication such as medroxyprogesterone) in an attempt to prevent any recurrent tissue from continued growth (37,38). Surgery consists of either reduction mammoplasty or subcutaneous mastectomy and nipple-areolar complex conservation with prosthetic reconstruction (Fig. 27.3B). An excellent summary of operations used for the treatment of macromastia is described by Corriveau and Jacobs (31). Some procedures for moderate hypertrophy may allow for future lactation in many patients, although surgery for extreme hypertrophy may require nipple excision and reimplantation (31). Recurrence after reduction mammoplasty is not uncommon, leading some authors to recommend subcutaneous mastectomy as the initial treatment (33).

There is a case report of a 41-year-old rheumatoid arthritis patient who, while taking *d*-penicillamine, had breast enlargement of unknown etiology. Danazol was successful in decreasing the size of the breast, although the mechanism of action could only be speculated as interfering with estrogen receptors in the breast (39). Its use in adolescent breast hypertrophy has not been reported.

Tuberous breast abnormality is a very rare condition described by Rees and Aston (40) in 1976. They describe an abnormality characterized by apparent overenlargement of the nipple-areolar complex in addition to underdevelopment of breast tissue. The nipple and areola appear to be on a thickened stalk. Plastic reconstruction with breast augmentation is the treatment of choice.

As mentioned earlier, primary breast hypoplasia may be idiopathic (due to injury or surgery) or it may be constitutional. Bilateral constitutional atrophy *(secondary hypoplasia)* may occur after aggressive dieting, in the setting of certain eating disorders (anorexia nervosa), and in the postpartum period.

Figure 27.4 shows an example of a young woman with bilateral *idiopathic hypoplasia*

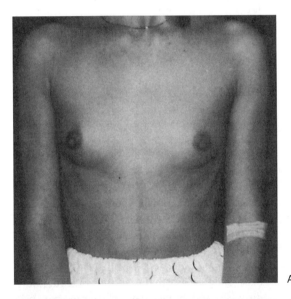

A

FIG. 27.4. A: A 30-year-old woman with idiopathic breast hypoplasia. **B:** Postoperative appearance after successful augmentation mammoplasty. (Courtesy of Sheri Slezak, M.D., University of Maryland Hospital.)

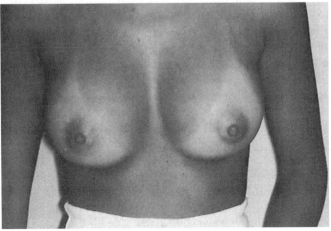

B

treated by augmentation mammoplasty. The breast tissue present functions normally, and lactation and nursing are unaffected. Menstruation is normal. Considerable psychological distress may result from small breasts, and surgical augmentation may be very beneficial.

Hypoplasia secondary to *delayed puberty* is rare. Delayed puberty is defined as puberty beginning after age 15 years. These conditions are divided into chromosomal defects, such as Turner's syndrome, or hormonal defects, such as end-organ unresponsiveness. Turner's syndrome is characterized by classic phenotypic features (webbed or short neck, short stature). The majority of affected females also have hypoplastic nipples and breasts associated with amenorrhea. The diagnosis is made on chromosomal analysis. Estrogen replacement effectively treats amenorrhea and may improve status of breast development if started early in the patient's teenage years (41).

DIAGNOSIS

History

As with any other organ system, the diagnosis of breast disease starts with a thorough history. It is important to remember, however, that the diagnosis of breast cancer cannot be excluded by any single finding in the patient's history. For example, factors such as the patient's young age, her race or ethnicity, her lack of risk factors for breast carcinoma, and benign-appearing symptoms associated with a breast mass cannot be used to exclude the diagnosis of breast carcinoma. In a study by Layfeld et al. (42) of adults with breast masses, modalities such as a finding on physical examination, radiologic procedures, and fine-needle aspiration (FNA) were found to be very sensitive in diagnosing breast carcinoma. History by itself is not sensitive enough to exclude carcinoma.

History assumes much greater importance in the diagnosis and treatment of benign conditions of the breast, including mastalgia and nipple discharge. Most children and adolescents seen by primary care physicians or breast clinics for breast complaints subsequently are found to have normal or benign conditions of the breast (43–45).

The history for patients with breast complaints should include detailed information about her chief complaint, as well as pertinent positive and negative symptoms related to the complaint. Risk factors for breast cancer, as well as results from previous breast diagnostic and surgical procedures, should be documented. As for all patient encounters, a review should be done of the patient's past medical reproductive and surgical history, as well as her current medication and social history (including educational level). In addition, a review of systems should be performed. Finally, knowing the patient's (or her family's) level of anxiety about whether her symptoms are due to breast cancer will be important when discussing the final assessment and plans.

Self Breast Examination

The literature on self breast examination (SBE) in adolescents is sparse and usually reflects opinions and theories. Even in adults, the literature is hampered by different SBE education strategies, different SBE performance, and different control groups used between studies. Among all women, sensitivity of SBE is 20% to 30%. Instruction increases SBE only over the short term. As sensitivity increased, specificity decreased (46). Baines (47) reviewed the adult literature on SBE and breast cancer. Tumor size was smaller, especially among optimal SBE performers, in the ten studies comparing controls with those practicing SBE. Data on the effect of SBE practice on breast cancer mortality vary, although some studies showed increased survival among women practicing SBE.

The hope that teaching adolescents the technique of SBE would familiarize the patients with their own breast (and thus allow recognition of changes) and get patients into the life-long habit of examining their breast has not been validated in appropriate clinical trials (48). Arguments for use of SBE in adolescents point to data showing that more than 80% of adolescent breast masses are discovered by the patient, although what percent of masses are found by accident rather than with SBE is unknown (49,50). The World Health Organization Consultation on Self-Examination in the Early Detection of Breast Cancer reported: "As breast cancer is very uncommon below the age of 35 or 40, it would be inappropriate and wasteful of resources to enroll younger women, unless it were shown that early training increased compliance at later ages, or that knowledge of SBE in younger women led to an increase in the extent to which older women practiced it by diffusion of knowledge from one generation to another. A disadvantage of educating young women is that harmless benign breast disease is more common in young women than in old, and identification of them by breast self examination might lead to an unnecessary increase in biopsies" (51). Current recommendations by the American College of Obstetricians and Gynecologists and the American Cancer Society are for SBE to be performed monthly beginning at age 20 years (52).

Any primary care provider can teach SBE successfully. Strategies that have improved frequency and competence include individual and group instruction of SBE technique, sometimes with the use of silicone models. The importance and benefits of early cancer detection can be imparted one-on-one by physicians, with accompanying literature and/or audiovisual equipment. Teaching the technique of SBE requires little extra time if it is done during a physician's clinical breast examination.

The technique of SBE mirrors that of the examination performed by physicians. Patients should learn to inspect their breast in various positions as well as to palpate the breast in the supine or standing position. Palpation is done with the fingers of the left hand palpating the right breast, and vice versa. All of the breast tissue, including the supraclavicular and axillary area, can be palpated in any fashion, with the exception of the "sliding finger palpation technique." This is because,

of all the different methods currently taught to patients, there is no significant difference in lump detection in silicone breast models, except a lower lump detection rate with the "sliding finger" method (53). Palpation in a circular manner seems to be the most common. For menstruating females, SBE is done 1 week after the completion of menses.

Clinical Breast Examination

A comprehensive breast examination is important in the evaluation of any breast complaint or in asymptomatic adolescents presenting for routine checkups. The exact technique used by the physician is not important. An interesting study by Fletcher et al. (54) tested the ability of physicians in different specialties to detect lumps in silicone breast models. The amount of time spent on the examination, not physician specialty, experience, or method, was found to be the most important variable associated with increased detection. Mitchell (55) has recommended spending 3 to 5 minutes on the clinical breast examination. Also important is detailed descriptive documentation of all findings, both positive and negative, in the medical record. Drawings often are very helpful and descriptive.

Physical examination of the breast is best done 1 to 2 weeks after the beginning of menses because of the following reasons: (a) luteal phase breast volume is increased by 20% because of vascular or lymph congestion; (b) breast tactile sensitivity is increased; and (c) there is a progesterone-influenced increase in cystic glandular tissue due to increased DNA production and cell division. The breast examination should take place in two positions: sitting and supine. Inspection of the breasts is done in the sitting position, and the physician should look for both dermatologic lesions and evidence of underlying breast pathology. Dermatologic lesions that can appear on the skin elsewhere on the body can, of course, occur on the skin of the breast. Pendulous breasts should be raised and the underlying skin examined.

Positions used for inspecting the skin include placing the hands behind the head with the elbows retracted, or placing the hands on the hips and contracting the pectoralis muscles. These will stretch the skin and may accentuate any masses present. Carcinoma that invades the Cooper's ligament can cause a deviation in the skin, and the invasion of a duct near the nipple can cause nipple deviation or retraction.

Palpation of the breast should be done in both the sitting and supine positions. During the examination, only the breast being examined should be exposed. Conversation should relate solely to the examination or to another issue involving the patient's breast. Extraneous conversation can be disconcerting to patients. Again, whether one uses a circular, up-and-down, or wheel-spoke pattern of palpation is less important than the time spent doing the examination.

The area palpated should include the axillary tail of Spence, the supraclavicular nodes, and the area under the nipple. Palpation of the axillary nodes is best accomplished with the patient sitting, her right arm resting on the physician's right arm, and the axilla palpated with the left hand. If there is a history of nipple discharge, a single finger around the areola in a clockwise fashion can help determine which quadrant's ducts are involved.

Mammography and Ultrasonography

Mammography has an extremely limited, if any, role in the diagnosis and management of child and adolescent breast disease. Although there is an earlier shift from dense mammograms to more lucent mammograms among ethnic groups with known lower incidence of breast cancer (e.g., Native Americans), adolescents of different ethnicities have similar dense mammograms (56). Because of this denseness, in young women the false-negative rate of mammography for benign and malignant lesions can be as high as 80% (57,58). For patients under age 30 years who had a mammogram in the evaluation of a palpable mass, almost 75% had no mass on mammogram, and the mammogram did not change the clinical management for any patient (59). For those referred for mammography for indications other than a mass, mammography did not contribute to their clinical management (59).

There are reported risks to mammography (60). One risk includes false-positive results, necessitating aspiration, surgical consultation, or biopsy for patients without abnormal breast disease or cancer. Another risk is the carcinogenic effect of the radiation from mammography (60–62). Although the dose from a mammogram is small (estimated to be 0.8×10^{-3} Gy [0.08 rad]), it has been estimated that, for example, one mammogram per year in women aged 40 to 49 years might be expected to cause 40 new breast cancers per one million women (60). Another risk is the false sense of security that a woman, or a physician, might have from a negative mammogram in light of other signs or symptoms of possible malignant breast disease (60). For these reasons, mammography in this young population was recommended only for the preoperative evaluation of the patient clinically suspected of having carcinoma (59).

Because of the limitations of mammography, ultrasonography is preferred over mammography in the evaluation of breast masses, if a radiologic procedure is to be used. Its use in the evaluation of a palpable mass remains controversial, as it is not sensitive enough to distinguish benign solid masses from malignant ones (63). It can differentiate solid from cystic lesions (64) and, therefore, might be of use in place of FNA when a simple cyst is seen. For malignant palpable masses, color Doppler sonography has a sensitivity of 87%, specificity of 70%, and positive predictive value of 82% in five published reports of women of all ages (65–69). The authors of one study concluded that results of color Doppler sonography most likely would not change the management of the palpable mass (65).

Fine-needle Aspiration

FNA has been recommended to routinely evaluate all palpable breast masses (70). In general textbooks, discussion of FNA, and the evaluation of a breast mass, does not use age to differentiate any difference in the protocol used (71–74). FNA has been studied extensively in the diagnosis of persistently palpable dominant breast masses (a thorough review is provided by Hindle (71) in his book, *Breast disease for gynecologists*). This method provides a cytology specimen for pathologic review. Drs. Hayes Martin and Edward Ellis (75) from Memorial Hospital in New York were the first to report on the use of FNA in the United States. FNA is a simple outpatient procedure, causes minimal discomfort, does not require anesthesia, has a negligible complication rate, has no absolute contraindications, can provide a means of rapid diagnosis, and, in the diagnosis of breast cysts, can be both diagnostic and therapeutic. In adults, FNA has an 8% to 11% false-negative rate and a 1% false-positive rate when used alone for the detection of breast carcinoma (76,77). FNA can be useful in confirming the clinical impression of both benign and malignant breast disease. However, a negative cytologic report, like a negative mammographic report, cannot be relied on to rule out cancer in a clinically suspicious lesion. Any clinically suspicious mass should be excised in spite of negative cytology (78).

The technique of FNA is simple; however, proper procedure and experience are important in obtaining adequate specimens (Fig. 27.5). Eisenhut et al. (43) have provided technical advice on FNA in this unique population. Infants can be restrained by a parent during the procedure. Toddlers up to age 4 years usually require manual restraint along with local anesthesia (using the MadaJet XL [Needle free injector, M.E.C., Carlstadt, NJ] followed by 1 mL or less of sodium bicarbonate buffered 2% lidocaine without epinephrine, administered by tuberculin syringe). Occasionally, this age group requires chloral hydrate suspension at a dose of 50 mg/kg (maximum dose of 1 g) to

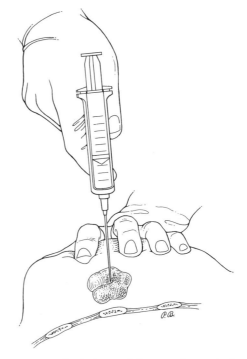

FIG. 27.5. Technique of fine-needle aspiration. The mass is stabilized with the nondominant hand (preferably over a rib). After the needle is inserted into the mass, negative pressure is applied.

perform multiple attempts. Children older than 4 years usually are compliant but frightened, and parental assistance, physician persistence, and local anesthesia are all that usually is needed (43).

After the procedure has been explained to the patient and/or family and consent has been obtained, the lesion is identified and stabilized between the fingers of the nondominant hand. The skin is cleaned with alcohol and wiped dry to prevent stinging when the needle is inserted. A 22-gauge, 1.5-inch needle with a clear hub attached to a 10- to 20-mL syringe is inserted into the mass (Fig. 27.5). The syringe can be placed in a pistol-grip holder, if desired (e.g., Caneco 20-mL PAD NR 3819091 syringe holder). Suction is applied, and the lesion is sampled by moving the needle back and forth within the mass several times in the same plane (moving at different angles may

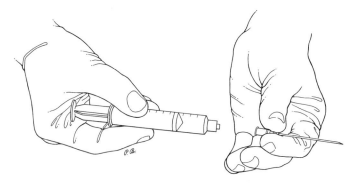

FIG. 27.6. Technique of the fine-needle aspiration—slide preparation. After the needle is removed from the mass, the needle is removed from the syringe and air is aspirated into the syringe. This avoids suctioning cellular material from the needle into the syringe; the cellular material should stay within the needle.

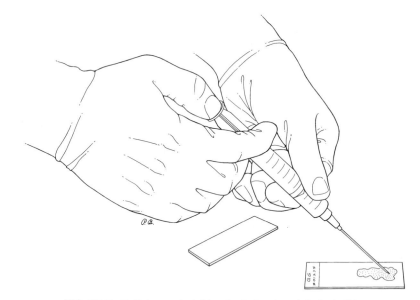

FIG. 27.7. Cellular material is ejected onto a labeled slide.

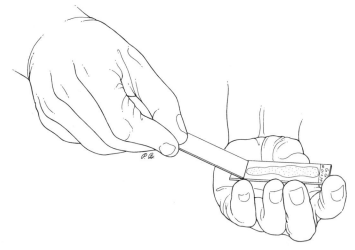

FIG. 27.8. A smear is made using another glass slide at a 45-degree angle. Note the position of the hand stabilizing the slide, which allows the smear to be made.

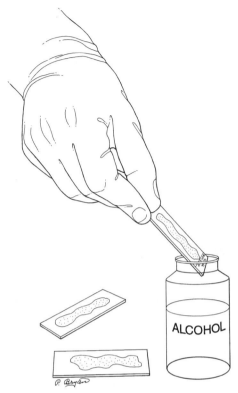

FIG. 27.9. Technique of the fine-needle aspiration—slide preparation. The slide is fixed as rapidly as possible to avoid air drying. Usually, two to three slides can be made from one fine-needle aspiration attempt. The technique chosen for slide preparation depends on the desire of the pathologist.

increase the chance of having excess blood in the needle or syringe). After ten up-and-down movements within the mass, or earlier if any tissue or blood is seen in the needle hub, suction is released and the needle removed from the lesion. Suction must be released before the needle is removed to prevent aspiration of cellular material into the syringe. Pressure is applied by having an assistant place a gauze pad over the site of aspiration for 2 minutes. The needle is detached, air is drawn into the syringe, the needle is reattached, and the cellular material is expelled onto a glass slide with the needle level side down (Figs. 27.6–27.9). A smear is made and the slide fixed. For Papanicolaou staining, immediate fixation with

95% ethanol or a spray fixative is crucial. If an alternative stain is used (such as Wright-Giemsa), the smear can air dry. Usually, one to three slides can be made from each aspiration, and multiple aspirations may be necessary to obtain adequate cytologic material.

To evaluate whether adequate cellular material has been obtained, the fixed slide can be examined microscopically with the aid of toluidine blue, one to two drops, and a cover slip, to identify ductal cells or cellular material. Large breast lesions may require more than one aspiration to adequately evaluate the entire mass. It is important that the clinician and cytopathologist work together in the interpretation of FNAs. An accurate clinical history, including age, clinical examination, and whether a patient is pregnant or lactating, is important in cytologic interpretation. Examples of FNA cytology are shown in Figs. 27.10–27.11.

MASTALGIA

Pain in the breasts can be divided between (a) physiologic swelling and tenderness; and (b) severe cyclic or noncyclic pain known as mastodynia or, more commonly, *mastalgia* (79). For the former, the lobular units of the adolescent breast undergo proliferate changes under the influence of hormones, especially symptomatic in some women close to the beginning of the menstrual cycle. Women can complain of increased fullness, discomfort, or lumpiness. Approximately half of all breast complaints in adolescent females are due to these physiologic changes (80). Once pathology has been ruled out, reassurance, analgesics, and a correctly fitted bra (for which the patient can be measured in a department or specialty store) may help symptoms.

Mastalgia in adolescents has not been adequately studied. Its incidence is unknown (80). In the adult literature, the histologic cause of mastalgia also is unknown. Although fibrocystic changes are seen in many women with mastalgia, there is no evidence that these changes cause mastalgia. The work of Preece

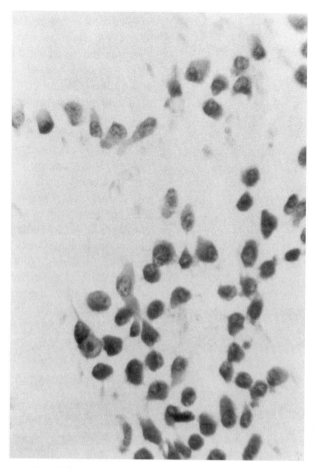

FIG. 27.10. High-power view of fine-needle aspiration cytology of ductal carcinoma. Note the cellular monomorphism and lack of stromal cells. The nuclei are enlarged, and the chromatin is coarse. Nucleoli are present in some cells. (Courtesy of George Birdsong, MD, Emory University School of Medicine, Atlanta, GA.)

et al. (81) disproved the long-held view that women with mastalgia were psychoneurotic.

Mastalgia can be classified as either as *cyclic* (usually associated with menses), *noncyclic,* or *nonbreast.* A careful history, including the use of pain charts documenting when pain occurs during the month, as well as a physical examination and radiologic procedures when appropriate, can differentiate the three groups. Studies of the treatment of breast pain are difficult to interpret because of the heterogeneous nature of the pain, because breast pain is usually a symptom that resolves spontaneously within a short time, and because one fifth of patients respond to placebo. Those with cyclic pain are more likely to respond to medical therapy than are those with noncyclic pain. For the overwhelming majority of patients without a dominant mass, however, only reassurance is required, and no further therapy is necessary (82). One must keep in mind that breast pain not originating from the breast includes such diverse causes as Tietze's syndrome (costochondral syndrome), fractured rib, cervical radiculopathy, and uncommon adolescent causes such as cholecystitis or cholelithiasis, hiatal hernia, peptic ulcer disease, or angina.

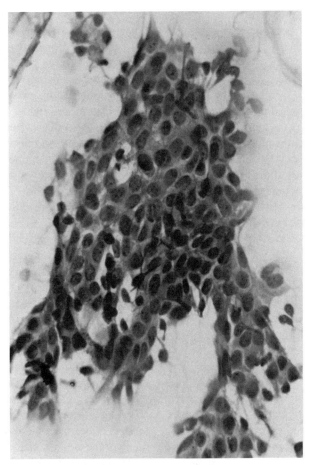

FIG. 27.11. High-power fragment of fine-needle aspiration cytology of benign ductal-epithelium from a fibroadenoma. Note the cohesiveness of the epithelial cells. The chromatin is homogeneous. Myo-epithelial cells (dark nuclei) are admixed with the ductal epithelium. (Couresy of George Birdsong, MD, Emory University School of Medicine, Atlanta, GA.)

Four medications have proved effective for treatment of mastalgia: danazol, bromocriptine, tamoxifen, and oil of evening primrose. There are no studies of the use of these medications in adolescents, and danazol (the only medication approved by the Food and Drug Administration for the treatment of mastalgia), bromocriptine, and tamoxifen are not recommended for use in this age group (80). Oil of evening primrose (3 to 4 g/day), which is available in health food stores, has the advantage of minimal side effects but may take up to 4 months to show an effect. Its mechanism of action is thought to be due to its high content of essential fatty acids acting via prostaglandin pathways (80). There are no scientific data confirming that taking vitamin E, progesterone, diuretics, or thyroid hormone, or decreasing methylxanthine (e.g., caffeine) intake, significantly alleviates breast pain.

NIPPLE DISCHARGE

Nipple discharge in females can be divided into endocrine and nonendocrine etiologies. Endocrine causes result in a milky discharge (galactorrhea). The majority of nonendocrine discharges, which may be purulent, bloody, or serous, are related to infections and benign conditions such as fibrocystic changes.

Galactorrhea

Galactorrhea is a term used to describe inappropriate lactation. Inappropriate lactation is lactation that (a) is not related to pregnancy or (b) continues postpartum in the absence of breastfeeding. Galactorrhea in newborns has already been discussed and seems to be related to maternal estrogen stimulation and withdrawal. In children and adolescents, however, other conditions are prevalent. Rohn (83) and Daughaday (84) classified the causes into six groups: neurogenic, hypothalamic, pituitary, hormonal/endocrine, drug-induced, and idiopathic.

Neurogenic causes are extremely uncommon and include chest wall disorders (traumatic, malignant, and infectious) resulting in local irritation or stimulation, chronic nipple manipulation, and psychiatric disorders. Presumably, with these etiologies, the hypothalamic-pituitary axis is stimulated. *Hypothalamic* causes are even more rare. *Pituitary* causes, however, are commonly reported and have received tremendous attention in the literature as interesting and treatable cases, especially in adults. The most common causative tumor of the pituitary is prolactinoma. The incidence of these tumors in children and adolescents is not well known but is presumably extremely low. Pituitary adenomas represent 1% to 10% of all intracranial tumors in the pediatric age group (83,85). In one report of 25 children and adolescents with these tumors, failure of sexual maturation and galactorrhea were the most common presenting symptoms (85). Visual problems and headaches were notably rare in contrast to adults. They were successfully treated by transsphenoidal resection. Currently, prolactinomas are effectively treated with bromocriptine. If prolactin levels are normal and no other cause of galactorrhea can be found, very close follow-up is necessary. A pathologic cause may declare itself. If prolactin levels are high and evaluation of the sella turcica unrevealing, then the child should have

yearly computed tomography or magnetic resonance imaging evaluation of the sella turcica until the end of puberty, even if the galactorrhea resolves (83).

Galactorrhea also may be caused by *hormonal* manipulation or *endocrine* disorders. Nipple discharge may result from estrogen withdrawal, such as that occurring on cessation of oral contraceptives, but this represents a tiny proportion of oral contraceptive users (32,83). Polycystic ovarian disease and tumors of the adrenal gland, or gonadal tumors, only rarely cause galactorrhea in children and adolescents (83). Hypothyroidism is a rare cause of galactorrhea in neonates and children, as documented by occasional case reports (86,87). Once hypothyroidism is documented as the likely cause of galactorrhea, return to the euthyroid state by the administration of exogenous thyroid hormone results in cessation of nipple discharge in most cases. Finally, certain *medications* may cause galactorrhea; but, again, this has generally been described in adults and not children. Galactorrhea has been ascribed to the use of neuroleptics, estrogens, opiates, and many other agents (32). A common denominator seems to be the antidopaminergic effects of many of these substances, as dopamine inhibits prolactin secretion. Withdrawal of the medication results in cessation of discharge.

The workup of galactorrhea in children and adolescents must be complete, because a pathologic etiology is common. This, again, contrasts with adult women, in whom the majority of galactorrhea occurs with normal menstruation and is, therefore, not likely to be pathologic. Amenorrhea and galactorrhea, on the other hand, require aggressive workup. The history must include drug use, including oral contraceptives, a menstrual and pregnancy history, a history of nipple manipulation, description of sexual maturation, headaches, visual disturbances, and findings suggestive of hypothyroidism. Pertinent physical findings would include goiter, visual field cuts, breast masses, quality of discharge, chest wall abnormalities, and extent of sexual maturation. Thyroid function and prolactin levels should be determined. If hyperprolactinemia is discovered, the sella should be evaluated by computed tomography or magnetic resonance imaging.

Treatment is directed by the results of this evaluation. Offending drugs should be stopped, hypothyroidism should be treated, and behavioral changes in the setting of nipple manipulation should be introduced. Prolactin-secreting pituitary adenomas currently are treated with bromocriptine which act as dopaminergic agonists. Rarely is surgery indicated. If the evaluation is unrevealing, these female patients should be followed closely for the development of prolactinoma, especially if sexual maturation is delayed.

Other Nipple Discharges

In contrast to galactorrhea, *nonmilky nipple discharges* often require surgical intervention. Infections can cause *purulent* discharge. Cultures should be obtained, and the infection usually can be treated with antibiotics. If the discharge fails to clear with antibiotics or is chronic, drainage and duct excision may be required (88). *Serous* discharge can be related to fibrocystic changes and usually is self-limited. *Bloody* or bloodstained discharge should make one suspicious of malignancy, but this is extremely rare in children and adolescents. Intraductal papillomata and duct ectasia are the usual cause of bleeding in children or adolescents and should be excised. An unusual, but easily overlooked, source of nipple discharges (serous, seropurulent, or serosanguineous) is from local irritation of the nipple by clothes, embroidery, or bra fabric (89). Finally, colored (viscous, dark) discharge from the areola has been reported in an adolescent (90). This colored sweat from the apocrine glands (apocrine chromhidrosis) may affect the face or axilla, first presents at adrenarche, and presents during exercise or with direct pressure to the glands. Treatment with topical capsaicin cream 0.025% may help decrease the discharge (90).

MASSES

Table 27.4 lists the common causes of breast masses in children and adolescents. The

TABLE 27.4. *Breast masses in children and adolescents*

Inflammatory
Mastitis
Abscess
Duct ectasia
Cystic abnormalities
Simple cyst
Papillomatosis
"Fibrocystic disease"
Neoplastic
Fibroadenomas
Juvenile or giant
Adult
Phyllodes tumors
Carcinoma
Secretory
Primary
Metastatic

categories for differential diagnoses include infections (mastitis and abscess), benign cystic diseases, benign neoplasms (fibroadenoma), and malignant neoplasms (phyllodes tumors and carcinoma). Other rarer causes are lipoma, lymphangioma, hemangioma, hematoma, lipoma, and fat cell necrosis (49). For children, differential diagnosis includes those mentioned plus the normal breast bud (which should not be excised) plus idiopathic asynchronous thelarche.

Previously, to establish the diagnosis of a solid mass in an adolescent, an excisional breast biopsy would be recommended (88,91). In recent literature, more authors are advocating a more conservative approach (49,70, 92,93).

The reasons are varied. First, and most importantly, the incidence of breast carcinoma, either primary or metastatic, is rare in the pediatric and adolescent population. A review of the adolescent literature since 1960 showed carcinoma to be 0.89% of breast lesions (80). No malignant lesions were found in many smaller series in which excisional breast biopsies were done for masses. Second, the regression rate of an adolescent breast mass is 10% to 40% (94,95).

Third, problems with excisional biopsies include intolerance of local anesthesia for some in the adolescent age group, as well as the potential for prominent, nonaesthetic surgical scars, asymmetry, hypoplasia, and incisional pain (45,96). Fourth, the use of FNA, in addition to clinical impression and radiologic study (if performed), has been shown in the adult and adolescent literature to correlate with excisional biopsy histology (43,96–98).

Fifth, the recommendation that excisional biopsy be done for all breast masses may be related to the fact that the relative risk for breast cancer of women who underwent a breast biopsy for benign disease increased when proliferative changes (such as sclerosing adenosis, papillomas, moderate or florid hyperplasia of the usual type) or atypia (such as atypical lobular or ductal hyperplasia) were seen histologically, as well as when these changes were present in patients with a family history of breast cancer (99). As well, increases in the relative risk of breast cancer occurred in women diagnosed with either so-called "complex" fibroadenomas (fibroadenomas with cysts, sclerosing adenosis, epithelial calcifications, or papillary apocrine changes), fibroadenomas associated with adjacent benign proliferative disease, or any fibroadenoma in a patient with a family history of breast cancer, and this increased risk continued for more than 20 years (100). Thus, without an excisional breast biopsy, the patient may not know her elevated relative risk for breast cancer. It is hoped that patients denoted as higher risk for breast cancer may have additional incentive to perform SBE, have regularly scheduled clinical breast examinations, and begin mammographic screening at age 35 to 40 years. The majority of women of all ages undergoing breast biopsy for benign disease, however, do not have these risk factors and are not at increased risk for breast cancer (99,100).

It appears that studies of breast masses from the general adolescent population find few, if any, carcinomas and thus recommend conservative (nonsurgical) approaches (43–45,96). Jonides et al. (92) recommend that if clinical breast examination and, if performed, ultrasound are consistent with a small fibroadenoma or cyst, the mass can be followed for 2 to 4 months. In study of 258 young women and adolescents with breast masses, no atypia or cancer was found using FNA; thus, they recommended open biopsy done only for persistent cytologic abnormalities (marked atypia, findings suspect for carcinoma) in this population, although they admitted that some cancers are found in women without atypia on FNA (70). Another study recommends that if a mass feels firm but not hard, discrete, and mobile, and the clinical diagnosis is fibroadenoma, up to a 6-month period of close observation can be done, with excision if the mass enlarges or has not regressed (93).

Other studies, especially those that concentrate on a series of adolescent patients with carcinoma, both primary and metastatic, point out that clinical examination does not always differentiate benign from malignant lesions (50,101), that physician delay in diagnosis will delay treatment and possibly decrease survival (101), and that lack of follow-up in the adolescent population is a significant concern (49).

Both approaches have their merits. Pediatric and adolescent patients are at a low, but not nil, risk for breast carcinoma. Clinical breast examination of adolescents, like that of adults, is not sensitive enough to exclude carcinoma. Even though a large majority of masses will resolve without treatment, evaluation of a breast mass with FNA is a cost-effective method for primary care physicians to easily triage masses (3,50). FNA can give an accurate and rapid diagnosis, without the concern that patients will not return for follow-up before diagnosis. This cytologic information, used with information taken from history and clinical breast examination, will help to differentiate those who must be referred for excisional biopsy from those who can be followed without surgery (or, for benign lesions, referred for excisional biopsy after breast maturation) (102,103). If any part of the history, physical examination, sonography, or FNA is not consistent with benign disease, or if the patient or her family remains concerned, the patient should be referred for excisional biopsy (92,97). This approach can help to decrease the number of excisional biopsies while still allowing for early diagnosis of malignant breast diseases.

Infections

Infections of the breast or areolar area may present as masses. In newborns, *mastitis* may present as a mass with overlying erythema. This often is caused by parental manipulation in the setting of hypertrophy or galactorrhea. The pathogenesis of neonatal mastitis is potentially pathogenic bacteria on the mucous membranes and skin (usually *Staphylococcus aureus*) interacting with the newborn's breast tissue under the influence of maternal hormones (104). The bacteria may move from the skin up the ducts, causing cellulitis and possible abscesses. Treatment includes cessation of manipulation, warm packs, and intravenous antibiotics, with incision and drainage for those cases where fluctuance is present (104).

Mastitis and *abscess* occur more commonly in females after thelarche. Often the etiology is unknown. Self-manipulation and breastfeeding are associated with some cases, but the majority are idiopathic. Mastitis initially may be treated with antibiotics that cover oral anaerobes and the staphylococci. Breastfeeding may continue during cases of mastitis that develop while nursing. Mastitis that progresses to frank abscess or that does not resolve on antibiotics should be surgically drained. Adipose loculations and septations in the breast make drainage difficult with local anesthesia, and most cases need to be performed under general anesthesia.

Duct Ectasia

Classically seen in the perimenopausal woman, *duct ectasia* (also known as nonpuerperal mastitis) is seen beginning at thelarche (105). Nipple discharge, breast mass, and possible nipple inversion can make the clinical picture similar to that of carcinoma (105), necessitating excisional biopsy in many to confirm the benign diagnosis. The etiology is unknown and has been reported to be a first symptom of hyperprolactinemia, even in patients without galactorrhea (105). Because the inflammation and surgery can induce a transient elevation of the prolactin level, a

prolactin level should be drawn 4 weeks after resolution of the inflammatory process to confirm an abnormality of the hypothalamic-pituitary region (105).

Cystic Diseases

Simple Cysts

Cystic disease of the breast occurs after the onset of breast development. Benign *simple cysts* are relatively common. They present as painless soft masses that are not fixed to surrounding breast tissue. They usually are single and unilateral. Needle aspiration of the cyst results in complete disappearance of the mass. The fluid may be serous or brown in color. The aspirate should not routinely be sent for cytologic examination, as the yield of this test is very low even in adults (106). Cytology should be sent only when blood-stained fluid is obtained, malignancy is clinically suspected on examination or radiologic study, or a mass remains or recurs after aspiration. A biopsy should be considered in these scenarios as well.

Juvenile Papillomatosis

Juvenile papillomatosis is a lesion of adolescents and young women first described in 1980 (107). It has received attention because certain histologic findings in juvenile papillomatosis may be considered premalignant in older women. There may be an increased risk of breast cancer developing in the patient with juvenile papillomatosis, as well as in her female relatives. Juvenile papillomatosis is uncommon. The presentation is of a painless mobile mass, initially felt to be a fibroadenoma. After excision, examination reveals multiple cysts. Histologic changes are varied and include papillomatosis, cysts, marked epithelial proliferation, and epithelial necrosis.

A report of 180 cases of juvenile papillomatosis revealed a mean age of 23 years; 96% were unilateral (108). Fifty patients (28%) reported the presence of breast cancer in one or more relatives. Additionally, seven patients

(4%) had concurrent breast cancer, and two developed breast cancer years later. Given the possible cancer association, treatment consists of wide excision and careful long-term follow-up.

Fibrocystic Changes

Fibrocystic changes of the breast, often a multifocal and bilateral problem, may present with breast masses and pain (88). It is the second most common diagnosis found from surgical biopsy in the adolescent age group (80). Although up to 90% of all women have histologic fibrocystic changes (formerly know as fibrocystic disease) (79,109), the number of adolescents with fibrocystic changes is unknown (80). Its etiology also is unknown, but it is characterized by ductal-lobular proliferation, duct dilation and elongation, and terminal duct cyst formation (110). Its clinical use has been questioned, because the term includes many breast processes, only some of which are pathologic. Excisional biopsy may be needed when symptoms are severe or there is a question of malignancy.

Neoplasms

Fibroadenomas

The most common masses of the breast in adolescents and young adults are *fibroadenomas*. These tumors are benign and have no malignant potential. They present as a single rubbery, round, mobile, and painless mass. Two types have been described; adult and juvenile. Adult fibroadenomas usually are small. Observation is appropriate (the regression rate is up to 10%) (111), with surgical excision reserved for growing lesions or when there is diagnostic uncertainty. Juvenile fibroadenomas are more rare, generally are much larger (greater than 5 cm), and occur in a slightly younger age group (8). These should not be observed. Early surgical excision is recommended to avoid significant asymmetry and deformity (28). There may be a relation between juvenile fibroadenomas and phyllodes tumors.

Phyllodes Tumors

Phyllodes tumors (formerly known as cystosarcoma phyllodes) are unusual tumors consisting of two important histologic features. Phyllodes tumors have both stromal hypercellularity and benign glandular elements, in contrast to fibroadenomas (112,113). Grossly, they may be large, but they usually remain well circumscribed. Generally considered benign lesions, many reports describe aggressive local recurrence after resection and even occasional metastases (114–119). These masses present as large, painless, rapidly growing lesions. The median age at time of diagnosis is 45 years, and very few present in women under age 25 years (113,120). The tumors feel multilobular and are not fixed. For a benign lesion, most physicians would recommend wide excision with a 2-cm margin.

For histologically malignant lesions, recommendation in adults is for mastectomy. This therapy appears too aggressive for the adolescent patient, and current strategies are for local excision of the mass only and close follow-up, regardless of the histology (115, 116,121). In a report of nine adolescents with this disorder, eight were treated by excision alone, with no recurrences (115). A review of the literature revealed 44 adolescents who had this tumor resected, with only three recurrences (115). Recurrent disease can be treated by local reexcision, often repeatedly (114–117,120).

Carcinoma

Carcinoma of the breast in children is rare, representing less than 1% of childhood cancers and less than 0.1% of all breast cancers (122,123). A carcinoma seen almost exclusively in the pediatric population, with a histology morphologically distinct from adult breast carcinoma, shows a prominent secretory pattern and has been termed secretory breast carcinoma. Serour et al. (124) reviewed all pediatric secretory breast carcinomas reported in the English literature. Twenty-two patients were described, ages 3 to 18 years. The most common presenting symptom was a long-standing breast lump, although local pain was seen in a minority of patients (122, 125,126). Nipple discharge was never present, and lymph node metastases were rare (127, 128). In general, reports confirm the less aggressive nature of these malignancies (122, 127,129).

Recommended therapy for breast cancer in childhood remains poorly defined. Some authors claim that secretory breast cancer, because of its benign course, should be treated by excisional biopsy only (125). Others believe that the 25% local recurrence rate after excision justifies simple mastectomy as initial therapy (122). Karl et al. (122) also urge that adjuvant therapy not be used for secretory breast cancer with axillary nodal metastases. Other authors find these recommendations untenable and recommend that children have aggressive therapy, as used in adults (127, 130). In reality, treatment of secretory carcinoma is controversial, but because various treatments have been used (from excisional biopsy to radical mastectomy) and there have been no reported deaths, Serour et al. (124) recommend wide excision with lymph node dissection.

Breast cancers of the nonsecretory histology are even more rare in children and adolescents. Descriptions in the literature consist of case reports only (130–134). Inflammatory breast cancer and infiltrating ductal cancer have been described (130,133,134). Patients with a previous history of radiation treatment for childhood or adolescent carcinomas are at increased risk for breast cancer. The treatments for Hodgkin's disease in children, chemotherapy and radiation, increase the risk of second malignancy (135), with young patients at especially high risk due to growth potential and hormonal factors at the time of the treatment (136). For second malignancy, the most common solid tumor in women treated as adolescents for Hodgkin's disease was breast cancer (135). In a study by Wolden et al. (35) of 16 patients with breast carcinoma occurring after Hodgkin's disease, the interval between Hodgkin's disease treatment and breast carcinoma was as short as 5 years.

The projected risk of an adolescent Hodgkin's disease survivor having subsequent breast carcinoma within 20 years is estimated to be 9.2% (135).

Currently, women with breast cancer primaries of smaller size (smaller than 5 cm) and favorable location (outer quadrants) are candidates for conservative excisional therapy (partial mastectomy), axillary sampling or dissection, and radiation of the breast. Table 27.5 shows the current TNM staging system for breast cancer. Numerous studies showed similar survival rates between adult patients undergoing modified radical mastectomy and those undergoing lumpectomy with axillary dissection plus radiation for stage I and stage II breast cancer (137,138). There is also a trend toward breast preservation for tumors with less favorable locations.

Children with breast cancer probably should be treated in a manner similar to identically staged adults. Such therapy consists of partial mastectomy, when feasible, with axillary sampling. Although the role of radiation therapy in children with breast cancer is unknown, it must be considered. Cases should be carefully staged and treatment strongly influenced by the histopathology. Likewise, there is no described experience of treating childhood breast cancer with axillary metastases with adjuvant therapy. In premenopausal women, additional chemotherapy is given, often consisting of cyclophos-

TABLE 27.5. *TNM staging system*

Stage	Findings		
	T	N	M
I	T1	N0	M0
II	T1 or T2	N1	M0
	T2	N0	M0
III	T1 or T2	N2	M0
	T3	Any N	M0
	T4	Any N	M0
IV	Any T	Any N	M1

T: 1, <2 cm in size; 2, 2–5 cm in size; 3, >5 cm in size; 4, any size tumor extending into chest wall or through skin. N: 0, no involved axillary nodes; 1, mobile ipsilateral nodes involved with tumor; 2, fixed ipsilateral nodes involved with tumor; 3, involved supraclavicular nodes or arm edema. M: 0, no evidence distant metastases; 1, distant metastases, including skin beyond breast.

phamide (Cytoxan), 5-fluorouracil, and doxo-rubicin (Adriamycin). Such use of adjuvant therapy should be considered carefully for children and adolescents with nonsecretory cancers. Therapy will need to be tailored to each child depending on age, sex, histology of tumor, markers of risk, and evidence of nodal metastases. Successful results from conservative therapy, if undertaken, will depend on close follow-up for extended periods of time. The rarity of such tumors in the adolescent female precludes prospective trials designed to evaluate different therapies.

Metastatic carcinoma is more common in this age group than primary breast carcinoma (64). The carcinomas most commonly found are rhabdomyosarcoma, leukemia, lymphoma, Ewing's sarcoma, neuroblastoma, synovial sarcoma, and yolk sac tumors (64,139). The masses of metastatic carcinoma to the breast in adolescents may be asymptomatic, and clinical examination may indicate benign disease, just as has been reported in adults (139–141). The metastatic mass in the breast may present before symptoms of the primary carcinoma, as is the case of granulocytic sarcoma, which can present before other signs or symptoms of leukemia (64), or, in the case of rhabdomyosarcoma of the breast, an entity almost entirely found in adolescent females (101).

ACKNOWLEDGMENT

Portions of this chapter are from Dolan MS, Glasser GA. Breast diseases: benign and malignant. In: Rock JA, Thompson, JD, eds. *Te Linde's operative gynecology,* 8th ed. Philadelphia: Lippincott–Raven Publishers, 1997:1239–1265.

REFERENCES

1. Osborne MP. Breast development and anatomy. In: Harris JR, Hellman S, Henderson IC, et al, eds. *Breast diseases.* Philadelphia: JB Lippincott, 1987:1–14.
2. Moore KL. *The developing human. Clinically oriented embryology.* Philadelphia: WB Saunders, 1973:354–356.
3. Snell RS. *Clinical embryology for medical students,* 3rd ed. Boston: Little, Brown and Company, 1983:340–341.
4. Freni-Titulaer LW, Cordero JF, Haddock L, et al. Premature thelarche in Puerto Rico. *Am J Dis Child* 1986;140:1263–1267.
5. Smith GMR, Greening WP. Carcinoma of aberrant breast tissue: a report of 3 cases. *Br J Surg* 1972;59:89–90.
6. Copeland MM, Beschickter CF. *Surg Clin North Am* 1950;30:1717.
7. Cutler M. *Tumors of the breast.* London: Pittman, 1961:33.
8. Greydanus DE, Parks DS, Farrell EG. Breast disorders in children and adolescents. *Pediatr Clin North Am* 1989;36:601–638.
9. Hersh JH, Bloom AS, Cromer AO, et al. Does a supernumerary nipple/renal field defect exist? *Am J Dis Child* 1987;141:989–991.
10. Ravitch MM. Poland's syndrome—a study of an eponym. *Plast Reconstr Surg* 1977;59:508–512.
11. McCauley RL, Beraja V, Rutan RL, et al. Longitudinal assessment of breast development in adolescent female patients with burns involving the nipple-areolar complex. *Plast Reconstr Surg* 1989;83:676–680.
12. Herman-Giddens ME, Slora EJ, Wasserman RC, et al. Secondary sexual characteristics and menses in young girls seen in office practice: a study from the pediatric research in office settings network. *Pediatrics* 1997;99:505–512.
13. Bacon G, Spencer M, Hopwood N, et al. *A practical approach to pediatric endocrinology.* Chicago: Year Book Medical Publishers, 1982:189.
14. Drife JO. Breast development in puberty. *Ann N Y Acad Sci* 1986;464:58–65.
15. Rosenfield RI, Furlanetto R, Bock D. Relationship of somatomedin-C concentrations to pubertal changes. *J Pediatr* 1983;103:723–728.
16. Sizonenko PC. Endocrinology in preadolescents and adolescents. *Am J Dis Child* 1978;132:704–712.
17. Marshall WA, Tanner JM. Variations in pattern of pubertal changes in girls. *Arch Dis Child* 1969;44:291–303.
18. Pescovitz OH, Hench KD, Barnes KM, et al. Premature thelarche and central precocious puberty: the relationship between clinical presentation and the gonadotropin response to luteinizing hormones-releasing hormone. *J Clin Endocrinol Metab* 1988;67:474–479.
19. Pasquino AM, Tebaldi L, Cioschi L, et al. Premature thelarche: a follow up study of 40 girls. *Arch Dis Child* 1985;60:1180–1192.
20. Mills JL, Stolley PD, Davies J, et al. Premature thelarche. Natural history and etiologic investigation. *Am J Dis Child* 1981;135:743–745.
21. Cutler GB. Precocious puberty. In: JW Hurst, ed. *Medicine for the practicing physician.* Boston: Butterworth, 1988:526–530.
22. Hermady ZS, Siler-khodr TM, Naijar S. Precocious puberty in juvenile hypothyroidism. *J Pediatr* 1978;92:55–59.
23. Costin G, Kershmar AK, Kogut MD, et al. Prolactin activity in juvenile hypothyroidism. *Pediatrics* 1972;50:881–889.
24. Mansfield MJ, Beardsworth DE, Loughlin JS, et al. Long-term treatment of central precocious puberty with a long-acting analogue of luteinizing hormone-releasing hormone. *N Engl J Med* 1983;309:1286–1290.
25. Pescovitz OH, Comite F, Hench K, et al. The NIH experience with precocious puberty: diagnostic sub-

groups and response to short-term luteinizing hormone releasing hormone analogue therapy. *J Pediatr* 1986; 108:47–54.

26. Comite F, Cassorla F, Barnes KM, et al. Luteinizing hormone releasing hormone analogue therapy for central precocious puberty. *JAMA* 1986;255:2613–2616.

27. Bryant WM, Archer RR. Unilateral breast enlargement in the adolescent. *Am Surg* 1972;38:560–562.

28. Davis C, Patel V. Surgical problems in the management of giant fibroadenoma of the breast. *Am J Obstet Gynecol* 1985;152:1010–1015.

29. Bauer BS, Jones KM, Talbot CW. Mammary masses in the adolescent female. *Surg Gynecol Obstet* 1987;165:63–65.

30. Stone AM, Shenker IR, McCarthy K. Adolescent breast masses. *Am J Surg* 1977;134:275–277.

31. Corriveau S, Jacobs JS. Macromastia in adolescence. *Clin Plast Surg* 1990;17:151–160.

32. Frantz AG, Wilson JD. Endocrine disorders of the breast. In: Wilson JD, Foster DW, eds. *Textbook of endocrinology*. Philadelphia: WB Saunders, 1985:402–421.

33. Samuelov R, Siplovich L. Juvenile gigantomastia. *J Pediatr Surg* 1988;23:1014–1015.

34. Marynick SP, Nisula BC, Pita JC, et al. Persistent pubertal macromastia. *Clin Endocrinol* 1980;50:128–130.

35. Fisher W, Smith JW. Macromastia during puberty. *Plast Reconstr Surg* 1971;47:445–451.

36. Lewison EF, Jones GS, Trimble FH, et al. Gigantomastia complicating pregnancy. *Surg Gynecol Obstet* 1960;110:215–223.

37. Sridhar GR, Sinha MJ. Macromastia in adolescent girls. *Indian Pediatr* 1995;32:496–499.

38. Mayl N, Vasconex LO, Jurkiewicz MJ. Treatment of macromastia in the actively enlarging breast. *Plastic Reconstr Surg* 1974;54:6–12.

39. Taylor PJ, Cumming DC. Successful treatment of d-penicillamine-induced breast gigantism with danazol. *BMJ* 1981;282:362–363.

40. Rees TD, Aston SJ. The tuberous breast. *Clin Plast Surg* 1976;3:339–345.

41. Hall JG, Gilchrist DM. Turner syndrome and its variants. *Pediatr Clin North Am* 1990;37:1421–1440.

42. Layfield LJ, Glasgow BJ, Cramer H. Fine needle aspiration in the management of breast masses. *Pathol Annu* 1989;24:23.

43. Eisenhut CC, King DE, Nelson WA, et al. Fine-needle biopsy of pediatric lesions: a three-year study in an outpatient biopsy clinic. *Diagn Cytopathol* 1996;14:43–50.

44. Meffiorini ML, Labi FL, Nusiner MP, et al. An overview of adolescent breast disorders. *Clin Exp Obstet Gynecol* 1991;18:265–269.

45. Siegal A, Kaufman ZVI, Siegal G. Breast masses in adolescent females. *J Surg Oncol* 1992;51:169–173.

46. O'Malley MS, Fletcher SW. Screening for breast cancer with breast self-examination. *JAMA* 1987;257:2196–2203.

47. Baines CJ. Breast self-examination. *Cancer* 1992;69:1942.

48. Goldbloom RB. Self-examination by adolescents. *Pediatrics* 1985;76:126–128.

49. Diehl T, Kaplan DW. Breast masses in adolescent females. *J Adolesc Health Care* 1985;6:353–357.

50. Hein K, Dell R, Cohen M. Self-detection of a breast mass in adolescent females. *J Adolesc Health Care* 1982;3:15–17.

51. Self-examination in the early detection of breast cancer: a report on a consultation on self-examination in breast cancer early detection programs. Geneva: World Health Organization, November 17–19, 1983.

52. American College of Obstetricians and Gynecologists. Carcinoma of the breast. *ACOG Technical Bulletin No. 158*. Washington, DC: American College of Obstetricians and Gynecologists, 1991.

53. Atkins E, Solomon LJ, Worden JK, et al. Relative effectiveness of methods of breast self-examination. *J Behav Med* 1991;14:357–367.

54. Fletcher SW, O'Malley MS, Bruce LA. Physician's abilities to detect lumps in silicone breast models. *JAMA* 1985;253:2224.

55. Mitchell GW Jr. History and physical examination. In: Mitchell GW Jr, Bassett LW, eds. *The female breast and its disorders*. Baltimore: Williams & Wilkins, 1990:22.

56. Hart BL, Steinbock TR, Mettler FA, et al. Age and race related changes in mammographic parenchymal patterns. *Cancer* 1989;63:2537–2539.

57. Sokol ES, Walker B, Terz JJ, et al. Role of mammography with palpable breast lesions. *Surgery* 1970;67:748–775.

58. Harper PA, Kelly-Fry E, Noe SJ. Ultrasound breast imaging: the method of choice for examining the young patient. *Ultrasound Med Biol* 1981;7:231–237.

59. Willaims SM, Kaplan PA, Petersen JC, et al. Mammography in women under age 30: is there clinical benefit? *Radiology* 1986;161:49–51

60. Eddy DM, Hasselblad V, McGivney W, et al. The value of mammography screening in women under age 50 years. *JAMA* 1988;259:1512–1519.

61. Fieg SA. Radiation risk from mammography: is it clinically significant. *AJR* 1984;143:469–475.

62. Baral E, Larsson LE, Mattsson B. Breast cancer following irradiation of the breast. *Cancer* 1977;40:2905–2910.

63. Kopans, DB. Imaging analysis of breast lesions. In: Harris JR, Lippman ME, Morrow M, et al, eds. *Diseases of the breast*. Philadelphia: Lippincott–Raven Publishers, 1996.

64. Ahrar K, McLeary MS, Young LW, et al. Granulocytic sarcoma (chloroma) of the breast in an adolescent patient: ultrasonographic findings. *J Ultrasound Med* 1998;17:383–384.

65. McNicholas MMJ, Mercer PM, Miller JC, et al. Color doppler sonography in the evaluation of palpable breast masses. *AJR* 1993;161:765–771.

66. Cosgrove DO, Bamber JC, Davey JB, et al. Color doppler signals from breast tumors. *Radiology* 1990;176:175–180.

67. Konishi Y. Clinical application of color doppler imaging in the diagnosis of breast disease. *Med Rev (Toshiba)* 1992;42:12–27.

68. Dixon M, Walsh J, Paterson D, et al. Color doppler ultrasonography studies of benign and malignant breast lesions. *Br J Surg* 1992;79:259–260.

69. Campi R, Carlotta M, Gorreta L, et al. Colour doppler sonography in the diagnosis for breast cancer. *Radiol Med (Torina)* 1990;79:182–184.

70. Markovic-Glamocak M, Sucic M, Boban D. Fine-needle aspiration and nipple discharge cytology in the diagnosis of breast lesions in adolescent and young women: cytologic findings as compared with those

obtained in older women. *Adolesc Pediatr Gynecol* 1994;7:205–209.

71. Hindle WH, ed. *Breast disease for gynecologists.* Norwalk, CT: Appleton & Lange, 1990.

72. Harris JR, Lippman ME, Morrow M, et al, eds. *Diseases of the breast.* Philadelphia: Lippincott–Raven Publishers, 1996.

73. Donegan WL, Spratt JS, eds. *Cancer of the breast,* 4th ed. Philadelphia: WB Saunders, 1995.

74. Bland KI, Copeland EM, eds. *The breast: comprehensive management of benign and malignant diseases,* 2nd ed. Philadelphia: WB Saunders, 1998.

75. Martin HE, Ellis EB. Biopsy by needle puncture and aspiration. *Ann Surg* 1930;92:169.

76. Aajicek J. The aspiration biopsy smear. In: Koss LG, ed. *Diagnostic cytology and its histological bases.* Philadelphia: JB Lippincott, 1979:1001.

77. Kern WH, Almas JP. Aspiration cytology in the diagnosis of breast cancer. *Diagn Gynecol Obstet* 1979;1: 295.

78. Hindle WH, Payne PA, Pan EY. The use of fine needle aspiration in the evaluation of persistent palpable dominant breast masses. *Am J Obstet Gynecol* 1993;168: 1814–1819.

79. Love SM. Fibrocystic disease: what's in a name. *Patient Care* 1990;24:65–82.

80. Neinstein LS. Review of breast masses in adolescents. *Adolesc Pediatr Gynecol* 1994;7:119–129.

81. Preece PE, Richards AR, Owen GM, et al. Mastalgia and the total body water. *BMJ* 1975;4:498.

82. Klimberg VS. Management of common breast disorders. In: Harris JR, Lippman ME, Morrow M, et al, *Diseases of the breast.* Philadelphia: Lippincott–Raven Publishers, 1996:99–106.

83. Rohn RD. Galactorrhea in the adolescent. *J Adolesc Health Care* 1984;5:37–49.

84. Daughaday WH. The adenohypophysis. In: Williams RH, ed. *Textbook of endocrinology,* 6th ed. Philadelphia: WB Saunders, 1981:73–116.

85. Richmond IL, Wilson CB. Pituitary adenomas in childhood and adolescence. *J Neurosurg* 1978;49:163–168.

86. Van Wyce JJ, Grumbach MM. Syndrome of precocious menstruation and galactorrhea in juvenile hypothyroidism: an example of hormonal overlap in pituitary feedback. *J Pediatr* 1960;57:416–435.

87. Macaron C. Galactorrhea and neonatal hypothyroidism. *J Pediatr* 1982;101:576–577.

88. Love SM, Schmitt SJ, Connolly JL, et al. Benign breast disorders. In: Harris JR, Hellman S, Henderson IC, et al, eds. *Breast diseases.* Philadelphia: JB Lippincott, 1987:15–53.

89. Casteels-VanDaele M, Wijndaele L, Reckles R, et al. Nipple discharge in children and adolescents: an irritating cause. *Clin Pediatr* 1990;January:53.

90. Saff DM, Owens R, Kahn TA. Apocrine chromhidrosis involving the areolae in a 15 year old amateur figure skater. *Pediatr Dermatol* 1995;12:48–50.

91. Weibke EA, Niederhuber JE. Disorders of the breast. In: Carpenter SE, Rock JA, eds. *Pediatric and adolescent gynecology.* Philadelphia: Lippincott–Raven Publishers, 1996:417–432.

92. Jonides L, Rudy C, Walsh S. Breast masses in adolescent girls. *J Pediatr Health Care* 1992;6[5 Pt 1]: 287–288.

93. Greydanus DE, Hofmann AD. The thorax. In: Hofmann

94. Neinstein LS, Atkinson J, Diament M. Prevalence and longitudinal study of breast masses in adolescents. *J Adolesc Health* 1993;13:277–281.

95. Seashore JH. Breast enlargements in infants and children. *Pediatr Ann* 1975;4:542–564.

96. Pacinda SJ, Ramzy I. Fine needle aspiration of breast masses. *J Adolesc Health* 1998;23:3–6.

97. Hindle WH, Payne PA, Pan EY. The use of fine-needle aspiration in the evaluation of persistent palpable dominant breast masses. *Am J Obstet Gynecol* 1993;168: 1814–1819.

98. Silverman JF, Gurley AM, Holbrook CT, et al. Pediatric fine needle aspiration biopsy. *Am J Clin Pathol* 1991; 95:653–659.

99. Dupont WD, Page DL, Risk factors for breast cancer in women with proliferative breast disease. *N Engl J Med* 1985;312:146–151.

100. Dupont WD, Page DL, Parl FF, et al. Long-term risk of breast cancer in women with fibroadenoma. *N Engl J Med* 1994;331:10–15.

101. Hays DM, Donaldson SS, Shimada H, et al. Primary and metastatic rhabdomyosarcoma in the breast: neoplasms of adolescent females, a report from the intergroup rhabdomyosarcoma study. *Med Pediatr Oncol* 1997;29:181–189.

102. Siegel A, Kufman Z, Siegal G. Breast masses in adolescent females. *J Surg Oncol* 1992;51:169–173.

103. West KW, Rescorla FJ, Scherer LR, et al. Diagnosis and treatment of symptomatic breasts masses in the pediatric population. *J Pediatr Surg* 1995;30:182–187.

104. Walsh M, McIntosh K. Neonatal mastitis. *Clin Pediatr* 1986;25:395–399.

105. Peters F, Schuth W. Hyperprolactinemia and non-puerperal mastitis (duct ectasia). *JAMA* 1989;261: 1618–1620.

106. Ciatto S, Cariaggi P, Bulgaresi P. The value of routine cytologic examination of breast cyst fluids. *Acta Cytol* 1987;31:301–304.

107. Rosen PP, Cantrell B, Mullen DL, et al. Juvenile papillomatosis (Swiss cheese disease) of the breast. *Am J Surg Pathol* 1980;4:3–12.

108. Rosen PP, Holmes G, Lesser ML, et al. Juvenile papillomatosis and breast cancer. *Cancer* 1985;55: 1345–1352.

109. Love SM, Gelman RS, Silen W. Fibrocystic disease of the breast—a nondisease? *N Engl J Med* 1982;307: 1010.

110. Vorherr H. Fibrocystic breast disease, pathophysiology, pathomorphology, clinical picture and management. *Am J Obstet Gynecol* 1986;154:161.

111. West KW, Rescorla FJ, Scherer LR, et al. Diagnosis and treatment of symptomatic breast masses in the pediatric population. *J Pediatr Surg* 1995;30:182–187.

112. Vorherr H, Vorherr UF, Key CR. Cystosarcoma phyllodes: epidemiology, pathohistology, pathobiology, diagnosis therapy, and survival. *Arch Gynecol* 1985; 236:173–181.

113. Rosai J. Breast. In: Rosai J, ed. *Ackerman's surgical pathology,* 7th ed. St. Louis: CV Mosby, 1989: 1246–1249.

114. Chua CI, Thomas A. Cystosarcoma phyllodes tumors. *Surg Gynecol Obstet* 1988;166:303–306.

115. Briggs RM, Walters M, Rosenthal D. Cystosarcoma

AD, ed. *Adolescent medicine.* Menlo Park: Addison Wesley, 1983:46–50.

phyllodes in adolescent female patients. *Am J Surg* 1983;146:712–714.

116. Stromberg BV, Golladay ES. Cystosarcoma phyllodes in the adolescent female. *J Pediatr Surg* 1978;13:423–425.

117. Hart J, Layfield LJ, Trumbull WE, et al. Practical aspects in the diagnosis of management of cystosarcoma phyllodes. *Arch Surg* 1988;123:1079–1083.

118. Hoover HL, Trestioreanu A, Ketcham AS. Metastatic cystosarcoma phyllodes in an adolescent girl: an unusually malignant tumor. *Ann Surg* 1975;181:279–282.

119. Gibbs BF, Roe RD, Thomas DF. Malignant cystosarcoma phyllodes in a pre-pubertal female. *Ann Surg* 1968;167:229–231.

120. Salvadori B, Cusumano F, del Bo R, et al. Surgical treatment of phyllodes tumors of the breast. *Cancer* 1989;63:2532–2536.

121. Mollitt DL, Golladay ES, Gloster ES, et al. Cystosarcoma phyllodes in the adolescent female. *J Pediatr Surg* 1987;22:907–910.

122. Karl SR, Ballatine TVN, Zaino R. Juvenile secretory carcinoma of the breast. *J Pediatr Surg* 1985;20:368–371.

123. Ferguson TB, McCarty KS, Filston HC. Juvenile secretory carcinoma and juvenile papillomatosis: diagnosis and treatment. *J Pediatr Surg* 1987;22:637–639.

124. Serour F, Gilad A, Kopolovic J, et al. Secretory breast cancer in childhood and adolescence: report of a case and review of the literature. *Med Pediatr Oncol* 1992;20:341–344.

125. McDivitt RW, Stewart FW. Breast carcinoma in children. *JAMA* 1966;195:144–146.

126. Byrne MP, Fahey MM, Gooselaw JG. Breast cancer with axillary metastasis in an eight and one-half-year-old girl. *Cancer* 1973;31:726–728.

127. Heydenrych JJ, Villet WT, Von Der Heyden L. Carcinoma of the breast in children. *S Afr Med J* 1980;57:1005–1008.

128. Masse SR, Rioux A, Beauchesne C. Juvenile carcinoma of the breast. *Hum Pathol* 1981;12:1044–1046.

129. Oberman HA, Stephens PJ. Carcinoma of the breast in children. *Cancer* 1972;30:470–474.

130. Close MB, Maximov NG. Carcinoma of the breast in young girls. *Arch Surg* 1965;91:386–389.

131. Byrne MP, Pahey MM, Gooselaw JG. Breast cancer with axillary metastasis in an eight and one half year old girl. *Cancer* 1973;31:726–728.

132. Hartman AW, Magrish P. Carcinoma of breast in children. Case report: six year old boy with adenocarcinoma. *Ann Surg* 1955;141:792–798.

133. Ramirez G, Ansfield FJ. Carcinoma of the breast in children. *Arch Surg* 1968;96:222–225.

134. Nichini FM, Goldman L, Lupayowker MS, et al. Inflammatory carcinoma of the breast in a 12 year old girl. *Arch Surg* 1972;105:505–508.

135. Wolden SL, Lamborn R, Cleary SF, et al. Second cancers following pediatric Hodgkin's disease. *J Clin Oncol* 1998;16:536–544.

136. Abrahamsen JF, Andersen A, Hannisdal E, et al. Second malignancies after treatment of Hodgkin's disease: the influence of treatment, follow-up time, and age. *J Clin Oncol* 1993;11:255–261.

137. Kinne DW. Primary treatment of breast cancer surgery. In: Harris JR, Hellman S, Henderson IC, et al, eds. *Breast diseases.* Philadelphia: JB Lippincott, 1987:259–284.

138. Harris JR, Hellman S. Primary treatment of breast cancer. Conservative surgery and radiotherapy. In: Harris JR, Hellman S, Henderson IC, et al, eds. *Breast diseases.* Philadelphia: JB Lippincott, 1987:299–324.

139. Kwan WH, Choi PHK, Li CK, et al. Breast metastasis in adolescents with alveolar rhabdomyosarcoma of the extremities: report of two cases. *Pediatr Hematol Oncol* 1996;13:277–285.

140. Toombs BD, Kalisher L. Metastatic disease to the breast: clinical, pathologic, and radiographic features. *AJR* 1977;129:673–676.

141. Bohman LG, Bassett LW, Gold RH, et al. Breast metastases from extramammary malignancies. *Radiology* 1982;144:309–312.

28

Child and Adolescent Sexual Abuse

Nancy N. Fajman

Sexual abuse involves the use of a child for the sexual stimulation or gratification of another individual who usually is older or developmentally more mature. Physical contact may include penetration by a finger, penis, or other object of the child's genital area, anus, or mouth. Fondling may occur on top of clothing or directly on the body, or a child may be encouraged to touch the perpetrator in a sexual manner. Noncontact abusive behaviors include exhibitionism, voyeurism, involvement with pornography, and facilitating prostitution.

EPIDEMIOLOGY

Incidence

The true incidence of sexual abuse is difficult to assess. Child and adolescent victims frequently delay reporting due to fear or confusion regarding the act. Case definitions for child sexual abuse also vary by state. The Third National Incidence Study of Child Abuse and Neglect (NIS-3) estimated that the number of newly identified sexually abused children rose from 133,600 in 1986 to 300,200 in 1993 (4.5 victims per 1,000 children). Girls were sexually abused three times more frequently than boys. The NIS-3 included children who had been physically injured by the abusive act as well as those children whose abuse put them at risk for harm (1).

Prevalence

Prevalence estimates of child sexual abuse, or the number of victims in the population at a given time, suggest an even larger problem. In a review of 19 prevalence studies, it was estimated that at least 20% of American women had been the victim of some form of sexual abuse as a child (2). A recent survey of 8,506 adults from a large health maintenance organization revealed a prevalence of 22% exposed to sexual abuse before the age of 18 years. The abuse included fondling and attempted or actual (oral, anal, or vaginal) intercourse (3). Because survey results depend on the recall and willingness of (usually) adult participants to respond to questions of a personal, potentially embarrassing nature, it is presumed that most prevalence statistics are underestimated (4).

Risk Factors

Most children know their perpetrator. In the NIS-3, 29% of perpetrators were a birth parent and 25% were stepparents or parent substitutes (e.g., boyfriend of the mother). The abusers are overwhelmingly male, although female perpetrators may represent up to 10% of the total. Children from lower income households are at increased risk for all forms of child maltreatment, including sexual abuse. Racial differences did not account for any risk factor, which was similar to the 1986 NIS-2 study (1). Children with physical disabilities or developmental delays may be at higher risk for sexual abuse from an attendant or care provider because of their increased dependence and/or inability to discern a dangerous situation (5).

PATIENT PRESENTATION

Children and adolescents who have been sexually abused present to the clinician in a variety of ways. An outcry of abuse may have already been made, and one may or may not find physical changes. Other children come to the physician because of a nonspecific physical complaint, usually referable to the gastrointestinal or genitourinary systems, with no discernible etiology. In this case, sexual abuse should be included in the differential diagnosis, and the doctor should ask about any inappropriate touch.

At times, the parent brings the child to medical attention because of significant behavioral changes that may reflect the child's response to a stressful situation. Some abused children act out in a sexual manner. Normal child sexual behaviors, such as self-stimulation, exhibitionism, or curiosity about genitals and bathroom activities, should not be misconstrued as indicative of abuse (6). The child who focuses on sexual behaviors, however, to the exclusion of usual childhood play or who is involved in explicit, forceful, or coercive sexual activity is in need of further evaluation (7).

TIMING OF ASSESSMENT

The purposes of the medical evaluation include identification and treatment of injuries, collection of forensic evidence, consideration of testing and treatment for sexually transmitted diseases (STDs), and guidance and reassurance of the patient and family.

The symptomatic child, or one who has been abused within a few days, should be assessed immediately by a medical practitioner. If the abuse occurred within 72 hours, collection of forensic evidence may be indicated. For the child whose abuse occurred more than 3 days before, but within the past 1 to 2 weeks, a medical appointment should be arranged as soon as possible to assess for any subtle or healing injuries. If the abuse occurred more than several weeks in the past and the child is asymptomatic, the evaluation may be scheduled for a time convenient to the patient and practitioner.

Although the medical evaluation frequently is not an emergency from the physical standpoint, it is an emotional emergency for many families. Only the clinical practitioner can provide the medical and emotional reassurance that the child will be physically all right. A prompt evaluation in the least traumatic setting, preferably not a hectic emergency room, is recommended.

HISTORY TAKING

A separate discussion with the parent should be held first to outline the concern. The patient's history is preferably taken privately as well, without the caretaker present. If this is not feasible, however, one should document who is present during the collection of the history, as this may influence the content of the information given. Important statements by the patient should be recorded verbatim and placed in quotation marks.

Developmentally appropriate, short, open-ended questions are recommended in talking about an abusive episode. Identify and use the child's words for the parts of her body, especially the genital and anal areas. Pictures or drawings may be helpful. Anatomically correct dolls, used for the purposes of demonstration or clarification of terminology, may be useful in understanding the child's history. Guidelines for the use of these dolls are available (8).

Avoid leading questions. Multiple choice questions, or questions that ask for a yes/no response, are to be discouraged, as children sometimes feel compelled to give an answer even if none of the options is appropriate, or they may consistently concur with the last option given.

If the child describes abusive genital contact, she may not truly know whether the object/finger/penis was placed *inside* her vagina. Although she may understand the general concept of inside/outside, a girl may easily misconstrue vulvar pressure for penile entry. Likewise, an adolescent who has never experienced intercourse, or who has never used a tampon, may not know whether a perpetrator fully penetrated her, although she may have felt painful pressure at the external genitalia.

The times of menarche and last menstrual period should be noted for the adolescent. Past history regarding prior consensual sexual activity may be important to providing optimum overall medical care, but generally is irrelevant to the specific case of abuse. Documentation of prior sexual activity by an adolescent is only indicated if the patient had consensual intercourse within a few days of the assault; in that case, an assault kit analysis may find DNA evidence of more than one contact. It is best to clarify what is meant by "having sex" or sexual "activity;" not all teens have the same understanding of these terms.

A complete Review of Systems is indicated; it may prove particularly helpful in the differential diagnosis. If the assault occurred within the past 72 hours and evidence will be collected, document what hygienic measures have been taken. Activities such as bathing or douching may diminish the amount of evidence available. Likewise, documentation of the use of a condom may later explain an absence of findings on DNA analysis.

Although the medical practitioner usually is not conducting an official forensic interview, these roles overlap somewhat and the medical history may be used for legal purposes. References are available for the practitioner who would like to pursue this area of history taking further (9,10). The history may be the most important "evidence" of abuse and should be addressed with great care.

PHYSICAL EVALUATION

The practitioner should convey a caring, confident manner to best reassure the patient as well as the parent. Some clinicians are concerned that the child will perceive the physical examination as another abusive encounter. For the practitioner who conducts the evaluation in a gentle, reassuring, confident manner, however, the physical examination may actually be a first step in the healing process (11).

Anesthesia and Analgesia

Children with active bleeding or suspected internal injuries will require an examination under anesthesia. Most children, however, do not require sedation. For the especially anxious child, oral midazolam may be helpful (12). Topical viscous lidocaine may be useful in minimizing discomfort in the child with vulvar trauma.

Equipment and Supplies

Equipment and supplies that are to be used for examination of the genital area should be demonstrated to the patient and parent before the examination. Allowing the child to touch a sample cotton swab, such as the type used for specimen collection, allows her to recognize its softness.

A good light source is necessary. A magnification device is helpful. An otoscope is available in most examination rooms; alternatively, a handheld magnifying glass can be used. A colposcope may be used to magnify the genital area and provide photodocumentation. Such documentation can be used for legal purposes and may obviate the need for a repeat examination when a finding is questioned (13).

Many parents are afraid that their young child will require a speculum examination to evaluate for abuse. Informing the parent of the preadolescent that this is not the case (unless anesthesia is used) will provide a great deal of reassurance. In the adolescent, however, this may be her first speculum examination, and the usual care and attention to patient concerns will be necessary.

A Foley catheter may be used to better evaluate the estrogenized hymen of the adolescent. The catheter is inserted into the vagina and the balloon is inflated with air. The balloon gently stretches the ruffled hymenal membrane and allows for enhanced visualization of small defects or tears (14). A moistened cotton swab may be helpful in discerning defects in the estrogenized hymen. The swab is positioned just inside the hymenal membrane at its attachment to the vaginal wall. By applying gentle outward pressure of the swab while moving it circumferentially, the full extent of the hymen can be observed. Some practitioners advocate the use of toluidine blue dye to enhance visualization of abraded skin or mucus membrane surfaces (15).

The collection of forensic evidence is facilitated by using a sexual assault (rape) kit. This topic is discussed further in the section on "Collection of Forensic Evidence."

Children can be encouraged to bring a favorite stuffed animal with them to the evaluation. It is helpful to have several distracter items available to occupy the patient's attention during the examination. A kaleidoscope or other small toys may divert the young child's attention. An older child may enjoy a handheld puzzle or listening through the stethoscope.

Patient Examination

In general, a full physical examination is performed. This allows the examiner to note any evidence of extragenital injury or findings that might be important in the differential diagnosis. Note the patient's demeanor, avoiding subjective descriptors such as "appropriate" or "inappropriate" because there is a wide variety of responses to a traumatic experience. Document the presence of bruises, bite marks, or "hickeys." Examine the oropharynx carefully

for signs of trauma or the presence of lesions compatible with human papillomavirus (HPV).

For examination of the genital area, an infant usually is placed in the supine position, hips abducted; it may help to mimic changing a diaper. An older child can assume a frog-leg or "butterfly" position, supine with knees bent and soles of the feet brought together. For the child who needs physical contact with a caregiver for reassurance, she can sit in the caregiver's lap, child's back resting against the caregiver's chest; with a caregiver arm under each knee of the child, the caregiver slowly draws the child's legs apart. The teenager or tall preteen usually can tolerate the lithotomy position.

With the patient in one of these positions, the practitioner first inspects the surfaces of the mons pubis, inner thighs, perineum, and labia for evidence of injury or any other dermatologic findings. The inguinal area is palpated for the presence of lymphadenopathy. The labia majora are gently grasped, spread a little bit laterally, and carefully pulled toward the examiner. This *traction* technique should overcome the moist adhesive forces of the hymenal membrane, allowing for adequate visualization (Fig. 28.1). Excessive lateral stretch can result in a painful, albeit slight, tear of the posterior fourchette in the presence of even a small posterior labial adhesion. The traction technique pro-

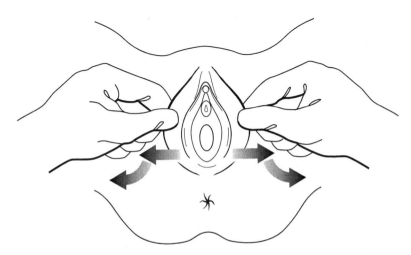

FIG. 28.1. Traction technique for examination of female genitalia.

vides better visualization of the vestibule than a simple separation technique wherein the practitioner uses the thumb and index finger of a single hand to separate the labia.

The knee-chest position, with the patient prone and buttocks elevated, may provide additional or supportive information, especially when there is redundant hymenal tissue. The examiner frequently can observe the posterior hymen with increased clarity as that edge unfolds. This position also may allow for better visualization of internal vaginal structures in the preadolescent (16).

Examination of the anus in the young child can be accomplished by pressing the knees to the chest while in the supine position. The lateral decubitus position is preferred for the older child. Young women who are tall enough to be in stirrups can be examined while in the lithotomy position. Note anal tone and the presence of any traumatic injury or lesions.

Specimen Collection

Specimen swabs are inserted through the vaginal orifice to collect samples as needed. The thin hymenal membrane is sensitive in the prepubescent girl, and care must be taken to avoid contact of the swab with the hymenal edge. The knee-chest position may provide a wider orifice in this age group. Thin, wire shafted swabs are more easily introduced than swabs with wooden or plastic handles, but some specimens require a specific type swab. It is always best to check first with your laboratory.

Moistened swabs are less irritating if there is contact with patient skin or mucus membrane. Vaginal washes may facilitate collection of multiple specimens (17). The use of nonbacteriostatic sterile water or saline is recommended for specimen collection so as not to inhibit the growth of microorganisms in culture.

CLINICAL FINDINGS

Normal Appearance

The genital examination in sexual abuse frequently is normal, even in cases where

there is legal proof of abuse (18–21). The nature of much abuse is not physically traumatic; fondling, rubbing, and even the gentle insertion of an object into the anus or vagina may leave no mark. In addition, children frequently do not give an outcry immediately after the molestation, allowing injuries to heal before the patient comes to medical attention (22,23). The medical practitioner must be familiar with the variety of normal findings and recognize that a normal examination does not preclude the possibility of abuse. Because of this, descriptive terms such as "virginal" or "intact" hymen can be misleading; many nonmedical people assume that such a hymen indicates no sexual contact at all. A glossary of standardized terms has been compiled to assist the clinician in providing clear, unambiguous documentation (24). Explanation of a simple diagram (Fig. 28.2), or demonstration during the physical examination, can be educational and reassuring.

Normal findings include the variety of hymenal configurations, hymenal tags or

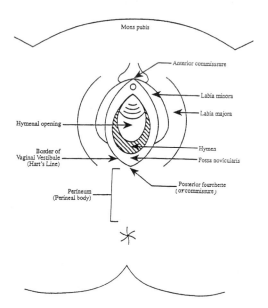

FIG. 28.2. Diagram of the genital anatomy of a prepubertal girl. A crescentic hymen is shown. (From Pokomy SF. *Pediatric and adolescent gynecology.* New York: Chapman and Hall, 1996, with permission.)

bumps, prominence of intravaginal ridges, perihymenal and periurethral bands, and septal bands or remnants (18,25–27). Findings in the midline that may be confused with a healed or healing injury include a prominent perineal raphe and a linea vestibularis (a pale vertical line found crossing the posterior fourchette and/or the fossa navicularis) (24). Failure of midline fusion is a congenital defect that can mimic abusive injury.

The appearance of the genital area changes with patient age. The newborn has a significant amount of transplacental estrogen from the mother. A small amount of withdrawal bleeding seen at the vaginal orifice, or on a diaper, within the first week of life may be misinterpreted by caregivers as an indication of abuse. Cervical ectropion, a normal finding in the adolescent, may have the appearance of an erythematous traumatic injury.

The size of the hymenal opening varies with the patient's age and examination position, her state of relaxation, and the examiner's technique. Despite researchers' attempts to document normal sizes for this orifice (25,26), caution is advised in using the finding of an apparently enlarged hymenal opening as the sole indicator of an abusive event (28).

Nonspecific Genital Findings

Nonspecific findings for child sexual abuse are those variations in the physical examination that may be seen in the abused as well as the nonabused child. Such findings should prompt the clinician to consider abuse in the early differential diagnosis. Examples include increased erythema or vascularity of the genital structures, labial adhesions, and small hymenal notches (18,25,27).

Genital discharge may be due to a variety of organisms, including STDs. Consideration of the Review of Systems may indicate a need to culture for respiratory or enteric organisms (29). Group A β-hemolytic streptococcus may be autoinnoculated to the anal or genital areas and produce erythematous skin findings and a discharge. Shigella can cause a bloody vaginal discharge. The presence of an intravaginal foreign body can result in a purulent or blood-tinged discharge.

Suspicious Genital Findings

Injury due to acute blunt force trauma may manifest as a few scratches or petechiae, or may demonstrate significant bruising and lacerations, depending on the force involved. The posterior portion of the hymenal rim and the posterior fourchette are at increased risk for traumatic injury in sexual assault. A significant tear of the hymen may result in scar tissue and/or a defect in the integrity of the hymenal contour (27,30). Victims may have narrowing of the inferior hymenal tissue at the 6 o'clock position (18,23); however, it can be difficult to assess the actual attachment site of the hymenal membrane to the vaginal floor for an accurate measurement (26).

Trauma to the genital area may occur during a sports activity or other nonabusive incident. Straddle mechanisms frequently cause crush injuries and bruises of the inner thighs or labia. The hymen is relatively recessed in the pelvis, and an accidental injury of the hymen should include a history of the child impaling herself on an object, otherwise abuse should be a concern (31).

Other considerations in the differential diagnosis of traumatic injury include urethral prolapse and congenital hemangioma. Lichen sclerosus et atrophicus may present with pale, shiny, atrophied skin around the genital and/ or anal areas. This skin is friable and may develop erosions, tears, or hematomas with even slight traumatic injury.

Chlamydia trachomatis or *Trichomonas vaginalis* infection beyond the neonatal period, or anogenital infections with herpes simplex virus (HSV) or HPV, is of great concern for the likelihood of child sexual abuse. Syphilis, gonorrhea, or human immunodeficiency virus (HIV) infections discovered beyond the neonatal period in a prepubertal girl most often are due to sexual contact with an infected perpetrator.

Definitive Findings

The presence of semen, sperm, or a pregnancy indicates exposure to sexual activity. For the safety of the child, significant genital injuries, such as lacerations, hymenal transections, and abrasions, in the absence of a reasonable explanation, should be assumed due to abuse unless proven otherwise.

Anal Findings

Traumatic injury to the anus may cause superficial scratches, stellate fissures, or deep lacerations depending on the force used, size of the object inserted, and use of lubrication. Internal injuries can cause life-threatening blood loss or peritonitis if bowel perforation has occurred. Superficial injuries, however, may heal within days, and the examination generally returns to normal within 1 to 2 weeks (22,32).

Normal findings at the anal examination include perianal erythema and hyperpigmentation, midline tags or flattening of rugae, and perianal venous engorgement after 2 to 3 minutes in the knee-chest position (27,33). The significance of earlier perianal venous congestion is unclear (30).

Anal dilatation larger than 15 mm in diameter that occurs early in the physical examination, in the absence of stool in the rectal ampulla, may be associated with sexual abuse (18,27). There is some debate, however, regarding the significance of this finding (30). One needs to assess the child's underlying neuromuscular tone, which may be decreased from a congenital or acquired disorder or from sedation. Anal tone should be reassessed when any anesthetic effect is past. One should always ask about (and document) a history of significant straining with bowel movements as a possible confounding factor, particularly in the child with rectal fissures or decreased anal tone. In children with decreased tone, the anal pectinate line may be apparent on examination and can be confused with traumatic injury.

Findings that may mimic anal sexual abuse include perianal streptococcal infection and lichen sclerosus. Rectal prolapse is a nonspecific finding.

COLLECTION OF FORENSIC EVIDENCE

By examining intimate parts of the patient's body, the clinician has the unique opportunity to collect evidence that may identify the perpetrator of a sexual assault. Forensic evidence relates to those medical findings that can be used in a legal proceeding. Rules of evidence collection and types of specimens requested vary by state ordinance. Most states have a preferred "Sexual Assault (Rape) Kit" that includes the appropriate collection materials. In general, the assault kit is collected if you are examining the victim within 72 hours of an abusive episode that potentially included intimate contact.

Clothing

Torn or stained clothing should be collected and stored in paper bags; plastic bags retain moisture and may be damaging to potential evidence. Underpants should be collected if there was a history of penis contact of the anogenital area. Even if the underwear was changed earlier, some small amounts of semen may drip from the anus or vaginal orifice. Some jurisdictions request that the victim undress over a large sheet of paper so that any trace evidence, such as fibers or hairs that may be linked to a perpetrator, falls on the paper; the paper subsequently is folded inward and preserved.

Sexual Assault (Rape) Kit

Biochemical Evidence

DNA and other biochemical markers provide the most specific evidence in cases of abuse. Swabs taken of the patient's body areas where the perpetrator's semen, saliva, or blood reportedly came into contact should be collected. A wet mount of vaginal secretions should be reviewed by the clinician for the presence of sperm. If sperm are identified, the presence or absence of motility should be noted.

The patient's whole body should be scanned with a Wood's lamp to identify areas with suspicious secretions. Although the Wood's lamp identifies nonspecific findings, semen, urine, and other secretions that are not otherwise obvious might be identified in this manner. If dried secretions are found, wipe with a moistened gauze pad or scrape into the provided container. Wet semen should be collected on a gauze pad and allowed to air dry.

When there is a history of penile/oral contact, take swabs from the upper and lower recesses of the mandibular ridges, where there is less turnover of saliva. When penile/genital contact has occurred, one should attempt to acquire specimens from the vagina or external genital area of the preadolescent. In the adolescent who can tolerate a speculum examination, specimens should be taken from the cervix as well as the vaginal pool, because sperm may survive longer in the cervix. Swabs taken from the anal area are indicated if the history includes penile/rectal contact. Swab the breasts if oral contact occurred there.

All moist specimens should be allowed to air dry before storage. A cool air fan may be used to hasten the process but warm air, such as from a hair dryer, may damage the evidence. Although the quantity of DNA evidence diminishes over time or with normal hygienic procedures, specimens should be collected even if the patient has voided, bathed, showered, douched, or brushed teeth, if she presents within 72 hours of the assault.

Fingernails

Fingernail scrapings and clippings are collected when there is obvious specimen present or there is a history of significant scratching of the perpetrator by the victim. Stained fingernails should be clipped close to the finger. Tweezers are used to place the fingernails into a storage container or envelope.

Pubic Hair

The pubic hair of the adolescent should be combed onto a clean sheet to collect trace evidence. Because patient hair may be mixed with perpetrator hair, a sample of known patient hair (head and pubic) may be needed, as many as 25 strands. Although plucked hair provides the most information to crime analysts, this is a painful and humiliating procedure for the patient. Some assault kits now include a fine-tooth comb to run through the patient's hair, assuming that some of her hair is ready to comb out easily. Others have suggested cutting the hair close to the base of the shaft, although this prevents collection of the hair root. Because of the more universal availability of DNA analysis, the reliance on hair samples for definitive evidence has diminished. It would seem that in the unlikely event that the success of a criminal case relies on plucked pubic hair, the victim could return to the physician at a later date, have a topical anesthetic applied, and the hair could be taken at that time. Such an approach should satisfy forensic needs and would be far better tolerated by the patient.

Chain of Evidence

All evidence collection must be done under a strict Chain of Evidence policy to document who collected, transported, and processed the specimens. The completed evidence collection kit should be sealed and given to local police authorities to arrange for analysis. The police officer should sign and date the Chain of Evidence form when taking the kit from the medical facility. A locked storage space with limited access should be available if police cannot take the kit immediately after its completion. A copy of the completed Chain of Evidence form should be placed on the patient's medical chart.

SEXUALLY TRANSMITTED DISEASES

Which Patients to Test

A sexually abused child or adolescent may be at increased risk for the acquisition of an

STD, depending on the type of abuse that occurred. Not all abused children, however, have been exposed to an STD; therefore, individual consideration is indicated in determining which children to screen.

The child who is at highest risk for an STD is the one with signs or symptoms of an infection that can be sexually transmitted, or whose history and/or physical findings are consistent with oral, genital, or anal penetration. The sexually active adolescent is already at increased risk for an STD. Situations that place a victim at high risk include a perpetrator with a known STD or who is at high risk for STDs (e.g., drug user, multiple sex partners), having a family member with an STD, high community prevalence of STDs, and the likelihood of poor patient follow-up (34,35).

Limiting the STD testing of preadolescents to those with one or more risk factors, as opposed to universal screening of all children with a complaint of sexual abuse, has been effective in some communities (36–38).

Timing of Sexually Transmitted Disease Evaluation

The optimum timing for the collection of specimens will depend on when the abuse occurred. For the victim of chronic abuse or whose last sexual encounter was more than 1 to 2 weeks prior, testing for gonococcal, chlamydial, and trichomonal infection can be accomplished at the time of presentation.

The patient who presents shortly after an assault, however, may not have an adequate concentration of organisms for accurate testing. In the prepubertal child who is at low risk for prior infection, deferral of nonserologic testing for 2 weeks is appropriate if follow-up is likely and prophylaxis is not given initially. In general, the adolescent or other patient at high risk for prior genital infection is tested at initial presentation after an acute assault, with follow-up evaluation in 2 weeks (35). Any patient who has a positive STD culture should have a repeat culture 10 to 14 days after treatment to assess for cure.

Serologic testing for antibody response to syphilis, HIV, and hepatitis B should be done at the time of initial presentation and again 12 weeks after the most recent sexual exposure (34). If HIV exposure is of particular concern, additional follow-up tests throughout the first year after exposure may be performed.

Neisseria Gonorrhoeae

Neisseria gonorrhoeae infection in the prepubertal child beyond the neonatal period is invariably associated with sexual abuse. In this age group, a genital infection usually is limited to the vagina. A purulent vaginal discharge may be found. Pharyngeal and rectal infections often are asymptomatic (39).

A gram stain can be helpful in forming a presumptive diagnosis, but it is not definitive. Other *Neisseria* species may be found in the vagina and oropharynx that are not related to sexual transmission. Culture is the gold standard for diagnosis in a case of suspected abuse. Specimens should be collected from the throat, rectum, and vagina of the child. A cervical specimen should replace the vaginal specimen in the adolescent. Direct plating of a specimen onto Thayer-Martin or chocolate agar media will provide optimum results (40). A positive culture should be laboratory confirmed by at least two other methods that use different analytic principles (34). Recently developed DNA probes and other rapid nonculture techniques have not been adequately tested in the preadolescent population and should not be substituted for a culture (39).

Centers for Disease Control and Prevention (CDC) Guidelines recommend that children who weigh less than 45 kg and who have uncomplicated gonococcal infection may be treated with ceftriaxone 125 mg IM. Preapplication with a topical analgesic 1 hour before treatment and/or mixture of the medication with 1% lidocaine decrease the associated pain of injection. Although cefixime has been approved for adult use in the prophylaxis and treatment of gonorrhea, there are no published reports of its effectiveness in the preadolescent population (34).

Children who weigh 45 kg or more are treated with one of the recommended adult regimens: ceftriaxone 125 mg IM × 1, cefixime 400 mg PO × 1, ciprofloxacin 500 mg PO × 1, or ofloxacin 400 mg PO × 1 (34).

Chlamydia Trachomatis

Chlamydial infection in the prepubertal child beyond infancy is suspicious for sexual abuse, although vertical transmission presumably can result in asymptomatic carriage for up to 3 years (35).

Only tissue culture is valid for the diagnosis of chlamydia in the evaluation for abuse; rapid nonculture diagnostic methods have not been tested adequately on children for the necessary scrutiny of a forensic procedure. Specimen swabs with plastic or wire shafts are used to obtain culture material; wooden shafts may be toxic to this organism. Because *C. trachomatis* is an intracellular pathogen, one should swab the mucosal surface to collect epithelial cells and not simply collect a specimen of the discharge (41). In the young child, specimens are collected from the anus and vagina. Anal and cervical specimens are preferred for the adolescent (34).

The CDC-recommended treatment for children with *C. trachomatis* who weigh less than 45 kg is erythromycin base 50 mg/kg/day PO divided into four doses per day for 10 to 14 days. Children who weigh 45 kg or more and who are less than 8 years of age should be treated with azithromycin 1 g PO × 1. For those children who weigh more than 45 kg and who are older than 8 years of age, the single oral dose of azithromycin 1 g still is appropriate; an alternative is doxycycline 100 mg PO b.i.d. × 7 days (34).

Syphilis

Syphilis in the preadolescent, beyond the neonatal period, generally is presumed to be sexually transmitted and should be evaluated as such (35). Some cases have been reported, however, of possible congenital transmission that were not identified until 6 months to 3 years of age (42,43).

A nontreponemal test (Rapid Plasma Reagin [RPR], Venereal Disease Research Laboratory [VDRL]) may be used to screen the patient. If the test is positive, the patient should have a confirmatory treponemal test (e.g., fluorescent treponemal antibody absorbed [FTA-ABS]) (40). Optimum treatment for syphilis is with penicillin; the form and dose of penicillin vary with the patient's age and stage of syphilis (34).

Human Immunodeficiency Virus

Although the likelihood of HIV acquisition from sexual abuse is low (44), the implications of acquiring this infection are devastating. Abuse victims generally are tested at presentation for baseline documentation of HIV status; this specimen may be frozen and analyzed later if subsequent tests are positive. Universal prophylaxis of patients at the time of presentation is not currently endorsed by the CDC. Medical discretion, however, is indicated in the victim who presents for evaluation shortly after an assault by a perpetrator with known HIV infection (45).

Hepatitis B

Hepatitis B is transmitted by sexual as well as nonsexual contact. Hepatitis B immunization currently is recommended for all children (46). There is insufficient data to support the routine prophylaxis of the nonimmunized child victim of sexual abuse with hepatitis B immune globulin; the risk of exposure to a perpetrator with active Hepatitis B must be considered (34). Initiation of the hepatitis B immunization series at the time of patient presentation is indicated, however, for the victim who has not been vaccinated.

Human Papillomavirus

Transmission of HPV is presumed to be by direct human contact. The incubation time for HPV in children is unknown. It is believed that infants exposed in the peripartum period may not manifest clinical signs of infection for up to 2 to 3 years, if ever. Given the close association of anogenital warts with sexual contact, however, it is recommended that all prepubertal children with condyloma acuminata beyond infancy be evaluated for possible sexual abuse (35). Although fomite or benign transmission of HPV theoretically is possible, there have been no documented cases of children acquiring the infection in this manner (47).

The diagnosis of HPV usually is made by clinical observation. Biopsy of a suspicious lesion is indicated if there is any question about its nature, because of the significant implications of possible abuse. Once the diagnosis of HPV is made, the investigation for abuse relies heavily on the history from the child and her caretakers. Although warts generally are site specific, this is not an absolute finding, and the diagnosis of a specific HPV biotype in the genital area neither proves nor disproves the diagnosis of abuse. Biotyping may, however, provide prognostic information.

Girls with external genital warts (48) and girls who have been sexually abused with or without external genital warts (49) appear to be at increased risk for intravaginal HPV infection. It is unclear what the potential is for dysplasia and malignancy in young girls exposed to HPV. Careful follow-up is indicated.

Treatment of anogenital warts does not eradicate the virus. Recurrent warts do not necessarily imply a repeat exposure but may be due to reactivation of latent virus.

Herpes Simplex Virus

There are two identified serotypes of HSV. Type 1 (HSV-1) is more commonly found in oral infections, whereas type 2 (HSV-2) typically is found in genital infections due to sexual transmission. The types are not site specific, however, and HSV-1 genital infections are not rare. Children may autoinnoculate their infected oral secretions to the genital area to establish a local infection (35). Abusive oral/genital contact may put a child at increased risk for HSV-1 genital infection.

The child who presents beyond the neonatal period with anal or genital lesions suggestive of a herpetic infection should be evaluated for sexual abuse, including tests for other STDs. Family history of HSV infection or recent cold sores should be documented. A culture from the base of a fresh lesion is the most specific test. Treatment with an antiviral medication may shorten the duration of symptoms. Serologic evaluation of alleged perpetrators is not helpful because of the high prevalence of HSV infection in the general population.

Trichomonas Vaginalis

Trichomonas vaginalis is a flagellated parasite that may be vertically transmitted in the peripartum period. Infants may present with vaginal discharge or with signs and symptoms of a urinary tract infection within the first few weeks of life. Trichomonas infection beyond the neonatal period is primarily sexually transmitted. The finding of this infection in the preadolescent should prompt a full investigation for sexual abuse and other STDs (50).

Single-dose treatment for the prepubertal girl can be accomplished with metronidazole 40 mg/kg (maximum 2 g). For adolescents and adults, a single oral dose of 2 g usually is adequate. Multidose regimens also are available (35).

Bacterial Vaginosis

The usual agent of bacterial vaginosis is *Gardnerella vaginalis*. The infection is seen most commonly in the sexually active teen or adult, but it has been reported in prepubertal girls with no other indicators of sexual activity or abuse (51). A careful history and evaluation for other STDs is indicated in the child who presents with this finding. Treatment is with metronidazole (35).

Implications of a Positive Test Result

The American Academy of Pediatrics has published guidelines advising when to report

TABLE 28.1. *Implications of commonly encountered sexually transmitted diseases for diagnosis and reporting of sexual abuse of prepubertal infants and children*

Sexually transmitted disease confirmed	Sexual abuse	Suggested action
Gonorrhea[a]	Certain	Report[b]
Syphilis[b]	Certain	Report
Chlamydia[a]	Probable[c]	Report
Condylomata acuminatum[a]	Probable	Report
Trichomonas vaginalis	Probable	Report
Herpes 1 (genital)	Possible	Report[d]
Herpes 2	Probable	Report
Bacterial vaginosis	Uncertain	Medical follow-up
Candida albicans	Unlikely	Medical follow-up

[a]If not perinatally acquired.
[b]To agency mandated in community to receive reports of suspected sexual abuse.
[c]Culture only reliable diagnostic method.
[d]Unless there is a clear history of autoinoculation.
From American Academy of Pediatrics Committee on Child Abuse and Neglect. Guidelines for the evaluation of sexual abuse of children. *Pediatrics* 1991;87:254–260, with permission.

possible abuse based on positive STD laboratory results (Table 28.1). Use of these guidelines and consultation with local experts in infectious disease or child sexual abuse should provide appropriate direction to the clinician faced with this concern.

Postexposure Prophylaxis

In the preadolescent, prophylactic treatment of an STD is based on the risk of exposure, concern of the parents, and time elapsed since the abusive event. Most of these patients do not receive prophylactic antibiotics. These children should be followed-up approximately 2 weeks after an acute assault to note interval development of signs or symptoms of infection and to reculture the patient who has been treated for a documented STD to assess cure.

Prophylactic treatment of the adolescent victim of sexual assault is similar to that for the adult. A full STD evaluation usually is performed on the patient at the time of presentation. In the acute situation, prophylaxis for gonococcal and chlamydial infection is provided. Additional prophylaxis with metronidazole often is included. Prophylaxis at the time of medical care, with medications that require a single dose, enables witnessed treatment and is more efficacious than prescriptions for multidose drugs. At the time of prophylactic treatment, it is helpful to advise the patient of the increased risk of a yeast infection secondary to the antibiotics. An over-the-counter azole cream can be recommended if the patient becomes symptomatic.

POSTCOITAL CONTRACEPTION

The provision of postcoital contraception should be discussed with the patient for whom there is a risk of pregnancy from the sexual assault. Options most commonly offered in the United States include combined estrogen-progestin pills, progestin-only pills, or insertion of a copper-releasing intrauterine device. Of these, most young women opt for the combination pills consisting of ethinyl estradiol 0.05 mg and norgestrel 0.5 mg, offered as Ovral oral contraceptives. The patient takes two tablets within 72 hours of the assault and two more tablets 12 hours later (52,53). Taken as directed, this method has an estimated efficacy rate of 75% to 80% (54). There are no known teratogenic effects to a preexisting fetus (55), but a baseline pregnancy test is advised before treatment. An antiemetic taken 1 hour before dosing is recommended due to the frequent side effects of nausea and vomiting. A repeat dose of Ovral should be taken if vomiting occurs within 1 hour of taking the medication. The patient should be advised that her next menses may be irregular. A follow-up pregnancy test is recommended in 2 to 3 weeks.

Several series have indicated that children and adolescent victims of sexual abuse are at increased risk for early pregnancy (56–58). This should be kept in mind as the patient follows-up for medical care so that appropriate contraceptive guidance can be considered.

see injuries with that type of abuse. A simple assessment of "normal examination," without further explanation, is not acceptable in the evaluation of sexual abuse.

MEDICAL ASSESSMENT

The assessment is a critical portion of the medical document. The physician should summarize any physical findings and comment about the likelihood of the findings being due to abuse. The absence of physical findings may still be compatible with a history of abuse; if so, a short explanation should be provided. For example, a history of oral/genital contact or genital fondling is compatible with a normal examination because you would not expect to

PLAN

A thorough plan for the patient, specimens, and evidence collection kit should conclude the medical document. Written instructions for home care should be given to the patient/family at the time of discharge to ensure they have proper information about follow-up and what to do if symptoms develop. Attention should be paid to medical as well as mental health needs. All children with a history of sexual abuse should be encouraged to undergo counseling, preferably with a professional skilled in addressing this issue. Parents also

TABLE 28.2. *Guidelines for making the decision to report sexual abuse of children*

Data available			Response	
History	Physical examination	Laboratory findings	Level of concern about sexual abuse	Report decision
None	Normal	None	None	No report
Behavioral changes[b]	Normal	None	Variable depending on behavior	Possible report;[a] follow closely (possible mental health referral)
None	Nonspecific findings	None	Low (worry)	Possible report;[a] follow closely
Nonspecific history by child or history by parent only	Nonspecific findings	None	Intermediate	Possible report;[a] follow closely
None	Specific findings[c]	None	High	Report
Clear statement	Normal	None	High	Report
Clear statement	Specific findings	None	High	Report
None	Normal, nonspecific or specific findings	Positive culture for gonorrhea; positive serologic test for human immuno-deficiency virus; syphilis; presence of semen, sperm acid phosphatase	Very high	Report
Behavior changes	Nonspecific findings	Other sexually transmitted diseases	High	Report

[a]A report may or may not be indicated. The decision to report should be based on discussion with local or regional experts and/or child protective services agencies.
[b]Some behavioral changes are nonspecific, and others are more worrisome (1).
[c]Other reasons for findings ruled out (13).
From American Academy of Pediatrics Committee on Child Abuse and Neglect. Guidelines for the evaluation of sexual abuse of children: subject review. *Pediatrics* 1999;103:186–191, with permission.

may benefit from such support, and referrals are appropriately made at the time of patient evaluation.

PROFESSIONAL LEGAL INVOLVEMENT

Each state cites its own legal definition for child sexual abuse. The legal age of consent varies, usually between 14 and 18 years of age. Medical care providers need to be familiar with their local laws and obligations.

Each state requires that any medical professional who has a reasonable suspicion of child abuse must report that concern to a designated agency for further investigation (59). Physical findings are not necessary. Medical professionals are not expected to *prove* that abuse has occurred. The American Academy of Pediatrics has published recommendations for when to report abuse based on the history and physical findings (Table 28.2).

Part of the professional's caring and advocacy for children may require testifying in court regarding the medical evaluation. Although a clinician may be intimidated by this possibility, one must remember that the role of the medical professional is to educate the court about the medical findings and their implications, not to win the case—there are plenty of lawyers to do that. Several references are available for medical professionals regarding court preparation (60–62).

REFERENCES

1. Sedlak AJ, Broadhurst DD. *The Third National Incidence Study of Child Abuse and Neglect.* Washington, DC: US Government Printing Office, 1996.
2. Finkelhor D. Current information on the scope and nature of child sexual abuse. *The Future of Children.* 1994;4:31.
3. Felitti VJ, Anda RF, Nordenberg D, et al. Relationship of childhood abuse and household dysfunction to many of the leading causes of death in adults. *Am J Prev Med* 1998;14:245.
4. Leventhal JM. Epidemiology of sexual abuse of children: old problems, new directions. *Child Abuse Negl* 1998;22:481.
5. Young ME, Nosek MA, Howland C, et al. Prevalence of abuse of women with physical disabilities. *Arch Phys Med Rehabil* 1997;78:S-34.
6. Friedrich WN, Fisher J, Broughton D, et al. Normative sexual behavior in children: a contemporary sample. *Pediatrics* 1998;101(4):e9.
7. Johnson, TC. Assessment of sexual behavior problems in preschool-aged and latency-aged children. *Child Adolesc Psych Clin North Am* 1993;2:431.
8. American Professional Society on the Abuse of Children. *Practice guidelines: use of anatomical dolls in child sexual abuse assessments.* Chicago: American Professional Society on the Abuse of Children, 1995.
9. Levitt CJ. The medical interview. In: Heger A, Emans SJ, eds. *Evaluation of the sexually abused child.* New York: Oxford University Press, 1992:31.
10. Saywitz KJ, Goodman GS. Interviewing children in and out of court. In: Briere J, Berliner L, Bulkley JA, et al, eds. *The APSAC handbook on child maltreatment.* Thousand Oaks: Sage Publications, 1996:297.
11. Heger AH. Twenty years in the evaluation of the sexually abused child: has medicine helped or hurt the child and the family? *Child Abuse Negl* 1996;20:893.
12. Hogan M. Oral midazolam for pediatric nonacute sexual abuse examinations. *Child Maltreatment* 1996;1:361.
13. Adams JA. The role of photo documentation of genital findings in medical evaluations of suspected child sexual abuse. *Child Maltreatment* 1997;2:341.
14. Persaud DI, Squires JE, Rubin-Remer D. Use of foley catheter to examine estrogenized hymens for evidence of sexual abuse. *J Pediatr Adolesc Gynecol* 1997;10:83.
15. McCauley J, Gorman RL, Guzinski G. Toluidine blue in the detection of perineal laceration in pediatric and adolescent sexual abuse victims. *Pediatrics* 1986;78:1039.
16. McCann J, Voris J, Simon M, et al. Comparison of genital examination techniques in prepubertal girls. *Pediatrics* 1990;85:182.
17. Embree JE, Lindsay D, Williams T, et al. Acceptability and usefulness of vaginal washes in premenarcheal girls as a diagnostic procedure for sexually transmitted diseases. *Pediatr Infect Dis J* 1996;15:662.
18. Adams JA, Harper K, Knudson S, et al. Examination findings in legally confirmed child sexual abuse: it's normal to be normal. *Pediatrics* 1994;94:310.
19. Muram D. Child sexual abuse: relationship between sexual acts and genital findings. *Child Abuse Negl* 1989:13:211.
20. De Jong AR, Rose M. Legal proof of child sexual abuse in the absence of physical evidence. *Pediatrics* 1991;88:506.
21. Adams JA, Knudson S. Genital findings in adolescent girls referred for suspected sexual abuse. *Arch Pediatr Adolesc Med* 1996;150:850.
22. Finkel MA. Anogenital trauma in sexually abused children. *Pediatrics* 1989;84:317.
23. McCann J, Voris J, Simon M. Genital injuries resulting from sexual abuse: a longitudinal study. *Pediatrics* 1992;89:307.
24. American Professional Society on the Abuse of Children. *Glossary of terms and the interpretations of findings for child sexual abuse evidentiary examinations.* Chicago: American Professional Society on the Abuse of Children, 1998.
25. McCann J, Wells R, Simon M, et al. Genital findings in prepubertal girls selected for nonabuse: a descriptive study. *Pediatrics* 1990;86:428.
26. Berenson AB, Heger AH, Hayes JM, et al. Appearance of the hymen in prepubertal girls. *Pediatrics* 1992;89:387.

27. Bays J, Chadwick D. Medical diagnosis of the sexually abused child. *Child Abuse Negl* 1993;17:91.

28. Heger A, Emans SJ. Introital diameter as the criterion for sexual abuse [Commentary]. *Pediatrics* 1990;85:222.

29. Koumantakis EE, Hassan EA, Deligeoroglou EK, et al. Vulvovaginitis during childhood and adolescence. *J Pediatr Adolesc Gynecol* 1997;10:39.

30. McCann J. The appearance of acute, healing, and healed anogenital trauma. *Child Abuse Negl* 1998;22:605.

31. Bond GR, Dowd MD, Landsman I, et al. Unintentional perineal injury in prepubescent girls: a multicenter, prospective report of 56 girls. *Pediatrics* 1995;95:628.

32. McCann J, Voris J. Perianal injuries resulting from sexual abuse: a longitudinal study. *Pediatrics* 1993;91:390.

33. McCann J, Voris J, Simon M, et al. Perianal findings in prepubertal children selected for nonabuse: a descriptive study. *Child Abuse Negl* 1989;13:179.

34. Centers for Disease Control and Prevention. 1998 Guidelines for treatment of sexually transmitted diseases. *MMWR* 1998;47(No. RR-1).

35. Peter G, ed. *1997 Red Book: Report of the Committee on Infectious Diseases,* 24th ed. Elk Grove Village: American Academy of Pediatrics, 1997.

36. Siegel RM, Schubert CJ, Myers PA, et al. The prevalence of sexually transmitted diseases in children and adolescents evaluated for sexual abuse in Cincinnati: rationale for limited STD testing in prepubertal girls. *Pediatrics* 1995;96:1090.

37. Ingram DL, Everett VD, Flick LAR, et al. Vaginal gonococcal cultures in sexual abuse evaluations: evaluation of selective criteria for preteenaged girls. *Pediatrics* 1997;99(6):e8.

38. Muram D, Speck PM, Dockter M. Child sexual abuse examination: is there a need for routine screening for N. gonorrhoeae? *J Pediatr Adolesc Gynecol* 1996;9:79.

39. Committee on Child Abuse and Neglect, American Academy of Pediatrics. Gonorrhea in prepubertal children. *Pediatrics* 1998;101:134.

40. Judson FN, Ehret J. Laboratory diagnosis of sexually transmitted infections. *Pediatr Ann* 1994;23:361.

41. Centers for Disease Control and Prevention. Recommendations for the prevention and management of chlamydia trachomatis infections. *MMWR* 1993;42(No. RR-12).

42. Connors JM, Schubert C, Shapiro R. Syphilis or abuse: making the diagnosis and understanding the implications. *Pediatr Emerg Care* 1998;14:139.

43. Christian CW, Lavelle J, Bell LM. Preschoolers with syphilis. *Pediatrics* 1999;103(1):e4.

44. Gellert GA, Durfee MJ, Berkowitz CD, et al. Situational and sociodemographic characteristics of children infected with human immunodeficiency virus from pediatric sexual abuse. *Pediatrics* 1993;91:39.

45. Centers for Disease Control and Prevention. Management of possible sexual, injecting-drug-use, or other nonoccupational exposure to HIV, including considerations related to antiretroviral therapy. *MMWR* 1998;47 (No. RR-17).

46. Committee on Infectious Diseases, American Academy of Pediatrics. Recommended childhood immunization schedule—United States, January–December 1999. *Pediatrics* 1999;103:182.

47. Gutman LT, Herman-Giddens ME, Phelps WC. Transmission of human genital papillomavirus disease: comparison of data from adults and children. *Pediatrics* 1993;91:31.

48. Gutman LT, St. Claire KK, Everett VD, et al. Cervical-vaginal and intraanal human papillomavirus infection of young girls with external genital warts. *J Infect Dis* 1994;170:339.

49. Gutman LT, St. Claire K, Herman-Giddens ME, et al. Evaluation of sexually abused and nonabused young girls for intravaginal human papillomavirus infection. *Am J Dis Child* 1992;146:694.

50. Jones JG, Yamauchi T, Lambert B. Trichomonas vaginalis infestation in sexually abused girls. *Am J Dis Child* 1985;139:846.

51. Ingram DL, White ST, Lyna PR, et al. Gardnerella vaginalis infection and sexual contact in female children. *Child Abuse Negl* 1992;16:847.

52. Van Look PFA, Stewart F. Emergency contraception. In: Kowal D, ed. *Contraceptive technology,* 16th rev ed. New York: Ardent Media, 1998:277.

53. Chiou VM, Shrier LY, Emans SJ. Emergency postcoital contraception. *J Pediatr Adolesc Gynecol* 1998;11:61.

54. Trussell J, Stewart F. The effectiveness of postcoital contraception. *Fam Plann Perspect* 1992;24:262.

55. Glasier A. Emergency postcoital contraception. *N Engl J Med* 1997;337:1058.

56. Boyer D, Fine D. Sexual abuse as a factor in adolescent pregnancy and child maltreatment. *Fam Plann Perspect* 1992;24:4.

57. Fergusson DM, Horwood LJ, Lynskey MT. Childhood sexual abuse, adolescent sexual behaviors and sexual revictimization. *Child Abuse Negl* 1997;21:789.

58. Fiscella K, Kitzman HJ, Cole RE, et al. Does child abuse predict adolescent pregnancy? *Pediatrics* 1998;101:620.

59. Kerns DL, Terman DL, Larson CS. The role of physicians in reporting and evaluating child sexual abuse cases. *The Future of Children.* 1994;4:119.

60. Chadwick DL. Preparation for court testimony in child abuse cases. *Pediatr Clin North Am* 1990;37:955.

61. Freeman KR. Testifying as an expert witness. In: Heger A, Emans SJ, eds. *Evaluation of the sexually abused child.* New York: Oxford University Press, 1992;171.

62. Stern P. *Preparing and presenting expert testimony in child abuse litigation.* Thousand Oaks: Sage Publications, 1997.

29

Gynecologic Care for the Mentally Handicapped Individual

Sue Ellen Koehler Carpenter

There is a great need to provide quality gynecologic care to mentally handicapped individuals. In general, these individuals now have greater life expectancy than previously. Those with mild-to-moderate retardation are being encouraged to fulfill their highest potential by living in society at large or in sheltered situations with a high degree of normalization. Severely affected individuals, who might have succumbed at a young age to the medical complications of their disorder, are living through puberty and surviving their parents. Issues of sexuality, contraception, menstrual hygiene, and premenstrual syndrome with severe behavioral disorders can become important. Management of common gynecologic disorders, such as vaginal discharge, dysfunctional uterine bleeding, and pelvic pain, becomes difficult due to limitations in communication and examination. In some institutions, multispecialty clinics have been created to serve these patients (1).

MENSTRUAL HYGIENE

Issues of menstrual hygiene are common. Frequently, behavior modification successfully trains mildly and moderately retarded women. These programs may be less successful for profoundly affected patients unless toilet training has been successful previously (2). Oral contraceptive pills can be useful for limiting the volume of menstrual flow. Alternatively, menstrual suppression with depot medroxyprogesterone acetate can be used. After 1 year of use, amenorrhea is induced in 50% of patients using the standard contraceptive dose of 150 mg every 3 months. A more frequent schedule can be used to induce amenorrhea more quickly. Long-term use of Depo-Provera carries the risk of bone mineral loss (3). The benefits of menstrual suppression must be weighed against this risk. Some patients may be able to cooperate with periodic bone mineral density assessments.

Vaginal hysterectomy has been reported as a means of menstrual management (4). In general, a less invasive form of therapy consistent with the patients' goals will be chosen. Hysterectomy will be reserved for patients with documented failure of training programs, gynecologic disease, severe anemia, or contraindications to hormonal therapy. A case of hepatitis-positive blood being splattered uncontrollably and posing a substantial threat to caregivers and housemates has been reported to justify a hysterectomy (5). Endometrial ablation may provide an acceptable alternative to hysterectomy (6,7).

Dysfunctional uterine bleeding certainly will exacerbate problems of hygiene. Accurate menstrual records should be kept. Alterations in previously normal cycles warrant investigation, as for any patient. Obesity and thyroid dysfunction, which occur commonly in patients with Down syndrome, may predispose this population in particular to abnormal bleeding.

PREMENSTRUAL SYNDROME

Premenstrual syndrome with exacerbation of autism, temper tantrums, irritability, restlessness, disobedient behavior, and seizure activity has been noted. The value of an accurate menstrual calendar for interpreting these behavioral changes is obvious. Some behavior problems reflect dysmenorrhea, which severely handicapped persons are unable to communicate. This will respond to timely, generous administration of nonsteroidal antiinflammatory drugs. Others may respond to oral contraceptive pills or Depo-Provera. Selective serotonin reuptake inhibitors can be used (see Chapter 16), but the collaboration of an interested psychiatrist may be required as the incidence of polypharmacy in these patients is quite high and the clinician's ability to assess a patient's progress and monitor side effects may be limited.

SEXUALITY

Issues surrounding sexual behavior are best dealt with in group educational and individual counseling sessions (8,9). Individuals who are integrated into the community often cannot interpret media representations of sexual behavior. They need help understanding the nature of appropriate relationships and learning to take responsibility for their actions. They must be taught to avoid situations that could lead to sexual abuse. Parent groups focus on helping parents learn to accept their children's sexuality and establish realistic goals for the maturing family member. More severely affected persons need limitations placed on unacceptable public displays of sexual behaviors and sexual self-abuse.

CONTRACEPTION

Providing adequate contraception can be difficult. Oral contraceptives and barrier methods demand a level of compliance that may be beyond the scope of an individual's abilities. However, oral contraceptives can be supervised by a caregiver. The risk of thromboembolism must be considered. Patients with impaired circulation or decreased mobility may be at increased risk. The intrauterine device may be appropriate in a few cases; however, it will be unacceptable to the extent that it increases dysmenorrhea and menstrual flow. Some patients will be unable to reliably report the symptoms that may accompany complications.

Depo-Provera is commonly used. The most common side effect is irregular bleeding during the first year of use. Thereafter, 50% of patients experience amenorrhea. Weight gain, abdominal bloating, headache, mood changes, and nervousness may occur, but usually are minor relative to the benefits of therapy. Bone mineral loss associated with long-term use has been reported, and clinicians need to be mindful of this potential effect (3). Norplant (subdermal levonorgestrel implants) provides protection for as long as 7 years. It does not carry the contraindications of estrogen-containing products. Although Norplant has been offered to patients with mental retardation, acceptance of the method has been limited (10).

STERILIZATION

The question of involuntary sterilization inevitably arises in a clinic where patients with mental retardation who are deemed incapable of giving informed consent are seen. The history of the procedure in the United States dates from the turn of the century, when the eugenics movement advocated involuntary sterilization to avoid genetic transmission of mental retardation. In 1927, the Supreme Court affirmed the constitutionality of eugenic sterilization in an opinion on *Buck v Bell* written by Justice Oliver Wendell Holmes: "It is better for all the world if instead of waiting to execute degenerative offspring for crime or let them starve of their imbecility, society can prevent those who are manifestly unfit from continuing their kind...three generations of imbeciles are enough" (11).

Today, most readers of the opinion of Justice Holmes would find it very disturbing. However, the decision set the stage for a 15-

year period during which 37 states passed eugenic sterilization legislation. In 1942, the Supreme Court, with a completely different membership, heard *Skinner v Oklahoma.* Skinner had been convicted three times of shoplifting and other similar offenses. Under the Oklahoma habitual criminal sterilization act, anyone convicted of specific crimes (including larceny) could be sterilized. The law excluded other equally serious offenses. Skinner argued that this differential treatment violated his right to equal protection. The opinion of the Supreme Court held the Oklahoma statute unconstitutional. In the words of Justice Douglas, "We are dealing here with legislation which involves one of the basic civil rights of man. Marriage and procreation are fundamental to the very existence and survival of the human race. The power to sterilize, if exercised, may have subtle, far reaching and devastating effects...there is no redemption for the individual whom the law touches...He is forever deprived of a basic liberty" (12).

The Skinner decision set the stage for the current debate on involuntary sterilization. The physician is placed in a difficult position when a patient and her family seem to have a reasonable request for sterilization because the individual cannot or does not wish to meet the demands of child rearing. Vining and Freeman (13) have appealed for a moderate approach that is guided by the level of retardation of the patient. In some cases, the level of supervision required for the severely affected patient makes sexual activity and, thus, the fear of pregnancy unreasonable. In the case of mildly retarded individuals who are able to marry and maintain themselves in the community, sterilization should not be an issue. For a middle group, living in a sheltered situation, increased efforts at normalization have led to acceptance of the right to sexual satisfaction, and sterilization may offer the best chance for normalcy. Advocacy for individual rights should include the possibility of obtaining sterilization under circumstances where the procedure allows patients to best fulfill their own potential.

Currently, the physician liability issues with regard to involuntary sterilization depend on state laws. There are three categories to consider: (a) potential liability when a state statute authorizes involuntary sterilization, (b) liability when a court orders sterilization at the request of the guardian without a specific statute, and (c) liability when there is no statute or court order (14). Approximately 19 states now have legislation enabling sterilization of mentally incompetent persons. The statutes generally have been upheld if they contain enough procedural protection for the patient. The New Jersey court invoked the *parens patriae* doctrine to order sterilization (15). The purpose of the doctrine is to protect the rights of mental incompetents. The judge interpreted sterilization as a procedure to which the patient had a right when it was clearly in her best interest. The court sought to protect that right. In some states where there is no statute, it may be possible to obtain a court order for sterilization when due process and equal protection under the law are emphasized. Other state courts have been unwilling to conclude that there is anything in their common law powers that enables them to mandate sterilization.

The substituted consent of parents alone, without a valid court order, will not suffice. The current attitude of the courts in such cases implies that physicians incur tremendous liability if they perform such procedures.

Rauh et al. (16) have advocated a moderate approach to the issue: a statute that would enable sterilization under specific circumstances. Applications would be reviewed by local courts or hospital review committees. Their proposed model statute would include the following:

1. The individual is presumed capable of procreation.
2. The individual is, or is likely to be, sexually active.
3. Pregnancy would not usually be intended by a competent person facing analogous choices.

4. All alternative contraceptive methods have proved unworkable or been shown inapplicable.
5. The individual's guardian agrees that sterilization is the best course of action in the case.
6. Comprehensive medical, psychological, and social evaluations recommend sterilization for the individual.
7. The individual is represented by independent legal counsel with demonstrated competence in dealing with medical, legal, social, and ethical issues involving sterilization.
8. The individual, regardless of her level of competence, has been informed in full by one able to make her understand and up to her level of competence shows awareness of the method of sterilization, the consequences of sterilization, the likelihood of success, alternative methods of sterilization and birth control, and the consequences of pregnancy and parenthood.

HYSTERECTOMY

Frequently, patients' families present to the clinic with requests for hysterectomy. This must be considered on an individual basis. The least harmful form of care consistent with the patients' best interest should be used. Families sometimes present with this request even before menstruation begins or when the patient is amenorrheic. Patients often have significant medical risks for surgery, which the family does not consider in their request. The family's specific concerns must be addressed with sensitivity, practical advice, and assurances of support. Questions of menstrual hygiene should be answered with adequate training programs and medication as needed. Contraception should be provided. Information that hysterectomy will not ameliorate premenstrual syndrome or prevent sexual abuse should be presented. Parent support groups and social work intervention may be encouraged. At times, a parent requests hysterectomy as part of a larger, sometimes overwhelming, agenda dealing with the physical, emotional, and financial demands that the maturing dependent places on the family.

McNeeley and Elkins (17) reported their experience with major gynecologic surgery in 15 mentally handicapped women. The indications for hysterectomy were menorrhagia (n = 3), leiomyomata (n = 9), and ovarian neoplasm (n = 3). All decisions for major surgery or sterilization in their clinic are presented to a societally based committee before admission (18). Six of the 13 women undergoing major abdominal surgery in this series developed significant complications. All three quadriplegic patients with cerebral palsy developed aspiration pneumonia. Pelvic cellulitis occurred in one case. Urinary tract infection and fecal impaction occurred in two others—one with associated small bowel obstruction. In this report, another 22 minor procedures (including dilatation and curettage, and laparoscopic sterilization) were performed without incident. Abdominal hysterectomy for sterilization alone certainly is contraindicated by its increased morbidity. Most of the patients in this series presented with advanced gynecologic pathology probably due to the difficulty of providing routine gynecologic examinations in this population.

ROUTINE CARE

The initial evaluation of patients with mental retardation who present for routine gynecologic care should include a complete medical history, gynecologic history with a menstrual calendar, if available, and physical examination. In this population, chronic illness and subnormal weights are not necessarily associated with amenorrhea (19). If a recent social work evaluation and psychological evaluation (with IQ testing) are available, they are helpful.

A pelvic examination should be performed, if possible, and a Pap smear obtained in patients with abnormal vaginal bleeding or vaginal discharge, patients over age 30 years, or patients who are sexually active. If a speculum examination is impossible, a Pap smear can be performed blindly using a moistened cotton-tipped swab directed to the cervix by an examiner's single finger. When a pelvic examination cannot be performed, a pelvic ultrasound may be a useful alternative. However, an examination under anesthesia will be required on some occasions. Office sedation may provide a convenient alternative to general anesthesia (20,21).

Routine complaints, such as vaginal discharge, require a practical approach. Urinary frequency, crying on urination, or foul-smelling urine suggest a urinary tract infection. Anal itching suggests the presence of pinworms. Vulvar irritation can result from or cause excessive masturbatory behavior. Hypoestrogenism may be a cause of discomfort, especially if hygiene is difficult. This responds to a regimen of frequent sitz baths, air drying, and soothing ointment such as Balmex. Hydrocortisone cream 1% may be used as well. Recent antibiotic use or a thick white discharge suggest *Candida* infection, and an empiric trial of an antifungal agent is appropriate. If the discharge is persistent or recurrent, a complete pelvic examination to rule out foreign body and to obtain complete cultures for *Candida,* gonorrhea, chlamydia, streptococcus, and fecal pathogens is required. A saline preparation should be examined for *Trichomonas* and *Gardnerella.* Appropriate treatment then is instituted. If cultures are positive for a sexually transmitted disease, rapid plasma reagin (RPR) and human immunodeficiency virus testing along with an investigation for sexual abuse may be required if consensual sexual activity cannot be confirmed.

In summary, the gynecologic care of mentally retarded adolescents requires special care. It is best provided by individuals with an interest in the field and the ability to consider the patient's unique medical and social circumstances when providing services. A commonsense approach to the patient's best interests is needed. The breadth of experience in the academic center clinics may be informative for those who provide community-based care for these special patients.

REFERENCES

1. Elkins TE, Gafford LS, Wilks CS, et al. A model clinic approach to the reproductive health concerns of the mentally handicapped. *Obstet Gynecol* 1986;68:185–188.
2. Kreutner AK. Sexuality, fertility and the problems of menstruation in mentally retarded adolescents. *Pediatr Clin North Am* 1981;28:275.
3. Cundy T, Evans M, Roberts H, et al. Bone density in women receiving depot medroxyprogesterone acetate for contraception. *Br Med J* 1991;27:220.
4. Sheth S, Malpani A. Vaginal hysterectomy for the management of menstruation in mentally retarded women. *Int J Gynecol Obstet* 1991;35:319–321.
5. Elkins TE, McNeeley SG, Punch M, et al. Reproductive health concerns in Down syndrome. *J Reprod Med* 1990; 35:745–750.
6. Wilson JE, Carlson GM, Taylor MT. Endometrial ablation: an option for the management of menstrual problems in the intellectually disabled. *Med J Aust* 1994;161:511–512.
7. Wingfield M, Healy DL, Nicholson A. Gynaecological care for women with intellectual disability. *Med J Aust* 1994;160:536–538.
8. Pincus S. Sexuality in the mentally retarded patient. *Am Fam Physician* 1988;37:319–323.
9. Saunders EJ. The mental health professional, the mentally retarded, and sex. *Hosp Commun Psychiatry* 1981; 32:717–721.
10. Haefner H, Elkins T. Contraceptive management for female adolescents with mental retardation and handicapping disabilities. *Curr Opin Obstet Gynecol* 1991;3: 820–824.
11. *Buck v Bell* 274 US 200, U.S. Supreme Court, 1927.
12. *Skinner v Oklahoma* 36 US 535, U.S. Supreme Court, 1942.
13. Vining EPG, Freeman JM. Sterilization and the retarded female: is advocacy depriving individuals of their rights? *Pediatrics* 1978;62:850–853.
14. Letterie GS, Fox WF. Legal aspects of involuntary sterilization. *Fertil Steril* 1990;53:391–398.
15. In *re Grady,* 85 NJ 235, 426 A. 2d. 467, 1981.
16. Rauh JL, Dine MS, Biro FM, et al. Sterilization for the mentally retarded adolescent. *J Adolesc Health Care* 1989;10:467–472.
17. McNeeley SG, Elkins TE. Gynecologic surgery and surgical morbidity in mentally handicapped women. *Obstet Gynecol* 1989;74:155–158.
18. Elkins TE, Strong C, Wolfe AR, et al. An ethics committee in a reproductive health clinic for mentally handicapped persons. *Hastings Cent Rep* 1986;16:20–22.
19. Furman LM. Institutionalized disabled adolescents: gynecologic care. The pediatrician's role. *Clin Pediatr* 1989;28:163–170.
20. Elkins TE, McNeeley SG, Rosen D. A clinical observation of a program to accomplish pelvic exams in difficult-to-manage patients with mental retardation. *Adolesc Pediatr Gynecol* 1988;1:195–198.
21. Rosen DA, Rosen KR, Elkins TE, et al. Outpatient sedation: an essential addition to gynecologic care for persons with mental retardation. *Am J Obstet Gynecol* 1991;164:825–828.

Subject Index